T0327445

Syncope:
Mechanisms and Management

To Barbara Straus, MD
Physician, teacher, mother, dancer,
community leader, soul mate and
source of all inspiration.

To Helen and Alex, two of
life's greatest and continuing joys

And to Paul B. Grubb (1924–1998)
father, friend, guide and source
of encouragement. May his memory
be for a blessing. . . .

B.P.G.

To Darlene Marie Postacchini Olshansky,
my loving wife, friend and advisor,
source of support, inspiration and
creativity.

B.O.

Syncope: Mechanisms and Management

SECOND EDITION

EDITED BY

Blair P. Grubb, MD

Professor of Medicine and Pediatrics
Director, Cardiac Electrophysiology Section
Medical College of Ohio
Toledo, OH

Brian Olshansky, MD

Professor of Medicine
Director, Cardiac Electrophysiology
University of Iowa Medical Center
Iowa City, IA

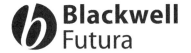

© 2005 by Blackwell Publishing
Blackwell Futura is an imprint of Blackwell Publishing

Blackwell Publishing, Inc., 350 Main Street, Malden, Massachusetts 02148-5018, USA
Blackwell Publishing Ltd, 9600 Garsington Road, Oxford OX4 2DQ, UK
Blackwell Science Asia Pty Ltd, 550 Swanston Street, Carlton, Victoria 3053, Australia

ISBN-13: 978-1-4051-2207-8
ISBN-10: 1-4051-2207-2

First published 1998
Second edition 2005

   Syncope : mechanisms and management / edited by Blair P. Grubb, Brian Olshansky. —
    2nd ed.
      p. ; cm.
    Includes bibliographical references and index.
    ISBN 1-4051-2207-2
    1. Syncope (Pathology)   I. Grubb, Blair P.   II. Olshansky, Brian.
    [DNLM: 1. Syncope.   WB 182 S9925 2005]
  RB150 .L67S96 2005
  616′ .047—dc22
    2004022822

A catalogue record for this title is available from the British Library

Acquisitions: Steve Korn
Development Editor: Vicki Donald
Set in 9.5/12pt Minion by Graphicraft Limited, Hong Kong

For further information on Blackwell Publishing, visit our website:
www.blackwellcardiology.com

The publisher's policy is to use permanent paper from mills that operate a sustainable forestry policy, and
which has been manufactured from pulp processed using acid-free and elementary chlorine-free practices.
Furthermore, the publisher ensures that the text paper and cover board used have met acceptable
environmental accreditation standards.

Notice: The indications and dosages of all drugs in this book have been recommended in the medical
literature and conform to the practices of the general community. The medications described do not
necessarily have specific approval by the Food and Drug Administration for use in the diseases and dosages
for which they are recommended. The package insert for each drug should be consulted for use and dosage
as approved by the FDA. Because standards for usage change, it is advisable to keep abreast of revised
recommendations, particularly those concerning new drugs.

Contents

Contributors

David G. Benditt, MD
Professor of Medicine
The University of Minnesota School of Medicine
Minneapolis, MN

Gerald J. Bloch, JD
Attorney at Law
Milwaukee, WI

Michele Brignole, MD, FESC
Department Head
Arrhythmia Center
Ospedali del Tigullio
Lavagna, Italy

Hugh Calkins, MD
Professor of Medicine
The Johns Hopkins Hospital
Baltimore, MD

N.A. Mark Estes III, MD
Professor of Medicine
Tufts – New England Medical Center
Boston, MA

Richard Friedman, MD
Associate Professor of Pediatrics
Texas Children's Hospital
Baylor College of Medicine
Houston, TX

Blair P. Grubb, MD
Professor of Medicine and Pediatrics
The Medical College of Ohio
Toledo, OH

Olaf Hedrich, MD
Tufts – New England Medical Center
Boston, MA

Munther K. Homoud, MD
Assistant Professor of Medicine
Tufts – New England Medical Center
Boston, MA

Yousuf Kanjwal, MD
Assistant Professor of Medicine
Medical College of Ohio
Toledo, OH

Rose Anne Kenny, MD
Professor of Cardiovascular Research
University of Newcastle School of Clinical Medical Sciences
Royal Victoria Infirmary
Newcastle upon Tyne, UK

George J. Klein, MD
Professor of Medicine
University of Western Ontario
London, Ontario, Canada

Daniel J. Kosinski, MD
Associate Professor of Medicine
Medical College of Ohio
Toledo, OH

Andrew D. Krahn, MD
Professor of Medicine
University of Western Ontario
London, Ontario, Canada

Mark S. Link, MD
Associate Professor of Medicine
Tufts – New England Medical Center
Boston, MA

Lewis Lipsitz, MD
Professor of Medicine
Harvard Medical School
Hebrew Rehabilitation Center for the Aged
Boston, MA

Phillip A. Low, MD
Professor of Neurology
The Mayo Clinic College of Medicine
Rochester, MN

Ronald McGinnis, MD
Professor of Psychiatry
The Medical College of Ohio
Toledo, OH

Angele McGrady, PhD, MEd, LPCC
Professor of Psychiatry
The Medical College of Ohio
Toledo, OH

Fred Morady, MD
Professor of Medicine
University of Michigan Medical Center
Ann Arbor, MI

Brian Olshansky, MD
Professor of Medicine
University of Iowa School of Medicine
Iowa City, IA

Steve W. Parry, MD
Senior Lecturer and Consultant Physician
University of Newcastle School of Clinical Medical Sciences
Royal Victoria Infirmary
Newcastle upon Tyne, UK

Frank Pelosi, Jr., MD
Assistant Professor of Medicine
University of Michigan Medical Center
Ann Arbor, MI

Peter C. Rowe, MD
Professor of Pediatrics
The Johns Hopkins Hospital
Baltimore, MD

Allan C. Skanes, MD
Assistant Professor of Medicine
University of Western Ontario
London, Ontario, Canada

Richard Sutton, DScMed
Professor of Cardiology
Royal Brompton and National Heart Hospital
London, UK

Edward A. Telfer, MD
Associate Professor of Medicine
Loyola University Medical Center
Maywood, IL

Raymond Yee, MD
Professor of Medicine
University of Western Ontario
London, Ontario, Canada

Mark J. Zucker, MD, JD, FACC
Associate Professor of Medicine
University of Medicine and Dentistry of New Jersey
Newark Beth Israel Medical Center
Newark, NJ

Foreword

Syncope remains one of the most common, yet frustrating, symptom complexes. It can occur at any age and it has no gender predisposition. There are multiple causes of this symptom complex, which can be quite innocent or presage sudden cardiac death. This latter concern results in the use of a variety of technologies at great expense, to attempt to delineate the cause and suggest appropriate therapy. Unfortunately, most of these tests are negative and, as a result, are extremely cost ineffective. Drs. Grubb and Olshansky's textbook, *Syncope: Mechanisms and Management* is the principal text in the field: the only one in the field devoted to providing pathophysiological, clinical diagnostic, and therapeutic information.

The book has several new chapters, including new data from the ISSUE trial, as well as results of multicenter trials using device therapy in patients with syncope and organic heart disease with demonstrated improved survival rate. Updated information about the mechanism of a neurocardiogenic syncope, carotid sinus hypersensitivity, syncope in childhood and adolescence, chronic fatigue, and orthostatic hypotension disorders is provided. The chapter on syncope in the athlete, as well as on the legal ramifications of managing patients with syncope, provides new information that is of increas-

ing interest. Most importantly, there have been updates on guidelines for device implantation for syncope from both the USA and Europe.

In sum, this unique book provides the reader with a wealth of practical information about the mechanisms, diagnosis, and consequences of syncope. Algorithms for work-up are provided, stressing the important aspects of the history and physical examination as the major initial aspects of dealing with the patient. As in the first edition, I think that the chapter on the overview of syncope by Olshansky is a masterpiece and should be read by all physicians in internal medicine, cardiology, and primary care.

In conclusion, *Syncope: Mechanisms and Management* is, in my opinion, the gold standard for information about this topic. It should be read by all.

Mark E. Josephson, MD
Herman C. Dana Professor of Medicine
Chief of the Cardiovascular Division
Director, Harvard – Thorndike Electrophysiology
Institute and Arrhythmia Service
Beth Israel Deaconess Medical Center
Boston, MA

Preface to the First Edition

Syncope, the transient loss of consciousness and postural tone with spontaneous recovery, is a common malady that has afflicted patients and challenged medical practitioners from the beginnings of recorded history. Since the time of Hippocrates, physicians have struggled to understand the complex and diverse etiologies that may culminate in syncope. The extreme diversity of causes and the similarities in presentation make the task of diagnosis a challenging one. Combined with the ever-present knowledge that "today's syncope may be tomorrow's sudden death," the evaluation and management of the patient with recurrent, unexplained syncope may seem truly overwhelming. The practitioner, seeking guidance in the approach to the patient with recurrent syncope, has been forced to search through a widely scattered medical literature belonging to a variety of medical specialties. This situation has been compounded by the extremely rapid growth of knowledge and research into many of the causes of syncope.

The aim of this book is to bring together in one volume a comprehensive yet usable reference source on syncope. This collaboration has brought together the skills and perspectives of internists, pediatricians, gerontologists, neurologists, cardiologists, and psychiatrists. In each aspect, we have attempted to provide a useful and complete body of information that not only provides a summary of the published literature, but also gives the personal insights and experiences of each author. The book has been organized to make this diverse quantity of information easy to assimilate, with each chapter designed to stand alone while also being part of a coherent whole. When appropriate, different perspectives on the same disorder have been presented. With this, we hope to help form a solid foundation for further development in this rapidly expanding and increasingly complex field.

Blair P. Grubb, MD
Toledo, OH

Brian Olshansky, MD
Iowa City, IA

Preface to the Second Edition

In this second edition, we have endeavored to provide, as in the first edition, a comprehensive reference for the diagnosis and treatment of a wide range of disorders that cause syncope. This edition incorporates the substantial advances that have occurred in the field since 1998. There has been extensive revision of most previous chapters as well as the incorporation of four new chapters. We are indebted to the wide range of international experts who have contributed to the second edition, who come from the USA, Canada, and Europe, and represent a variety of disciplines including cardiology, internal medicine, neurology, pediatrics, gerontology, psychiatry, and law. The book has been made more comprehensive in scope with the addition of chapters on cardiac obstructive and inherited arrhythmic causes of syncope, as well as chapters on tilt table testing and use of implantable cardioverter defibrillators in patients with syncope. The chapter on syncope in the child and adolescent has been significantly expanded, as have the sections on dysautonomic, neurologic, and psychiatric causes of syncope. A section on the postural tachycardia syndrome and orthostatic intolerance has been added to the chapter on chronic fatigue syndrome. As in the first edition, each chapter can be read in a stand-alone fashion or as part of a comprehensive whole. Differing perspectives are presented on the same disorders, as well as the experiences, insights, and opinions of each author. In summary, this expanded and updated edition continues the goal of the first: to provide a comprehensive, rational guide for those who seek information on the causes, evaluation, and management of syncope.

Blair P. Grubb, MD
Toledo, OH

Brian Olshansky, MD
Iowa City, IA

Acknowledgments

No book would be possible without the efforts of many people. We offer deep thanks to all our patients, as well as to the many physicians from around the world who have sent them to us. We would like, in particular, to thank Steven Korn, Gina Almond, Katrina Chandler, and Alice Nelson from Blackwell Publishing for working so closely and amicably with us. We would also like to express our gratitude to Barbara Straus, MD, for patiently and critically reading most chapters for style, grammar, and content, while keeping me (B.P.G.) steadily on track towards the book's completion; to Laura Goodwin for her superb transcription of my (B.P.G.) multiple scrawled notes into a coherent whole; to Sam Khouri, MD, for his help in preparing multiple echocardiographic images; to the staff of the MCO Cardiology and Syncope Clinics for their dedication and care; to Helen Grubb for her assistance in illustration; and to Darlene Olshansky for having patience with me (B.O.) during the book's completion. We would finally like to thank each of the contributors for sacrificing the time and effort necessary to write each of their chapters, without which this book would not be possible.

B.P.G.
B.O.

Web Resources

The National Dysautonomic Research Association:
www.ndrf.org

Dysautonomia Youth Network of America:
www.dynakids.org

Long QT syndrome website:
www.sads.org

Syncope Trust and Anoxic Reflex Seizure Group:
www.stars.org.uk

Hypertrophic Cardiomyopathy Association:
www.4hcm.org

Right Ventricular Dysplasia:
www.arvd.org

Those who suffer from frequent and severe fainting often die suddenly.

Hippocrates
Aphorisms 2.41
1000 B.C.E.

Only if one knows the causes of syncope will he be able to recognize its onset and combat the cause.

Maimonides
1135–1205 C.E.

If you save one human life
It is as if you had saved
The whole of humanity.

Sura Maida
Chapter 5, Verse 32
The Koran

They shall renew their strength
They shall mount up with wings like eagles
They shall run and not be weary
They shall walk and not faint.

Isaiah 40:31
The Bible

CHAPTER 1

Syncope: Overview and approach to management

Brian Olshansky, MD

Introduction

Syncope is a common, important medical problem caused by many conditions, ranging from benign and self-limiting to chronic, recurrent, and potentially fatal causes. Unfortunately, differentiation between benign and malignant causes can be difficult and challenging. Even with knowledge of common syndromes and conditions that cause syncope, and guidelines [1], an effective approach to the problem requires careful integration of clues provided in the history and physical examination combined with keen clinical acumen. Management of this baffling problem can be frustrating, confusing, and often unrewarding. Treatment can be impossible to prescribe without a clear understanding of the cause, and treatments may be directed to risk as well as symptom reduction.

Fortunately, experienced, astute, circumspect clinicians can deliver effective care when careful attention is paid to detail. This chapter considers a general overview of the problem of syncope and provides guidelines on how to approach management. Reference is given to other chapters in this book that provide more detail on specific topics.

Definitions

Syncope is often considered with several more vague symptoms that are manifestations of many clinical conditions. "Spells," transient confusion or weakness, dizziness, loss of memory, lightheadedness, near loss of consciousness ("presyncope" or

"near-syncope"), falling episodes, and coma are often confused with, and inappropriately labeled as, "true" syncope. Distinction between sleeping, confusion, intoxication, and fainting may not be completely clear. To make matters more difficult, an elderly patient, already confused, may fall and pass out with only vague recall of the event. Such a patient may even think he or she passed out when nothing of the sort occurred. This diverse collection of clinical presentations perplexes the patient and the physician. Episodes can be difficult to define even with careful observation, and the mechanism may be confusing even with extensive monitoring.

True syncope is an abrupt but transient loss of consciousness associated with absence of postural tone followed by rapid, usually complete, recovery without the need for intervention to stop the episode. A prodrome may be present. While alarming, this *symptom* is non-specific. It is generally triggered by a process that results in abrupt, transient (5–20 s) interruption of cerebral blood flow, specifically to the reticular activating system.

Collapse, associated with syncope, can be misinterpreted. In one study of 121 patients admitted to the emergency room with "collapse" as the admitting diagnosis, 19 had cardiac arrest, four were brought in dead and one was asleep [2]. Only 15 were ultimately diagnosed as having fainted. The final diagnosis in eight was still "collapse." Primary neurological or metabolic derangements can also mimic, but rarely cause, true syncope. Also, syncope can mimic a seizure or a metabolic derangement.

Importance of syncope

*"The only difference between syncope and
sudden death is that in one you wake up."*
[3] (vive la différence) [4]

*Syncope can be the premonitory sign of a serious
cardiac problem including cardiac arrest.* Generally,
syncope is benign and self-limited but it can mimic
a cardiac arrest and even be its precursor. Several
causes for syncope, generally cardiac, are potentially fatal. When syncope is caused by hemodynamic
collapse from critical aortic stenosis, ventricular
tachycardia, AV block, dissecting aortic aneurysm,
or pulmonary embolus, an aggressive evaluation
and treatment regimen is needed to forestall death.
A potentially lethal cause should always be suspected, especially in elderly patients, or it will be
missed [5,6]. While less common, even younger
individuals with syncope can be at risk of death [7].
For this age group, the congenital long QT interval syndrome, hypertrophic cardiomyopathy, right
ventricular dysplasia, Brugada syndrome, polymorphic ventricular tachycardia with associated short
or normal QT interval, congenital aortic stenosis,
among other causes, must be considered. Even apparently healthy individuals can die suddenly after
a syncopal episode (consider the death of basketball
star Reggie Lewis [8]).

Syncope can have a major impact on lifestyle.
Patients' reactions to syncope can vary from complete lack of recognition and concern, to fear and
difficulty returning to previous level of activities
with complete disability. Even if syncope is benign,
it can have a major impact on quality of life and
may change lifestyle dramatically, independent of
physicians' concerns and recommendations. The
degree of functional impairment from syncope can
match that of other chronic diseases, including
rheumatoid arthritis, chronic back pain, or chronic
obstructive lung disease [9]. Patients can have fear
of recurrence and excessive fear of dying. There
can be imposed limitations on driving and work
(see Chapter 20). Restrictions can be self-imposed,
imposed by the family, by the physician, or by legal
constraints (see Chapter 21). Up to 76% of patients
will change some activities of daily living, 64% will
restrict their driving, and 39% will change their

employment [9]. Seventy-three percent become
anxious or depressed, especially if a cause is not
found and treated [10,11].

Syncope can cause injuries. Injuries from syncope
occur in 17–35% of patients [12–16]. When injuries
occur, syncope is often suspected to be caused by
a serious, life-threatening, or cardiac cause, but
data conflict [16,17]. Sudden, *unexpected* loss of
consciousness (sometimes referred to as "Stokes–
Adams" attacks) can have many causes. The circumstances that surround the episode and absence
of a warning prodrome cause most injuries. Injury
itself does not necessarily indicate a life-threatening, cardiac, or arrhythmic cause for syncope,
although sudden collapse with injury has been
associated with an arrhythmic cause. While an
arrhythmic cause is often suspected when serious
injury results from syncope, few compelling data
support the need for a more aggressive approach to
evaluate or to treat syncope in injured patients.
Minor injuries occur in 10–29%, fractures occur
in 5–7% (more severe in the elderly), and traffic
accidents in 1–5% of syncope patients [18,19].

Syncope is expensive. Up to one million patients
annually are evaluated for syncope in the USA, with
500,000 new cases each year. Approximately 3–5%
of emergency room visits are to evaluate syncope
[14,20], emergency room visits leading to hospital
admission [13]. Between 1 and 6% of acute hospital
admissions are for syncope. The cost to evaluate
and treat syncope exceeds $750 million/year. The
cost for the average admission is more than $5500
[20] and hospitalization is helpful in only 10% of
patients admitted in whom the etiology was not
clear by the admitting history, physical examination, and electrocardiogram (ECG). The cost
expended to determine one syncope diagnosis in
patients diagnosed in 1982 was $23,000 [20] after a
mean hospital stay of 9.1 days. When vasodepressor
syncope is not recognized, evaluations can lead to
tremendous expense [21]. The costs per diagnosis
can be as high as $78,000, depending on the tests
performed and the diagnostic accuracy. The average patient with syncope makes 10.2 visits/year to a
physician and sees an average of 3.2 specialists for
the problem [22].

Approximately 10% of falls in the elderly are

caused by syncope [23]. Serious injury is more frequent when syncope precedes the fall [24–30]. Falls occur in 20% of the population over 65 years old. The cost to treat falls in the elderly exceeds $7 billion/year in the USA [23]. It is a common cause for disability.

Epidemiology

The frequency of syncope and its associated mortality varies with age, gender, and cause. In one large series, 60% of syncope patients were women [14], but in the Framingham study more younger syncope patients were women while more elderly syncope patients were men [24]. In the Framingham study, syncope had occurred in 3% of men and 3.5% of women, based on biannual examinations [24], with the highest frequency in the elderly. In the Framingham population, the annual incidence of syncope for those over 75 years old was 6% and the prevalence of syncope in the elderly was 5.6%, compared with a low of 0.7% in the 35–44-year-old male population [24]. The elderly are most likely to have syncope, to be injured from syncope, to seek medical advice, and to be admitted to a hospital [31,32] (see Chapter 18).

Of 3000 US Air Force personnel queried (mean age 29.1 years), 2.7% (82 of 3000) had at least one episode of syncope [33]. Other retrospective studies of healthy individuals suggest that up to 40% will pass out [34,35]. The population evaluated (outpatients, emergency room patients, hospitalized patients, the elderly), the definition of syncope, and the criteria for diagnosis (by examination or questionnaire), contribute to wide variations in published data. Probably, 20–30% of the population will pass out sometime in their lifetime [14,36,37]. Most individuals with syncope do not seek medical advice but the actual percentage of those who do is unknown. It is suspected that most individuals who do not seek medical attention have a low recurrence rate and probably have an excellent long-term survival. Outpatients evaluated or never admitted for their episodes *may* also be at lower risk for recurrence and *may* have a more benign long-term prognosis. Patients in these subgroups probably have neurocardiogenic syncope or some other autonomically mediated or situational cause for collapse.

Forty to eighty-five percent of those who come for evaluation of syncope will not have a recurrence [38]. Isolated episodes are common: 90% will have only one episode in 2 years, yet 54% with two episodes have recurrence over the same time period [39]. The recurrence rate of syncope remains similar despite widely different suspected causes (severe cardiovascular disease or not) and despite apparently effective treatment [38]. The fact that syncope is frequently an isolated occurrence can make it difficult to diagnose and difficult to assess the need for treatment (it may or may not recur). An apparent therapeutic effect of any intervention may instead be related to the sporadic nature of the symptom and not to treatment of the underlying process [38,40,41]. An older report suggested that tonsillar enlargement caused tachycardia and syncope [42]. Following tonsillectomy, syncope did not recur. Therefore, tonsillectomy was assumed to prevent recurrent syncope. While ludicrous, it is important to recognize the similarity to modern thinking on this same topic.

Even without treatment, syncope can remain dormant for a protracted period or "respond" to the apparent effect of the evaluation itself. Indeed, many benign forms of syncope seem to be heavily influenced by placebo. However, the goal of therapy, to reduce the frequency and severity of episodes, is achievable. It appears that syncope is less likely to recur when its cause is diagnosed properly and treated effectively [43–45].

The differential diagnosis

With so many potential causes for syncope, it is difficult, if not impossible, to provide a complete reference list of all common and uncommon causes (Tables 1.1 and 1.2). New and creative ways to pass out are always possible [46–53], and some syncope is not really syncope at all [54–56]. Syncope has its fads [57–62]; consider the "mess trick" (the fainting lark [61,62]) of the Valsalva maneuver during hyperventilation. This rarely causes syncope now but mass fainting at rock concerts is possible [59]. Syncope has even been reported with sushi ingestion [63].

An old, retrospective study [57], representing a large collection of patients with syncope, provides insight into the most common causes and myths

Table 1.1 Common causes for syncope.

Cardiovascular disease	Non-cardiovascular disease	Other
Arrhythmic	Reflex mechanisms	Syncope of unknown origin
AV block with bradycardia	Vasodepressor "neurocardiogenic"	About 50% of all syncope patients
Sinus pauses/bradycardia	Micturition	Undiagnosed seizures
Ventricular tachycardia and	Deglutition	Improperly diagnosed syncope
structural heart disease	Orthostatic hypotension	Confusional states due to
Non-arrhythmic – hemodynamic	Dysautonomia	hypoglycemia, stroke, etc.
Hypertrophic cardiomyopathy	Fluid depletion	Drug induced
Aortic stenosis	Illness, bed rest	Alcohol
	Drugs	Illicit drugs
	Psychogenic	Prescribed drugs (esp. the elderly)
	Hysterical	
	Panic disorder	
	Anxiety disorder	

Table 1.2 Uncommon causes for syncope.

Cardiovascular disease	Non-cardiovascular disease
Arrhythmic etiology	Reflexes
Supraventricular tachycardia	Post-tussive
Long QT interval syndrome	Defecation
Brugada syndrome	Glossopharyngeal
Arrhythmogenic right ventricular cardiomyopathy	Postprandial
Idiopathic ventricular tachycardia(s)	Carotid sinus hypersensitivity
Myocardial infarction (and bradycardia/tachycardia)	Hyperventilation
Non-arrhythmic etiology	Migraine
Pulmonary embolus	Carcinoid syndrome
Pulmonary hypertension	Systemic mastocytosis
Dissecting aortic aneurysm	Metabolic
Subclavian steal	Hypoglycemia
Atrial myxoma	Hypoxia
Cardiac tamponade	Multivessel cerebrovascular disease

regarding syncope. Between 1945 and 1957, of a total cohort of approximately 1000 syncope patients, data from 510 patients were evaluated [57]. The remaining patient charts were "unsatisfactory for analysis." In contrast to more recent data, a cause for syncope was diagnosed in nearly all (96%) of the patients (Table 1.3). Is this amazing clinical acumen? Perhaps. More likely, though, the diagnoses were a "best guess" with few, if any, confirmatory data.

Data from the Framingham study provide new insights into the differential diagnosis of syncope in the modern era and provide the outcome of these patients [64]. Of 727 patients with syncope, the cause was vasovagal in 21%, orthostatic hypotension in 9.4%, cardiac causes in 9.5%, seizures in 4.9%, stroke or transient ischemic attack in 4.1%, medication related in 6.8%, and other in 7.5%. Of importance, even with modern methods to assess cause, syncope was a result of an unknown cause in 36.6% (31% of men and 41% of women) [64].

In a report of five pooled studies, the etiology of syncope was vasovagal in 18%, situational in 5%, orthostatic in 8%, cardiac in 18%, medication related in 3%, psychiatric in 2%, neurological in 10%, carotid sinus hypersensitivity related in 1%, and

Table 1.3 Breakdown of various causes of syncope in an older retrospective study of 510 patients. Although an accurate cause for syncope may not be diagnosed from the data, interesting conclusions may be drawn. (Data from [57].)

Presumed cause for syncope	Number
Vasovagal	298
Orthostatic hypotension	28
Epilepsy	26
Cerebrovascular disease	24
Unknown etiology	23
Postmicturition	17
Stokes–Adams attacks	17
Hyperventilation	15
Hypersensitive carotid sinus	15
Tussive	13
Aortic stenosis	9
Paroxysmal tachycardia	8
Angina	4
Hysteria	4
Myocardial infarction	3
Pulmonary hypertension	2
Migraine	2
Hypertensive encephalopathy	2

unknown in 34% [65,66]. The presence of cardiac disease does not indicate the cause for syncope is cardiac or is even known [67].

Common causes for syncope

Neurocardiogenic (vasovagal) syncope

A vasovagal episode is the most common cause for syncope [57,64,66] (Table 1.3). Vasovagal (neurocardiogenic) mechanisms may account for, or contribute to (in the presence of other clinical conditions), 30–80% of all syncopal episodes [13,15,33,35,37,68–71]. Recent data from several studies confirm that neurocardiogenic syncope is the most common etiology of syncope.

Neurocardiogenic syncope can be caused by, or provoked by, several inciting, often noxious, stimuli. The specific stimulus can be difficult to characterize, can be highly individualized, and can vary by physical and emotional state [3]. Emotional stresses alone (danger, real or perceived, fear, or anxiety) are common triggers [3,72] and distinctly human [73]. The responsible reflex causing syncope can be "normal" and may be self-limited.

When a specific set of conditions initiates syncope, it is termed "situational syncope" [71]. For example, the vasovagal (neurocardiogenic) reflex can occur with severe volume loss resulting from diarrhea or blood loss and may never recur. Complete evaluation and long-term drug therapy is indicated only when episodes recur frequently and cannot be explained by a precipitating cause (see Chapter 2). Sometimes it is difficult to discover an initiating factor responsible for the complex vasovagal reflex so that the diagnosis is not clear. This may explain, in part, the wide variation in the frequency of the diagnosis of neurocardiogenic syncope between reports.

While neurocardiogenic causes for syncope are generally benign, a syndrome of "malignant" vasovagal syncope has been used to describe patients who have frequent and recurrent episodes, who have episodes without obvious prodrome, who have prolonged asystole, and/or who have spells without an apparent triggering stimulus [74–78]. The specific implications of having this form of neurocardiogenic syncope are unclear regarding prognosis and treatment but these patients do not necessarily require more aggressive therapy [79,80]. Testing the response to orthostatic stress (tilt table testing) can secure the diagnosis for these individuals [81] (see Chapters 2, 7 and 13). An even more malignant, poorly understood, vasovagal reflex might also (rarely) cause death by asystole in some patients with severely impaired left ventricular function [6,82] and in others [83].

Orthostatic hypotension

The second most common cause of syncope is orthostatic hypotension [57] (Table 1.3). This problem is often overlooked, underdiagnosed, and incompletely evaluated. Orthostatic hypotension [84–92] has many etiologies (see Chapters 3 and 13) but is generally caused by a dysautonomic syndrome, drugs, volume depletion (e.g., blood loss), or a combination of factors each of which, alone, would have no effect. Peripheral autonomic (sympathetic) denervation, resulting from systemic diseases including diabetes and amyloidosis [93,94], can prevent needed peripheral vasoconstriction with standing. Additional specific disease states besides, most commonly diabetes [95], that can cause this condition include Parkinsonism [96], Addison's disease [97], porphyria [98], tabes dorsalis [99], syringomyelia [100], spinal cord transection [101], Guillian–Barré syndrome [102], Riley–Day syndrome [103], surgically induced sympathectomy [104], pheochromocytoma [105], multisystem atrophy [106], Bradbury–Eggleston syndrome [107], and the Shy–Drager syndrome (also known as idiopathic orthostatic hypotension) [108–113]. It can even occur with anorexia nervosa [114].

The elderly are most susceptible to conditions that test the resiliency of their response to orthostatic stress [115–117], particularly if there is another trigger (such as a non-sustained tachyarrhythmia or a vasodilator, even if the patient is otherwise hypertensive). Elderly patients frequently have difficulty with effective autoregulation of peripheral and cerebral blood flow and are highly susceptible to symptomatic orthostatic hypotension [85, 118–123]. The elderly tend to have slower heart rates at baseline [122,124] and they tend to be more hypertension at night [125]. Orthostatic hypotension and its treatment are discussed in Chapters 3 and 13.

Medications can cause syncope by a variety of mechanisms, including, commonly, orthostatic hypotension. Nearly 13% of syncopal and presyncopal spells in patients who presented to an ambulatory clinic were caused by an adverse drug reaction [126]. Vasodilators (hydralazine, nitrates, angiotensin-converting enzyme inhibitors), α_1- and β-adrenergic blockers and α_2-adrenergic stimulants, diuretics, tricyclic antidepressants and phenothiazines, and others, can cause orthostatic hypotension [126]. Nitrates can also trigger a hypotensive, vagal, or other autonomic response [127–129]; to wit, they may be used in the tilt table laboratory. Non-steroidal anti-inflammatory drugs can decrease peripheral vascular resistance and its response to orthostatic stress [126,130]. Hypokalemia can impair reactivity of vascular smooth muscle and limit increase in peripheral vascular resistance.

Volume depletion from blood loss or diuretic use commonly causes orthostatic hypotension. Prolonged bed rest or chronic illness can provoke or exacerbate transient orthostatic hypotension in vulnerable patients, such as the elderly or those with diabetes. Even normal individuals at prolonged bed rest, especially if volume depleted, may pass out abruptly on rising. Water ingestion or even eating a meal can help by several mechanisms including, but not limited to, fluid repletion [131–133]. Rarely, inherent circulating vasodilators present in a vasoactive intestinal peptide tumor (VIPoma), the carcinoid syndrome, a prolactinoma, or systemic mastocytosis can cause orthostatic hypotension and, rarely, syncope [134–141]. Of note, prolactin levels can be elevated after syncope or a seizure [142,143].

The response to changes in position can be immediate or delayed. As part of the physical examination, orthostatic signs should always be obtained but change in blood pressure may be seen soon after standing in fluid depletion, or may require several minutes of standing for dysautonomic conditions. An orthostatic change (lowering) in blood pressure, without a compensatory change (increase) in heart rate, suggests an autonomic neuropathy.

Arrhythmic causes

Surprisingly, "paroxysmal tachycardia" and "Stokes–Adams attacks" were suspected as a rare cause for syncope in older studies [57] (Table 1.3). Cardiac and cardiac arrhythmic causes are now suspected to be more common [64]. However, Donzelot described syncope resulting from ventricular tachycardia in 1914 [144] and Barnes [42] described cerebral symptoms of paroxysmal tachycardia in 1926. Cardiac rhythm disturbances, bradycardias, and tachycardias are now well known to be a common cause for syncope [44]. The arrhythmias can be benign (not associated with death) or malignant (associated with increased risk of death). In earlier studies, techniques to detect cardiac arrhythmias were lacking [57]. Now, with more sophisticated diagnostic tools (prolonged monitoring techniques and electrophysiologic tests), a primary arrhythmic etiology can be more easily identified. Common rhythm disturbances associated with syncope include paroxysms of ventricular tachycardia, AV block associated with bradycardia, and marked sinus bradycardia (sick sinus syndrome and tachy-brady syndrome).

Organic heart disease, especially in association with impaired left ventricular function, a bundle branch block, a long QT interval, or pre-excitation (Wolff–Parkinson–White syndrome) should raise suspicions of an arrhythmic etiology for syncope.

Arrhythmic syncope, caused by AV block (generally second or third degree) or ventricular tachycardia, tends to have an abrupt onset with no prodrome ("Stokes–Adams" attack, not *specific* for arrhythmic etiology for syncope). It may have a malignant course (associated with cardiac arrest) and be distinguishable from neurocardiogenic syncope [145], or mimic other causes for syncope.

Supraventricular tachycardia (AV nodal re-entry or AV reciprocating tachycardia), atrial flutter, and fibrillation, while generally benign, can occasionally cause syncope but there is usually a history of palpitations or tachycardia [146]. Up to 15% of patients with supraventricular tachycardia will have syncope or near-syncope brought about by the tachycardia [147].

Atrial fibrillation rarely causes syncope unless the ventricular rate is excessively fast or slow. Slow rates tend to occur in the elderly because of autonomic changes [120–124] or AV nodal dysfunction, whereas fast rates can occur in younger patients with Wolff–Parkinson–White syndrome or with enhanced AV nodal conduction [148].

There are special subgroups of arrhythmias that are important to consider. Short paroxysms of asymptomatic, non-sustained, ventricular tachycardia can be problematic and, while sometimes ascribed to be the cause for syncope [15], the two may be unrelated. Sinus arrest can cause syncope. While generally resulting from intrinsic sinus node disease causing sick sinus syndrome or tachy-brady syndrome, it can be difficult to distinguish intrinsic sinus node disease from accentuated vagal tone. Ventricular bigeminy can be associated with hypotension and a slow pulse but almost never with syncope. Ventricular pacing may cause dizziness and weakness but rarely loss of consciousness [149]. However, patients with pacemakers may have syncope from abrupt pacemaker failure or other, unrelated causes, including malignant neurocardiogenic syncope [149–151].

A special subgroup includes patients who have implanted defibrillators. When a patient with an implanted cardioverter defibrillator (ICD) passes out, a recurrent ventricular arrhythmia must be suspected. Careful assessment of the functioning of the ICD and of the underlying rhythm is required. There may be a need to restrict the patient with an ICD if the syncope is caused by an arrhythmia.

Physiologically, tachycardias are less well tolerated hemodynamically than bradycardias, whether or not AV synchrony is present. The *abrupt onset* of the arrhythmia, even when otherwise tolerated, can cause syncope [152,153]. Ventricular tachycardia is usually less well tolerated than supraventricular tachycardia, even at the same heart rate, but hemodynamics worsen with increasing rates [154]. Syncope, however, is most directly related to an abrupt change in the rate, caused by lack of effective reflex peripheral vascular vasoconstriction and ineffective accommodation of cerebral blood flow [42,152].

Chronic sinus bradycardia is much less of a problem than is sinus rhythm with abrupt sinus arrest. Persistent atrial flutter or ventricular tachycardia is less likely to cause syncope than is a paroxysm of the same tachycardia, even at the same rate. It is common for the blood pressure to drop at the onset of tachycardia causing syncope but, over several seconds, the blood pressure can rise and syncope can resolve despite continuation of tachycardia [155–157], resulting from reflex vasoconstriction and elevation in catecholamine levels. Ventricular function, body position, and medications all influence the hemodynamic response to and presence of changes in heart rate, and the presence and length of syncope [158]. The presence of sustained ventricular tachycardia alone does not always explain syncope because it does not always cause syncope. In one series, only 15% of patients who presented to an emergency room with sustained ventricular tachycardia had syncope associated with tachycardia [40].

An arrhythmia present at the time of syncope may be a secondary phenomenon or unrelated and may not be explanatory. Treatment of the arrhythmia would therefore not treat syncope effectively. An example is a patient with a vasovagal spell who develops a "relative" bradycardia after hypotension and after syncope had already started. Treating the bradycardia (with a pacemaker) would not be expected to correct a primary peripheral hemodynamic or central nervous system problem but each case must be considered individually [159]. In neurocardiogenic syncope, when bradycardia is a secondary issue, it is not surprising that its treatment may not help syncope recurrence.

Case 1

A 50-year-old avid bicyclist has recurrent syncope at rest (after exercise) with associated AV block and > 8-s pauses but the sinus rate did not slow. Carotid sinus massage was negative. A tilt table test was positive for hypotension and relative. On the treadmill, his heart rate exceeded 180 b min^{-1}. He refused to stop exercising. The cause for his AV block was unclear but may have been autonomically mediated.

Therapy. A permanent dual chamber pacemaker was placed with complete improvement in symptoms.

Case 2

A 45-year-old woman has recurrent syncope and on a Holter monitor had 8-s pauses resulting from sinus arrest. A permanent pacemaker was placed but she continued to pass out. A tilt table test was subsequently positive for hypotension and syncope despite AV pacing.

Seizures

Seizures can be mistaken for syncope and vice versa [57,160–167] (Table 1.3). Generally, it is not difficult to distinguish seizures from syncope [166]. When there is confusion, it is most likely that neurocardiogenic syncope is confused with seizures ("convulsive syncope"). A possible exception to this rule is akinetic seizures. The episodes are manifest by abrupt loss of consciousness and dropping to the ground. The episodes may be so violent that the patient appears to be thrown to the ground. As opposed to generalized seizures, at the end of an episode, the patient appears normal and has no postictal drowsiness. The seizures themselves are quite brief but their sudden and unpredictable nature may lead to injury. Myoclonic jerks may precede the attacks and the episodes tend to occur while going to sleep at night or on awakening in the morning. This type of seizure is most common in the 2–5 year pediatric age range but cases have been observed in older children. The electroencephalogram (EEG) is usually markedly abnormal, demonstrating either generalized or multifocal epileptiform discharges. This form of seizure is exceedingly difficult to treat. The usual antiseizure medications are often ineffective, although some patients may respond to valproic acid or a benzodiazepine. Some authors have recommended section of the corpus callosum in patients with medically intractable seizures that result in repeated injury [168], but this is controversial. Some patients have responded to a medium-chain triglyceride (MCT 3) variant of the ketogenic diet [169].

The incidence of seizure diagnoses as cause for syncope varies widely between reports [13,16]. Hofnagels *et al.* [162] noted that only 31% of physicians caring for patients with "spells" could agree whether or not seizure was the cause. The distinction can be especially difficult if seizures are atypical or episodes are unwitnessed. This problem is compounded by the lack of sensitivity and specificity of the EEG as it is generally performed.

An EEG, by itself, cannot be relied upon to diagnose a seizure disorder. Up to 50% of patients who have a seizure focus will have a negative EEG unless sleep deprivation is used or unless nasopharyngeal leads or deep brainstem leads are placed [161,170–173] (see Chapter 9). To complicate matters, up to 40% of asymptomatic elderly individuals will have asymptomatic electroencephalographic abnormalities. These abnormalities do not imply seizure is the cause for the episode. Nevertheless, seizures likely account for 10–15% of apparent syncopal episodes [16,57]. However, patients with seizures rarely have episodes with sudden onset and abrupt, rapid recovery. Instead, the postictal state is slow and lingering. The tilt table test may be useful to distinguish seizure from syncope [160] and creatine kinase measurements may also be helpful [174].

Alternatively, syncope, with loss of cerebral blood flow, can cause tonic–clonic movements and can mimic a seizure [175]. This apparent seizure activity is associated with slowing of the brain waves not with epileptiform spikes on the EEG. Sometimes, a video EEG is required to determine if a seizure is indeed present.

Case 3

A 27-year-old woman with primary pulmonary hypertension has prolonged and frequent episodes of loss of consciousness. Tonic–clonic movements are noted and recovery is prolonged. A video EEG showed a flat recording during an episode. During combined hemodynamic and video EEG recordings, it was discovered that she has apnea, hypotension followed by sinus tachycardia, and asystole with an episode. The "seizure" is syncope. This is a fairly typical autonomic response for a patient with this condition.

Temporal lobe epilepsy can rarely trigger neuro-cardiogenic syncope [176]. Also, asystole can masquerade as temporal lobe epilepsy [177].

Micturition syncope and syncope resulting from other autonomic causes

Micturition syncope is one of several variations of autonomically mediated syncope which include deglutition syncope, carotid sinus hypersensitivity, post-tussive syncope, defecation syncope, and trumpet player's syncope [33,57,178]. The mechanism for these forms of syncope are related to abrupt changes in autonomic tone, in intravascular volume, and in cerebrospinal fluid pressure. Specifically, micturition syncope is a result of an abrupt change in position combined with a strong vagal stimulus. Micturition syncope can occur in either sex. Kapoor *et al.* [179] reported that women (in contrast to previous studies suggesting a clear male predominance) have a higher incidence of syncope caused by evening micturition.

While the exact mechanisms for these entities may not be identical, the autonomic nervous system appears to be critically involved in the initiation of the episode. Generally, all causes for syncope appear to involve a poorly tolerated hemodynamic response to specific autonomic cardiovascular reflexes. Autonomic reflexes are often critical in the initiation and termination of syncope, or the presence of the pre-existing problems would allow patients to lose consciousness continuously.

Case 4 [56]

A 72-year-old man passes out after drinking cold, carbonated beverages. Syncope causes a major motor vehicle accident. He has a complete evaluation by cardiologists and internists, including a cardiac catheterization, tilt table test, treadmill test, EEG, and magnetic resonance imaging (MRI) of the brain. The diagnosis was secured by observing him and his heart rhythm while he drank a cold can of soda.

Diagnosis. Deglutition syncope resulting from cold, carbonated beverages.

Therapy. Avoidance of cold, carbonated beverages eliminated the problem.

Case 5

A 52-year-old man with reactive airways disease and chronic aspiration caused by gastroesophageal reflux has recurrent syncope after prolonged episodes of coughing. Syncope resolved after effective therapy for his pulmonary problems.

Diagnosis. Post-tussive syncope.

Case 6

A 58-year-old man became asystolic during abdominal surgery during peritoneal manipulation. He gives a history of syncope when he drinks cold liquids and was noted to become asystolic (AV block and sinus arrest are both noted on different occasions) while drinking iced water. Carotid massage caused 7 s of symptomatic asystole. Temporary ventricular pacing during carotid massage was associated with hypotension, but with dual chamber pacing the blood pressure remained above 100 mmHg systolic.

Diagnosis. Deglutition syncope.

Therapy. With permanent pacing, he remained asymptomatic for 7 years.

Case 7

An 85-year-old man with a history of coronary artery disease and benign prostatic hypertrophy has taken furosemide, digoxin, and captopril for mild congestive heart failure. He passed out suddenly when awakening to urinate. There was a 15-mmHg drop in blood pressure with standing.

Diagnosis. Micturition syncope.

Therapy. The patient was warned to arise slowly before urinating in the evening and to sit when urinating.

Uncommon, but important, causes for syncope

Cerebrovascular disease

Cerebrovascular disease is an uncommon and probably overdiagnosed cause for syncope. Stroke and transient ischemic attacks tend to cause focal neurologic deficits from which recovery is slow and incomplete. If posterior cerebral circulation is impaired, symptoms such as nausea or dizziness are more likely than transient loss of consciousness. If the anterior circulation is impaired, a focal neurologic defect will occur. Severe, obstructive, multivessel cerebrovascular disease can cause syncope but other neurologic findings will likely occur first and will likely persist after syncope.

Myocardial ischemia and myocardial infarction

Syncope is often suspected to be caused by myocardial infarction or ischemia, thus resulting in hospital admission to "rule out" myocardial infarction and assess ischemia. This process is usually unnecessary and unwarranted because myocardial infarction rarely causes syncope [57,180]. If myocardial infarction or ischemia is the cause for syncope, there are generally obvious clues from the history and from the ECG [180]. One potential cause for syncope is bradycardia and hypotension from the Bezold–Jarisch reflex [181], but other arrhythmic and non-arrhythmic causes related to ischemia and infarction are possible.

Other cardiac causes for syncope

Obstructive valvular lesions, such as aortic stenosis and hypertrophic cardiomyopathy, are well-recognized but relatively rare causes of syncope [13,16,182–184]. Other obstructive valvular lesions, such as atrial myxoma and atrial ball valve thrombus, are even rarer. Obstructive lesions such as aortic stenosis tend to cause an exaggerated and malignant form of an exercise-induced vasovagal response leading to syncope and perhaps even death [185]. Other forms of syncope can be confused with obstructive hemodynamic problems [186]. The obstruction itself may not be the direct cause for collapse. When aortic stenosis causes syncope, the episodes tend to be markedly prolonged. Episodes can be triggered by exertion.

Metabolic causes

Syncope, characterized by abrupt onset and complete, brisk recovery, is rarely a result of a toxic or metabolic cause. Hypoglycemia, hypoxia, meningitis, encephalitis, and sepsis can cause coma, stupor, and confusion, but rarely syncope [187]. Hypoxia can, however, influence vascular tone [188]. If a patient does not recall the history surrounding the

event or if the event was unwitnessed, coma and syncope can be hard to distinguish.

Neurologic and psychiatric causes

Neurally mediated (neurocardiogenic) syncope can mimic transient ischemic attacks [189]. Psychiatric causes for syncope can mimic neurocardiogenic syncope [190]. There are several neurologic and psychiatric causes for syncope, which are discussed in detail in Chapters 9 and 12 [191,192].

Case 8

A 32-year-old woman was referred for a tilt table test for recurrent episodes of loss of consciousness associated with a prodrome of nausea and vomiting. Upon further questioning, the patient described quadriparesis with near-blindness after the episode while awake.

Diagnosis. Migraine headaches.

Syncope of unknown origin

In older studies, hardly any patients had syncope of unknown origin (SUO) [57]. In contrast, most contemporary data would indicate that in nearly 50% of patients presenting with syncope (even evaluated by a meticulous history, physical examination, and proper diagnostic testing), no cause will be found, making this a critically important and large patient subgroup [13–16,64,67]. The marked discrepancy between different studies relates partly to the level of certainty tolerated for a diagnosis. Perhaps a low degree of accuracy or "clinical judgment" alone was sufficient to clinch the diagnosis in an older, retrospective analysis. Differences may also be related to selection bias, to inclusion and exclusion criteria, and to physicians' assumptions made in diagnosing the causes for syncope [193].

Thus, the assumed cause for syncope is often based on flawed methods and incorrect assumptions. It may only be possible to know the definite cause for syncope if the episode is witnessed with an ECG, arterial line, oximeter, and EEG attached to the patient. Even then, the causal mechanism may not be clear. Therefore, even in the best of circumstances, the diagnosis of syncope is often a "leap of faith."

Various definitions exist for SUO but perhaps the best accepted is syncope without an apparent cause despite a meticulous history and physical examination and monitoring but no involved diagnostic testing. In reality, *all* patients have SUO, even if testing shows possible causes, as long as the relationship between the abnormality and the episode is not proven.

Because almost all diagnoses are presumptive, SUO has been used to describe different types of patients. This is important when considering diagnostic evaluation and assessment of the prognosis of these patients. Those who undergo electrophysiologic testing for syncope, for example, do not have a cause diagnosed although an arrhythmic cause for syncope is usually suspected. If the tests show induced ventricular tachycardia, did ventricular tachycardia cause syncope or is the cause still unknown? If there are episodes of asymptomatic, non-sustained ventricular tachycardia on Holter monitoring, is this enough evidence to consider that it caused syncope [13]? If all testing is unrevealing, and the patient has no obvious underlying disease, it is likely that syncope under these circumstances results from a neurocardiogenic or dysautonomic origin.

Case 9

A 45-year-old woman develops abdominal pain, and severe nausea and vomiting. She develops gross hematemesis and passes out at home. The paramedics are called.

Presumed diagnosis. Gastrointestinal bleed or vagal-induced bradycardia/hypotension.

Actual diagnosis. In the ambulance she is noted to have long runs of hemodynamically intolerable wide QRS complex tachycardia causing recurrent syncope.

Case 10: Is it really syncope?

A 52-year-old Cambodian man collapsed three times at home while working in his garden and standing in the kitchen. He injured himself. On monitoring at night he had 5-s pauses but he also had sleep apnea. On evaluation, he complained of generalized weakness, edema, cold intolerance, difficulty swallowing, changes in his voice, and weight gain. He had bradycardia and a slightly prolonged QT interval. The thyroid-stimulating hormone level was markedly elevated at 55 uIU/ml. The creatine kinase was markedly elevated.

Myxedema explained his "collapse"; it mimicked syncope. The sinus pauses were "red herrings."

Classification

Based on a long differential diagnostic list of potential causes, it has become fashionable to subclassify the etiology of syncope into three broad categories: cardiovascular, non-cardiovascular, and unknown [13,14,68,184]. Several contemporary reports have lent support to this approach. Considering patients who are admitted to hospitals or are seen in emergency rooms, approximately 30% will have a cardiovascular cause for syncope found [13,14,68]. Approximately 50% of patients with suspected cardiovascular disease will have an arrhythmia diagnosed, although it may not be the cause of syncope [14].

There is a high sudden and total death rate, despite therapy, for patients with underlying cardiovascular disease, even if the presumed problem responsible is corrected [14]. The 5-year mortality in patients with syncope and a diagnosed cardiovascular cause approaches 50%, with a 30% incidence of death in the first year [14,15]. When a cardiovascular cause is diagnosed, treatment, including specific treatment of hemodynamically unstable and life-threatening arrhythmias, can improve the long-term outcome. Perhaps the treatment that prevents death also prevents recurrent syncope. This becomes difficult to determine because, in comparative trials, the recurrence rate of syncope is similar whether or not a cardiovascular cause was found and treated [38].

Twenty to thirty percent of patients have a non-cardiovascular cause for syncope [14,15]: neurologic causes (see Chapter 9), vasodepressor syncope (see Chapter 2), and orthostatic hypotension (see Chapters 3 and 13). Although the mortality in this group is lower (less than 10% in 1 year, and 30% over a 5-year period), there is nevertheless a substantial risk to the welfare of the patient [13,14].

In nearly half of the patients with syncope, a cause is suspected but not diagnosed, despite a complete evaluation [14,15]. These patients with SUO generally have a benign course, with a low (6 to < 10%) 3-year risk and a modest 5-year risk (24%) of death at one center [14,15], but not all agree that SUO has such a benign prognosis [16].

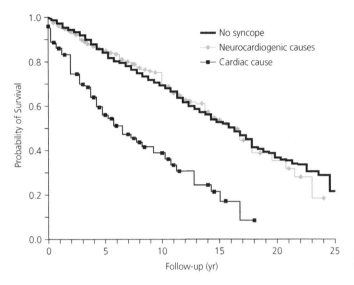

Fig. 1.1 Syncope: Outcome by condition. (Adapted from [64].)

Table 1.4 Common causes of syncope by patient age.

Young (< 35 years)	Middle-aged (35–65 years)	Elderly (> 65 years)
Neurocardiogenic	Neurocardiogenic	Multifactorial
Situational	Cardiac	Cardiac
Psychiatric	Arrhythmic	Mechanical/obstructive
(Undiagnosed seizures)	Mechanical/obstructive	Arrhythmic
(Long QT syndrome)		Orthostatic hypotension
(Wolff–Parkinson–White syndrome, other SVT)		Drug-induced
(Hypertrophy cardiomyopathy)		Neurally mediated
		(Neurocardiogenic)

Less common, but important and potentially life-threatening causes are in brackets.
SVT, supraventricular tachycardia.

It *appears* helpful to consider the simple sub-classification of syncope into three main causes: cardiovascular, non-cardiovascular, or unknown origin. The advantage of patient categorization is that it allows clinical assessment of the prognostic meaning of syncope. Recent data from the Framingham Study indicates mortality by cause for syncope [64] (Fig. 1.1). Classification by patient age may also be helpful (Table 1.4). The elderly are at highest risk of death, with a 2-year mortality of 27% compared with 8% in the younger age group, but the presence of syncope has not been shown to influence mortality independently in the elderly [31,32,194,195].

There are, nevertheless, several caveats concerning this classification. The non-cardiovascular group is not really totally non-cardiovascular. Vasodepressor syncope, often considered a non-cardiovascular cause, is actually a cardiovascular reflex that could just as well be considered a cardiovascular cause for syncope. If this entity were considered to be a cardiovascular cause for syncope, the prognostic categorization would lose its meaning, because most episodes of vasovagal syncope have a benign prognosis. Pulmonary emboli and dissecting aortic aneurysms, often considered to be cardiovascular causes, could actually be con-sidered non-cardiac. If these were considered non-cardiovascular, the prognostic value of this subclassification would change [196]. Also, the presence or absence of a cardiovascular cause did not influence survival of patients admitted with syncope [197].

Syncope is not always related to the cause of death. Syncope patients with dissecting aortic aneurysm, aortic stenosis, ventricular tachycardia, or pulmonary emboli have a high risk of dying even if syncope is not present. Syncope is not clearly an *independent* predictor of death, although for specific conditions, such as dilated cardiomyopathy, arrhythmogenic right ventricular cardiomyopathy, congenital long QT interval syndrome, and Brugada syndrome, it may be. For patients with syncope caused by, or associated with, structural heart disease, the incidence of sudden and total death may be high. It remains unclear whether syncope itself augments the risk of death further [198,199]. It is not surprising that syncope patients with cardiovascular disease have a higher mortality than syncope patients without cardiovascular disease. The subgroups, cardiovascular and non-cardiovascular, are not comparable by age, underlying disease, or prognosis otherwise. The long-term prognosis may be related more to the underlying cardiac disease than to syncope.

To evaluate this further, Silverstein *et al.* [200] stratified patients with and without syncope who were admitted to an intensive care unit. He found that the prognosis was independent of syncope but depended on the severity of the underlying disease. Similarly, the Framingham study did not indicate that patients with cardiovascular disease and syncope were any more likely to die than those with cardiovascular disease without syncope [24]. Others have found a similar result [201]. Even when the cause for syncope is diagnosed and treated in patients with cardiovascular disease, the mortality remains higher than in patients without known cardiovascular disease [14,15].

Patients admitted to hospital with syncope, especially if cardiovascular disease is diagnosed, tend to be sicker and older, and tend to have a higher mortality independent of syncope or its cause. Syncope does not place an extremely elderly (or even young) patient at higher risk of death than other individuals of the same age [32,121,194]. Syncope is probably not a prognostic indicator for patients with the Wolff–Parkinson–White syndrome [202,203] or hypertrophic cardiomyopathy [203,204] (although this is debated), even in younger patients. The presence or absence of a cardiovascular cause for syncope does not necessarily predict long-term survival.

Patients with syncope with an arrhythmic or hemodynamic cause may have a high mortality. It is an especially important prognostic indicator if impaired left ventricular function, ventricular ectopy, and induced ventricular tachycardia at electrophysiologic testing are all present [17,35,43–45,206–215]. Such patients have a prognosis as poor as those who have had a cardiac arrest or sustained ventricular tachycardia [197]. Other examples include syncope associated with the hereditary long QT interval syndrome (see Chapters 8 and 11), aortic stenosis [216] (even if syncope is caused by alteration in autonomic response [217]), or an atrial myxoma [218]. Treatment of these conditions can improve prognosis and prevent recurrence of syncope. Similarly, repair of an aortic valve for aortic stenosis or removal of an atrial tumor will improve long-term prognosis and *may* treat the cause of syncope [219].

Middlekauff *et al.* [220,221] and Tchou *et al.* [222] found syncope to be an important prognostic predictor for specific patient subgroups: those with impaired left ventricular function and congestive heart failure. In patients with advanced heart failure and syncope, the 1-year mortality was 45% compared with 12% without syncope [220,221]. Patients with idiopathic dilated cardiomyopathy have a 56% 4-year mortality in contrast with a 4% 4-year mortality in patients with dilated cardiomyopathy who do not have syncope [222]. Using electrophysiologic testing, several investigators have shown in separate studies that the mortality in patients with induced ventricular tachycardia was lowered if the tachycardia was treated properly [44,45,197]. Another report using electrophysiologic testing showed that there was a 5% recurrence rate of syncope for treated patients versus a 24% recurrence rate in those with untreated syncope [43].

The prognostic impact of syncope is clearly disease-specific but prompt, aggressive treatment of syncope in patients with malignant ventricular arrhythmias is required and can be life-saving. For other conditions, including various cardiovascular etiologies, the cause of death and syncope are not clearly directly linked. In this regard, categorization into cardiovascular, non-cardiovascular, and unknown etiologies, while potentially useful, represents an oversimplification of an extraordinarily complex issue.

It is possible that syncope and mortality are unrelated. Further, treatment can alter mortality and syncope recurrence but this is disease dependent. The two are not necessarily linked. For example, an ICD may prevent cardiac arrest in a patient with the congenital long QT interval syndrome but it may not prevent syncope. Repair of an aortic valve may prevent syncope but the patient may still have a significant cardiovascular mortality resulting from associated conditions.

Initial approach to the patient with syncope

The proper diagnostic and therapeutic approach requires careful analysis of the symptoms and clinical findings, and integration of all the clues in the history, from the patient and others present. No specific battery of tests is ever indicated or is always useful. Extensive diagnostic evaluation is generally unnecessary, expensive, and risky. Repeated evaluation and hospital admission after an initial negative assessment tends to be unrewarding. If this point is reached, consider exploring the history in more detail with the patient, witnesses, and family.

With present technology it is clearly impractical to monitor all episodes of syncope to arrive at a diagnosis, although it is useful to implant and electrocardiographically monitor selected patients [223] (see Chapter 19). Clinicians must base their decisions on historical features, with the presumption that the description of the episode is accurate and complete [14,16,20,36,57,224–226].

Diagnostic evaluation must be guided from the history. Common sense cannot be underestimated, even if it is difficult to describe [56]. Listen to the patient. The proper evaluation requires a balance of the judicious use of inpatient and outpatient diagnostic modalities. The expense and risk of the procedures and hospitalization are intensified by the possibility of causing iatrogenic harm from a diagnostic or therapeutic mishap.

The location of the evaluation is important. In the emergency room, immediate decisions are crucial concerning the need for admission, assessment of risk, and the need for restriction and follow-up. For the hospitalized patient, early decisions are encouraged concerning types of inpatient management approach. Discharge planning for further outpatient evaluation, if necessary, should begin early in the hospitalization. Surprisingly few patients admitted with syncope, without some kind of plan

before admission, will benefit from hospitalization. Arguably, patients admitted are their own subgroup and have a different, perhaps higher risk of death [197]. The outpatient with a vague or distant history of syncope can be evaluated more leisurely, in contrast to the patient hospitalized in the intensive care unit with impaired left ventricular function. For each circumstance, the cause for and prognosis of syncope will differ and the approach to diagnosis and therapy will differ concomitantly.

Various clinical algorithms have been developed but, because of the diverse nature of syncope, it becomes impossible to implement an evaluation stratagem that will succeed in all circumstances and for all patients. Indeed, algorithms can confuse more than clarify. Consider the complexity of one such algorithm published in a neurology text (Fig. 1.2). Such an approach, even if understandable, or readable, has not been shown to improve outcome.

The history

To evaluate syncope, sound clinical decisions are based on a carefully performed history with great attention to detail. The history, with its proper interpretation, and a directed physical examination are the only appropriate ways to guide further diagnostic evaluation. The history and physical examination alone can be diagnostic in 25–35% of patients [13,14,16,20,67,200,226] (Table 1.5). Of those for whom a cause is found, the history and physical examination alone were sufficient in 75–85% of patients [13]. If the history does not provide diagnostic clues, it is much more likely that no diagnosis will be reached even with an extensive battery of tests.

Symptoms and several historical features, summarized in Tables 1.6 and 1.7, can help to direct further diagnostic procedures. Specific attention should be directed toward:

1 characteristics and length of the episode;

2 patient's and witnesses' accounts;

3 patient age;

4 concomitant (especially cardiac) disease;

5 associated, temporally related, symptoms (e.g., neurologic symptoms, angina, palpitations, and heart failure);

6 premonitory (prodromal) symptoms;

7 symptoms on awakening (postsyncope symptoms);

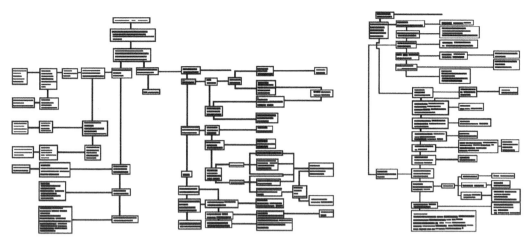

Fig. 1.2 An algorithm for management of syncope. This may confuse more than help.

Table 1.5 Evaluation of syncope. How often is the cause found by history and physical? (Modified from [209].)

	Patient type	Patient number	Diagnosis "found"	History and physical helped
Kapoor [20]	Admitted (SUO)	121	13	—
Day [13]	ER	198	173	147
Silverstein [200]	MICU	108	57	42
Kapoor [14]	All comers	204	107	52
Eagle [16]	Admitted	100	61	52
Martin [226]	ER	170	106	90

History and physical will provide clues to the diagnosis in 30–75% of patients. Diagnosis based on history and physical may be (and often is) inaccurate. ER, emergency room; MICU, medical intensive care unit; SUO, syncope of unknown origin.

8 circumstances, situations surrounding the episode;

9 exercise, body position, posture, and emotional state;

10 number, frequency, and timing of previous syncopal episodes;

11 medications;

12 family history.

As part of the initial assessment, early determination of the presence of heart disease is especially crucial because these patients are at highest risk of death. Make sure that it is indeed syncope that has occurred. Obtain information from other hospitals and doctors, talk with others who have cared for the patient, and to family members.

Consider characteristics of the event itself, the patient, and length of the episodes. One reason for the differ-ent outcomes for syncope patients relates to the nature of the episodes. Contrast an elderly male who has had a series of syncopal attacks, spaced by short episodes of recovery, to a young woman with multiple episodes spaced over several years. Based on this information alone, the woman is likely to have neurocardiogenic syncope and the man an arrhythmic or orthostatic cause. A patient who is witnessed to collapse and then noted to be pulse-less, apneic, and *appears* to require cardiopul-monary resuscitation is probably at higher risk for a malignant arrhythmia or a cardiac cause for syncope. Sudden unexpected collapse ("Stokes–Adams attacks") suggests, but does not prove, an arrhythmic cause for syncope.

The patient may not remember events surround-ing the episode, have retrograde amnesia, or other-wise be incapable of providing an adequate history

Table 1.6 History: symptoms related to syncopal spell.

Symptom	Probable cause
Nausea, diaphoresis, fear	Neurocardiogenic
Aura	Seizure
Palpitations	Tachycardia (non-specific finding]
Exercise-related	Ventricular or supraventricular tachycardia, hypotension/bradycardia
Posture-related	Orthostatic hypotension, volume depletion, dysautonomia
Urination, defecation, eating, coughing	Vagal-induced hypotension, bradycardia
Diarrhea, vomiting	Hypovolemia, hypokalemic-induced arrhythmia, vagal-induced hypotension, bradycardia
Melena	Gastrointestinal bleed
Visual change, neurologic abnormality	Stroke (unlikely presentation), seizure, migraine
Headaches	Migraine, intracerebral bleed
Chest pain	Ischemia-induced arrhythmia
Dyspnea	Pulmonary embolus, pneumothorax, hyperventilation (hysteria)
Abdominal pain	Aortic aneurysm, gastrointestinal bleed, peritonitis acute abdomen, trauma
Back pain	Dissecting aneurysm, trauma
Flushing	Carcinoid syndrome
Prolonged syncope	Aortic stenosis, seizure, neurologic or metabolic cause
Slow recovery	Seizure, drug, ethanol intoxication, hypoglycemia, sepsis
Injury	Arrhythmia, cardiac cause, neurocardiogenic
Confusion	Stroke, transient ischemic attack, intoxication, hypoglycemia
Prolonged weakness	Neurocardiogenic syncope
Skin color	Pallor – neurocardiogenic; blue – cardiac; red – carbon monoxide

Table 1.7 History: important data to obtain.

Witnesses	The entire event from multiple viewpoints
Situation	Was there a "trigger"?
Age elderly (> 65 years)	Multifactorial – rule out heart disease. Consider medications
Age young (< 40 years)	Neurocardiogenic most likely cause
Heart disease	Could indicate a poor long-term prognosis
Family history of sudden death	Increased predisposition for malignant arrhythmia or cardiac cause
Number of episodes	< 3, possibly malignant and life-threatening
	> 3, more likely to be benign and a continued problem
Previous evaluation	Obtain results from previous evaluation
Medications	Possible proarrhythmia, bradycardia, hypotension

[227,228]. Therefore, witnesses' accounts are of major importance but, while often heavily relied upon, may be inaccurate. The pulse appearing to be absent may not have been properly taken; there are also several reasons why a patient may be (or appears) pulseless. Inherent biases are always possible by the historian and those listening to the story.

Try to define the episodes as completely as possible. The patient may remember very little of the episode, deny it, or remember it inaccurately. Always

suspect that aspects of the history reported by the patient or witnesses are incomplete, misinterpreted, or are overblown because of the startling nature of the symptom. Paramedics may ignore witnesses' accounts and misinterpret the responses of an individual who appears healthy, alert, and talking by the time they arrive. The importance of a serious problem can be under- or overestimated.

Consider events that trigger the episodes. Emotions can trigger syncope by a variety of mechanisms

[3,229]. An emotional trigger raises the suspicion of neurocardiogenic syncope; it also may indicate a psychiatric cause. Chest pain can indicate the presence of ischemic heart disease or coronary vasospasm. Abrupt collapse, without premonitory symptoms, may indicate a cardiac arrhythmia, but triggers can be misleading and may be non-specific. Fatigue may be associated with neurocardiogenic syncope [230]. Other associated symptoms with neurocardiogenic syncope include pallor and diaphoresis. Other triggers for neurocardiogenic collapse include coughing [231], exercise [232], cold, carbonated beverages [56], but no history related to these issues is specific.

Consider situations surrounding and preceding syncope. Syncope is often related to the situation in which it occurs. Vasovagal (neurocardiogenic) episodes are often provoked by noxious stimuli such as a strong emotional outburst, blood loss, or pain. If the trigger is situational, episodes may be avoided by simply avoiding the situation.

Sometimes it is difficult, if not impossible, to discover the initiating factor. Slow recovery from symptoms is common in neurocardiogenic syncope, as it is after a seizure. Slow recovery is not common in orthostatic hypotension or after a long sinus pause. Consider that patients may try to explain circumstances, such as a motor vehicle accident, with syncope, when in fact they did not pass out.

Consider specific aspects of the history. Upper extremity exercise preceding syncope suggests subclavian steal. Back pain raises the suspicion of a dissecting aortic aneurysm. Dyspnea may indicate a cardiac or pulmonary cause. Pulmonary emboli can cause syncope but only with a large embolus. Associated tachypnea, cyanosis, hypotension, and acute right heart failure clarify the diagnosis. Similarly, the presence of angina may indicate the presence of an ischemically mediated arrhythmia or the Bezold–Jarisch reflex (bradycardia and hypotension from inferior wall ischemia) [181].

Assess the relationship to meals, alcohol, and drugs. A large meal can cause peripheral vasodilation and hypotension and syncope by a vagal or dysautonomic mechanism [118]. When episodes begin with slow onset and gradual recovery, consider a toxic or metabolic cause such as hypoglycemia, hyperventilation, alcohol, or drugs (illicit or prescribed). Alcohol and illicit drugs can cause syncope by several mechanisms including exacerbation of a supraventricular or ventricular tachyarrhythmia. Alcohol can also trigger syncope by abrupt change in hemodynamics and other mechanisms [233–239]. Alternatively, what might appear to be syncope from alcohol may instead be intoxication. In such a case, syncope can be used by a patient as a ready explanation for a motor vehicle accident or other adverse consequences related directly to the drinking itself.

Consider the relation to exercise, position, posture, and events. If the episode begins after a coughing bout, consider post-tussive syncope. In this case, there is a Valsalva physiology, associated increased intracerebral pressure, and a vagal response. If the episodes occur after awakening to urinate, consider micturition syncope. If the episode occurs during athletic competition or immediately after exercise, it may be completely explained by a neurocardiogenic response, but be careful not to ignore a potentially more severe, underlying cause [3,232,240–242]. Even in a young patient, consider potentially malignant causes: hypertrophic cardiomyopathy, congenital aortic valve disease, or even exercise-induced, idiopathic, right ventricular, left ventricular or bi-directional ventricular tachycardia [243,244]. Exercise-induced supraventricular tachycardias, atrial flutter, or atrial fibrillation rarely cause syncope but when they do, there is usually a history of palpitations or tachycardia. Seizures are often associated with muscular jerks, incontinence, and tongue biting, and there may be postictal confusion or a preictal aura.

If syncope occurs on abrupt rise from a prone position, consider orthostatic hypotension. Even if there is no evidence on examination, orthostatic hypotension may still be a possible cause of syncope if other precipitating contributors are considered. Orthostatic hypotension should be suspected in the elderly and in those with diabetes, if there is prolonged bed rest, and even when the patient is euvolemic. If the episodes occur after intense exposure to heat, consider heat syncope. If there are paresthesias, lip tingling, and anxiety, consider hyperventilation. If loud noises precede the episode, consider an autonomic mechanism or an arrhythmia resulting from long QT interval syndrome [245].

Prodromal symptoms can help secure a diagnosis. Premonitory (prodromal) symptoms including diaphoresis, cold sweat, nausea, anxiety, dizziness, lightheadedness, impending doom, and pallor are common in vasovagal (neurocardiogenic) syncope. Yawning, pallor, nausea, visual blurring, darkening of the vision, sweating, and weakness are also consistent with vagal cause (neurocardiogenic syncope). If the episode is associated with a strong emotional reaction, nausea, diaphoresis, and sense of impeding doom, a neurocardiogenic cause is highly likely. These symptoms may also occur independent of syncope but be neurocardiogenic in origin.

If palpitations precede the episode, suspect an arrhythmic etiology. Unfortunately, palpitations are vague and non-specific, and do not diagnose a specific etiology. Palpitations are of several types: sustained rapid, irregular, or pounding. Each type may provide some clues regarding a possible arrhythmic cause for syncope. By themselves, palpations are unreliable but suggestive for further evaluation.

An aura immediately preceding the episodes is consistent with a seizure. If the episode begins during exercise consider aortic stenosis, hypertrophic cardiomyopathy, or an exercise-induced arrhythmia. If the episode begins after exercise, consider a strong vagal response to exercise.

Symptoms on awakening (postsyncopal symptoms) can be helpful. The recovery phase from the syncopal episode can also provide important diagnostic clues. If there is confusion, headache, or dizziness, consider migraines, seizure, or another neurologic cause.

Consider the number and frequency of episodes. The frequency of occurrence of syncope at initial presentation can be used to assess risk. Patients with recurrent episodes are unlikely to have a malignant arrhythmia as the cause, particularly if the episodes are distributed over several months to years. Patients with multiple syncope recurrences, especially if they are spread out over a long time period, are at

lower risk of cardiac mortality [246]. These episodes are most likely neurocardiogenic, autonomically mediated, or resulting from a psychiatric cause (see Chapters 2, 3 and 12). In contrast, patients with isolated episodes (less than three) of syncope or with a short history of recurrence are at risk for a cardiac death [210,246]. Even if only one episode is present, it can presage a cardiac arrest. Patients with new-onset syncope, even if multiple episodes over a short time period, may have an underlying new cardiovascular cause for syncope that could be a serious premonitory sign.

Consider cardiac history. The most worrisome patient is one with left ventricular dysfunction and coronary artery disease. If such a patient presents for evaluation of syncope for which no other cause is obvious, immediate admission should be arranged for further inpatient evaluation. However, other forms of cardiac disease, not even associated with left ventricular dysfunction, can predict a malignant course. These include patients with right ventricular dysplasia or a prolonged QT interval (congenital or drug-induced). Both may occur in young patients and may lead to a malignant outcome. A cardiac history, however, does not prove a cardiac cause for syncope. It is still possible that the patient with underlying heart disease has a non-cardiac cause for syncope including a neurocardiogenic or an unknown cause [67].

Pay attention to associated, temporally related, symptoms. Angina in association with the episode suggests an ischemic etiology; heart failure may suggest a hemodynamic or arrhythmic cause; a coughing bout suggests a pulmonary cause; jerking of the hand suggests a neurologic etiology; melena suggests a gastrointestinal etiology, etc. The symptoms may not be obvious or directly related. This includes fever causing hypotension by sepsis, constipation causing straining, and a Valsalva maneuver leading to hypotension and bradycardia.

Consider medications. Medications and medication combinations, particularly in the elderly, may be contributory, if not causal, for syncope in a substantial number of patients. Assess changes in medications preceding syncope. Check for antihypertensives, antiarrhythmic drugs, diuretics, and psychotropic drugs in particular, and check dosage. Check for electrolyte (e.g., potassium) abnormalities. A patient may develop torsade de pointes if taking a class IA antiarrhythmic drug, especially if hypokalemia is present. Consider the additive effects of drugs. For example, digoxin and amiodarone may cause bradycardia or lead to digoxin toxicity. Several antihypertensive drugs may not control blood pressure adequately but trigger profound hypotension at another time because of marked vasodilation. Some drugs can cause torsade de pointes by lengthening the QT interval. This may be more apparent in the elderly and in women. Recently, we saw a case of gatifloxicin causing torsade de pointes associated with marked QT prolongation in an elderly woman.

Consider the family history of death or syncope. Syncope patients with a family history of congenital long QT interval syncope or right ventricular dysplasia have a higher risk of arrhythmic death, especially if other family members died of the problem. Patients with hypertrophic cardiomyopathy or the Wolff–Parkinson–White syndrome who have a family history of sudden death related to the same presumed diagnosis also have a high risk of cardiac arrest. There may be a familial history of neurocardiogenic syncope [247].

Consider risk factors for sudden death. Recent data indicate that selected patient can benefit from an ICD implant even if syncope is not present. Regardless of the evaluation performed for syncope, keep in mind the possibility that an ICD may improve the prognosis in patients with left ventricular dysfunction and heart failure symptoms [248–250].

Talk to previous doctors. The more information you have to assess the patient's medical problems the better.

Case 11
A 65-year-old woman with a 20-year history of neurocardiogenic syncope passes out again. As my patient, I suggested that she was checked out locally. I was expecting a call from the doctor who evaluated her in the emergency room to review her history. Instead, he admitted her and did the following: ruled out a myocardial infarction, per-

formed carotid Doppler testing, performed a computerized tomography (CT) scan of the brain, and an EEG. All this could have been avoided by a call to the treating doctor.

As indicated in Table 1.4, the differential diagnosis for patients with syncope varies with age. While the middle aged (40–65 years), the elderly (65–80 years), and the very elderly (80 years and over) have an incremental risk for mortality (see Chapter 18), the young and pediatric age groups are also at risk for specific serious underlying causes. Based on these and other historical findings, the patient can be targeted for further diagnostic evaluation. Response to treatment of a condition such as neurocardiogenic syncope can also vary with age.

Physical examination
The physical examination can provide important supporting clues to a diagnosis suspected by the history. Attention should be directed to the vital signs, the cardiovascular examination, and the neurological examination (Table 1.8).

Patients' orthostatic vital signs should be obtained. This includes blood pressure taken supine, sitting and standing, initially and after several minutes, with attention to change in the heart rate (if present) and to symptoms. Evidence for an abrupt drop in blood pressure with standing, especially with reproduction of symptoms, suggests volume depletion as a potential cause. The heart rate should rise with standing in a volume-depleted patient with the anatomic nervous system intact. In patients with idiopathic orthostatic hypotension, diabetes, amyloidosis, or autonomic insufficiency, the blood pressure can drop over several minutes in the standing position but the heart rate may not change. If the heart rate increases > 30 b min^{-1} with minor blood pressure drop, consider postural orthostatic tachycardia syndrome (see Chapter 13).

Respiratory rate and pattern may indicate a pulmonary cause. Hyperventilation may be the cause of syncope [251,252]. Tachypnea may indicate pneumonia, pulmonary embolus, or congestive heart failure.

Temperature changes. These may indicate sepsis, hypothyroidism, or renal insufficiency.

Table 1.8 Physical findings: key points.

Finding	Implication
Heart rate – slow, fast	Arrhythmic cause for syncope, acute illness, gastrointestinal bleed
Respiration rate – slow, fast	Hyper-/hypoventilation, pneumothorax, heart failure
Carotid massage	Carotid hypersensitivity
Blood pressure	Orthostatic hypotension, drug-induced hypotension, volume depletion
Neck vein distension	Pulmonary embolus, congestive failure, cardiac causes
Skin pallor	Blood loss, neurocardiogenic cause
Carotid bruits	Concomitant heart disease. Unlikely, primary cause for syncope
Heart murmur	Obstructive or other cardiac syncope
Left ventricular lift	Heart failure with cardiac syncope
S3 gallop	Heart failure with cardiac syncope
Rash	Anaphylaxis causing syncope
Abdominal tenderness	Blood loss, or hypotensive cause for syncope
Absent or variable pulses	Dissecting aneurysm, subclavian steal
Neurologic findings	Seizure, stroke, transient ischemic attack
Stool guaiac	Blood loss

Carotid sinus massage. This can give insight into carotid sinus hypersensitivity (see Chapter 14). The use of carotid sinus massage in older patients with syncope has recently been emphasized [253–256]. The SAFE PACE trial suggests that a pacemaker implant with a positive carotid sinus massage may be of benefit for elderly patients.

There are no firm standards for performing the carotid sinus massage and, not surprisingly, the results can therefore be highly variable. Even if it is positive (i.e., a long sinus pause or prolonged AV block, blood pressure decreases 50 mmHg, sinus pause > 3 s), as it is frequently in the elderly even without symptoms, other causes for syncope should be explored. A carotid massage is an integral part of the physical examination of the syncope patient but the results cannot be relied upon to diagnose the cause of syncope. It is a diagnosis of exclusion. It should be considered if there is a suggestive history, such as the onset of symptoms with neck compression from position or shaving.

An evaluation of the pulses can provide insight into the presence of a dissecting aneurysm or subclavian steal. The carotid impulse may reveal evidence for aortic stenosis but a carotid bruit does not provide a direct cause for syncope. However, it may indicate the presence of other atherosclerotic lesions such as coronary artery disease (cardiac cause for syncope) or subclavian artery occlusion (subclavian steal related syncope).

The cardiovascular examination is crucial. This may reveal murmurs consistent with hypertrophic cardiomyopathy, aortic stenosis, mitral valve prolapse, or pulmonary hypertension. Tricuspid regurgitation may indicate carcinoid syndrome or endocarditis (two rare causes for syncope). If the baseline murmur is provoked by a Valsalva maneuver, this may indicate that hypertrophic cardiomyopathy is present and is the cause of syncope. Evaluate the presence of an LV lift, abnormal impulse, an S4 and an S3 gallop, all potential indicators of cardiac disease that may be responsible for syncope. An S3 gallop could indicate the presence of congestive heart failure. Consider complete evaluation for congestive heart failure. Evidence of Eisenmenger's syndrome, pulmonic stenosis, prosthetic valve dysfunction, presence of a permanent pacemaker or implantable defibrillator, aortic stenosis, or a tumor plop (atrial myxoma) can provide further clues to the diagnosis of syncope and the risk for the patient.

Lung examination may reveal congestive heart failure. If present, suspect a potentially serious cardiac cause for syncope and consider the need for further inpatient evaluation. While a pulmonary embolus may be missed, a pneumothorax could be found. Wheezing may indicate post-tussive syncope or a hypoxic cause for syncope.

An abdominal examination may reveal evidence of a gastrointestinal catastrophe. Specifically, a vagal response to a ruptured viscous or a gastro-intestinal bleed are possibilities. The abdominal examination may reveal tenderness consistent with an acute abdomen or an ulcer. The stool guaiac can reveal the presence of a gastrointestinal bleed.

A neurological evaluation may indicate focal or localizing signs or evidence for a systemic neuro-logic process such as Parkinson's disease. Assess for evidence of a tremor, unilateral weakness, and visual changes. Changing neurological signs are also important. A new neurological deficit in a patient with syncope should be considered a pre-monitory sign for a cerebrovascular accident.

The complexion may indicate anemia or shift in blood flow [257]. Pallor occurring transiently during an episode may indicate neurocardiogenic syncope, but if it persists after awakening consider blood loss as the cause. Marked bradycardia can also cause a dusky or pale appearance. Bright red pallor may indicate carbon monoxide intoxication. Cyanosis can indicate a cardiopulmonary process such as a right-to-left shunt with Eisenmenger's physiology. The extremities may demonstrate clubbing.

The physical examination and history remain the cornerstones for initial evaluation of the patient with syncope. This approach is cost-effective and may help to prescribe other necessary, and help avoid unnecessary, diagnostic procedures. Unfortunately, for most patients, the physical examination is negative and further evaluation will be needed to help to understand the cause for syncope.

Diagnostic testing

The proper diagnostic approach requires careful analysis of syncope in light of all available clinical findings. Diagnostic tests need to be used sparingly. Often inappropriate and expensive evaluations are undertaken (Table 1.9). When used properly, they will increase the diagnostic yield compared with the history and physical examination alone. No specific test is always helpful and no specific battery of tests is ever indicated or always useful. All testing must be tailored to the individual patient, based on the findings of the history and physical examinations and with knowledge of the sensitivity and spe-cificity of each test to identify the cause for syncope. An abnormal test result does not necessarily indic-ate the cause for syncope and does not necessarily sanction a "wild goose chase." An abnormal tilt

Table 1.9 Initial evaluation after admission.

Should these be routine?
Computed tomography scan
Carotid Doppler
Electroencephalogram
Cardiac enzymes
Neurology consult
Cardiac catheterization
Exercise test
NO!

table test result or the presence of inducible mono-morphic ventricular tachycardia on electrophysio-logic testing must be interpreted carefully in light of the clinical situation.

Extensive and repeated diagnostic evaluations are generally unrewarding, expensive, painful, and possibly risky. Repeat inpatient evaluations are discouraged unless new clues are uncovered. If the patient is evaluated for syncope but no cause can be diagnosed initially, further admissions are highly unlikely to arrive at a diagnosis and benefit the patient.

Even with appropriate diagnostic testing, a likely cause for syncope may not be found in many pati-ents. Fortunately, most patients with an undiag-nosed cause for syncope will not have a recurrence but if they do, they tend to have a benign long-term prognosis. As part of a proper evaluation, it is important to know when to stop testing.

Occasionally, laboratory (blood) tests can iden-tify the cause for syncope. However, a routine battery of blood tests is rarely productive. The hemoglobin may provide a diagnosis of acute blood loss as a cause for syncope in approximately 5% of patients [14]. An SMA-6 has an even smaller diagnostic yield. It may help to detect a seizure if metabolic acidosis is present [149,258]. An elevated blood urea nitrogen (BUN), creatinine, or sodium level may indicate fluid depletion. An abnormal potassium value may indicate an arrhy-thmic cause for syncope. Oxygen desaturation may indicate a pulmonary embolus. As part of a general screening evaluation, it is probably useful and cost-effective to obtain a hemoglobin and perhaps an SMA-6, but it is not clear that even this evaluation is worthwhile. Drug levels (such as digoxin), and other blood tests should be obtained based on the history.

Use of diagnostic testing

Several tests should be considered: ECG, tilt table test, echocardiogram, electrophysiologic test, treadmill test, or a monitor. The more tests, the more abnormalities will be found. Some clinicians use a "routine" battery of tests that are useless, expensive, and misleading (Table 1.9). It is not clear how some tests and approaches (such as use of carotid Doppler testing, EEG, MRI scans, CT scans, neurology consultations) emerged.

All patients should have an ECG. An ECG is simple, inexpensive, risk free, and may provide helpful information in 5–10% of patients (Table 1.10). Twenty to eighty percent of patients will have an abnormal, but non-diagnostic ECG, which is useful in 7%. The presence of a bundle branch block in a patient with syncope indicates the presence of His–Purkinje disease and may indicate the possibility of complete heart block [259,260]. Bundle branch block can also be an indication of organic heart disease. Up to 30% of patients with syncope and bundle branch block will have the induction of sustained monomorphic ventricular tachycardia on electrophysiologic testing [261–264]. A patient with undiagnosed syncope and a bundle branch block should therefore be considered for an electrophysiologic test. The ECG can also show ventricular pre-excitation (Wolff–Parkinson–White syndrome), ectopic beats, heart block, ventricular hypertrophy, atrial fibrillation, a myocardial infarction (new or old), a long QT interval (arguably, > 0.500 s), or sustained ventricular tachycardia. An abnormal ECG can point towards a diagnosis and a normal ECG may help exclude the need for an aggressive evaluation approach [265].

The signal-averaged ECG is not particularly useful in patients with syncope but may have a specific role to determine if a patient with intact left ventricular function (LVEF ≥ 0.40), but underlying coronary artery disease (with no bundle branch block), has a risk for ventricular tachycardia or arrhythmic death, and would otherwise benefit from electrophysiologic testing [266–268].

An echocardiogram may be appropriate to evaluate ventricular function and valvular heart disease but, if the ECG is normal, there is no cardiac history, and there are no abnormalities found on physical examination, this does not need to be obtained urgently. Younger patients, without a history of heart disease and with a normal physical examination, will be unlikely to benefit from an echocardiogram. Patients with suspected neurocardiogenic syncope do not need an echocardiogram. A chest X-ray may show cardiomegaly or pulmon-

Table 1.10 The electrocardiogram: to evaluate syncope.

Finding	Significance
Normal or non-specific	Common, does not rule out serious cause
Complete heart block	Pacemaker indicated
Second-degree heart block	Correlate with symptoms. Pacemaker may be indicated
First-degree heart block	No obvious significance in most cases
Delta waves	Wolff–Parkinson–White pattern. Possible supraventricular tachycardia
Sinus bradycardia	Non-specific – may indicate sick sinus syndrome
Myocardial infarction	Acute: arrhythmia, hemodynamic problem
	Old: risk for death, arrhythmia
Epsilon waves	Right ventricular dysplasia
Bundle branch block	Possible heart block, or ventricular tachycardia
QT prolongation (> 0.500)	Possible torsade de pointes
Ectopic beats	No known significance
Atrial fibrillation	May indicate underlying structural heart disease, arrhythmic cause
Supraventricular tachycardia	Rare. Likely cause for syncope
Ventricular tachycardia	Rare. Likely cause for syncope
Paced rhythm	Pacemaker malfunction

ary edema and should be obtained if there is other evidence on examination but, as a routine screen, it adds little but an increase in cost. No other tests are required as part of the initial evaluation.

The use of monitoring is described in more detail in other chapters but includes the use of external loop recorders and implanted monitors. The use of these devices depends on the clinical scenario, the capability of the patient to push the button on an external recorder for an episode, and the risk the patient has for recurrence. The use of implanted monitors is described in detail in Chapter 19.

What to do after the initial evaluation

When to hospitalize the patient

A key aspect in the evaluation and treatment is syncope is to decide whether and when to admit a patient who has had syncope. Based on the information collected as part of the history, physical examination, and initial evaluation, appropriate decisions can be made regarding hospitalization (Table 1.11) [269,270]. This has become increasingly important in a time of managed medical care. With the costs of hospital admissions escalating, prudent admission criteria are required. Many hospitals are developing practice guidelines to care for patients with syncope (Fig. 1.3a,b). The SEEDS study [271] showed that a syncope unit may facilitate proper management, decrease costs, shorten length-of-stay, and improve outcomes compared to patients managed in the hospital in a standard fashion.

There are some potential benefits of hospitalization. It can be useful to diagnose and treat the cause for syncope, to prevent death, injury and symptoms, and to satisfy medicolegal requirements

Table 1.11 Criteria for hospitalization.

Malignant arrhythmia or cardiovascular cause suspected
New neurologic abnormality present
Severe injury present
Multiple frequent episodes
Severe orthostatic hypotension
Uncontrolled "malignant" vasovagal syncope
Elderly patient
Treatment plans not possible as an outpatient

(the "standard-of-care"). However, in most cases, hospitalization is unnecessary. It can be associated with iatrogenic complications for syncope patients. Despite hospitalization, syncope often remains undiagnosed. The prognosis and recurrence rates may not change. If a patient has previously been hospitalized, repeated hospitalizations for recurrent syncope are rarely productive (and helpful in < 15% of such patients). Clearly, considering the scope of the problem of syncope, the lack of benefit of admission, and the present medical environment, hospital admission for syncope should be considered carefully and used prudently.

The reasons given to hospitalize are as follow:
1 to monitor the patient suspected of having a serious, poorly tolerated arrhythmia;
2 to perform tests not readily performed as an outpatient;
3 to formulate and undertake specific treatment plans not possible as an outpatient (cardiac catheterization or electrophysiologic testing when a life-threatening arrhythmia is suspected);
4 for medicolegal purposes;
5 when the patient is having multiple, closely spaced episodes;
6 when there is a new neurologic abnormality or a suspected neurologic cause, new seizure disorder, transient ischemic attack, or stroke;
7 when the patient is elderly, has been injured, or is at risk for serious injury;
8 when there is a severe abnormality on physical examination;
9 when any cardiovascular cause is suspected (resulting from an arrhythmia or caused by a hemodynamic problem);
10 when there is symptomatic orthostatic hypotension;
11 for the patient with suspected "malignant" vasovagal syncope or vasovagal syncope that is difficult to control and causes severe symptoms.

Often, the reason to admit is to make sure the patient does not have frequent and recurrent symptoms, or is on the verge of developing a more serious problem. If the risk of discharge from the emergency room is low, there is little reason to admit a patient (Figs 1.3 & 1.4). Besides protecting a patient from a life-threatening risk, expected results of hospitalization include finding the cause for syncope and initiating a treatment that cannot be performed on an outpatient basis. This could

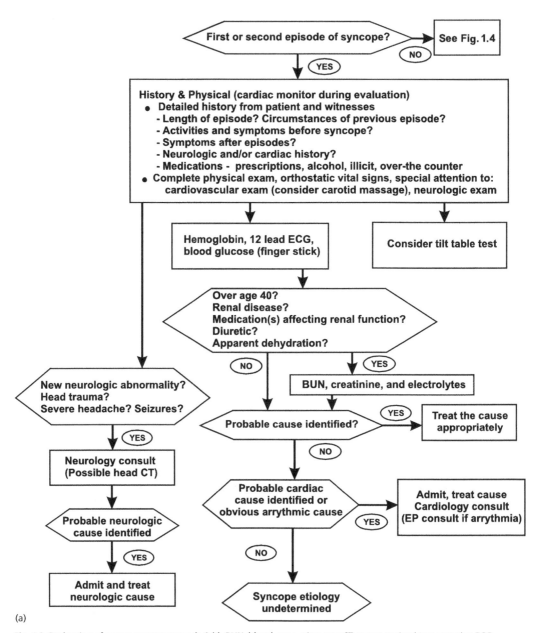

(a)

Fig. 1.3 Evaluation of recent onset syncope (a & b). BUN, blood, urea, nitrogen; CT, computerized tomography; ECG, electrocardiogram; EP, electrophysiology; LVEF, left ventricular ejection fraction; MUGA, multiple gated acquisition.

include treatment of a cardiac arrhythmia with drugs, surgery, or implanted devices. Patients who are suspected to have a new neurologic event may benefit from close inpatient observation for worsening of their condition. Hospital admission is also based on patient concerns.

When considering hospital admission, several additional factors must be appraised: patient age,

cardiac risk factors, circumstances of the episodes, history from the patient and witnesses, underlying medical conditions, and results of the physical examination. Hospitalization should be considered to formulate and undertake specific diagnostic and therapeutic plans that cannot be performed as an outpatient. The goals for hospitalization must be clear before admission because non-directed

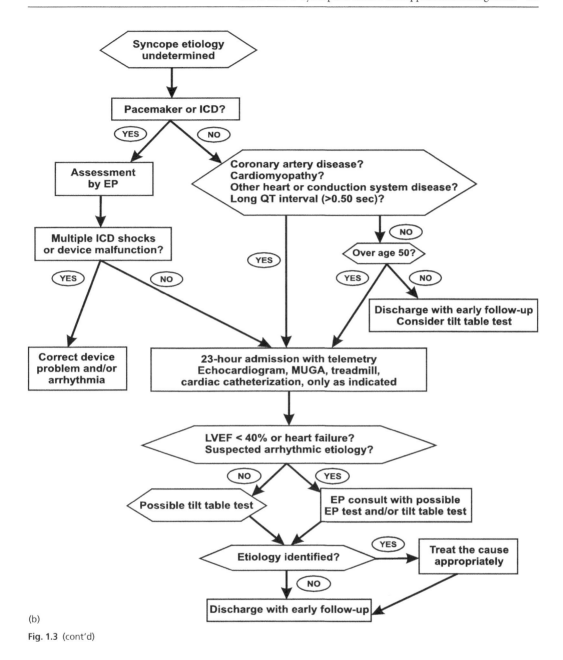

(b)

Fig. 1.3 (cont'd)

admissions for syncope are generally non-productive. The prognosis and recurrence rate of syncope may not change. Patients who do not benefit from hospitalization include those with isolated episodes of syncope and no apparent heart disease, those with recurrent episodes but normal physical examination, echocardiogram, ECG and no cardiac risk factors, and those who have undergone a previous complete evaluation as repeat hospitalizations to evaluate such patients is generally unrewarding.

Mozes *et al.* [272] found that prolonged inpatient monitoring was rarely productive. In this study, for patients hospitalized with syncope, a diagnostic evaluation, leading to an appropriate therapeutic intervention was present in 24%, consistent with other reports. With admission based on

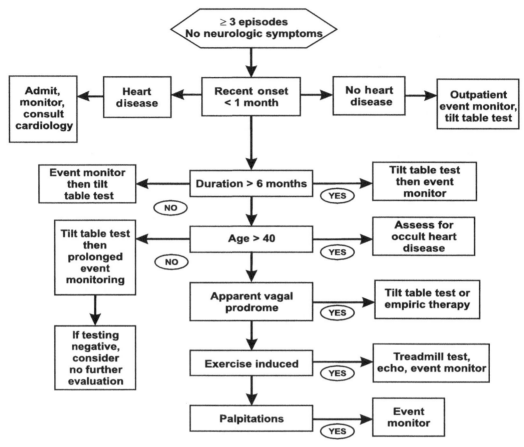

Fig. 1.4 Recurrent undiagnosed syncope.

the history, physical examination, and the ECG, 85% of hospitalizations could be avoided.

In a study of 350 patients, clinical judgment was compared with "objective" diagnosis-related group (DRG) criteria to evaluate the need for and benefit of hospitalization [273]. This study included patients with syncope. In this report, physicians' clinical judgment outperformed objective DRG data in identifying that patients needed and benefited from acute-care hospitalization.

Medicode ICD-9-CM codes for syncope under 780, "general symptoms". Medicode ICD-9-CM 780.2: "syncope and collapse" includes blackouts, fainting, vasovagal attacks, "near" or "pre" syncope but excludes carotid sinus syncope, heat syncope, neurocirculatory asthenia, orthostatic hypotension, or shock. ICD-9-CM 780.4 codes: "dizziness and giddiness" includes "lightheadedness and vertigo". Sometimes, syncope coding includes DRG 427.89,

"cardiac dysrhythmia," 427.9, "cardiac dysrhythmia, unspecified."

At my prior institution, over 1 year, 236 syncope patients were admitted with these diagnoses. The average length of stay was 3.7 days. Third party payers applied less pressure for discharge during hospitalization as long as a treatment plan was in place, which is appropriate because for hospitalization to be worthwhile, a plan needs to be in place at the time of admission.

Unless a new diagnostic assessment plan is established, in one report of 161 patients admitted (Ferrick PACE 1997), 75% did not benefit from admission. Repeated admissions are even less useful.

When to consult a specialist
Patients often visit primary care physicians, appropriately so, for initial episodes of syncope in an

emergency room or in a clinical setting. While internists, emergency physicians, and family practitioners see the bulk of syncope patients, consultation can become necessary. A consultant should be considered after the complete initial evaluation has been undertaken and an etiology is suspected that requires disease-specific evaluation and treatment. The history and physical examination provide the best clues to the diagnosis and to decide when to call in a consultant.

The first step in evaluating syncope is *not* to call a neurologic or an electrophysiologic consult, although both can be helpful for specific patients. A neurologic consult will rarely provide useful guidance unless there are no specific clues in the history or physical examination. An electrophysiologist will help to:

1 assess the risk of an arrhythmic cause for syncope using electrophysiologic testing;
2 provide information concerning the prognostic risk of syncope;
3 evaluate potential autonomic causes for syncope, including neurocardiogenic causes;
4 perform tilt table testing and evaluate the results;
5 manage (diagnose and treat) arrhythmic causes of syncope.

Because the electrophysiologist can help to manage the patient with potential arrhythmic causes for syncope, he or she should be called early when there is organic heart disease, bundle branch block, or a history of arrhythmia. A cardiologist should be called to help to evaluate the patient with suspected cardiovascular disease causing syncope including aortic valve disease, hypertrophic cardiomyopathy, other cardiomyopathies, or coronary artery disease.

A psychiatrist may be needed when a psychiatric etiology seems likely. A good consultant will help to direct the evaluation of the patient with syncope promptly, properly, and efficiently, without inappropriate testing. In this way, the consultant should actually improve the quality of care and lower the total costs. Electrophysiologists are likely not called often enough to see patients with syncope. Neurologists are often called too early to help with the management and should be called only if there are neurologic signs. Any neurologic testing should be performed with the aid of a neurologist. Autonomic medicine is rapidly emerging as a separate medical specialty that deals with patients with

difficult to treat neurocardiogenic and dysautonomic syncope.

When to carry out diagnostic tests

A variety of tests are used to evaluate patients with syncope, as described in the European guidelines [1]. Frequently, the following "complete" work-up is planned (Table 1.9): carotid Doppler examination, cardiac enzymes, prolonged inpatient telemetric monitoring, echocardiogram, treadmill test, head CT scan, and neurology consult. It is not clear where this "shotgun" approach originated but it has no scientific basis and it is not advocated because it will almost never lead to a diagnostic cause for syncope. It is expensive and time consuming but ubiquitous.

CT and MRI brain scans are almost never warranted, especially if there are no neurologic findings. While an abnormality may be found, such as tumor or cerebrovascular accident, this may be concomitant (and, perhaps, asymptomatic) rather than a cause for syncope.

The EEG has been used as a screen in several reports that evaluate syncope. The routine and undirected use of the EEG for undiagnosed syncope has not been helpful and cannot be recommended without other suggestive clinical information. On one occasion I found the test to be useful when a patient had a neurocardiogenic episode on the EEG as a result of the electrodes and appeared to seize.

Several diagnostic tests can help to evaluate syncope but it is important to consider the sensitivity, specificity, and diagnostic accuracy of any test used. An abnormality found does not necessarily indicate that it caused syncope. Induction of ventricular tachycardia on electrophysiologic testing or a hypotensive bradycardic episode on a tilt table test is suggestive, but not indicative, of the cause for syncope. Any finding must be considered in light of all clinical findings and must be interpreted before using the results to initiate therapy. The test must be evaluated on its own merits and chosen based on the finding uncovered from the history and physical examination.

Tilt table testing

The tilt table test is used to evaluate neurocardiogenic causes for syncope, especially if the cause for syncope is otherwise unclear [81,273–275]. The tilt table test has been in use since before the 1950s to evaluate syncope [33]. It helps to assess a reflex mechanism that is only now beginning to be understood [276–280]. Over the past decade, the use of, and indications for, tilt table testing have expanded tremendously. It has changed the evaluation and treatment of patients with suspected neurocardiogenic and dysautonomic syncope (see Chapters 2, 3 and 7).

Not all patients with possible neurocardiogenic syncope require a tilt table test. If a patient has a clear history of neurocardiogenic syncope or has episodes related to a specific situation, the test may not be needed. Sensitivity and specificity issues may influence use of the tilt table but there is no other "gold standard" method to evaluate the presence of neurocardiogenic reflexes implicated as cause for syncope (the reflex itself may not be abnormal) [281]. A negative test can occur even in the presence of an obvious cause for neurocardiogenic syncope and a positive test can occur when syncope clearly results from other causes [282]. As with electrophysiology, testing a positive test (especially if "borderline" positive) may potentially be misleading. Always consider that there may be other (or multiple) causes for syncope. This problem was well illustrated in the case of the basketball player, Reggie Lewis, who had syncope and a positive tilt table test but died suddenly of ventricular fibrillation while playing basketball. When syncope clearly appears to be a result of neurocardiogenic causes, treatment plans can potentially begin without a tilt table test (although some authors wish to determine exact response patterns during tilt table testing as a guide to therapy). Guidelines for tilt table testing have been published [281]. The tilt table is best considered when there is suspected neurocardiogenic syncope in patients in whom the cause is not obvious (see Chapters 2 and 7) or in those with syncope of otherwise unknown origin.

Holter monitoring

Holter monitoring is often ordered for patients with syncope but it rarely diagnoses a serious underlying arrhythmic cause and rarely provides useful information unless the patient has an episode with the monitor attached. In several large studies using Holter monitoring, the correlation between arrhythmic abnormalities and symptoms, including syncope, was < 5% [283–287]. If an asymptomatic abnormality is detected, it may not be the cause for syncope and may lead to further unnecessary diagnostic and, perhaps, therapeutic interventions [288]. Asymptomatic non-sustained ventricular tachycardia, premature ventricular beats, sinus pauses, or sinus bradycardia may have no specific meaning in this setting and may confuse, rather than reveal the cause for the syncope. The only reason to consider a Holter monitor is when a patient has multiple or frequent episodes of syncope or related symptoms over a short period of time (Fig. 1.5). Prolonged Holter monitoring is an option to evaluate selected patients but there are now better methods to monitor for arrhythmias in the long term.

Endless-loop recorders – event recorders

External endless-loop recorders have emerged as highly prescribed, quite useful devices to manage syncope and assess its potential arrhythmic causes [289] (Table 1.12). The newer devices are technologically superior, smaller, and with a larger battery capacity. They can be used to capture and save episodes even minutes after they have occurred. These devices can be attached to the patient for weeks or months at a time.

A tape continuously records the ECG so that if a patient passes out, the episode can be saved by pushing a button on the recorder after awakening. Therefore, the episodes could be recorded and played back by the patient over the phone or by other knowledgeable individuals. The time interval recorded before the button is pushed is often programmable but acceptably long compared with the length of routine syncope episodes. Few data are published on this technology, which is now used routinely to evaluate syncopal episodes. This technique is quite useful to diagnose a potentially syncopal arrhythmia cost-effectively. Outpatient use of this device should be reserved for patients who are responsible and intelligent enough to learn how to use the device and who are willing to do so.

Implanted loop recorders can help to diagnose the cause for syncope when it is difficult to capture an episode with an external loop recorder or if the episodes are quite far apart. This small implanted

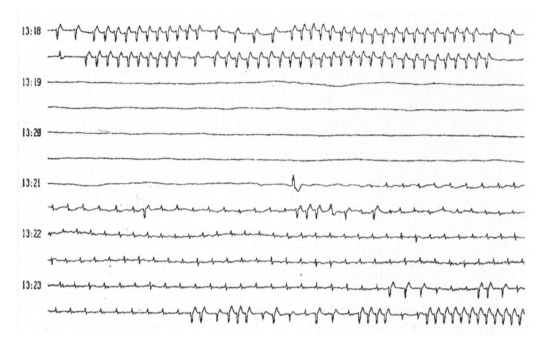

Fig. 1.5 A Holter monitor performed on a patient with recurrent, frequent episodes of syncope. The patient was admitted to the hospital and had a Holter monitor placed. The patient had more than 2 min of asystole.

Table 1.12 Holter monitor versus endless-loop recorder.

To assess	AV block, sinus node dysfunction supraventricular/ventricular tachycardia
Holter	
Advantage	For patients unable to comply with event recorder, or frequent episodes
Disadvantage	Rare correlation of rhythm to symptoms for Holter
Endless-loop recorder	
Advantage	Long-term evaluation to correlate symptoms with rhythm
Disadvantage	Requires knowledge of how and when to use

device can automatically detect rapid and slow rhythms and can be triggered by the patient to save an event. There is evidence that implantable recorders may be useful before other technology in the diagnosis of an arrhythmic cause for syncope [5,290] (Fig. 1.6) (see Chapter 19).

Electrophysiologic testing

Most arrhythmias that cause syncope are paroxysmal, infrequent, and unpredictable. They can be difficult, if not impossible, to diagnose. Electrophysiologic testing has emerged as a useful method to assess arrhythmic causes for syncope (Table 1.13) (see Chapter 6) and to assess the risk for arrhythmic death. A consensus document outlines the recommendations on the use of electrophysiologic testing for syncope [291]. Various arrhythmias and clinical conditions can be evaluated by electrophysiologic testing but the test has differing capabilities to assess each rhythm disturbance (Table 1.14). A compilation of electrophysiologic test results are shown in Fig. 1.7 and Table 1.15. Abnormal test results are seen in 7–50% of patients selected for study [17,41,43−45,206−208,212−214,262−264,292−298].

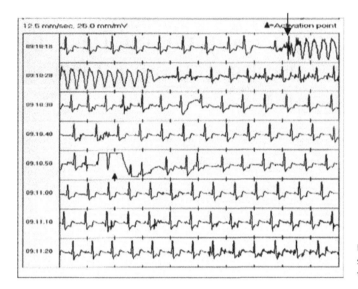

Fig. 1.6 Implantable loop recorder showing non-sustained ventricular tachycardia in a syncope patient.

Table 1.13 When to perform electrophysiologic testing.

Coronary artery disease with left ventricular dysfunction*
Dilated cardiomyopathy
Valvular cardiomyopathy*
Bundle branch block*
Congestive heart failure, any cause*
Supraventricular tachycardia but not temporally associated syncope
Wolff–Parkinson–White syndrome
Possible, for undiagnosed syncope multiple recurrence

---

* Cardiac catheterization, may need to be performed first, on a case-by-case basis.

Table 1.14 Electrophysiologic testing: to evaluate syncope.

Sustained ventricular tachycardia (also to assess risk for death)
Supraventricular tachycardia (rare finding at electrophysiologic testing)
Bradycardia – fair → poor to evaluate the sinus node
Heart block – fair → poor to evaluate the AV node

Caveats
May not find the cause for syncope
Not predictive for all populations
Multiple abnormalities common
Not clearly indicative for cause for syncope
Patients may need an ICD or pacemaker for another indication

This wide range of results reflects patient selection. The electrophysiologic test is an invasive method to try to initiate an arrhythmia by stimulation of the atria and ventricles (see Chapter 6). The goal is to try to uncover a clinically important arrhythmia that caused syncope.

The main use for electrophysiologic testing in patients with syncope is to evaluate the presence of monomorphic ventricular tachycardia. It can provide the cause for syncope and will help to determine the long-term prognosis. (The two might not be related.) Induction of sustained monomorphic ventricular tachycardia is the most common abnormality seen in patients selected for electrophysiologic testing, higher than would be expected in a matched non-syncopal population with similar structural heart disease. Induction of sustained ventricular tachycardia likely indicates that it was the cause for syncope but a negative test does not rule out ventricular tachycardia.

Results are disease-specific. The electrophysiologic test has the highest sensitivity and specificity to detect sustained monomorphic ventricular tachycardia and the cause for syncope in patients with coronary artery disease who are not acutely ischemic. Another group with a high incidence of inducible ventricular tachycardia are patients with an underlying bundle branch block. Up to 30% of these patients will have ventricular tachycardia induced.

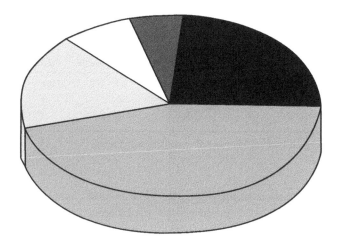

Fig. 1.7 Electrophysiologic testing. Patients with syncope of undetermined origin (12% of patients had multiple abnormalities). AVN/HP, AV node/His–Purkinje; SND, sinus node disease; SVT, supraventricular tachycardia; VT, ventricular tachycardia.

■ VT ▦ SVT ☐ SND ▨ AVN/HP ▨ Normal

Table 1.15 Electrophysiologic testing for syncope-selected studies.

Study	All patients	Positive test	VT	SVT	SND	AVB	Other
Bass [207]	70	37	31	3	0	3	0
Denes [293]	89	53	13	13	15	58	0
DiMarco [214]	25	17	9	0	1	3	4
Doherty [294]	119	78	31	6	4	5	32
Gulamhusein [297]	34	6	0	3	3	0	2
Hess [41]	32	18	11	0	5	1	1
Kall [45]	175	52	29	4	9	11	0
Krol [210]	104	31	22	2	2	6	0
Morady [215]	53	30	24	0	2	0	4
Olshansky [44]	105	41	28	13	1	3	5
Reiffel [299]	59	29	8	3	15	13	0
Teichman [213]	105	112	36	16	19	69	20

AVB, atrioventricular block; SND, sinus node dysfunction; SVT, supraventricular tachycardia; VT, ventricular tachycardia.

Several conditions can place patients at risk for malignant arrhythmia but cannot be effectively evaluated by electrophysiologic testing. The ejection fraction can further select which patients will have an abnormal electrophysiologic test result. In one report [210], 31 of 104 syncope patients had ventricular tachycardia induced on electrophysiologic testing. If the left ventricular ejection fraction was < 0.40, ventricular tachycardia was induced in 35% of the patients, whereas for those with an ejection fraction > 0.40, only 3% had ventricular tachycardia induced. Patients with normal or near normal left ventricular ejection, even in the presence of structural heart disease, will likely have a normal electrophysiologic test unless other evidence is present (e.g., idiopathic ventricular tachycardia). The test is now not generally recommended as a first-line test for patients with a left ventricular

Table 1.16 Electrophysiologic testing. Does therapy prevent recurrent syncope and sudden death?

Study	Patients	Follow-up	Syncope Effective Rx	Sudden death Effective Rx	Syncope Ineffective Rx	Sudden death Ineffective Rx
Bass [207]	70	30	20	31	50	47
Kall [45]	175	24	0	3	27	25
Olshansky [44]	87	26	12% (14%)	0% (8%)	30% (54%)	16%

Figures in brackets indicate lack of compliance with therapy.

ejection fraction > 0.40; however, it may be useful if other testing is negative, if syncope recurs, if there is a late potential on signal-averaged ECG, or if there are prolonged episodes of non-sustained ventricular tachycardia on monitoring. The Holter monitor, however, does not appear to be a good method to assess which patients will benefit from electrophysiologic testing [44,299,300].

The test can miss a tachycardia that is responsible for syncope. Non-sustained ventricular tachycardia can cause syncope but the sensitivity of the electrophysiologic test to evaluate this rhythm is low. Electrophysiologic testing can miss ventricular tachycardia such as in patients with dilated or valvular cardiomyopathy. The electrophysiologic test cannot assess the "clinical" arrhythmia accurately for patients with polymorphic ventricular tachycardia, hypertrophic cardiomyopathy, or the long QT interval syndrome.

Occasionally, the electrophysiologic test should be considered for a patient with frequent episodes of syncope when no other cause can be found even if the ejection fraction is intact. In such a patient with recurrent episodes, the tilt table test should be performed first. If negative, an electrophysiologic test may be diagnostic but a negative result would be expected in over 70% of such patients. One possible abnormality that may be found is an idiopathic monomorphic ventricular tachycardia which can be cured by radiofrequency ablation during testing. Another is a poorly tolerated supraventricular tachycardia, even possible in patients without apparent structural heart disease. In one study of syncope patients, 13 of 105 had a supraventricular tachycardia induced (four of these patients had ventricular tachycardia induced also) [44]. The incidence of supraventricular tachycardia induction varies between studies but is relatively

rare. Induction of supraventricular tachycardia is rare in previously asymptomatic patients. Therefore, if induced and associated with hypotension or hemodynamic collapse, it should be considered a cause for syncope and treated, perhaps with radiofrequency ablation. The electrophysiologic test is not adequate to assess atrial flutter or fibrillation, or to assess the ability of the AV node to conduct very rapidly or very slowly under all conditions.

The use of electrophysiologic testing to evaluate tachycardia in syncope patients appears warranted. Patients who have therapy guided by electrophysiologic testing appear to have less syncope recurrence and reduced mortality (Table 1.16), although no prospective, randomized trials have been performed. Olshansky et al. [44] have shown that if tachycardia is induced and is suppressible by medication, 14% had recurrent syncope or cardiac arrest if they took medications that appear to be effective versus 54% who were non-compliant with medications in a 25.8-month follow-up. However, there are studies suggesting that electrophysiologic testing is useful in syncope patients.

Electrophysiologic testing is fair, at best, to evaluate sinus bradycardia and AV block in patients with syncope [296,299,301]. An abnormal sinus node recovery time is relatively specific to detect sinus node disease but its presence does not indicate that sinus node dysfunction caused the syncope; also sensitivity is low. If the sinus node recovery time is more than 3 s and there is no other apparent cause for syncope, sinus node dysfunction is the likely cause for syncope and a pacemaker should be implanted. His–Purkinje conduction can be evaluated by the electrophysiologic test but rarely is an abnormal finding noted and significant infra-Hisian block can be missed. An HV interval > 100 ms is a probable cause for syncope if no other cause can be found. If there is a bundle branch block, pacing-induced infra-Hisian block can be seen. Procainamide or other class IA antiarrhythmic drugs can be used to "stress" the His–Purkinje system and determine the presence of pacing-induced infra-Hisian block [302,303]. Fujimura *et al.* [296] found that only two of 13 patients had the correct diagnosis of infra-Hisian block determined be electrophysiologic testing. If present, it is the likely cause for syncope and a pacemaker should be implanted. Atrioventricular block in the AV node as cause for syncope cannot be evaluated accurately.

The electrophysiologic results derived must be interpreted in light of the clinical situation and are not always helpful [304]. An induced arrhythmia may not be the cause of syncope, but simply a laboratory artefact [305]. Induction of ventricular fibrillation only has little, if any, clinical significance in syncope patients. Patients generally do not pass out from ventricular fibrillation; they die [306]. Induction of non-sustained, monomorphic, ventricular tachycardia is similarly difficult to interpret.

We found several years ago that 21% of our primary electrophysiologic tests had been to evaluate and diagnose a potential cause for syncope. The test was performed on outpatients with a history of syncope and during an acute hospitalization for a recent episode of syncope. We still advocate the use of electrophysiologic testing in patients with heart disease and syncope, although the test is being used less and less in lieu of empiric ICD implantation.

While electrophysiologic testing is useful for a subset of syncope patients, there are several concerns:

1 not all arrhythmias are diagnosed accurately;

2 multiple "soft" abnormalities may be found, none of which may be responsible for syncope;

3 autonomic effects influencing a tachycardia are not adequately evaluated;

4 sinus node and AV node dysfunction cannot be evaluated fully.

Other testing

Cardiac echo. The echocardiogram is useful but cannot be recommended as an initial screening tool unless the history or physical examination warrants its use [307]. Pericardial tamponade, valvular abnormalities, aortic valve disease, and hypertrophic cardiomyopathy can all cause syncope and these abnormalities can be quantitated by the echocardiogram. The main reason to perform an echocardiogram, even without obvious physical findings, is to assess the presence of left ventricular dysfunction or right ventricular enlargement (resulting from right ventricular dysplasia) that may suggest the presence of a ventricular arrhythmia. The test should be considered to evaluate left ventricular function in patients over 50 years old even if there is no history consistent with heart disease and even if the ECG is normal. It adds expense but is safe and unlikely to lead to therapeutic mishap.

Signal-averaged ECG. The signal-averaged ECG is useful to detect risk for cardiac arrest and monomorphic ventricular tachycardia in syncope patients with apparent heart disease and is therefore useful in some patients with syncope [308–310]. An abnormal result consists of the presence of a "late potential" or a prolonged QRS complex. The chance of finding the presence of ventricular tachycardia is related to the extent of the abnormalities observed (i.e., if three out of the three observed criteria: QRS duration, amplitude of the last 40 ms of the QRS complex, and length of the low amplitude signal at the end of the QRS complex).

This non-invasive test has its highest predictive accuracy when coronary artery disease is present. The main use of the signal-averaged ECG is for patients who have coronary artery disease and syncope but have preserved ventricular function (ejection fraction > 0.40). If the ejection fraction is < 0.40, proceeding directly to electrophysiologic testing is recommended.

The signal-averaged ECG, however, may provide some adjunctive information in patients with coronary artery disease and ejection fraction < 0.40 should the electrophysiologic test be negative. The test may be falsely negative (and may miss the risk of ventricular tachycardia) if there has been an inferior myocardial infarction. Also, the test lacks predictive accuracy in patients who do not have coronary artery disease. It may be falsely positive when a bundle branch block is present.

The use of other non-invasive tests as general screen for syncope, including T-wave alternans and heart rate variability, are of uncertain utility to predict the need for ICDs.

Cardiac catheterization

Cardiac catheterization is advocated for patients with suspected heart disease and syncope. Cardiac catheterization may find an underlying structural heart problem but the test is not justified unless there is a history suggestive of a significant valvular problem or adequate suspicion for an ischemically mediated arrhythmia. The blanket use of cardiac catheterization in syncope patients, even when heart disease is diagnosed, is certainly not warranted, is probably overused, and can only be recommended on a case-by-case basis.

Treatment

Once a cause for syncope has been identified, treatment should be *considered*. Treatment for all the conditions mentioned is beyond the scope of this chapter and is discussed elsewhere. Not all patients who pass out require treatment even if the cause is identified. For example, a patient who has an isolated vasovagal episode resulting from a specific situation unlikely to be reproduced does not require therapy.

Case 12
A 52-year-old woman had a viral syndrome associated with diarrhea, nausea, and vomiting. Fluid intake was inadequate. After abruptly standing up from bed, she developed nausea and lightheadedness. Several minutes later she became diaphoretic and collapsed, waking up on the floor. After hydration and recovery from her viral infection, no further therapy was indicated.

Management of recurrent syncope, no cause identified

Proper evaluation of the syncope patient, before evaluation becomes futile and excessive, depends on patient age, underlying medical conditions, and ensuing physical limitations imposed upon the patient. For patients with an unidentified cause for syncope, no specific therapy can be prescribed and no studies clearly document a valid, rational treatment plan. In many such patients, syncope will not recur or episodes will be rare and nothing more needs to be done, but, depending on the patient, an aggressive approach may be needed. The prognosis

for patients with syncope of undetermined etiology using appropriate methods to evaluate the cause is relatively good in the short term. The recurrence rate of syncope can be up to 30% [15,38].

For patients with recurrent syncope, reassessment may be necessary. Even *after* further extensive or repeated evaluation, however, no cause for syncope is ever found in up to 85% of these patients. Hospitalizations for repeat monitoring, tilt table testing, and electrophysiologic testing are therefore rarely indicated. Perhaps certain aspects of the history were not completely considered and should be revisited. It is likely that the majority of patients with SUO have an autonomically mediated cause and are likely to have neurocardiogenic syncope. Always consider psychological causes as well (see Chapter 12). While such patients with undiagnosed syncope generally have a good prognosis [15,282], specific patient subgroups fare poorly (e.g., patients with dilated cardiomyopathy) and syncope recurrence is always possible. For some patients with recurrent, debilitating episodes, a trial of empiric therapy may be warranted.

In the elderly, the empiric placement of a pacemaker has been considered an option but this remains highly controversial [311–315]. It has been shown with extensive monitoring that transient bradyarrhythmias can be diagnosed as the cause for syncope when no other cause can be found [223].

While some patients with undiagnosed syncope appear to benefit from pacing, it is always best to have good justification for a pacemaker. With newer techniques for monitoring, this is now possible.

Empiric therapy for SUO is usually no better and can even be worse than no therapy at all [211,316,317]. Moazez *et al.* [211] found that the recurrence rate of syncope was even worse if empiric therapy was given. Therapy guided by electrophysiologic testing may have helped prevent syncope recurrence [211,316].

Recent data suggest that an adenosine triphosphate (ATP) infusion may provide information regarding the need for a pacemaker in patients aged over 60 years [318]. If the infusion of ATP causes a > 10-s pause, this suggests highly active muscarinic vagal receptors and indicates that a pacemaker may eliminate syncopal episodes if no other cause is diagnosed.

Case 13

An 85-year-old man with recurrent syncope collapses with increasing frequency. The initial evaluation was negative. An electrophysiologic consult was called to rule out an arrhythmic cause for syncope. Further history was obtained. The patient collapsed in the morning at breakfast. Apparently the patient was being treated with increasing dosage of acetaminophen with codeine for arthritis and haloperidol at night for sleep. The patient was seen to be confused in the morning and did not really have syncope. After the drugs were stopped the "syncope" stopped.

Case 14

A 51-year-old New York Heart Association functional class I woman with dilated cardiomyopathy, ejection fraction of 0.25, and left bundle branch block, plowed her car into a truck, destroying it, after she passed out. When she awoke, she did not remember anything. History and physical examination were otherwise negative. On the monitor, she had a three-beat run of ventricular tachycardia. An electrophysiologic test was negative. She had passed out a year before but did not see a doctor.

Therapy. An empiric implantable defibrillator was placed.

Case 15

A 17-year-old woman with more than 10 episodes of syncope, once when driving a car, has no history of medical problems, a normal physical examination (except sinus bradycardia and occasional junctional rhythm), a normal ECG, and a normal tilt table test. She has seasonal asthma. An event monitor was not helpful.

Therapy. Theophylline was started for presumed neurocardiogenic syncope and she remains asymptomatic for 3 years.

Case 16

An 80-year-old male patient who lives in a nursing home falls frequently. He takes amlodipine and hydrochlorothiazide for hypertension. He collapsed at the nursing home and broke his right hip. Initially, upon attaching a monitor, he was found to be in atrial fibrillation with a rate of 50 and an associated blood pressure when awake of 165/70 mmHg

without orthostatic signs. An echocardiogram showed left ventricular hypertrophy and intact left ventricular function.

Therapy. An empiric pacemaker was placed and he remains symptom-free.

Case 17

A 39-year-old woman with history of mitral valve prolapse passed out suddenly without warning on two occasions. She takes no medication.

Physical. No orthostatic signs, a midsystolic click was present. ECG was normal. Echocardiogram showed mitral valve prolapse. A tilt table test was negative. An event monitor was given for 1 month but she had no symptoms.

Therapy. No further evaluation was performed and no therapy was given.

Case 18

A 52-year-old hypertensive woman without known history collapsed at home and came to the emergency room with a rapid rate in atrial fibrillation, evidence for Wolff–Parkinson–White syndrome, and a blood pressure of 90/60 mmHg. She remained slightly lethargic even after DC cardioversion. Her sister stated that she had the worst headache of her life before collapsing at home. A CT scan revealed a subarachnoid bleed.

Therapy. After resection of her berry aneurysm, and with no further therapy for Wolff–Parkinson– White syndrome, she recovered without incident.

A protocol to evaluate syncope in the emergency room (see also Figs. 1.3a,b & 1.4, pp. 24–26)

After an initial history (including evaluation of prodrome, palpitations, cardiovascular disease, seizures, and medications) and physical examination (including orthostatic vital signs, a complete cardiac and neurologic examination, carotid massage as needed) in the emergency room or other outpatient setting, an ECG, a hemoglobin test, a blood glucose test, and cardiac monitoring are obtained (during evaluation in the emergency room). If the patient is older than 40 years, is taking a diuretic or a vasodilator, has evidence for dehydration or renal disease, a BUN, creatinine and electrolytes are ordered. If there is history of a new neurologic abnormality, head trauma, or a severe headache, a head CT scan is considered in conjunction with a neurology consult; otherwise, a CT scan is not ordered. If no specific etiology of syncope is identified, attention is directed to categorization by age and underlying medical conditions. Is there pacemaker or implanted defibrillator present, is there potential for malfunction? Did the implanted defibrillator discharge? Is there a long QT or corrected QT interval, either continuously or intermittently (> 0.500 s)? Is there a bundle branch block? Is there a known or suspected heart condition? If the answer to any of these questions is "yes," the patient is admitted. If there is an implanted defibrillator or a pacemaker, it is interrogated immediately, even before admission. If the patient is older than

50 years, but the answer to the above questions is "no," the patient is either discharged with early follow-up by the following physical or an internist or is admitted for a 23-h ("outpatient") admission with a bedside cardiac monitor. In the hospital, an electrophysiologic consult is obtained if there is a history of heart disease, impaired left ventricular function, bundle branch block, pacemaker, or ICD. Testing directed at the specific cause of syncope is planned and performed in the hospital or as an outpatient. If no cause is identified, the patient is discharged, often with an event monitor. A tilt table test is considered.

An algorithm to manage syncope

A valid universal algorithmic approach to syncope is shown in Fig. 1.8. Such an approach can be applied to the great majority of patients who have syncope. Specific intricacies of each patient's problems must

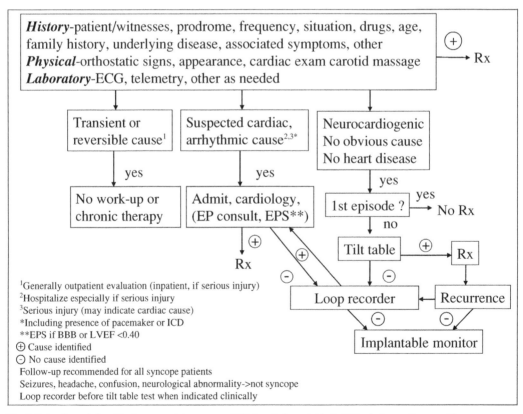

Fig. 1.8 A universal algorithmic approach to syncope. BBB, bundle branch block; ECG, electrocardiogram; EP, electrophysiology; EPS, electrophysiology studies; ICD, implantable cardioverter defibrillator; LVEF, left ventricular ejection fraction.

be considered. These intricacies may further direct proper diagnostic approaches and therapeutic strategies.

Summary

This chapter reviews an initial approach to patients who present with syncope. It is not meant to be inclusive. Throughout the chapter, the reader is referred to other chapters for more in-depth coverage of the many topics presented.

Conclusions

Syncope is a common manifestation of many disease processes. The problem is recurrent and handicapping in a minority of cases. Patients with syncope and heart disease, particularly when there is impaired left ventricular function, bundle branch block, evidence for congestive heart failure, or a positive family history, appear to be at particularly high risk of death and require an aggressive initial approach. Patients who benefit most from hospitalization include those with suspected cardiac disease, the elderly, those with serious injuries, and those with new neurologic findings.

Diagnostic tests should be used sparingly, directed by a carefully performed history and physical examination. No series of tests is universally applicable. Extensive, undirected testing and repeat hospital admissions are usually unrewarding and expensive.

Over the past few decades, there have been advances in the ability to evaluate the syncope patient properly. The initial management is best directed by the savvy clinician who can discern clues from the history and physical examination to direct further diagnostic evaluation when needed. Up to half of patients with syncope remain undiagnosed, indicating that while we have come a long way we still have a long way to go.

Acknowledgment

Thanks to Wishwa Kapoor for his suggestions and comments.

References

1 Brignole M, Alboni P, Benditt DG, *et al.* Guidelines on management (diagnosis and treatment) of syncope: update 2004. *Eur Heart J* 2004;**25**:2054–72.

2 McLaren AJ, Lear J, Daniels RG. Collapse in an accident and emergency department. *J R Soc Med* 1994;**87**:138–9.

3 Engel GL. Psychologic stress, vasodepressor (vasovagal) syncope, and sudden death. *Ann Intern Med* 1978;**89**:403–12.

4 Olshansky B. Is syncope the same thing as sudden death except that you wake up? *J Cardiovasc Electrophysiol* 1997;**8**:1098–101.

5 Olshansky B. Syncope evaluation at a crossroad: for which patients? *Circulation* 2001;**104**:7–8.

6 Olshansky B. For whom does the bell toll? *J Cardiovasc Electrophysiol* 2001;**12**:1002–3.

7 Liberthson R. Sudden death from cardiac causes in children and young adults. *N Engl J Med* 1996;**334**:1039–40.

8 Futterman LG, Lemberg L. Unexplained syncope: diagnostic value of tilt-table testing. *Am J Crit Care* 1994;**3**:322–5.

9 Linzer M, Pontinen M, Gold DT, Divine GW, Felder A, Brooks WB. Impairment of physical and psychosocial function in recurrent syncope. *J Clin Epidemiol* 1991;**44**:1037–43.

10 Linzer M, Gold DT, Pontinen M, Divine GW, Felder A, Brooks WB. Recurrent syncope as a chronic disease: preliminary validation of a disease-specific measure of functional impairment. *J Gen Intern Med* 1994;**9**:181–6.

11 Linzer M, Varia I, Pontinen M, Divine GW, Grubb BP, Estes NA III. Medically unexplained syncope: relationship to psychiatric illness. *Am J Med* 1992;**92**:18S–25S.

12 Hori S. Diagnosis of patients with syncope in emergency medicine. *Keio J Med* 1994;**43**:185–91.

13 Day S. Evaluation and outcome of emergency room patients with transient loss of consciousness. *Am J Med* 1982;**73**:15–23.

14 Kapoor WN. Evaluation and outcome of patients with syncope. *Medicine (Baltimore)* 1990;**69**:160–75.

15 Kapoor WN, Karpf M, Wieand S, Peterson JR, Levey GS. A prospective evaluation and follow-up of patients with syncope. *N Engl J Med* 1983;**309**:197–204.

16 Eagle KA, Black HR, Cook EF, Goldman L. Evaluation of prognostic classifications for patients with syncope. *Am J Med* 1985;**79**:455–60.

17 Morady F, Shen E, Schwartz A, *et al.* Long-term follow-up of patients with recurrent unexplained syncope evaluated by electrophysiologic testing. *J Am Coll Cardiol* 1983;**2**:1053–9.

18 Kapoor WN. Evaluation of syncope in the elderly. *J Am Geriatr Soc* 1987;**35**:826–8.

19 Blanc JJ, Genet L, Forneiro I, *et al.* Short loss of consciousness: etiology and diagnostic approach: results of a prospective study. *Presse Med* 1989;**18**:923–6.

20 Kapoor WN, Karpf M, Maher Y, Miller RA, Levey GS. Syncope of unknown origin: the need for a more cost-effective approach to its diagnosis evaluation. *JAMA* 1982;**247**:2687–91.

21 Calkins H, Byrne M, el-Atassi R, Kalbfleisch S, Langberg JJ, Morady F. The economic burden of unrecognized vasodepressor syncope. *Am J Med* 1993;**95**:473–9.

22 Linzer M, Prystowsky EN, Divine GW, *et al.* Predicting the outcomes of electrophysiologic studies of patients with unexplained syncope: preliminary validation of a derived model. *J Gen Intern Med* 1991;**6**:113–20.

23 Campbell AJ, Reinken J, Allan BC, Martinez GS. Falls in old age: a study of frequency and related clinical factors. *Age Ageing* 1981;**10**:264–70.

24 Savage DD, Corwin L, McGee DL, Kannel WB, Wolf PA. Epidemiologic features of isolated syncope: the Framingham Study. *Stroke* 1985;**16**:626–9.

25 Davies AJ, Kenny RA. Falls presenting to the accident and emergency department: types of presentation and risk factor profile. *Age Ageing* 1996;**25**:362–6.

26 Dey AB, Bexton RS, Tyman MM, Charles RG, Kenny RA. The impact of a dedicated "syncope and falls" clinic on pacing practice in northeastern England. *Pacing Clin Electrophysiol* 1997;**20**:815–7.

27 Gordon M. Falls in the elderly: more common, more dangerous. *Geriatrics* 1982;**37**:117–20.

28 Kenny RA, O'Shea D. Falls and syncope in elderly patients. *Clin Geriatr Med* 2002;**18**:xiii–xiv.

29 Mahoney JE. Falls in the elderly: office-based evaluation, prevention, and treatment. *Cleve Clin J Med* 1999;**66**:181–9.

30 Rubenstein LZ, Josephson KR. The epidemiology of falls and syncope. *Clin Geriatr Med* 2002;**18**:141–58.

31 Lipsitz LA, Wei JY, Rowe JW. Syncope in an elderly, institutionalized population: prevalence, incidence, and associated risk. *Q J Med* 1985;**55**:45–54.

32 Lipsitz LA. Syncope in the elderly. *Ann Intern Med* 1983;**99**:92–105.

33 Dermksian G, Lamb LE. Syncope in a population of healthy young adults: incidence, mechanisms, and significance. *JAMA* 1958;**168**:1200–7.

34 Murdoch BD. Loss of consciousness in healthy South African men: incidence, causes and relationship to EEG abnormality. *S Afr Med J* 1980;**57**:771–4.

35 Williams RL, Allen PD. Loss of consciousness: incidence, causes and electroencephalographic findings. *Aeromed Acta* 1962;**33**:545–51.

36 Manolis AS, Linzer M, Salem D, Estes NA III. Syncope: current diagnostic evaluation and management. *Ann Intern Med* 1990;**112**:850–63.

37 Schaal SF, Nelson SD, Boudoulas H, Lewis RP. Syncope. *Curr Probl Cardiol* 1992;**17**:205–64.

38 Kapoor WN, Peterson J, Wieand HS, Karpf M. Diagnostic and prognostic implications of recurrences in patients with syncope. *Am J Med* 1987;**83**:700–8.

39 Grimm W, Langenfeld H, Maisch B, Kochsiek K. Symptoms, cardiovascular risk profile and spontaneous ECG in paced patients: a five-year follow-up study. *Pacing Clin Electrophysiol* 1990;**13**:2086–90.

40 Morady F, Shen EN, Bhandari A, Schwartz AB, Scheinman MM. Clinical symptoms in patients with sustained ventricular tachycardia. *West J Med* 1985;**142**:341–4.

41 Hess DS, Morady F, Scheinman MM. Electrophysiologic testing in the evaluation of patients with syncope of undetermined origin. *Am J Cardiol* 1982;**50**:1309–15.

42 Barnes A. Cerebral manifestations of paroxysmal tachycardia. *Am J Med Sci* 1926;**171**:489–95.

43 Denniss AR, Ross DL, Richards DA, Uther JB. Electrophysiologic studies in patients with unexplained syncope. *Int J Cardiol* 1992;**35**:211–7.

44 Olshansky B, Mazuz M, Martins JB. Significance of inducible tachycardia in patients with syncope of unknown origin: a long-term follow-up. *J Am Coll Cardiol* 1985;**5**:216–23.

45 Kall JG, Olshansky B, Wilber D. Sudden death and recurrent syncope in patients presenting with syncope of unknown origin: predictive value of electrophysiologic testing. *PACE* 1991;**14**:387A.

46 Esber EJ, Davis WR, Mullen KD, McCullough AJ. Toothpick in ano: an unusual cause of syncope. *Am J Gastroenterol* 1994;**89**:941–2.

47 Epstein AM, Shupack JL. Syncope associated with liquid nitrogen therapy. *Arch Dermatol* 1977;**113**:847.

48 Elejalde JI, Louis CJ, Elcuaz R, Pinillos MA. Drug abuse with inhalated xylazine. *Eur J Emerg Med* 2003;**10**:252–3.

49 Vates GE, Wang KC, Bonovich D, Dowd CF, Lawton MT. Bow hunter stroke caused by cervical disc herniation: case report. *J Neurosurg* 2002;**96**:90–3.

50 Sheth RD, Bodensteiner JB. Effective utilization of home-video recordings for the evaluation of paroxysmal events in pediatrics. *Clin Pediatr (Phila)* 1994;**33**:578–82.

51 Inoue N, Ohkusa T, Nitta T, Harada M, Murata K, Matsuzaki M. Syncope induced by tobacco smoking in the head-up position. *Jpn Circ J* 2001;**65**:1001–3.

52 Birkinshaw RI, Gleeson A, Gray AJ. Hairdryer syncope. *Br J Clin Pract* 1996;**50**:398–9.

53 Carbon monoxide poisoning associated with a propane-powered floor burnisher – Vermont, 1992. *MMWR Morb Mortal Wkly Rep* 1993;**42**:726–8.

54 Lau G. Did he drown or was he murdered? *Med Sci Law* 2002;**42**:172–80.

55 Igarashi M, Boehm RM Jr, May WN, Bornhofen JH. Syncope associated with hair-grooming. *Brain Dev* 1988;**10**:249–51.

56 Olshansky B. A Pepsi challenge. *N Engl J Med* 1999;**340**:2006.

57 Wayne HH. Syncope: physiological considerations and an analysis of the clinical characteristics in 510 patients. *Am J Med* 1961;**30**:418–38.

58 Hecker J. Die tanswut, eine volkrankheit im mittelalter, Berlin, Germany. *TCF.* 1832.

59 Lempert T, Bauer M. Mass fainting at rock concerts. *N Engl J Med* 1995;**332**:1721.

60 Morens DM. Mass fainting at medieval rock concerts. *N Engl J Med* 1995;**333**:1361.

61 Rumball A. Pulmonary oedema with neurological symptoms after the fainting lark and mess trick. *BMJ* 1963;**5349**:80–3.

62 Wieling W, van Lieshout JJ. The fainting lark. *Clin Auton Res* 2002;**12**:207.

63 Spitzer DE. Horseradish horrors: sushi syncope. *JAMA* 1988;**259**:218–9.

64 Soteriades ES, Evans JC, Larson MG, *et al.* Incidence and prognosis of syncope. *N Engl J Med* 2002;**347**:878–85.

65 Linzer M, Yang EH, Estes NA III, Wang P, Vorperian VR, Kapoor WN. Diagnosing syncope. Part 2: Unexplained syncope. Clinical Efficacy Assessment Project of the American College of Physicians. *Ann Intern Med* 1997;**127**:76–86.

66 Linzer M, Yang EH, Estes NA III, Wang P, Vorperian VR, Kapoor WN. Diagnosing syncope. Part 1: Value of history, physical examination, and electrocardiography. Clinical Efficacy Assessment Project of the American College of Physicians. *Ann Intern Med* 1997;**126**:989–96.

67 Alboni P, Brignole M, Menozzi C, *et al.* Diagnostic value of history in patients with syncope with or without heart disease. *J Am Coll Cardiol* 2001;**37**:1921–8.

68 Eagle KA, Mulley AG, Skates SJ, *et al.* Length of stay in the intensive care unit: effects of practice guidelines and feedback. *JAMA* 1990;**264**:992–7.

69 Kapoor WN. Syncope. *N Engl J Med* 2000;**343**:1856–62.

70 Wright KE Jr, McIntosh HD. Syncope: a review of pathophysiological mechanisms. *Prog Cardiovasc Dis* 1971;**13**:580–94.

71 Brignole M, Alboni P, Benditt D, *et al.* Task force on syncope, European Society of Cardiology. Part 1. The initial evaluation of patients with syncope. *Europace* 2001;**3**:253–60.

72 Alboni P, Brignole M, Menozzi C, *et al.* Clinical spectrum of neurally mediated reflex syncopes. *Europace* 2004;**6**:55–62.

73 van Dijk JG. Fainting in animals. *Clin Auton Res* 2003;**13**:247–55.

74 Maloney JD, Jaeger FJ, Fouad-Tarazi FM, Morris HH. Malignant vasovagal syncope: prolonged asystole provoked by head-up tilt. Case report and review of diagnosis, pathophysiology, and therapy. *Cleve Clin J Med* 1988;**55**:542–8.

75 Abe H, Iwami Y, Nagatomo T, Miura Y, Nakashima Y. Treatment of malignant neurocardiogenic vasovagal syncope with a rate drop algorithm in dual chamber cardiac pacing. *Pacing Clin Electrophysiol* 1998;**21**:1473–5.

76 Biffi M, Boriani G, Sabbatani P, *et al.* Malignant vasovagal syncope: a randomised trial of metoprolol and clonidine. *Heart* 1997;**77**:268–72.

77 Fitzpatrick A, Theodorakis G, Vardas P, *et al.* The incidence of malignant vasovagal syndrome in patients with recurrent syncope. *Eur Heart J* 1991;**12**:389–94.

78 Pentousis D, Cooper JP, Cobbe SM. Prolonged asystole induced by head-up tilt test: report of four cases and brief review of the prognostic significance and medical management. *Heart* 1997;**77**:273–5.

79 Reybrouck T, Heidbuchel H, Van de Werf F, Ector H. Tilt training: a treatment for malignant and recurrent neurocardiogenic syncope. *Pacing Clin Electrophysiol* 2000;**23**:493–8.

80 Riffee-Landa R. Determining if vasovagal syncope is "malignant" not as important as treatment. *Crit Care Nurse* 1994;**14**:25–6.

81 Fitzpatrick A, Sutton R. Tilting towards a diagnosis in recurrent unexplained syncope. *Lancet* 1989;**1**:658–60.

82 Luu M, Stevenson WG, Stevenson LW, Baron K, Walden J. Diverse mechanisms of unexpected cardiac arrest in advanced heart failure. *Circulation* 1989;**80**:1675–80.

83 Grubb BP, Wolfe DA, Nelson LA, Hennessy JR. Malignant vasovagally mediated hypotension and bradycardia: a possible cause of sudden death in young patients with asthma. *Pediatrics* 1992;**90**:983–6.

84 Grubb BP, Kosinski DJ, Kanjwal Y. Orthostatic hypotension: causes, classification, and treatment. *Pacing Clin Electrophysiol* 2003;**26**:892–901.

85 Hickler RB. Orthostatic hypotension and syncope. *N Engl J Med* 1977;**296**:336–7.

86 Hermosillo AG, Marquez MF, Jauregui-Renaud K, Cardenas M. Orthostatic hypotension, 2001. *Cardiol Rev* 2001;**9**:339–47.

87 Mukai S, Lipsitz LA. Orthostatic hypotension. *Clin Geriatr Med* 2002;**18**:253–68.

88 Thomas JE, Schirger A, Fealey RD, Sheps SG. Orthostatic hypotension. *Mayo Clin Proc* 1981;**56**:117–25.

89 Bradshaw MJ, Edwards RT. Postural hypotension: pathophysiology and management. *Q J Med* 1986;**60**:643–57.

90 Ibrahim MM, Tarazi RC, Dustan HP. Orthostatic hypotension: mechanisms and management. *Am Heart J* 1975;**90**:513–20.

91 Ibrahim MM, Tarazi RC, Dustan HP, Bravo EL. Idiopathic orthostatic hypotension: circulatory dynamics in chronic autonomic insufficiency. *Am J Cardiol* 1974;**34**:288–94.

92 Bradley JG, Davis KA. Orthostatic hypotension. *Am Fam Physician* 2003;**68**:2393–8.

93 Suzuki T, Higa S, Sakoda S, *et al.* Orthostatic hypotension in familial amyloid polyneuropathy: treatment

with DL-threo-3,4-dihydroxyphenylserine. *Neurology* 1981;**31**:1323–6.

94 Cohen JA, Gross KF. Autonomic neuropathy: clinical presentation and differential diagnosis. *Geriatrics* 1990;**45**:33–7, 41–2.

95 Vinik AI, Maser RE, Mitchell BD, Freeman R. Diabetic autonomic neuropathy. *Diabetes Care* 2003;**26**:1553–79.

96 Senard JM, Rai S, Lapeyre-Mestre M, *et al.* Prevalence of orthostatic hypotension in Parkinson's disease. *J Neurol Neurosurg Psychiatry* 1997;**63**:584–9.

97 Kloehn S, Arendt T, Kohler W, Folsch UR, Monig H. Primary adrenal cortex insufficiency and subclinical neurological changes in a young man. Primary adrenal cortex insufficiency (Addison disease) in X-chromosome linked adrenoleukodystrophy. *Internist (Berl)* 2000;**41**:218–22.

98 Schirger A, Martin WJ, Goldstein NP, Huizenga KA. Orthostatic hypotension in association with acute exacerbations of porphyria. *Mayo Clin Proc* 1962;**37**:7–11.

99 Spalding JM. Some disorders of the circulation due to neurological disease. *Mod Trends Neurol* 1967;**4**:193–208.

100 Aminoff MJ, Wilcox CS. Autonomic dysfunction in syringomyelia. *Postgrad Med J* 1972;**48**:113–5.

101 Baliga RR, Catz AB, Watson LD, Short DJ, Frankel HL, Mathias CJ. Cardiovascular and hormonal responses to food ingestion in humans with spinal cord transection. *Clin Auton Res* 1997;**7**:137–41.

102 Inoue K, Kohriyama T, Ikeda J, Maruyama H, Nakamura S. A case of Guillain–Barre syndrome complicated with severe autonomic failure and presented elevated anti-GD1b and anti-GQ1b antibody. *Rinsho Shinkeigaku* 2002;**42**:13–7.

103 Kita K. Riley–Day syndrome (familial dysautonomia). *Nippon Rinsho* 1992;**50**:846–51.

104 van Lieshout JJ, Wieling W, Wesseling KH, Endert E, Karemaker JM. Orthostatic hypotension caused by sympathectomies performed for hyperhidrosis. *Neth J Med* 1990;**36**:53–7.

105 Fouad FM, Tadena-Thome L, Bravo EL, Tarazi RC. Idiopathic hypovolemia. *Ann Intern Med* 1986;**104**:298–303.

106 Wenning GK, Geser F. Multiple system atrophy. *Rev Neurol (Paris)* 2003;**159**:3S31–8.

107 Bradbury SEC. Postural hypotension. *Am Heart J* 1925;**1**:73.

108 Bannister R, Ardill L, Fentem P. Defective autonomic control of blood vessels in idiopathic orthostatic hypotension. *Brain* 1967;**90**:725–46.

109 Hart RG, Kanter MC. Acute autonomic neuropathy: two cases and a clinical review. *Arch Intern Med* 1990;**150**:2373–6.

110 Zweiker R, Tiemann M, Eber B, *et al.* Bradydysrhythmia-related presyncope secondary to pheochromocytoma. *J Intern Med* 1997;**242**:249–53.

111 Shimizu K, Miura Y, Meguro Y, *et al.* QT prolongation with torsade de pointes in pheochromocytoma. *Am Heart J* 1992;**124**:235–9.

112 Hodder J. Shy–Drager syndrome. *Axone* 1997;**18**:75–9.

113 Russo R, Permutti B, Crociani P, Bortolotti U, Fernandez P, Schivazappa L. Idiopathic orthostatic hypotension (Shy–Drager syndrome). Clinical and hemodynamic studies of a case. *Minerva Med* 1981;**72**:2621–4.

114 Davani S, Bouhaddi M, Nezelof S, Vandel S, Regnard J, Kantelip JP. Orthostatic hypotension and anorexia nervosa: is there a treatment? *Therapie* 2003;**58**:170–2.

115 Wohrle J, Kochs M. Syncope in the elderly. *Z Gerontol Geriatr* 2003;**36**:2–9.

116 Brady PA, Shen WK. Syncope evaluation in the elderly. *Am J Geriatr Cardiol* 1999;**8**:115–24.

117 Maurer MS, Karmally W, Rivadeneira H, Parides MK, Bloomfield DM. Upright posture and postprandial hypotension in elderly persons. *Ann Intern Med* 2000;**133**:533–6.

118 Lipsitz LA. Syncope in the elderly patient. *Hosp Pract (Off Ed)* 1986;**21**:33–44.

119 Lipsitz LA, Nyquist RP Jr, Wei JY, Rowe JW. Postprandial reduction in blood pressure in the elderly. *N Engl J Med* 1983;**309**:81–3.

120 Wehrmacher W. Syncope among the aging population. *Am J Geriatric Cardiol* 1993;**1**:50–7.

121 Whiteside-Yim C. Syncope in the elderly: a clinical approach. *Geriatrics* 1987;**42**:37–41.

122 McIntosh H. Evaluating elderly patients with syncope. *Cardiovasc Rev Rep* 1988;**9**:54–8.

123 Collins KJ, Exton-Smith AN, James MH, Oliver DJ. Functional changes in autonomic nervous responses with ageing. *Age Ageing* 1980;**9**:17–24.

124 Camm AJ, Evans KE, Ward DE, Martin A. The rhythm of the heart in active elderly subjects. *Am Heart J* 1980;**99**:598–603.

125 Carmona J, Amado P, Vasconcelos N, *et al.* Does orthostatic hypotension predict the occurrence of nocturnal arterial hypertension in the elderly patient? *Rev Port Cardiol* 2003;**22**:607–15.

126 Hanlon JT, Linzer M, MacMillan JP, Lewis IK, Felder AA. Syncope and presyncope associated with probable adverse drug reactions. *Arch Intern Med* 1990;**150**:2309–12.

127 Ma SX SP, Long JP. Noradrenergic mechanisms and the cardiovascular actions of nitroglycerin. *Life Sci* 1994;**55**:1595–603.

128 Coperchini ML, Kreeger LC. Postural hypotension from topical glyceryl trinitrate ointment for anal pain. *J Pain Symptom Manage* 1997;**14**:263–4.

129 Raviele A, Menozzi C, Brignole M, *et al.* Value of head-up tilt testing potentiated with sublingual nitroglycerin to assess the origin of unexplained syncope. *Am J Cardiol* 1995;**76**:267–72.

130 Richards CJ, Mark AL, Van Orden DE, Kaloyanides GJ. Effects of indomethacin on the vascular abnormalities of Bartter's syndrome. *Circulation* 1978;**58**:544–9.

131 Imai C, Muratani H, Kimura Y, Kanzato N, Takishita S, Fukiyama K. Effects of meal ingestion and active standing on blood pressure in patients > or = 60 years of age. *Am J Cardiol* 1998;**81**:1310–4.

132 Schroeder C, Bush VE, Norcliffe LJ, *et al.* Water drinking acutely improves orthostatic tolerance in healthy subjects. *Circulation* 2002;**106**:2806–11.

133 Lu CC, Diedrich A, Tung CS, *et al.* Water ingestion as prophylaxis against syncope. *Circulation* 2003;**108**:2660–5.

134 Kunert H, Kuhn FM, Schwemmle K, Ottenjann R. VIP and GIP-producing pancreatic tumour: relationship to the Verner–Morrison syndrome. *Dtsch Med Wochenschr* 1976;**101**:920–3.

135 Delsignore JL, Dvoretsky PM, Hicks DG, O'Keefe RJ, Rosier RN. Mastocytosis presenting as a skeletal disorder. *Iowa Orthop J* 1996;**16**:126–34.

136 Aldrich LB, Moattari AR, Vinik AI. Distinguishing features of idiopathic flushing and carcinoid syndrome. *Arch Intern Med* 1988;**148**:2614–8.

137 Seiler L, Braune S, Borm K, *et al.* Autonomic failure mimicking dopamine agonist induced vertigo in a patient with macroprolactinoma. *Exp Clin Endocrinol Diabetes* 2002;**110**:364–9.

138 Zaina AS, Horn IE, Haj M. Ten years of recurrent syncope due to mastocytosis. *Isr Med Assoc J* 2001;**3**:712.

139 Koide T, Nakajima T, Makifuchi T, Fukuhara N. Systemic mastocytosis and recurrent anaphylactic shock. *Lancet* 2002;**359**:2084.

140 Castells M, Austen KF. Mastocytosis: mediator-related signs and symptoms. *Int Arch Allergy Immunol* 2002;**127**:147–52.

141 Suchard JR. Recurrent near-syncope with flushing. *Acad Emerg Med* 1997;**4**:718–24.

142 Lusic I, Pintaric I, Hozo I, Boic L, Capkun V. Serum prolactin levels after seizure and syncopal attacks. *Seizure* 1999;**8**:218–22.

143 Oribe E, Amini R, Nissenbaum E, Boal B. Serum prolactin concentrations are elevated after syncope. *Neurology* 1996;**47**:60–2.

144 Donzelot & Esmein. Le forme syncope de la tachycardie paroxystique. *La Presse Médicale* 1914;**xxii**:489.

145 Calkins H, Shyr Y, Frumin H, Schork A, Morady F. The value of the clinical history in the differentiation of syncope due to ventricular tachycardia, atrioventricular block, and neurocardiogenic syncope. *Am J Med* 1995;**98**:365–73.

146 Leitch JW, Klein GJ, Yee R, Leather RA, Kim YH. Syncope associated with supraventricular tachycardia: an expression of tachycardia rate or vasomotor response? *Circulation* 1992;**85**:1064–71.

147 Dhala A, Bremner S, Blanck Z, *et al.* Impairment of driving abilities in patients with supraventricular tachycardias. *Am J Cardiol* 1995;**75**:516–8.

148 Benditt DG, Klein GJ, Kriett JM, Dunnigan A, Benson DW, Jr. Enhanced atrioventricular nodal conduction in man: electrophysiologic effects of pharmacologic autonomic blockade. *Circulation* 1984;**69**:1088–95.

149 Fitzpatrick AP, Travill CM, Vardas PE, *et al.* Recurrent symptoms after ventricular pacing in unexplained syncope. *Pacing Clin Electrophysiol* 1990;**13**:619–24.

150 Morley CA, Perrins EJ, Grant P, Chan SL, McBrien DJ, Sutton R. Carotid sinus syncope treated by pacing: analysis of persistent symptoms and role of atrioventricular sequential pacing. *Br Heart J* 1982;**47**:411–8.

151 Sgarbossa EB, Pinski SL, Jaeger FJ, Trohman RG, Maloney JD. Incidence and predictors of syncope in paced patients with sick sinus syndrome. *Pacing Clin Electrophysiol* 1992;**15**:2055–60.

152 Esmein D. Le forme syncopale a tachycardie paroxystique. *Presse Med* 1914;**27**:489–90.

153 Ross R. *Syncope*. London, UK: W.B. Saunders, 1988.

154 Hamer AW, Rubin SA, Peter T, Mandel WJ. Factors that predict syncope during ventricular tachycardia in patients. *Am Heart J* 1984;**107**:997–1005.

155 Waxman MB, Cameron DA. The reflex effects of tachycardias on autonomic tone. *Ann N Y Acad Sci* 1990;**601**:378–93.

156 Waxman MB, Cameron D. Interactions between the autonomic nervous system and tachycardias in man. *Cardiol Clin* 1983;**1**:143–85.

157 Waxman MB, Sharma AD, Cameron DA, Huerta F, Wald RW. Reflex mechanisms responsible for early spontaneous termination of paroxysmal supraventricular tachycardia. *Am J Cardiol* 1982;**49**:259–72.

158 Daoud EG, Dimitrijevic R, Morady F. Syncope mediated by posturally induced ventricular tachycardia. *Ann Intern Med* 1995;**123**:431–2.

159 Sra JS, Akhtar M. Cardiac pacing during neurocardiogenic (vasovagal) syncope. *J Cardiovasc Electrophysiol* 1995;**6**:751–60.

160 Grubb BP, Gerard G, Roush K, *et al.* Differentiation of convulsive syncope and epilepsy with head-up tilt testing. *Ann Intern Med* 1991;**115**:871–6.

161 Hofnagels WA, Padberg GW, Overweg J, *et al.* Syncope or seizure? The diagnostic value of the EEG and hyperventilation test in transient loss of consciousness. *J Neurol Neurosurg Psychiatry* 1991;**54**:953–6.

162 Hofnagels WA, Padberg GW, Overweg J, Roos RA. Syncope or seizure? A matter of opinion. *Clin Neurol Neurosurg* 1992;**94**:153–6.

163 Hofnagels WA, Padberg GW, Overweg J, van der Velde EA, Roos RA. Transient loss of consciousness: the value of the history for distinguishing seizure from syncope. *J Neurol* 1991;**238**:39–43.

164 Zaidi A, Clough P, Scheepers B, Fitzpatrick A. Treatment resistant epilepsy or convulsive syncope? *BMJ* 1998;**317**:869–70.

165 Zaidi A, Clough P, Mawer G, Fitzpatrick A. Accurate diagnosis of convulsive syncope: role of an implantable subcutaneous ECG monitor. *Seizure* 1999;**8**:184–6.

166 Zaidi A, Clough P, Cooper P, Scheepers B, Fitzpatrick AP. Misdiagnosis of epilepsy: many seizure-like attacks have a cardiovascular cause. *J Am Coll Cardiol* 2000;**36**:181–4.

167 Wiederholt W. Seizure disorders. Philadelphia, PA: W.B. Saunders, 1995.

168 Maehara T, Shimizu H. Surgical outcome of corpus callosotomy in patients with drop attacks. *Epilepsia* 2001;**42**:67–71.

169 Nebeling LC, Lerner E. Implementing a ketogenic diet based on medium-chain triglyceride oil in pediatric patients with cancer. *J Am Diet Assoc* 1995;**95**:693–7.

170 Samuel MDJ. Use of the hand held video camcorder in the evaluation of seizures. *J Neurol Neurosurg Psychiatry* 1994;**57**:1417–8.

171 VanNess P. Invasive electrocenphalography in the evaluation of supplementary motor area seizer. *Adv Neurol* 1996;**70**:319–40.

172 Verity C. The place of the EEG and imaging in the management of seizures. *Arch Dis Child* 1995;**73**:557–62.

173 Swoboda KJ. Seizure disorder: syndromes, diagnosis and management. *Compr Ther* 1994;**20**:67–73.

174 Libman MD, Potvin L, Coupal L, Grover SA. Seizure vs. syncope: measuring serum creatine kinase in the emergency department. *J Gen Intern Med* 1991;**6**:408–12.

175 Aminoff MJ, Scheinman MM, Griffin JC, Herre JM. Electrocerebral accompaniments of syncope associated with malignant ventricular arrhythmias. *Ann Intern Med* 1988;**108**:791–6.

176 Constantin L, Martins JB, Fincham RW, Dagli RD. Bradycardia and syncope as manifestations of partial epilepsy. *J Am Coll Cardiol* 1990;**15**:900–5.

177 Ficker DM, Cascino GD, Clements IP. Cardiac asystole masquerading as temporal lobe epilepsy. *Mayo Clin Proc* 1998;**73**:784–6.

178 Manolis AS. The clinical spectrum and diagnosis of syncope. *Herz* 1993;**18**:143–54.

179 Kapoor WN, Peterson JR, Karpf M. Micturition syncope: a reappraisal. *JAMA* 1985;**253**:796–8.

180 Georgeson S, Linzer M, Griffith JL, Weld L, Selker HP. Acute cardiac ischemia in patients with syncope: importance of the initial electrocardiogram. *J Gen Intern Med* 1992;**7**:379–86.

181 Mark AL. The Bezold–Jarisch reflex revisited: clinical implications of inhibitory reflexes originating in the heart. *J Am Coll Cardiol* 1983;**1**:90–102.

182 Benditt D. Syncope. In: Willerson JT, Cohn JN, eds. *Cardiovascular Medicine.* 1995: 1404–21.

183 Chang-Sing P, Peter CT. Syncope: evaluation and management – a review of current approaches to this multifaceted and complex clinical problem. *Cardiol Clin* 1991;**9**:641–51.

184 Farrehi PM, Santinga JT, Eagle KA. Syncope: diagnosis of cardiac and noncardiac causes. *Geriatrics* 1995;**50**:24–30.

185 Mark AL, Kioschos JM, Abboud FM, Heistad DD, Schmid PG. Abnormal vascular responses to exercise in patients with aortic stenosis. *J Clin Invest* 1973;**52**:1138–46.

186 White CW, Zimmerman TJ, Ahmad M. Idiopathic hypertrophic subaortic stenosis presenting as cough syncope. *Chest* 1975;**68**:250–3.

187 Weisberg L. Differential diagnosis of coma: a step-by-step strategy. *J Crit Illness* 1989;**4**:97–108.

188 Heistad DD, Abboud FM, Mark AL, Schmid PG. Impaired reflex vasoconstriction in chronically hypoxemic patients. *J Clin Invest* 1972;**51**:331–7.

189 Grubb BP, Temesy-Armos P, Samoi P, Habn H, Elliott L. Episodic periods of neurally mediated hypotension and bradycardia mimicking transient ischemic attacks in the elderly: identification with head-up tilt-table testing. *Cardiol Elderly* 1993;**1**:221–5.

190 Mathias CJ, Deguchi K, Bleasdale-Barr K, Smith S. Familial vasovagal syncope and pseudosyncope: observations in a case with both natural and adopted siblings. *Clin Auton Res* 2000;**10**:43–5.

191 Shihabuddin L, Shehadeh A, Agle D. Syncope as a conversion mechanism. *Psychosomatics* 1994;**35**:496–8.

192 Kapoor WN, Fortunato M, Hanusa BH, Schulberg HC. Psychiatric illnesses in patients with syncope. *Am J Med* 1995;**99**:505–12.

193 Benditt DG, Brignole M. Syncope: is a diagnosis a diagnosis? *J Am Coll Cardiol* 2003;**41**:791–4.

194 Kapoor W, Snustad D, Peterson J, Wieand HS, Cha R, Karpf M. Syncope in the elderly. *Am J Med* 1986;**80**:419–28.

195 Lipsitz LA. What's different about syncope in the aged? *Am J Geriatr Cardiol* 1993;**2**:37–41.

196 Johnson R. Evaluation of patients with syncope (Letter). *N Engl J Med* 1983;**309**:1650.

197 Getchell WS, Larsen GC, Morris CD, McAnulty JH. Epidemiology of syncope in hospitalized patients. *J Gen Intern Med* 1999;**14**:677–87.

198 Olshansky B, Hahn EA, Hartz VL, Prater SP, Mason JW. Clinical significance of syncope in the electrophysiologic study versus electrocardiographic monitoring (ESVEM) trial. The ESVEM Investigators. *Am Heart J* 1999;**137**:878–86.

199 Steinberg JS, Beckman K, Greene HL, *et al.* Follow-up of patients with unexplained syncope and inducible ventricular tachyarrhythmias: analysis of the AVID registry

and an AVID substudy. Antiarrhythmics versus implantable defibrillators. *J Cardiovasc Electrophysiol* 2001;**12**: 996–1001.

200 Silverstein MD, Singer DE, Mulley AG, Thibault GE, Barnett GO. Patients with syncope admitted to medical intensive care units. *JAMA* 1982;**248**:1185–9.

201 Kapoor WN, Hanusa BH. Is syncope a risk factor for poor outcomes? Comparison of patients with and without syncope. *Am J Med* 1996;**100**:646–55.

202 Yee R, Klein GJ. Syncope in the Wolff–Parkinson–White syndrome: incidence and electrophysiologic correlates. *Pacing Clin Electrophysiol* 1984;**7**:381–8.

203 Auricchio A, Klein H, Trappe HJ, Wenzlaff P. Lack of prognostic value of syncope in patients with Wolff–Parkinson–White syndrome. *J Am Coll Cardiol* 1991;**17**:152–8.

204 Nienaber CA, Hiller S, Spielmann RP, Geiger M, Kuck KH. Syncope in hypertrophic cardiomyopathy: multivariate analysis of prognostic determinants. *J Am Coll Cardiol* 1990;**15**:948–55.

205 Cecchi F, Olivotto I, Montereggi A, Santoro G, Dolara A, Maron BJ. Hypertrophic cardiomyopathy in Tuscany: clinical course and outcome in an unselected regional population. *J Am Coll Cardiol* 1995;**26**:1529–36.

206 Bachinsky WB, Linzer M, Weld L, Estes NA III. Usefulness of clinical characteristics in predicting the outcome of electrophysiologic studies in unexplained syncope. *Am J Cardiol* 1992;**69**:1044–9.

207 Bass EB, Elson JJ, Fogoros RN, Peterson J, Arena VC, Kapoor WN. Long-term prognosis of patients undergoing electrophysiologic studies for syncope of unknown origin. *Am J Cardiol* 1988;**62**:1186–91.

208 Denes P, Uretz E, Ezri MD, Borbola J. Clinical predictors of electrophysiologic findings in patients with syncope of unknown origin. *Arch Intern Med* 1988;**148**:1922–8.

209 Kapoor WN, Hammill SC, Gersh BJ. Diagnosis and natural history of syncope and the role of invasive electrophysiologic testing. *Am J Cardiol* 1989;**63**:730–4.

210 Krol RB, Morady F, Flaker GC, *et al.* Electrophysiologic testing in patients with unexplained syncope: clinical and noninvasive predictors of outcome. *J Am Coll Cardiol* 1987;**10**:358–63.

211 Moazez F, Peter T, Simonson J, Mandel WJ, Vaughn C, Gang E. Syncope of unknown origin: clinical, noninvasive, and electrophysiologic determinants of arrhythmia induction and symptom recurrence during long-term follow-up. *Am Heart J* 1991;**121**:81–8.

212 Prystowsky EN, Evans JJ. Diagnostic evaluation and treatment strategies for patients at risk for serious cardiac arrhythmias, Part 1: Syncope of unknown origin. *Mod Concepts Cardiovasc Dis* 1991;**1991**:49–54.

213 Teichman SL, Felder SD, Matos JA, Kim SG, Waspe LE, Fisher JD. The value of electrophysiologic studies in

syncope of undetermined origin: report of 150 cases. *Am Heart J* 1985;**110**:469–79.

214 DiMarco JP, Garan H, Harthorne JW, Ruskin JN. Intracardiac electrophysiologic techniques in recurrent syncope of unknown case. *Ann Intern Med* 1981;**95**: 542–8.

215 Morady F. The evaluation of syncope with electrophysiologic studies. *Cardiol Clin* 1986;**4**:515–26.

216 Olsson M, Rosenqvist M, Forssell G. Unnecessary deaths from valvular aortic stenosis. *J Intern Med* 1990; **228**:591–6.

217 Grech ED, Ramsdale DR. Exertional syncope in aortic stenosis: evidence to support inappropriate left ventricular baroreceptor response. *Am Heart J* 1991;**121**: 603–6.

218 Reynen K. Cardiac myxomas. *N Engl J Med* 1995;**333**: 1610–7.

219 Wilmshurst PT, Willicombe PR, Webb-Peploe MM. Effect of aortic valve replacement on syncope in patients with aortic stenosis. *Br Heart J* 1993;**70**:542–3.

220 Middlekauff HR, Stevenson WG, Saxon LA. Prognosis after syncope: impact of left ventricular function. *Am Heart J* 1993;**125**:121–7.

221 Middlekauff HR, Stevenson WG, Stevenson LW, Saxon LA. Syncope in advanced heart failure: high risk of sudden death regardless of origin of syncope. *J Am Coll Cardiol* 1993;**21**:110–6.

222 Tchou PJ, Krebs AC, Sra J, *et al.* Syncope: a warning sign of sudden death in idiopathic dilated cardiomyopathy patients. *J Am Coll Cardiol* 1991;**17**:196A.

223 Krahn AD, Klein GJ, Norris C, Yee R. The etiology of syncope in patients with negative tilt table and electrophysiologic testing. *Circulation* 1995;**92**:1819–24.

224 Haddad RM, Sellers TD. Syncope as a symptom: a practical approach to etiologic diagnosis. *Postgrad Med* 1986;**79**:48–53, 56–7, 61–2.

225 Noble RJ. The patient with syncope. *JAMA* 1977; **237**:1372–6.

226 Martin GJ, Adams SL, Martin HG, Mathews J, Zull D, Scanlon PJ. Prospective evaluation of syncope. *Ann Emerg Med* 1984;**13**:499–504.

227 Kenny RA. Syncope. History may be inaccurate in elderly people. *BMJ* 1994;**309**:474–5.

228 Sutton R, Nathan A, Perrins J, Skehan D, Davies W. Syncope: a good history is not enough. *BMJ* 1994; **309**:474.

229 Taggart P, Carruthers M, Somerville W. Some effects of emotion on the normal and abnormal heart. *Curr Probl Cardiol* 1983;**7**:1–29.

230 Rowe PC, Bou-Holaigah I, Kan JS, Calkins H. Is neurally mediated hypotension an unrecognised cause of chronic fatigue? *Lancet* 1995;**345**:623–4.

231 Sharpey-Schafer EP. The mechanism of syncope after coughing. *BMJ* 1953;**4841**:860–3.

232 Sakaguchi S, Shultz JJ, Remole SC, Adler SW, Lurie KG, Benditt DG. Syncope associated with exercise, a manifestation of neurally mediated syncope. *Am J Cardiol* 1995;**75**:476–81.

233 Tsutsui M, Matsuguchi T, Tsutsui H, *et al.* Alcohol-induced sinus bradycardia and hypotension in patients with syncope. *Jpn Heart J* 1992;**33**:875–9.

234 Kirkman E, Marshall HW, Banks JR, Little RA. Ethanol augments the baroreflex-inhibitory effects of sciatic nerve stimulation in the anaesthetized dog. *Exp Physiol* 1994;**79**:81–91.

235 Kettunen RV, Timisjarvi J, Heikkila J, Saukko P. The acute dose-dependent effects of ethanol on canine myocardial perfusion. *Alcohol* 1994;**11**:351–4.

236 Chaudhuri KR, Maule S, Thomaides T, Pavitt D, Mathias CJ. Alcohol ingestion lowers supine blood pressure, causes splanchnic vasodilatation and worsens postural hypotension in primary autonomic failure. *J Neurol* 1994;**241**:145–52.

237 Brackett DJ, Gauvin DV, Lerner MR, Holloway FA, Wilson MF. Dose- and time-dependent cardiovascular responses induced by ethanol. *J Pharmacol Exp Ther* 1994;**268**:78–84.

238 Lu CY, Wang DX, Yu SB. Effects of acute ingestion of ethanol on hemodynamics and hypoxic pulmonary vasoconstriction in dogs: role of leukotrienes. *J Tongji Med Univ* 1992;**12**:253–6.

239 Freedland ES, McMicken DB. Alcohol-related seizures. Part I: Pathophysiology, differential diagnosis, and evaluation. *J Emerg Med* 1993;**11**:463–73.

240 Byrne JM, Marais HJ, Cheek GA. Exercise-induced complete heart block in a patient with chronic bifascicular block. *J Electrocardiol* 1994;**27**:339–42.

241 Williams CC, Bernhardt DT. Syncope in athletes. *Sports Med* 1995;**19**:223–34.

242 Calkins H, Seifert M, Morady F. Clinical presentation and long-term follow-up of athletes with exercise-induced vasodepressor syncope. *Am Heart J* 1995;**129**:1159–64.

243 Leenhardt A, Lucet V, Denjoy I, Grau F, Ngoc DD, Coumel P. Catecholaminergic polymorphic ventricular tachycardia in children: a 7-year follow-up of 21 patients. *Circulation* 1995;**91**:1512–9.

244 Freed MD. Advances in the diagnosis and therapy of syncope and palpitations in children. *Curr Opin Pediatr* 1994;**6**:368–72.

245 Nakajima T, Misu K, Iwasawa K, *et al.* Auditory stimuli as a major cause of syncope in a patient with idiopathic long QT syndrome. *Jpn Circ J* 1995;**59**:241–6.

246 Kushner JA, Kou WH, Kadish AH, Morady F. Natural history of patients with unexplained syncope and a non-diagnostic electrophysiologic study. *J Am Coll Cardiol* 1989;**14**:391–6.

247 Cooper CJ, Ridker P, Shea J, Creager MA. Familial occurrence of neurocardiogenic syncope. *N Engl J Med* 1994;**331**:205.

248 Grimm W, Alter P, Maisch B. Arrhythmia risk stratification with regard to prophylactic implantable defibrillator therapy in patients with dilated cardiomyopathy-results of MACAS, DEFINITE, and SCD-HeFT. *Herz* 2004;**29**:348–52.

249 Moss AJ, Zareba W, Hall WJ, *et al.* Prophylactic implantation of a defibrillator in patients with myocardial infarction and reduced ejection fraction. *N Engl J Med* 2002;**346**:877–83.

250 Bristow MR, Saxon LA, Boehmer J, *et al.* Cardiac-resynchronization therapy with or without an implantable defibrillator in advanced chronic heart failure. *N Engl J Med* 2004;**350**:2140–50.

251 Evans RW. Neurologic aspects of hyperventilation syndrome. *Semin Neurol* 1995;**15**:115–25.

252 Nixon G. Hyperventilation and cardiac symptoms. *Intern Med* 1989;**10**:67–84.

253 Morillo CA, Camacho ME, Wood MA, Gilligan DM, Ellenbogen KA. Diagnostic utility of mechanical, pharmacological and orthostatic stimulation of the carotid sinus in patients with unexplained syncope. *J Am Coll Cardiol* 1999;**34**:1587–94.

254 Kenny RA. SAFE PACE 2: Syncope and falls in the elderly – pacing and carotid sinus evaluation: a randomized controlled trial of cardiac pacing in older patients with falls and carotid sinus hypersensitivity. *Europace* 1999;**1**:69–72.

255 Kenny RA, Dunn HM. Carotid sinus massage in carotid sinus syndrome. *Ulster Med J* 1990;**59**:93–5.

256 Kenny RA, Richardson DA, Steen N, Bexton RS, Shaw FE, Bond J. Carotid sinus syndrome: a modifiable risk factor for nonaccidental falls in older adults (SAFE PACE). *J Am Coll Cardiol* 2001;**38**:1491–6.

257 Aita JF. Etiology of syncope in 100 patients with associated pale facial appearance. *Nebr Med J* 1993;**78**:182–3.

258 Martin GJ AS, Martin HG. Evaluation of patients with syncope (Letter). *N Engl J Med* 1983;**309**:1650.

259 Dhingra RC, Denes P, Wu D, *et al.* Syncope in patients with chronic bifascicular block: significance, causative mechanisms, and clinical implications. *Ann Intern Med* 1974;**81**:302–6.

260 McAnulty JH, Rahimtoola SH, Murphy E, *et al.* Natural history "high-risk" bundle-branch block: final report of a prospective study. *N Engl J Med* 1982;**307**:137–43.

261 Morady F, Higgins J, Peters RW, *et al.* Electrophysiologic testing in bundle branch block and unexplained syncope. *Am J Cardiol* 1984;**54**:587–91.

262 Click RL, Gersh BJ, Sugrue DD, *et al.* Role of invasive electrophysiologic testing in patients with symptomatic bundle branch block. *Am J Cardiol* 1987; **59**:817–23.

263 Ezri M, Lerman BB, Marchlinski FE, Buxton AE, Josephson ME. Electrophysiologic evaluation of syncope in patients with bifascicular block. *Am Heart J* 1983;**106**:693–7.

264 Englund A, Bergfeldt L, Rehnqvist N, Astrom H, Rosenqvist M. Diagnostic value of programmed ventricular stimulation in patients with bifascicular block: a prospective study of patients with and without syncope. *J Am Coll Cardiol* 1995;**26**:1508–15.

265 Sarasin FP, Louis-Simonet M, Carballo D, *et al.* Prospective evaluation of patients with syncope: a population-based study. *Am J Med* 2001;**111**:177–84.

266 Gang ES, Peter T, Rosenthal ME, Mandel WJ, Lass Y. Detection of late potentials on the surface electrocardiogram in unexplained syncope. *Am J Cardiol* 1986;**58**: 1014–20.

267 Winters SL, Stewart D, Gomes JA. Signal averaging of the surface QRS complex predicts inducibility of ventricular tachycardia in patients with syncope of unknown origin: a prospective study. *J Am Coll Cardiol* 1987;**10**:775–81.

268 Kuchar DL, Thorburn CW, Sammel NL. Signal-averaged electrocardiogram for evaluation of recurrent syncope. *Am J Cardiol* 1986;**58**:949–53.

269 Ben-Chetrit E, Flugelman M, Eliakim M. Syncope: a retrospective study of 101 hospitalized patients. *Isr J Med Sci* 1985;**21**:950–3.

270 Graff L, Mucci D, Radford MJ. Decision to hospitalize: objective diagnosis-related group criteria versus clinical judgment. *Ann Emerg Med* 1988;**17**:943–52.

271 Shen WK, Decker WW, Smars PA, *et al.* Syncope evaluation in the emergency department study (SEEDS): a multidisciplinary approach to syncope management. *Circulation* 2004;**110**:3636–45.

272 Mozes B, Confino-Choen R, Halkin H. Cost-effectiveness of in-hospital evlaluation of patients with syncope. *Isr J Med Sci* 1988;**24**:302–6.

273 Fitzpatrick AP, Sutton R. Tilt-induced syncope. *N Engl J Med* 1989;**321**:331.

274 Kenny RA, Ingram A, Bayliss J, Sutton R. Head-up tilt: a useful test for investigating unexplained syncope. *Lancet* 1986;**1**:1352–5.

275 Almquist A, Goldenberg IF, Milstein S, *et al.* Provocation of bradycardia and hypotension by isoproterenol and upright posture in patients with unexplained syncope. *N Engl J Med* 1989;**320**:346–51.

276 Abboud FM. Ventricular syncope: is the heart a sensory organ? *N Engl J Med* 1989;**320**:390–2.

277 Rea RF, Thames MD. Neural control mechanisms and vasovagal syncope. *J Cardiovasc Electrophysiol* 1993;**4**: 587–95.

278 Kosinski DWD, Grubb BP. Neurocardiogenic syncope: a review of pathophysiology, diagnosis and treatment. *Cardiovasc Rev Rep* 1993;**363**:21–3.

279 Samoil D, Grubb BP. Vasovagal syncope: current concepts in diagnosis and treatment. *Heart Dis Stroke* 1993;**2**:247–9.

280 Wiley TM ODS, Platia EV, *et al.* Neurocardiogenic syncope: evaluation and treatment. *Cardiovasc Rev Rep* 1993;**14**:12–25.

281 Benditt DG, Ferguson DW, Grubb BP, *et al.* Tilt table testing for assessing syncope. American College of Cardiology. *J Am Coll Cardiol* 1996;**28**:263–75.

282 Kapoor WN, Brant N. Evaluation of syncope by upright tilt testing with isoproterenol: a nonspecific test. *Ann Intern Med* 1992;**116**:358–63.

283 Boudoulas H, Geleris P, Schaal SF, Leier CV, Lewis RP. Comparison between electrophysiologic studies and ambulatory monitoring in patients with syncope. *J Electrocardiol* 1983;**16**:91–6.

284 Clark PI, Glasser SP, Spoto E Jr. Arrhythmias detected by ambulatory monitoring: lack of correlation with symptoms of dizziness and syncope. *Chest* 1980;**77**: 722–5.

285 Gibson TC, Heitzman MR. Diagnostic efficacy of 24-hour electrocardiographic monitoring for syncope. *Am J Cardiol* 1984;**53**:1013–7.

286 Lacroix D, Dubuc M, Kus T, Savard P, Shenasa M, Nadeau R. Evaluation of arrhythmic causes of syncope: correlation between Holter monitoring, electrophysiologic testing, and body surface potential mapping. *Am Heart J* 1991;**122**:1346–54.

287 Zeldis SM, Levine BJ, Michelson EL, Morganroth J. Cardiovascular complaints: correlation with cardiac arrhythmias on 24-hour electrocardiographic monitoring. *Chest* 1980;**78**:456–61.

288 Gordon M, Huang M, Gryfe CI. An evaluation of falls, syncope, and dizziness by prolonged ambulatory cardiographic monitoring in a geriatric institutional setting. *J Am Geriatr Soc* 1982;**30**:6–12.

289 Linzer M, Prystowsky EN, Brunetti LL, Varia IM, German LD. Recurrent syncope of unknown origin diagnosed by ambulatory continuous loop ECG recording. *Am Heart J* 1988;**116**:1632–4.

290 Krahn AD, Klein GJ, Skanes AC, Yee R. Use of the implantable loop recorder in evaluation of patients with unexplained syncope. *J Cardiovasc Electrophysiol* 2003;**14**:S70–3.

291 Rahimtoola SH, Zipes DP, Akhtar M, *et al.* Consensus statement of the conference on the state of the art of electrophysiologic testing in the diagnosis and treatment of patients with cardiac arrhythmias. *Circulation* 1987;**75**:III-3–11.

292 Akhtar M, Shenasa M, Denker S, Gilbert CJ, Rizwi N. Role of cardiac electrophysiologic studies in patients with unexplained recurrent syncope. *Pacing Clin Electrophysiol* 1983;**6**:192–201.

293 Denes P, Ezri MD. The role of electrophysiologic studies in the management of patients with unexplained syncope. *Pacing Clin Electrophysiol* 1985;**8**:424–35.

294 Doherty JU, Pembrook-Rogers D, Grogan EW, *et al.* Electrophysiologic evaluation and follow-up characteristics of patients with recurrent unexplained syncope and presyncope. *Am J Cardiol* 1985;**55**:703–8.

295 Fisher JD. Role of electrophysiologic testing in the diagnosis and treatment of patients with known and suspected bradycardias and tachycardias. *Prog Cardiovasc Dis* 1981;**24**:25–90.

296 Fujimura O, Yee R, Klein GJ, Sharma AD, Boahene KA. The diagnostic sensitivity of electrophysiologic testing in patients with syncope caused by transient bradycardia. *N Engl J Med* 1989;**321**:1703–7.

297 Gulamhusein S, Naccarelli GV, Ko PT, *et al.* Value and limitations of clinical electrophysiologic study in assessment of patients with unexplained syncope. *Am J Med* 1982;**73**:700–5.

298 Lu J, Lu Z, Voss F, Schoels W. Results of invasive electrophysiologic evaluation in 268 patients with unexplained syncope. *J Huazhong Univ Sci Technol Med Sci* 2003; **23**:278–9.

299 Reiffel JA, Wang P, Bower R, *et al.* Electrophysiologic testing in patients with recurrent syncope: are results predicted by prior ambulatory monitoring? *Am Heart J* 1985;**110**:1146–53.

300 Boudoulas H, Schaal SF, Lewis RP. Electrophysiologic risk factors of syncope. *J Electrocardiol* 1978;**11**:339–42.

301 Gann D, Tolentino A, Samet P. Electrophysiologic evaluation of elderly patients with sinus bradycardia: a long-term follow-up study. *Ann Intern Med* 1979; **90**:24–9.

302 Kaul U, Dev V, Narula J, Malhotra AK, Talwar KK, Bhatia ML. Evaluation of patients with bundle branch block and "unexplained" syncope: a study based on comprehensive electrophysiologic testing and ajmaline stress. *Pacing Clin Electrophysiol* 1988;**11**:289–97.

303 Wilber DW, Kall J, Olshansky B, Scanlon P. Pacing induced infra-Hisian block in patients with syncope of unknown origin: incidence and clinical significance. *PACE* 1990; **13**:562A.

304 Klein GJ, Gersh BJ, Yee R. Electrophysiologic testing: the final court of appeal for diagnosis of syncope? *Circulation* 1995;**92**:1332–5.

305 Aonuma K, Iesaka Y, Gosselin AJ, Rozanski JJ, Lister JW. Cardiac syncope: a case exhibiting dichotomy between clinical impression and electrophysiologic evaluation. *Pacing Clin Electrophysiol* 1986;**9**:178–87.

306 Masrani K, Cowley C, Bekheit S, el-Sherif N. Recurrent syncope for over a decade due to idiopathic ventricular fibrillation. *Chest* 1994;**106**:1601–3.

307 Recchia D, Barzilai B. Echocardiography in the evaluation of patients with syncope. *J Gen Intern Med* 1995;**10**:649–55.

308 Kuchar DL, Thorburn CW, Sammel NL. The role of signal averaged electrocardiography in the investigation of unselected patients with syncope. *Aust N Z J Med* 1985;**15**:697–703.

309 Turitto G, el-Sherif N. The signal averaged electrocardiogram and programmed stimulation in patients with complex ventricular arrhythmias. *Pacing Clin Electrophysiol* 1990;**13**:2156–9.

310 Masaki R, Watanabe I, Nakai T, *et al.* Role of signal-averaged electrocardiograms for predicting the inducibility of ventricular fibrillation in the syndrome consisting of right bundle branch block and ST segment elevation in leads V1-V3. *Jpn Heart J* 2002;**43**:367–78.

311 Kwoh CK, Beck JR, Pauker SG. Repeated syncope with negative diagnostic evaluation: to pace or not to pace? *Med Decis Making* 1984;**4**:351–77.

312 Rattes MF, Klein GJ, Sharma AD, Boone JA, Kerr C, Milstein S. Efficacy of empirical cardiac pacing in syncope of unknown cause. *CMAJ* 1989;**140**:381–5.

313 Shaw DB, Kekwick CA, Veale D, Whistance TW. Unexplained syncope: a diagnostic pacemaker? *Pacing Clin Electrophysiol* 1983;**6**:720–5.

314 Fisher M, Cotter L. Recurrent syncope of unknown origin: value of permanent pacemaker insertion. *Int J Cardiol* 1995;**51**:93–5, discussion 96–7.

315 Proclemer A, Sternotti G, *et al.* Value of pacemaker treatment in patients with syncope of unkown origin. *New Trends Arrhyth* 1990;**6**:323–32.

316 Muller T, Roy D, Talajic M, Lemery R, Nattel S, Cassidy D. Electrophysiologic evaluation and outcome of patients with syncope of unknown origin. *Eur Heart J* 1991; **12**:139–43.

317 Raviele A, Gasparini G, Di Pede F, Delise P, Bonso A, Piccolo E. Usefulness of head-up tilt test in evaluating patients with syncope of unknown origin and negative electrophysiologic study. *Am J Cardiol* 1990;**65**:1322–7.

318 Flammang D, Erickson M, McCarville S, Church T, Hamani D, Donal E. Contribution of head-up tilt testing and ATP testing in assessing the mechanisms of vasovagal syndrome: preliminary results and potential therapeutic implications. *Circulation* 1999;**99**:2427–33.

CHAPTER 2

Neurocardiogenic syncope

Blair P. Grubb, MD

Introduction

The term neurocardiogenic syncope (also called vasovagal or neurally mediated syncope) is used to describe episodes of transient, centrally mediated hypotension and bradycardia that ultimately lead to loss of consciousness. Neurocardiogenic syncope may take many forms, ranging from the common faint to a sudden dramatic loss of consciousness indistinguishable from Stokes–Adams attacks, and possibly even to sudden death. Often, the individuals who suffer from these disorders exhibit no evidence of underlying structural heart disease or of abnormalities in the cardiac conducting system.

Until relatively recently, patients with recurrent unexplained syncope were routinely subjected to a long and expensive battery of tests which often included glucose tolerance testing, Holter monitoring, cranial computed tomography, electroencephalography, exercise tolerance testing, and electrophysiological studies [1]. Yet, despite these extensive evaluations (costing up to $16,000 per patient), in up to 50% of patients a diagnosis was never arrived at [2,3]. Linzer *et al.* [4] report that the degree of functional impairment suffered by these individuals with recurrent unexplained syncope is not dissimilar to that observed in chronic debilitating disorders such as rheumatoid arthritis. Recurrent syncopal episodes also placed the patient at risk for bodily trauma secondary to falls, and syncope while driving a motor vehicle could have disastrous consequences [5]. In the elderly, a single syncopal episode may result in injuries sufficiently profound that the patient may require permanent nursing home placement, at a tremendous cost to the individual and to society as a whole.

A number of investigators had, for some time, postulated that transient episodes of centrally mediated hypotension and bradycardia could be responsible for many of these episodes. However, until recently there was no effective means of reproducing these episodes and thereby confirming the diagnosis. In addition, many aspects of these disorders were shrouded in mystery because of the relative inability to consistently observe spontaneous events.

To uncover an individual's predisposition to these episodes of centrally mediated hypotension and bradycardia, investigators proposed that a strong orthostatic stimulus such as prolonged upright posture be used. Since the landmark study in 1986 by Kenny *et al.* [6], numerous centers around the world have reported that head-upright tilt table testing appears to be a safe and effective means of revealing an individual's predisposition to neurocardiogenic events. At the same time, the ability to provoke these episodes in a controlled setting has afforded a unique opportunity to directly observe and record the events that occur during syncope, allowing for a marked enhancement in our knowledge of this disorder [7]. This chapter deals with our current understanding of the pathophysiology of neurocardiogenic syncope, its clinical manifestations, and the use of tilt table testing in diagnosis, as well as potential therapeutic options available for the treatment of these disorders.

Pathophysiology of neurocardiogenic syncope

Fainting has been observed in all peoples throughout history, and speculations as to its origins are centuries old. In 1773, John Hunter [8] observed patients who would faint during phlebotomy (a common practice at the time) and suggested that vasodilation may have an important role. In 1888, a brilliant report by Foster [9] noted that during spontaneous syncopal spells, profound bradycardia sometimes occurred, which he felt lowered cerebral blood flow to a level inadequate to maintain consciousness. In 1932, Sir Thomas Lewis [10] observed that although the bradycardia associated with syncope could be reversed by the administration of atropine, hypotension and loss of consciousness would still occur. The concurrence of both a vasodilatory and bradycardic component led to his use of the neurological "vasovagal" to describe this phenomenon.

Starting in the 1940s, physiologists began to explore the human body's response to changes in position, with later investigators focusing on the body's response to the stresses of aviation and the microgravity environment of space travel. During this period, head upright tilt table testing came into use in order to provide a controlled setting in which the body's responses to incremental changes in position could be carefully observed and recorded [11]. Based on these observations, it has become well established that in the normal subject, the assumption of upright posture leads to a gravity-mediated displacement of blood downward, with pooling in the lower extremities. This has been found to be accompanied by a compensatory increase in both heart rate and peripheral vascular resistance [12]. Several investigations have confirmed these observations. Mehdirah *et al.* [13] performed echocardiography during tilt table testing on 17 subjects. They noted no differences in left ventricular volume or cardiac output between subjects at rest. After upright tilt, significant changes began to appear after 10 min. Subjects who went on to develop syncope also went on to develop marked decrease in left ventricular end-systolic and end-diastolic volumes when compared to non-syncopal subjects, an observation consistent with peripheral venous pooling. Similar findings are reported by El-Bedawi and Hainsworth [14,15] by use of a combination of head-up tilt and lower body negative pressure on a series of patients. Here tilt table testing produced a decrease in cardiac output of approximately 1.4 L/min, again suggesting peripheral sequestration of blood.

The reduction in blood pressure produced by this downward displacement of blood is sensed by arterial baroreceptors, which are scattered throughout the vasculature but located principally in the aortic arch and carotid sinus [16]. These receptors send afferent signals to the medulla, where they communicate with the nucleus ambiguous and dorsal motor nucleus of the vagus nerve (governing parasympathetic activity) and the costal ventromedial and ventrolateral medulla (governing sympathetic activity) [17]. During increased arterial pressure, there is a greater degree of stretch on these receptors with an increase in receptor afferent transmission, leading to a centrally mediated decrease in sympathetic tone with a subsequent reduction in heart rate. Reductions in arterial blood pressure have the opposite effect. The heart itself functions as a part of this baroreflex activity by virtue of the presence of mechanoreceptors (or C-fibers), consisting of unmyelinated fibers found in the atria, ventricles (particularly in the inferoposterior aspect of the left ventricle), and the pulmonary artery [18]. Although C-fibers seem to respond to either stretch or pressure, stretch activations appear to be more important. These fibers send afferent projections centrally to the dorsal vagal nucleus of the brainstem. As with arterial baroreceptors, a decrease in C-fiber output results in a reflex increase in sympathetic stimulation. Therefore, the normal response to upright posture is an increase in heart rate, an increase in diastolic pressure, and an unchanged or slightly decreased systolic blood pressure [12].

Although the exact processes involved in the production of neurocardiogenic syncope remain the subject of considerable debate, some basic mechanisms have been elaborated [7]. To date, most investigators have felt that excessive venous pooling associated with upright posture results in central hypovolemia, causing an abrupt fall in venous return to the heart. This sudden reduction in ventricular volume is thought to result in extremely vigorous ventricular contractions, which in turn cause the activation of a large number of C-fibers that would normally respond to mechanical stretch. The resultant surge in afferent neural traffic to the medulla is thought to mimic the conditions seen during hypertension, thereby resulting in an apparent "paradoxic" sympathetic withdrawal with bradycardia and hypotension. Studies by use of echocardiography during tilt have tended to support this contention [19].

Some investigators, however, have voiced reservations concerning this hypothesis. In animal studies, surgical denervation of the heart did not prevent sudden sympathetic withdrawal during sudden blood volume reduction [20]. In addition, both Lightfoot et al. [21] and Fitzpatrick et al. [22] reported neurocardiogenic hypotension and bradycardia during orthostatic stress in patients who had received orthotopic heart transplants. Because mechanoreceptor C-fibers have also been identified in the atria and pulmonary arteries, these observations do not exclude their contribution to neurocardiogenic syncope. Waxman et al. [23] and Rudas et al. [24] also pointed out that vagal afferent reinnervation of the donor hearts may have occurred. Vasodilators have also been reported to provoke syncope in transplant recipients [25]. The most important challenge to the cardiac mechanoreceptor hypothesis has come from Wright et al. [26] who, using a dog model, reported that after separation of coronary afferents of the baroreflex from ventricular receptor action, provocation of Bezold–Jarisch reflex activity becomes quite difficult under physiologically achievable conditions.

In considering these observations, it is important to realize that activation of ventricular mechanoreceptors is not the only mechanism that has been shown to provoke neurocardiogenic syncope. Using a cat model, Lofring [27] found that direct electrical stimulation of the anterior cingulated gyrus of the limbic system can trigger a vasovagal response. In humans, syncope is well known to be provoked by strong emotion or by a stimulus such as the sight of blood. Temporal lobe epilepsy has been shown to provoke vasovagal episodes [28]. These observations suggest that higher neural centers may also participate in the provocation of neurocardiogenic syncope.

An alternative hypothesis concerning the mechanism of neurocardiogenic syncope was recently advanced by Dickinson [29]. Previous observations have demonstrated that when the intraluminal pressure within the carotid artery falls to near zero, the rate of discharge of the carotid sinus baroreceptors increases [30]. Dickinson postulates that a similar process may occur in the atria and great veins; when the fall in intrathoracic pressure exceeds atrial and venous filling pressure, the venoarterial stretch receptors exhibit a comparable "collapse

firing." This sudden increase in afferent nerve traffic could thereby elicit a similar type of "paradoxic" sympathetic withdrawal. Evidence supporting this theory has come from a study of eight heart–lung transplant patients (in whom afferent nerve projections have been severed), none of whom had vasovagal reactions during tilt [31]. However, this observation may have resulted from the use of a less aggressive tilt protocol than that of other studies.

The term "vasovagal" was initially applied to the process of fainting because of the perception that parasympathetic activity was felt to predominate [10]. Although parasympathetic activity does appear to increase somewhat during syncope (and is responsible for the observed bradycardia), the principal phenomenon responsible for loss of consciousness is vasodilation resulting in hypotension [32]. Several studies have reported that while the administration of atropine or cardiac pacing will eliminate bradycardia, it will seldom prevent syncope [10,33].

The first detailed investigations into the neurophysiological mechanisms involved in neurocardiogenic syncope were reported by Oberg and Thoren [34]. They used an open-chest cat preparation and caused sudden hemorrhagic hypovolemia. A marked initial tachycardia was found to be an essential component of ventricular C-fiber stimulation. Later, Wallin and Sundlof [35] were able to record peripheral autonomic nervous system activity during neurocardiogenic syncope from peroneal nerve fascicles by use of microelectrodes. Sympathetic activity was initially noted to increase, followed by a dramatic decrease at the onset of syncope. Sra et al. [36] have demonstrated that during the initial phases of upright tilt-induced syncope, both norepinephrine and epinephrine increase. Consistent with the previous observations, at the onset of syncope, plasma epinephrine levels were noted to increase while norepinephrine levels fell. Lewis et al. [37] also report that peripheral sympathetic inhibition was demonstrated prior to syncope induced by either head-up tilt or lower-body negative pressure.

A recent series of studies by Goldstein et al. [38,39] have evaluated the degree to which cardiac sympathetic function is affected in neurocardiogenic syncope. In one study, patients with postural tachycardia syndrome or neurocardiogenic syncope underwent measurements of neurochemical indices of cardiac release, reuptake, and synthesis of the sympathetic neurotransmitter norepinephrine based on entry of norepinephrine into the cardiac venous drainage (cardiac norepinephrine spill-over) [38]. Cardiac extraction of circulating ^{3}H-norepinephrine, and cardiac production of dihydroxyphenylalanine and measurement of left ventricular myocardial innervation density using 6-[^{18}F] fluorodopamine positron emission tomographic scanning. In marked contrast to patients with postural orthostatic tachycardia syndrome (POTS), patients with neurocardiogenic syncope had abnormal tonically decreased cardiac norepinephrine release. They concluded that these findings reflected a decrease in cardiac nerve traffic as the basis for reduced cardiac norepinephrine spillover in neurocardiogenic syncope, and suggested that neurocardiogenic syncope entails both tonic restraint of cardiac sympathetic outflow as well as attenuated increments in sympathetic outflow to skeletal muscle during orthostasis. A second equally insightful paper by Goldstein's group [39] looked at forearm blood flow using impedance plethysmography during tilt-induced syncope while at the same time measuring plasma catecholamines serially. Patients with tilt-induced syncope showed progressive marked increases in plasma epinephrine levels to a mean value 11 times baseline. Simultaneously obtained norepinephrine increased to a much lesser degree than did epinephrine levels, producing a "sympathoadrenal imbalance." In the same patients, forearm vascular resistance decreased by 21% before syncope, suggesting that sympathoadrenal imbalance precedes tilt-invoked and spontaneous neurocardiogenic syncope and correlates with concurrent skeletal muscle vasodilation. They concluded that sympathoadrenal imbalance may contribute to the hemodynamic alterations that precipitate neurocardiogenic syncope.

Therefore, the initial fall in central blood volume resulting from peripheral venous pooling provokes a reflex increase in sympathetic output with resultant tachycardia and vasoconstrictions, in an apparent effort to maintain normal hemodynamics. Yet this very increase in sympathetic tone may both sensitize and facilitate activation of the cardiac mechanoreceptors that have been implicated in the production of vasovagal events [40]. The paroxysmal increase in neural traffic seen during vigorous ventricular contraction (or from C-fiber activation by myocardial ischemia and reperfusion) leads to a sudden, centrally mediated, sympathetic withdrawal with peripheral sympathetic inhibition followed by vasodilation [41]. There may also be some aspect of decreased α-receptor responsiveness or increased β-receptor responsiveness involved [18,32].

The central mechanisms that contribute to the production of neurocardiogenic syncope are still unclear, but have been the subject of several recent investigations [42,43]. Studies on the hemodynamic and neuroendocrine responses to acute hypovolemia in conscious mammals (a condition most investigators feel is roughly analogous to neurocardiogenic syncope) have tended to focus on the contributions of two substances: endogenous opioids and serotonin [7]. By use of a rat model, evidence appears to suggest that the vasodepressor response to hemorrhage is centrally mediated by endogenous opiates [32]. Inhibition of renal sympathetic nerve activity occurs if opiate receptor antagonists are given during hypotensive hemorrhage in rabbits [44]. It has also been reported that the intracisternal administration of naloxone (an opiate receptor antagonist) can block the vasodilatory response seen during acute hemorrhage in rabbits [45]. Ferguson [46] reported that in humans, naloxone augments the cardiopulmonary baroreflex activation of sympathetic activity. In addition, two studies have found significant increases in plasma β-endorphin levels prior to tile-induced syncope [47,48]. Unfortunately, in humans, opiate antagonists have not been reported to prevent vasodepressor syncope during lower-body negative pressure; however, this may, in part, be because the dosages of naloxone used were proportionally many times lower than those used during animal studies [49,50].

Serotonin (5-hydroxyltryptamine or 5-HT) is a biologic amine widely distributed throughout the nervous system [51]. Serotonin has long been recognized to have an important role in blood pressure regulation [52]. The application of serotonin directly to the brain (through the lateral ventricle) results in inhibition of efferent sympathetic activity, whereas the direct administration of serotonin into the nucleus tractus solitarii causes parasympathetic stimulation and bradycardia as well as sympathetic withdrawal [53,54]. Abboud [55] reports that the administration of intracerebroventricular serotonin induces hypotension, inhibition of renal sympathetic nerve activity, and excitation of adrenal sympathetic nerve activity. In normal volunteers, the administration of 5-HT1 receptor-activating compounds results in profound sympathetic blockage [56]. Serotonin has also been shown to be an important modulator of the responses seen during acute hemorrhage. Using a cat model, Elam et al. [57] found that depletion of serotonin stores blunts the vasodilatory response to hemorrhage. Other studies have found that the administration of the serotonin receptor blocker methysergide during acute blood loss produces a marked pressor effect. Hasser et al. [58] reports that methylsergide can increase blood pressure when administered to conscious animals made hypotensive during acute hemorrhage. Based on these and other observations, Morgan et al. [59] suggests that sympathoinhibitory mechanisms in the central nervous system may be stimulated during acute hemorrhage.

Data confirming the role of serotonergic activity in neurocardiogenic syncope are provided by Theodorakis et al. [60]. Based on the fact that changes in central serotonergic activity influence the release of prolactin and cortisol, they measured the serum content of these hormones in 28 patients with recurrent syncope who underwent tilt table testing. Nine patients experienced syncope during the test while 19 did not. Cortisol and prolactin levels were significantly increased only in the tilt-positive patients. Interestingly, they note that the patterns of release of these hormones during syncope appeared quite similar to those caused by drugs that activate central serotonergic neurons (clomipramine and fenfluramine), suggesting an important role for serotonin in neurocardiogenic syncope.

There are at least 14 distinct types of serotonin receptors in the central nervous system, with different receptors postulated to govern various functions. Matzen et al. [61] evaluated the effects of various specific serotonin receptor blockers during upright tilt-induced syncope. They found that methysergide (a 5-HT1 + 2 receptor antagonist) and ondansetron (a 5-HT3 receptor antagonist)

attenuate the sympathetic response to head-up tilt as reflected in the blunting in the increase in plasma catecholamine levels.

Grubb and associates [62,63] and DiGirolamo et al. [64] have found that the use of serotonin reuptake inhibitors can be an effective treatment for patients with severe recurrent neurocardiogenic syncope. These agents, as opposed to the tricyclic antidepressant compounds, are characterized by highly selective serotonin reuptake inhibition with little or no affinity for adrenergic, cholinergic, or histamine receptors. As extracellular serotonin levels increase, 5-HT neuronal release is attenuated and impulse transmission velocity increases, both contributing to a progressive decrease in postsynaptic receptor density ("downregulation") [63]. This downregulation in postsynaptic receptor density is thought to blunt the potential responses to rapid shifts in central serotonin levels and thereby reduce the ability for such surges to result in abrupt sympathetic withdrawal.

Several other humoral agents have been implicated in the pathogenesis of neurocardiogenic syncope. A rise in serum levels of renin [65], vasopressin [66], endothelin [67], and nitric oxide [68] have all been noted to occur prior to the onset of syncope. However, at present there are insufficient data to comment fully on the role of these agents in producing syncope. The potential role of the responses of the cerebral vasculature during neurocardiogenic syncope has also been explored. It was previously believed that cerebral autoregulation of cerebral blood flow occurred solely at the local arteriolar level in response to arterial pressure changes; arteriolar vasoconstriction during peripheral blood pressure increases and vasodilation following systemic pressure decreases. However, recent studies by Grubb et al. [69], Janasik et al. [70], Gomez et al. [71], and Njemanze [72] using transcranial Doppler ultrasonography (TCD) have generated considerable evidence that during upright tilt-induced neurocardiogenic syncope, a paradoxic intense cerebral vasoconstriction (rather than the expected vasodilation) occurs in the face of increasing hypotension. Kaminer et al. [73] also demonstrate significant abnormalities in cerebral hemodynamics in children during head-up tilt-induced syncope. These apparently "paradoxic" changes would suggest that sudden alterations in cerebral vascular resistance (arteriolar vasocon-striction) might have a significant role in the pro-duction of neurocardiogenic syncope. Others have questioned these findings, suggesting that they occur as a consequence of a rapid fall in cerebrovas-cular perfusion [74,75]. However, Gomez *et al.* [71] reported that sudden cerebral vasoconstriction alone (as measured by TCD) in the absence of systemic hypotension or bradycardia could cause loss of consciousness during tilt table testing. Daffertshafer and Hemmerici [76] made similar observations of syncope associated with cerebral blood flow alterations alone, calling it "normo-tensive orthostatic syncope" and referred to the phenomenon in general as "cerebrovascular dysautoregulation syndrome." Friedman *et al.* [77] and Obara *et al.* [78] also reported cases of tilt-induced syncope with TCD-measured cere-bral vasoconstriction in the absence of systemic hypotension. Grubb *et al.* [79] reported on five patients with tilt-induced loss of consciousness (confirmed by electroencephalographic monitor-ing) associated with TCD-recorded vasoconstric-tion without systemic hypotension, and referred to this entity as "cerebral syncope." Further studies are necessary to clarify this phenomenon.

Recently, Asensio and Oseguera [80] have pro-posed a possible link between reactive hypogly-cemia and neurocardiogenic syncope. Evidence exists that repeated hypoglycemic episodes in patients with type 1 diabetes may lead to autonomic dysfunction [81]. This in turn causes a blunted response to the symptoms of hypoglycemia and possible syncope. In relation to neurocardiogenic syncope, it is unclear as to whether there is a causal relationship or merely a tendency for these two disorders to occur together. Further investigations will help to explore this potential relationship.

Clinical aspects of neurocardiogenic syncope

Neurocardiogenic syncope may have a wide variety of presentations. Indeed, there seem to exist a number of triggers that may all ultimately result in neurocardiogenically mediated hypotension and bradycardia. The postprandial state, upright pos-ture, vigorous exercise in warm environments, sodium restriction or diuretic use, and emotional or stressful situations are a few of the important triggers to consider. Alcohol is well recognized to increase predisposition to these events. Rapid changes in time zones during air travel (jet lag) also seem to exacerbate these tendencies.

There are typically three identifiable phases to an event: presyncope or aura, the actual loss of con-sciousness, and the postsyncopal period. Patients with the more classic forms of vasovagal syncope will often give a longstanding history of recurrent events ("easy fainters"). The situations that pro-voke fainting in this group are those that are most likely to cause fear, emotional distress, anxiety, and anticipation (the very events that are most likely to result in increased sympathetic nervous system stimulation). A somewhat similar response is seen in some animal species when they are placed in life-threatening situations in which neither "fight" nor "flight" is possible. These animals have then been observed to experience loss of sympathetic tone, leading to vasodilation, bradycardia, and resultant loss of motion; in effect they "play dead" [82].

During the aura phase, the typical warning phenomena often include weakness, diaphoresis, epigastric discomfort, dizziness/vertigo, visual blur-ring, palpitations, headache, nausea, and vomit-ing. These prodromal symptoms may last from less than 1 s to several minutes, giving the patient who recognizes them an opportunity to lie down and ward off (or lessen the severity of) an event. Linzer *et al.* [83] have analyzed the frequency of pre-syncopal symptoms in a large number of pati-ents, finding that the most common were dizziness (44%), weakness (44%), blurred vision (33%), sweating (33%), nausea (29%), and abdominal discomfort (11%).

The actual loss of consciousness is usually not remembered by the patient. Observers who witness a syncopal episode will often report that the patient appeared pale or ashen in color, with cold skin and profuse sweating, dilated pupils, and rarely urinary (or even fecal) incontinence [84]. The sign that often seems to make the greatest impression on observers is the appearance of tonic and/or clonic movements. The appearance of convulsions indic-ates that the cerebral anoxic threshold has been reached, allowing an acute "decortication" to occur. These movements usually (but not always) begin after loss of consciousness with a tonic contraction of extended legs, extended arms in adduction, and elevation and backward throw of the head (opisthotonos) [85]. These are in contrast to the sequence of decreasing frequency and increasing amplitude that are characteristic of the tonic–clonic grand mal seizures of epilepsy. The loss of consciousness itself is usually short, with rapid recovery and little, if any, postictal period of confusion. Although mentally clear during the postsyncopal period, patients may complain of nervousness, nausea, headache, or dizziness [86].

While this description holds for many patients with neurocardiogenic syncopal episodes, it is important to realize that many patients will have atypical presentations. Some patients (particularly many older ones) will give no history of any prodrome whatsoever, describing a "drop attack" that may mimic Stokes–Adams syncope secondary to atrioventricular block. The abruptness of these episodes may lead to severe injury as a result of the trauma associated with falling. This is of particular concern in older patients, where falls are an important cause of both morbidity and mortality. Even though the majority of patients are unconscious for a brief period of time (seconds), in some patients the period of loss of consciousness may be prolonged, lasting up to 15 min. In occasional patients, the convulsive movements seen during the syncopal episode may be remarkably similar to those of an epileptic seizure, and episodes may be associated with incontinence or a prolonged postictal period [87–89].

There are patients in whom the sudden vagally mediated fall in blood pressure and heart rate will be sufficient to produce symptoms of cerebral hypoperfusion, but will not be sufficient to produce full loss of consciousness. These individuals often present with complaints of severe dizziness, lightheadedness, vertigo, and disequilibrium, and are frequently referred to an otolaryngologist for evaluation [90]. In elderly patients, neurocardiogenic hypotension may cause periods of focal neurological dysfunction that can appear remarkably similar to transient ischemic attacks [91]. Patients may experience disorientation, dysarthria, and even visual field cuts.

Controversy exists over whether neurocardiogenic syncope can be lethal. In Europe, the term "malignant" is applied to episodes of neurocar-

diogenic syncope that occur without warning and result in bodily injury [92]. In North America, the term "malignant" is applied to episodes of neurocardiogenic syncope associated with prolonged cardiac asystole [93]. Both spontaneous and tilt-induced episodes of neurocardiogenic asystole have lasted as long as 73 s, and there is at least one reported episode of sustained polymorphic ventricular tachycardia induced during upright tilt [94]. Episodes of near-fatal cardiac asystole have occurred during tilt table testing [95]. Engle [96] and others have postulated that prolonged asystole may degenerate into ventricular fibrillation and death, particularly in those individuals with preexistent coronary disease and myocardial dysfunction [96]. At the Medical College of Ohio, we have seen several patients who were resuscitated from apparent sudden death episodes, in whom the only abnormality found (despite extensive evaluations) was reproducible neurocardiogenic asystole.

In general, younger patients – adolescents in particular – tend to have more classic presentations, whereas atypical presentations are more frequent in older patients. In adolescents, there is often a history of a rapid growth spurt in the period just preceding the first syncopal episode. It is not uncommon for these tendencies to run in families. Often, even frequent and severe syncopal spells that begin in adolescence will spontaneously abate by the time the patient reaches his or her midtwenties. In young women there is a definite tendency for these episodes to be more frequent around the time of the menstrual cycle, in particular during the premenstrual period. Patients who had recurrent syncope during adolescence, which later resolved, may begin to experience recurrences during or immediately following pregnancy.

Linzer *et al.* [97] described an increased incidence of neuropsychiatric disorders in patients with recurrent neurocardiogenic syncope. The three most common disorders are major depression, somatization disorder, and panic disorders (the latter being more common among female patients). Patients with recurrent neurocardiogenic syncope have also been noted to have an increased incidence of neurosomatic disorders such as chronic vascular headaches or migraine headaches as well as functional gastrointestinal conditions such as peptic ulcer disease, unstable bowel syndrome, and indigestion. Recent reports provide evidence for a link between neurocardiogenic hypotension and chronic fatigue syndrome [98]. Indeed, one of the more common complaints of the patients with neurocardiogenic syncope at our institution is fatigue.

Clinical reproduction of the syncopal or near-syncopal event is important in establishing the diagnosis and the responses to therapy. Over the years, a number of maneuvers have been used to trigger vagal reactions including carotid sinus compression, Weber and Valsalva maneuvers, hyperventilation, and ocular compression. However, these techniques were ultimately abandoned because of their relatively low sensitivity and weak correlation with clinical events.

Head-up tilt table testing

Until the mid-1980s, the diagnosis of neurocardiogenic syncope was made principally by history and a process of exclusion, mainly because there was no effective laboratory technique for reproducing episodes and thereby confirming the diagnosis. To address this difficulty, it was reasoned that a potent orthostatic stimulus, such as prolonged upright posture, could be used to produce a state of maximal venous pooling, thus provoking the previously described responses in susceptible individuals. Tilt tables were first used by physiologists to study compensatory changes produced during movement from the supine to the head-upright position. During the course of these studies, it was noted that a small proportion of the subjects studied developed hypotension and bradycardia of a degree sufficient to result in fainting [99]. Despite these observations, tilt table testing was not used as a potential diagnostic modality for neurocardiogenic syncope until the groundbreaking report by Kenny et al. [6] in 1986. Since then, a number of reports have appeared, attesting to the utility of the test to reproduce syncopal episodes in patients who are prone to neurocardiogenic hypotension and bradycardia.

Several observations can be cited to support the concept that a "positive head-up tilt table test" is for the most part equivalent to spontaneously occurring episodes [100]. Principal among these observations is that both spontaneous and tilt-induced syncopal episodes are associated with virtually identical signs, as well as symptoms such as nausea, lightheadedness, pallor, diaphoresis, and loss of postural tone. In addition, the temporal sequence of heart rate and blood pressure changes noted during tilt-induced syncope are for the most part the same as those reported during spontaneous episodes. The plasma catecholamine changes alluded to previously are similar in both spontaneous and tilt-induced episodes, with rapid surges in plasma epinephrine occurring prior to loss of consciousness. Finally, tilt table testing has been able to reproduce spontaneously occurring episodes of asystole in patients with negative electrophysiologic studies (see Fig. 2.4) [93].

Two principal methods of tilt table testing have evolved, both of which are simple, safe, and inexpensive. The first uses a passive tilt for a period of 45 min at an angle between 60° and 80° (most centers now use 70°). No provocative pharmacological agents are used [101]. The second method frequently uses a shorter period of upright tilt in association with a variety of provocative agents to facilitate the induction of syncope. A number of agents have been used, including isoproterenol, nitroglycerin, edrophonium, and adenosine.

Early studies indicated that the use of a tilt angle of less than 60° is associated with a loss of sensitivity, while angles of 80° or more are believed to produce a loss of specificity [101]. Initial studies using tilt table testing revealed that the test only rarely provoked syncope in normal subjects. Shvartz [102] and Shvartz and Meyerstein [103] note only three syncopal episodes among a total of 36 subjects tilted at an angle of 70° for 20 min, while Vogt et al. note only two episodes of syncope during 64 tilts at 70° among nine healthy male volunteers [102–104]. Fitzpatrick et al. [101] note only two (7%) episodes of syncope among 27 normal control subjects tilted at 60° for 60 min, while only five (15%) of 34 patients with syncope known to be caused by conduction system disease had positive tests [101]. The use of a 60° tilt for 60 min has become known as the Westminster protocol, and has an apparent specificity of 91% and a positive yield of 27–75%, with a mean of approximately 50% [105].

The response to head-up tilt of patients with a history of recurrent syncope thought to be neurocardiogenic in nature is quite different. The initial report by Kenny et al. [6] found that 10 of 15 patients (67%) suffering from unexplained syncope had a positive response after a mean of 29 ± 19 min upright. Strasberg et al. [106] studied 40 patients with recurrent unexplained syncope (as well as 10 normal controls) with a 60° tilt for 60 min. Syncope that was the same as that experienced clinically was produced in 15 patients (38%) after a mean tilt time of 42 ± 12 min. Similar results were obtained by Raviele et al. [107] in 30 patients with unexplained syncope, also using a 60° tilt for 60 min. Fifteen patients (50%) had syncope similar to the clinical episodes provoked, whereas eight concomitant controls were asymptomatic. A larger study by Abi-Samra et al. [108] reports reproduction of syncope similar to that experienced clinically in 63 of 154 patients undergoing tilt table testing.

Following observations that endogenous catecholamine levels increase prior to syncope, some investigators postulate that the infusion of the catecholamine-like substance isoproterenol may increase the sensitivity of the test. This concept was first evaluated by Almquist et al. [109]. In this study, only five of 24 patients with recurrent idiopathic syncope had positive responses during the initial baseline tilt. However, after retilt with a concomitant isoproterenol infusion, an additional nine patients had positive responses. Comparable results are reported by Grubb et al. [110] and Pongiglione et al. [111]. Sheldon and Killam [112] have used a single upright tilt with a concomitant isoproterenol infusion of 5 µg/min for 10 min, with similar outcomes. However, Kapoor and Brant [113] raise questions as to whether the potential increase in sensitivity seen with isoproterenol use may result in a decrease in sensitivity.

Several recent studies have sought to address this point. Morillo et al. [114] evaluated 120 patients with recurrent syncope, 30 healthy controls, and 30 patients with documented syncope not related to a vasodepressor reaction. Each underwent a 60° head-up tilt for 15 min, followed by an infusion of isoproterenol sufficient to increase the heart rate by 25%. The false-positive rate in both the control group and the documented syncope group was 6.6%. The initial tilt was positive in 30 (25%) of the 120 patients, with an additional 43 (36%) demonstrating positive responses during isoproterenol in-

fusion. Overall, "sensitivity," specificity, and reproducibility were 61%, 93% and 86%, respectively.

A more comprehensive evaluation was undertaken by Natale et al. [115]. Here 150 normal subjects were randomized into two groups of 75. One group was further randomized to a 60°, 70°, and 80° tilt followed by a second tilt with an isoproterenol infusion that increased the heart rate by 20%. The second group underwent tilt at 70° with either a low dose, 3 µg/min, or 5 µg/min isoproterenol infusion. They found that tilt table testing at a 60° or 70° angle with or without low dose isoproterenol provided a specificity of approximately 88–92%. They also reported that higher angles of tilt or higher dosages of isoproterenol were less specific.

Over the last several years the tilt protocol we have used has undergone considerable evolution. Based on the aforementioned observations and those of our own group, we currently use a two-stage tilt table protocol. Studies are performed in the morning after an overnight fast and an intravenous line is established. After a 15-min rest period, the patient is positioned on a tilt table with footboard support and inclined to an angle of 70° for a period of 45 min (Fig. 2.1). Heart rate and rhythm are monitored continuously via a defibrillator monitor, and blood pressures are taken using a sphygmomanometer every 3 min or by continuous tomographic recording. Cardiopulmonary resuscitation equipment is present and a registered nurse and a physician are present. If symptomatic hypotension and bradycardia occur, reproducing the patient's symptoms, the patient is then lowered to the supine position and the test ended. If no syncope occurs during this initial phase, the patient is lowered to the supine position and an intravenous infusion of isoproterenol is started. The dose is then titrated to increase the heart rate to 20–25% above the initial supine value. Upright tilt is then performed as previously described. Isoproterenol infusions are not used in the presence of known severe coronary artery disease or hypertrophic cardiomyopathy. A second approach is to administer 0.4 mg of sublingual nitroglycerine instead of isoproterenol (see Chapter 7).

The exact sensitivity of head-up tilt table testing is difficult to ascertain because of a lack of a "gold standard" with which to compare it. Reported estimates of the accuracy of tilt table testing range

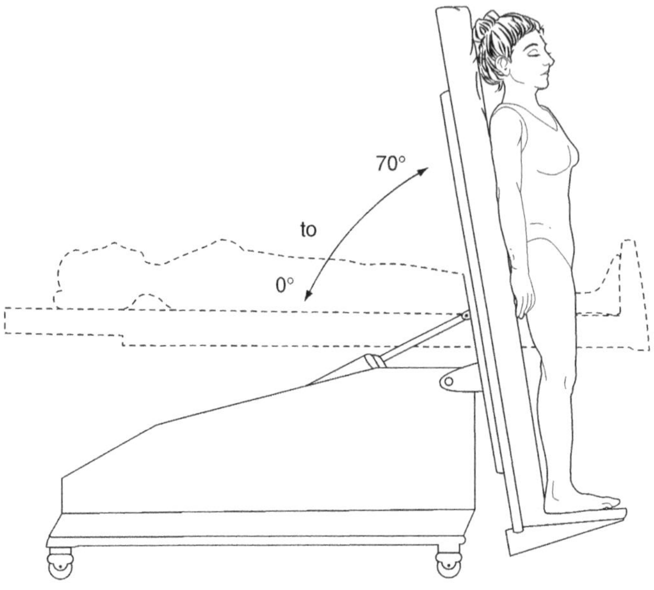

Fig. 2.1 A 70° tilt table test. After 15 min of rest, the patient is positioned on a tilt table and inclinded to an angle of 70° for 45 min.

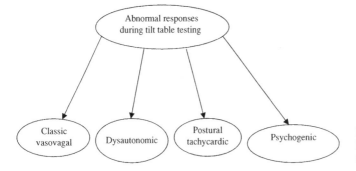

Fig. 2.2 Positive response patterns to head-up tilt table testing are divided into four groups.

between 30% and 80% [101]. However, it should be kept in mind that the exact specificity of tilt table is, to a great extent, dependent on the physiological processes that result in neurocardiogenic syncope. The sequence of reflex events alluded to previously appears to be a normal (albeit paradoxic) response that could potentially be produced in most (if not all) people, given the right amount of stimulation. Therefore, tilt table testing cannot be thought to identify an underlying pathology, rather it determines an exaggerated susceptibility to this normal reflex. The actual specificity might thus be underestimated because healthy asymptomatic subjects who have positive tilt tests may be more susceptible than other individuals and could potentially experience clinical syncopal episodes. A study by Grubb *et al.* [116] found that a control subject with tilt-induced syncope later experienced a spontaneous neurocardiogenic clinical syncope.

There are various positive response patterns seen during head-up tilt table testing. We tend to group these into four groups (Figs 2.2 and 2.3). The first is the "classic vasovagal" (or neurocardiogenic) described in detail previously, which is characterized by the sudden onset of hypotension with or without coexistent bradycardia. In between episodes of syncope these patients appear perfectly healthy and normal, with few if any other complaints. For the most part, these patients tend to be younger (although we have observed this response in virtually all age groups). A second pattern has been termed a "dysautonomic response," characterized by gradual parallel declines in systolic and diastolic blood pressure, leading to loss of consciousness

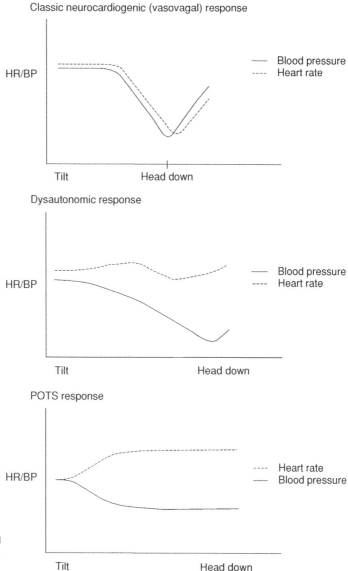

Fig. 2.3 Blood pressure and heart rate patterns observed in abnormal responses to tilt table testing. BP, blood pressure; HR, heart rate; POTS, postural orthostatic tachycardia syndrome.

(also called delayed orthostatic hypotension). This pattern has been reported to be associated with low levels of circulating catecholamines [117]. These patients are often noted to have other signs of autonomic dysfunction such as abnormal sweating and thermoregulatory control as well as orthostatic hypotension, and syncope itself is but one manifestation of a general state of autonomic failure (primary autonomic failure) [118]. Unlike patients with the more classic vasovagal form, these patients never really feel "well" and are much more disabled by their illness. We call the third pattern a psychogenic or psychosomatic response. These patients experience syncope during tilt table testing with no ascertainable alteration in heart rate, blood pressure, electroencephalographic, or transcranial blood flow patterns [119]. This group of patients usually has underlying psychiatric disturbances which range from somatoform disorders (or conversion reactions) to anxiety disorders and major depression. Interestingly, serum catecholamines in these patients are quite high prior to, during, and after syncope (in contrast to the low levels seen in dysautonomic patients and the abrupt decline in catecholamines seen in the classic vasovagal pattern).

We have recently realized that a fourth tilt pattern exists. We have termed this tilt pattern the postural orthostatic tachycardia syndrome (POTS) [120]. This pattern is characterized by an increase in heart rate of at least 30 b min^{-1} (or a maximum heart rate of 120 b min^{-1}) within the first 10 min upright during the baseline tilt. The tachycardia is not associated with profound hypotension. Several investigators have reported that these patients demonstrate a mild form of autonomic dysfunction in which a deficiency in peripheral vascular function (peripheral blood pooling) results in an excessive compensatory postural tachycardia. These patients also demonstrate exaggerated heart rate responses to the infusion of isoproterenol. Streeten [121] postulates that this may represent the earliest and most sensitive sign of autonomic dysfunction. In this group of patients, near-syncope tends to occur more frequently than does full syncope. Many of these patients will complain of exercise intolerance, dizziness, and chronic disabling fatigue. These patients are often referred for evaluation of a persistent sinus tachycardia. Approximately 50% of these patients will report the onset of symptoms following a severe viral illness, suggesting a possible autoimmune etiology. A more comprehensive discussion of POTS can be found in Chapter 13.

An alternative classification system has been developed by Sutton et al. [122], which basically divides responses into cardioinhibitory, vasodepressor, and mixed types. The cardioinhibitory response was further divided into those where the arterial pressure falls before heart rate, and those where the fall in heart rate appears to pull the pressure down with it.

The reproducibility of tilt table testing has been assessed by several studies. With use of prolonged passive head-up tilt alone, the reproducibility of a positive test is 62–77% over a period of 3–7 days [123,124]. When using isoproterenol infusions with tilt table testing, the clinical reproducibility is reported to range between 67% and 88% when performed over periods of 30 min to 2 weeks [125,126]. Interestingly, the reproducibility of

negative tests is 85–100% over the same period. Overall, the results of the first test are 80% reproducible on subsequent testing, suggesting that there may be little to be achieved by performing a second tilt on a patient suffering from recurrent unexplained syncope who has an initial normal test result. More detailed information on use of an indications for tilt table testing can be found in Chapter 7.

Therapeutic approaches

The therapeutic approach to any patient who suffers from recurrent neurocardiogenic syncope must be individualized. In many of these patients, syncope occurs infrequently and only under exceptional circumstances. Therefore, the cornerstone of any therapy is the eduction of the patient and their family as to the nature of the disorder and counseling to avoid any known predisposing factors (such as extreme heat or dehydration). Drugs that could potentially enhance a person's predisposition to syncope should be identified and, if possible, discontinued. Agents such as alcohol, angiotensin-converting enzyme (ACE) inhibitors, hydralazine, some calcium-channel blockers, and benzodiazepine may all worsen the tendency toward syncope (most probably because of the vasodilatory effect enhancing the tendency to peripheral venous pooling; see Table 2.1). Patients should also be advised to lie down at the onset of any premonitory symptoms and not remain standing or sitting. If

Table 2.1 Agents that may exacerbate syncope.

Alcohol

Angiotensin-converting enzyme inhibitors

Calcium-channel blockers

Methyldopa

Reserpine

Barbiturates

Prazosin

Anesthetics

Beta-blockers

Hydralazine

Diuretics

Sildenafil citrate

Vardenafil HCl

another person is present during a spontaneous syncopal episode, he or she should place the affected individual supine (with the feet elevated and the head down) until a stable blood pressure and pulse rate returns. A common error is to attempt to have the patient try to sit up moments after he or she has regained consciousness; this will only provoke another episode. Once the patient has regained consciousness in the supine position, it is best to allow at least 5–10 min to elapse before allowing him or her to sit up. Patients who begin to experience warning signs will often experience a strong urge to get up and walk (probably reflecting an unconscious desire to increase venous return through skeletal muscle contraction), thereby increasing the degree of orthostatic stress and precipitating a syncopal event. When given a choice between falling down or lying down, most informed patients will choose the latter.

Recently, Kerdiet *et al.* [127] reported that leg crossing and muscle tensing during the prodromal phase of syncope can activate the skeletal muscle pump and raise blood pressure sufficiently so as to control or even abort the episode. One retired physician related to me that patients were once told to keep a "darning egg" or golf ball in their pockets and to squeeze it tightly at the onset of prodromal symptoms.

The initial management of patients should consist of encouraging an increase in oral fluid intake and salt consumption [128,129]. We also encourage patients to become physically conditioned, working toward a goal of performing at least 30 min of continuous aerobic activity three times a week. At the same time we encourage developing leg muscle strength with physical resistance training (i.e., weight training). Several groups have reported that "tilt training" can often be an effective therapy in preventing further syncopal episodes [130]. To do this we ask patients to stand with their back against a wall with their feet placed approximately 30 cm (12 in) away from the wall. This appears to "desensitize" the system to the effects of orthostatic stress. While effective, long-term compliance with this technique is sometimes poor.

For some individuals, however, the prodromal phase is either quite brief or absent altogether (a finding more common in older patients). Patients in whom syncope is sudden, recurrent, and without

warning will usually require some type of prophylactic therapy (especially those who experience repeated bodily injury resulting from a syncopal event). However, before beginning any form of treatment, it must be kept in mind that drug therapy for these disorders (like most chronic illness) is palliative rather than curative in nature. Thus, even well-controlled patients may, on occasion, experience recurrences resulting from exceptional stressor non-compliance.

If patients do not respond to these conservative measures, the mineral corticoid fludrocortisone is frequently employed [131]. While used extensively in the treatment of young people, it has not been subjected to placebo controlled trials. Although it was initially believed that its principal effect was an increase in blood volume, fludrocortisone also appears to increase the sensitivity of blood vessels to the vasoconstrictive effects of norepinephrine. Grubb *et al.* [132] reported on 21 pediatric patients with syncope and positive tilt table test results, 10 of whom were rendered tilt-negative. Over a 20-month follow-up period, 20 of the 21 had no further syncopal episodes. Later, Scott *et al.* [133] evaluated 58 pediatric patients with syncope, randomizing them to either treatment with atenolol (25–50 mg/day) or fludrocortisone (0.1 mg/day). Over a 6-month follow-up period, there was little difference between the two groups, with a total of 48 patients having no further syncopal events. However, the dose of fludrocortisone was low (usual dosage 0.2 mg/day) and no placebo group was used.

Fludrocortisone is safe and has a low side-effect profile. Some patients will become severely hypokalemic or hypomagnesemic on fludrocortisone and may require potassium or magnesium supplementation. On occasion, the drug may cause hair loss, peripheral edema, exacerbate acne, and even cause depression [131]. The usual dosage is 0.2 mg/day, and we never exceed 0.4 mg/day so as to avoid any adrenal suppressive effects. The drug is commonly used to treat orthostatic hypotension in adults, with favorable results. An alternative volume-expanding agent is oral vasopressin (or DDAVP); however, it may cause headaches and hyponatremia.

The agents most widely used in the treatment of neurocardiogenic syncope are the β_1-adrenergic blockers [134]. These agents are presumed to exert their effects via their negative inotropic actions, which are thought to diminish the degree of cardiac mechanoreceptor activation [135]. However, studies by Hjorth and Sharp [136] and Hjorth [137] have demonstrated that beta-blockers have powerful central serotonin-blocking activities (principally at the 5-HT1A + B receptors) that may somehow contribute to their therapeutic effects. Additionally, beta-blockers may blunt the effects of high circulating levels of epinephrine and norepinephrine. Beta-blockers have been reported to be useful in a number of uncontrolled studies and in one controlled trial [135,138–142]. However, in five of six controlled trials they failed to be of benefit [143–149]. These results must be interpreted with some caution because of the wide variance of methodology employed. For example, most studies have determined that major predictors of beta-blocker success in neurocardiogenic syncope include presence of tachycardia during tilt table testing, the need for isoproterenol to induce syncope, and an acute response to beta-blockers. Most studies have used a positive tilt table study as a criterion for inclusion. A study by Madrid *et al.* [146] that showed no benefit of atenolol over placebo included a high proportion of tilt-negative patients (approximately 60%), thereby diluting any potential therapeutic benefit. In addition, Fitzpatrick *et al.* [149] have suggested that the lipophilic properties of metoprolol (which allows for a greater degree of central nervous system penetration), as opposed to atenolol, may in part be responsible for the discrepancies seen between different studies. It has been noted that beta-blocking agents may on occasion worsen the tendency toward syncope rather than reduce it (resulting in a phenomena that we call "pro-syncope") [150]. While the data are conflicting, beta-blocking agents appear useful in some patients (especially those with concomitant migraines) and are safe and relatively inexpensive. A recent study presented by Sheldon [151] has shed some further light on the use of beta-blockers in syncope. The Prevention of Syncope Trial (POST) was a randomized, placebo controlled trial of metoprolol versus placebo in 208 patients with recurrent syncope and positive tilt table tests. Interestingly, in those patients under 42 years of age, metoprolol was no better than placebo, while in those over 42 years of age, treatment with meto-

prolol produced a significant reduction in the syncopal recurrence rate. The reason for this discrepancy is not known. They also found that requiring isoproterenol during tilt table testing to induce syncope was not predictive of a beneficial effect from isoproterenol. Further studies are planned to better define the role of beta-blockade in treatment of neurocardiogenic syncope.

Transdermal scopolamine has been reported useful in treating neurocardiogenic syncope [152]. It has been thought to block the vagally mediated decline in blood pressure and heart rate; however, the physiologic process is not an increase in parasympathetic tone, but rather a sudden sympathetic withdrawal. Nearly 70 years ago, Lewis noted that while atropine could prevent bradycardia it did little to prevent syncope. A placebo controlled trial by Lee *et al.* [153] showed little difference between scopolamine and placebo. Propantheline, another anticholinergic agent, has been reported to be effective in several small uncontrolled trials [154]. Side-effects from these drugs are common and include dry mouth, visual blurring, constipation, urinary retention, and, on rare occasions, confusion. In addition, tachyphylaxis often occurs.

Milstein *et al.* [155] have reported that disopyramide, an agent possessing negative inotropic, anticholinergic, and direct peripheral vasoconstrictive effects is useful in preventing recurrent neurocardiogenic syncope. However, both Morillo *et al.* [156] and Kelly *et al.* [157] have reported that disopyramide is no more effective than placebo. Others have reported that oral theophylline, presumably because of its adenosine antagonistic effects. However, frequent side-effects limit its utility.

Because vasodilation has such a prominent role in neurocardiogenic syncope, it would seem logical to use vasoconstrictors in its management. Both α_1- and α_2-adrenergic agents have been employed. Strieper and Campbell [158] evaluated the use of pseudoephedrine in pediatric patients and found it to be effective, as did Janosik *et al.* [159] using ephedrine. However, the effect of these agents rapidly diminishes with chronic use. Susmano *et al.* [160] found that dextroamphetamine (an α- and β-receptor agonist) was effective in preventing neurocardiogenic syncope in a small number of patients. Although useful, the drug has a number of side-effects and a high potential for abuse. This led our group to explore the use of the chemically similar agent methylphenidate in patients who were refractory to other forms of therapy [161]. We found it to be a reasonably well-tolerated and effective therapy in this otherwise refractory group. The drug also has the advantage of coming in several sustained-release preparations that allow it to be given once daily.

The direct α_1-receptor agonist midodrine HCl was released in the USA for the treatment of orthostatic hypotension. Both Sra et al. [162] and Grubb et al. [163] reported on the use of midodrine in open labeled, non-randomized trials. Later, in a placebo controlled, crossover trial, Ward et al. [164] evaluated 16 patients with recurrent neurocardiogenic syncope over a 2-month period and found that 10 of 16 (63%) showed improvement. Shortly thereafter Perez-Lugones et al. [165], in a randomized controlled trial, compared midodrine to salt and fluid therapy in 61 patients over a period of 6 months. In the midodrine group, the recurrence rate was significantly lower than in the salt and fluid group. Interestingly, Moya et al. [166] evaluated etilefrine, an α-agonist; a double blind, crossover study of 30 patients showed that it was no better than placebo. A similar study by Raviele et al. [167] showed a similar lack of efficacy.

Clonidine, an agent with selective α_2-agonist, is felt to decrease venous capacitance, possibly because of the large number of α_2-receptors present there. However, Biffi et al. [168] found that it was not superior to metoprolol in a randomized study.

Interestingly, a study by Zeng et al. [169] showed that the ACE inhibitor enalapril was effective in preventing neurocardiogenic syncope in a randomized, placebo controlled, acute evaluation performed by tilt table testing. The mechanisms by which this may act is unclear, and no subsequent trials have been performed.

Based on the observations on the role of serotonin in the pathophysiologic processes that result in neurocardiogenic syncope, the use of the serotonin-altering drugs as a potential therapy have been explored [63]. The serotonin reuptake inhibitors (SSRIs) prevent the reuptake of serotonin in the synaptic cleft, thereby increasing intrasynaptic serotonin concentrations and producing a down-regulation in post-synaptic serotonin receptor density [51]. Following anecdotal observations that

some patients with both neurocardiogenic syncope and depression had a marked improvement in both conditions after receiving fluoxetine, we began to explore the possibility of using the SSRIs as a therapy in neurocardiogenic syncope. We published several open labeled, non-randomized trials demonstrating that both fluoxetine hydrochloride and sertraline hydrochloride were effective therapies for patients who were refractory to or intolerant of other agents, with response rates of 50% [170,171]. In a double blind, randomized, placebo controlled study of paroxetine, 68 patients received either study drug or placebo. On repeat tilt table testing after 1 month, 62% of the patients on paroxetine became tilt-negative compared with 38% of placebo patients [64]. Over a follow-up period of 25 months, 82% of patients on the study drug remained syncope-free, whereas 53% on placebo had recurrent syncopal episodes ($P < 0.0001$). While effective patients can experience side-effects such as tremor, insomnia, headache, nausea, and diarrhea. Paradoxic depression and hyperagitated states have also been reported, as has sexual dysfunction. Newer, subselective agents may have fewer side-effects.

For those patients in whom there are known situations that can provoke syncope (e.g., the sight of blood or a needle), biofeedback has been very successfully used to help "desensitize" the individual to the psychological trigger, thereby blunting its effects [172,173].

During an episode of syncope, some patients may demonstrate significant bradycardia or asystole (Fig. 2.4). There is perhaps no other treatment modality that is more controversial than the role of permanent cardiac pacing. The first reports on the use of permanent pacing for neurocardiogenic syncope demonstrated that VVI mode pacing is almost always ineffective and may actually aggravate syncope because of retrograde ventriculoatrial conduction [174]. In their original paper on tilt table testing, Kenny et al. [6] also reported the successful use of dual-chamber cardiac pacing for neurocardiogenic syncope. Later, Fitzpatrick and Sutton [175] reported the results of pacing in 20 tilt-positive patients with induced symptomatic bradycardia (< 60 b min^{-1}). Syncope was eliminated in about half of the patients, while the remainder experienced fewer syncopal episodes of a lesser

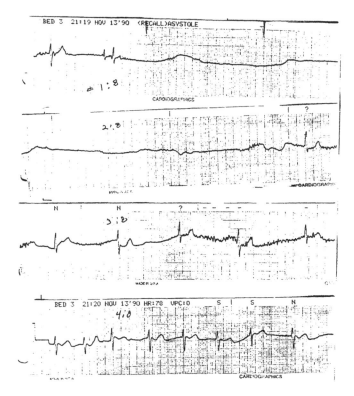

Fig. 2.4 A "malignant" episode of neurocardiogenic syncope.

severity. Fitzpatrick *et al.* [176] then investigated tilt table testing performed with a temporary dual-chamber pacemaker in place. He found that temporary DVI pacing with hysteresis could abort approximately 85% of the cases of neurocardiogenic syncope, induced by 60° head-up tilt. Both McGuinn *et al.* [177] and Samoil *et al.* [178] also found that in a small number of patients, temporary dual-chamber pacing could prevent tilt-induced syncope or at least prolong the time from onset of symptoms to syncope. These findings are in contrast to those of Sra *et al.* [33], who studied the effects of temporary pacing in 22 patients: 20 with sinus rhythm during AV sequential pacing and two with atrial fibrillation who had ventricular pacing alone. All 22 patients had an initial positive baseline tilt test after repeating the tilt with pacing (at a rate 20% higher than the supine resting heart rate): one patient remained asymptomatic, one had dizziness without hypotension, and 15 experienced

presyncope rather than syncope. Only five patients had syncope during the following tilt. Afterward, all patients had repeat tilt table testing while on pharmacological therapy: metoprolol was effective in 10 of 22 patients, theophylline in three of 12 patients, and disopyramide in six of nine patients. From this, they concluded that pacing was of little benefit, although it can also be concluded that pacing offered a clear benefit for some patients.

Finally, Petersen *et al.* [179] presented data on the long-term effects of permanent pacing in patients with severe recurrent syncope and reproducible tilt-induced neurocardiogenic syncope (with a pronounced bradycardic component). Dual-chamber permanent pacemakers were implanted in 37 patients who were then followed for 50 ± 24 months. Approximately 89% had a marked reduction in symptoms, while 27% had complete elimination of symptoms. There was a reduction in the overall frequency of syncopal episodes from 136 to

11 episodes/year. Interestingly, the clinical features that best predicted the usefulness of permanent pacing included a young age (56 years compared with 76 years) and the absence of a prodrome before spontaneous syncopal episodes [180].

The first randomized controlled trial that appeared was the North American Vasovagal Pacemaker Study (the VPS1) trial [181]. The study had planned to recruit 280 patients randomized to pacemaker placement or previous therapy. However, the study was stopped after recruitment of only 54 patients because of the dramatic difference between time to syncopal recurrence of the two groups. Shortly thereafter the VASIS trial reported similar results, despite the fact that there were a number of significant differences [182]. Patients in the VASIS trial tended to be older and had fewer symptoms than those in the VPS1 study, and the follow-up was longer. The difference in syncope recurrence between the paced group and the no-therapy group was quite significant in terms of syncope recurrence.

The potential benefit of a rate drop response pacemaker was evaluated by Ammirati *et al.* (the SYDIT trial) [183]. They studied a total of 20 patients over a 17 ± 4 month follow-up period and found that the rate drop pacing algorithm was better than rate hysteresis. Ammirati *et al.* [184] later reported the results of a multicenter, randomized trial of medical therapy with atenolol compared with dual-chamber cardiac pacing. The paced group had a significantly lower syncope recurrence rate than did the atenolol group.

Two recent trials have cast some doubt on the efficacy of pacing in neurocardiogenic syncope. One was the VPS2 trial, which consisted of 100 patients who received dual-chamber pacemakers randomized to being "ON" (DDD mode) or "OFF" (ODO; sensing without pacing) [185]. Patients included had six or more episodes during the course of their lifetime or had at least three episodes during the prior 2 years. They also had positive tilt table tests; however, no standardized test protocol was employed and provocation was with either nitroglycerine or isoproterenol. Interestingly, only 15–23% of patients had recorded heart rates of less than 40 b min^{-1}. No significant difference was observed in time to first syncopal recurrence

between the two groups over a 6-month follow-up period (the pacing "ON" group had a relative risk reduction of 30%). It is interesting to speculate if this trend may have become more significant had the study continued for a longer period of time; however, at 6 months the groups were then changed to rate drop response versus conventional rate hysteresis.

A similar study was the SYNPACE trial, which compared 29 patients with pacemakers turned "ON" versus those turned "OFF" [186]. While there was no significant difference to syncope recurrence between the two groups, those patients who had asystolic preimplant tilt table tests showed a significant increase in the time to recurrence compared with those who only experienced bradycardia (91 days vs. 11 days). Interestingly, in the VASIS trial, 85% of patients had tilt-induced asystole and in the SYDIT trial 60% had asystole. This raises the possibility that asystole during tilt table testing may be a predictor of response to permanent cardiac pacing. Also, patients in the VASIS and SYDIT trials were older, raising the question as to whether age may be a predictor of pacing response. Where does this leave us? As Sutton [187] eloquently noted, "When the final judgment is made it will be necessary to take into account that we appear to have in dual chamber pacing a very effective means of symptom control, and there is no doubt that it works in some patients," and "Our role as physicians is to relieve symptoms." Based on the physiologic processes at play in neurocardiogenic syncope, it should be kept in mind that a fall in blood pressure usually precedes the fall in heart rate. Thus, pacing determined by rate criteria alone often represents "too little too late." The development of newer sensor technologies that allow for the direct or indirect measurement of blood pressure would permit for the onset of pacing at the earliest point in the syncopal episode.

At present we do not employ pacing as first-line therapy because many patients will respond to conservative measures or pharmacotherapy. However, for patients who demonstrate a significant bradycardic or asystolic component of their syncope, cardiac pacing may significantly prolong the time from onset of symptoms to loss of consciousness. For patients who experience little or no warning prior to syncope (drop attacks), cardiac pacing may cause a more gradual fall in blood pressure that can be perceived by the patient as a prodrome, thereby allowing him or her to take appropriate evasive actions (such as lying down).

Sra [188] has noted that evaluation of any therapy in neurocardiogenic syncope "has been undermined by a variety of factors, including difficulty in demonstrating efficacy of therapy under controlled conditions, unrealistic endpoints (i.e., a goal of entirely eliminating all symptoms) and inadequate understanding of the natural history of the problem."

The wide range of treatment options outlined and the debates concerning their efficacy often tend to leave one confused over how to initiate a rational treatment plan. Indeed, at present, treatment seems somewhat more of an art than a science. This having been said, we offer these suggestions (based both on evidence and personal experience) for the treatment of patients with recurrent neurocardiogenic syncope [189]. First, we institute conservative measures such as avoidance of situations that provoke syncope, hydration, and increased salt intake (two glasses of water with meals is a reasonable amount). At the same time, we ask the patient to build strength in their lower extremities through a combination of aerobic and resistance training, thereby enhancing their skeletal muscle pump. We ask patients to work toward a goal of doing a minimum of 20 min of aerobic activity three times a week. Patients are also instructed on various physical counter-maneuvers (such as one leg over the other at thigh level while standing or sitting) to perform when they experience a prodrome. Patients are also asked to stand with their backs against the wall with their feet slightly forward (often referred to as "tilt training"), for at least 10–20 min each day. Long-term compliance with this technique is often poor, particularly in young people. In patients with situational syncope resulting from psychologic stimuli (such as the sight of blood or a needle), a combination of biofeedback and deconditioning can be most helpful.

Pharmacotherapy is started when conservative measures are inadequate, or when there is little or no prodrome and syncope is associated with severe bodily injury. Prior to starting any medication, one must consider any concomitant illness or conditions present in the patient to be sure that any potential therapy will be compatible. In children and adolescents we often begin with fludrocortisone 0.1 mg/day p.o., increasing by 0.1 mg at 2-week intervals up to a dose of 0.3 mg (if needed). The pressor effects of the agent are seen to occur gradually over a number of days. A serum potassium level should be obtained 2 weeks after each dosing increment to check for hypokalemia. If only a modest response is seen after 2–3 weeks, we will usually add a second agent to it. Midodrine is often started at this point at doses of 2.5–10 mg p.o. three times daily. An alternative if midodrine is not tolerated is methylphenidate. This may be particularly attractive in young or very active people as the drug comes in a number of sustained release preparations that can be administered once daily (greatly enhancing compliance). In patients who are refractory to or intolerant of the above, we will use an SSRI (e.g., citalopram or escitalopram). It has been our experience that the use of two or three different agents (that work through different mechanisms) at lower dosages is often more effective and better tolerated than huge dosages of a single agent. Also keep in mind that the human body is a dynamic entity that changes over time. Thus, therapies that were initially effective may become less so over the course of years, especially if concomitant medical disorders develop.

Prognosis

Data on the long-term outcomes of patients are quite limited; however, some general trends have been observed. One of the most important is that adolescents who develop recurrent syncope will usually "grow out of it" by the time they are in their twenties. Thus, the philosophy of treatment should be to get them through the "bad years" and then discontinue therapy. For this reason we are extremely reluctant to consider permanent pacing in this group, and we use it only when the life of the patient is considered to be in jeopardy. Our usual practice in adolescents is to treat for 1–2 years and then, if the patient has remained completely symptom-free during that time, to discontinue therapy. Approximately 80% of adolescents will not require further therapy, while the remaining 20% will experience recurrent symptoms and need to be placed back on treatment. The majority of these will be able to discontinue therapy after an additional 1–2 years. Older patients with recurrent neurocardiogenic syncope are a different matter. For this group, it may be necessary to continue therapy indefinitely, as we have observed a high recurrence rate when treatments are stopped.

Concurrent conditions seem to either reactivate a prior tendency toward syncope or exacerbate a previously unrecognized predisposition toward it. Principal among these conditions are pregnancy and the postpartum period (see Chapter 13).

Other conditions that seem to reactivate a prior tendency toward syncope are severe viral infections and treatment with chemotherapeutic agents (in particular *cis*-platinum and vincristine). We have also noted the return of syncope following trauma or severe emotional stress, and following exposure to extreme heat.

Summary

The disorder now known as neurocardiogenic syncope is a complex one with a wide clinical spectrum of presentations. Indeed, it often seems more like a group of related disorders rather than a single clinical entity. Currently understood as an exaggerated form of an otherwise normal response, the mechanism seems to involve sudden mechanoreceptor activation following a rapid increase in peripheral vascular pooling. Tilt table testing has emerged as an invaluable tool for reproducing episodes of neurocardiogenic syncope, allowing not only for the confirmation of the diagnosis, but also for more detailed investigations into the pathophysiology of the condition. Furthermore, detailed studies will be necessary to better understand this common, fascinating, and yet enigmatic condition and to elaborate optimal diagnostic and therapeutic modalities.

References

1 Kapoor W, Karpf M, Wieand S, *et al*. A prospective evaluation and follow-up of patients with syncope. *N Engl J Med* 1983;**309**:197–204.

2 Calkins H, Byrne M, El-Atassi R, *et al*. The economic burden of unrecognized vasodepressor syncope. *Am J Med* 1993;**95**:473–9.

3 Eagle KA, Black HR, Cook EF, Goldman L. Evaluation of prognostic classification for patients with syncope. *Am J Med* 1985;**79**:455–60.

4 Linzer M, Pontinen M, Gold GT. Impairment of physical and psychosocial function in recurrent syncope. *J Clin Epidemiol* 1991;**44**:1037–43.

5 Decter BM, Goldner B, Cohen TJ. Vasovagal syncope as a cause of motor vehicle accidents. *Am Heart J* 1994;**127**:1619–21.

6 Kenny RA, Ingram A, Bayless J, Sutton R. Head up tilt: a useful test for investigating unexplained syncope. *Lancet* 1989;**1**:1352–5.

7 Kosinski D, Grubb BP, Temesy-Armos P. Pathophysiological aspects of neurocardiogenic syncope. *Pacing Clin Electrophysiol* 1995;**18**:716–21.

8 Hunter J. *Works of John Hunter*, Vol. 3. London: J.F. Palmer, 1837.

9 Foster M. *Textbook of Physiology*. London: Macmillan, 1888: 297, 345.

10 Lewis T. A lecture on vasovagal syncope and the carotid sinus mechanism: with comments on Gower's and Nothnagel's syndrome. *BMJ* 1932;**1**:873–6.

11 Allen SC, Taylor CL, Hall VE. A study of orthostatic insufficiency by the tilt board method. *Am J Physiol* 1945;**143**:11–20.

12 Wieling W, Lieshout J. Maintenance of postural normotension in humans. In: Low P, ed. *Clinical Autonomic Disorders*. Boston: Little, Brown and Company, 1993: 69–73.

13 Mehdirah AA, Janosik D, Fredman C. Mechanisms of tilt table-induced hypotension and bradycardia in patients with neurally mediated syncope (Abstract). *J Am Coll Cardiol* 1993;**17**:216A.

14 El-Bedawi KM, Hainsworth R. Combined head-up tilt and lower body suction: a test of orthostatic intolerance. *Clin Auton Res* 1994;**4**:41–7.

15 Hainsworth R, El-Bedawi KM. Orthostatic intolerance in patients with unexplained syncope. *Clin Auton Res* 1994;**4**:239–44.

16 Tseng CJ, Tung CS. Brainstem and cardiovascular regulation. In: Robertson D, Biaggioni I, eds. *Disorders of the Autonomic Nervous System*. London: Harwood Academic, 1995: 9–24.

17 Benarroch E. The central autonomic network: functional organization, dysfunction, and perspective. *Mayo Clin Proc* 1993;**68**:988–1001.

18 Smith ML, Carlson MD, Thames MD. Reflex control of the heart and circulation: implications for cardiovascular electrophysiology. *J Cardiovasc Electrophysiol* 1991; **2**:441–9.

19 Fitzpatrick A, Williams T, Ahmed R, *et al.* Echocardiographic and endocrine changes during vasovagal syncope induced by prolonged head up tilt. *Eur J Cardiac Pacing Electrophysiol* 1992;**2**:121–8.

20 Morita H, Vatner SF. Effects of haemorrhage on renal nerve activity in conscious dogs. *Circ Res* 1985;**57**:788–93.

21 Lightfoot JT, Rowe SA, Fortney SM. Occurrence of presyncope in subjects without ventricular innervation. *Clin Sci* 1993;**85**:695–700.

22 Fitzpatrick AP, Banner N, Cheng A, *et al.* Vasovagal syncope may occur after orthotopic heart transplantation. *J Am Coll Cardiol* 1993;**21**:1132–7.

23 Waxman MB, Cameron DA, Wald RW. Role of ventricular afferents in vasovagal reactions. *J Am Coll Cardiol* 1993;**21**:1138–41.

24 Rudas L, Pflugfelder PW, Kostuk WJ. Vasodepressor syncope in a cardiac transplant recipient: a case of vagal re-innervation? *Can J Cardiol* 1992;**8**:403–5.

25 Scherrer U, Vissing S, Morgan BJ, *et al.* Vasovagal syncope after infusion of a vasodilator in a heart transplant patient. *N Engl J Med* 1990;**322**:602–4.

26 Wright C, Drinkhill MJ, Hainsworth R. Reflex effects of independent stimulation of coronary and left ventricular mechanoreceptors in anaesthetized dogs. *J Physiol* 2000;**528**:349–58.

27 Lofring V. Cardiovascular adjustments induced from the rostral cingulated gyrus: with specific reference to sympatho-inhibiting mechanisms. *Acta Physiol Scand* 1961;**51**(Suppl. 184):5–82.

28 Constantin L, Martins JB, Fincham RW, *et al.* Bradycardia and syncope as manifestations of partial epilepsy. *J Am Coll Cardiol* 1990;**15**:900–15.

29 Dickinson CJ. Fainting precipitated by collapse firing of venous baroreceptors. *Lancet* 1993;**342**:970–2.

30 Landgren S. On the excitation mechanism of carotid baroreceptors. *Acta Physiol Scand* 1952;**26**:1–34.

31 Banner NR, Williams M, Patel N, *et al.* Altered cardiovascular and neurohumoral response to head up tilt after heart–lung transplantation. *Circulation* 1990;**82**: 863–71.

32 Rea R, Thames M. Neural control mechanisms and vasovagal syncope. *J Cardiovasc Electrophysiol* 1993;**4**:587–95.

33 Sra J, Jazayeri M, Avitall B, *et al.* Comparison of cardiac pacing with drug therapy in the treatment of neurocardiogenic syncope with bradycardia or asystole. *N Engl J Med* 1993;**328**:1085–90.

34 Oberg B, Thoren P. Increased activity in left ventricular receptors during hemorrhage or occlusion of caval veins in the cat: a possible cause of the vasovagal reaction. *Acta Physiol Scand* 1972;**85**:164–73.

35 Wallin BG, Sundlof G. Sympathetic outflow to the muscles during vasovagal syncope. *J Auton Nerv Syst* 1982;**6**:284–91.

36 Sra J, Jazayeri M, Murthy V, *et al.* Sequential catecholamine changes during upright tilt: possible hormonal mechanisms responsible for pathogenesis of neurocardiogenic syncope. *J Am Coll Cardiol* 1991;**17**:216A.

37 Lewis W, Smith M, Carlson M. Peripheral sympatho-inhibition precedes hypotension and bradycardia during neurally mediated vasovagal syncope. *Pacing Clin Electrophysiol* 1994;**17**:747.

38 Goldstein D, Holmes C, Frank S, *et al.* Cardiac sympathetic dysautonomia in chronic orthostatic intolerance syndromes. *Circulation* 2002;**106**:2358–65.

39 Goldstein DS, Holmes C, Frank S, *et al.* Sympathorenal imbalance before neurocardiogenic syncope. *Am J Cardiol* 2003;**9**:53–8.

40 Waxman MB, Asta JA, Cameron DA. Vasodepressor reaction induced by inferior vena cava occlusion and isoproterenol in the rat. *Circulation* 1994;**89**:2401–11.

41 Chosy JJ, Graham DT. Catecholamines in vasovagal fainting. *J Psychosom Res* 1965;**9**:189–94.

42 Mosqueda-Garcia R, Furlan R, Tank J, Fernandez-Violante R. The elusive pathophysiology of neurally mediated syncope. *Circulation* 2000;**102**:2898–906.

43 Kaufman H, Hainsworth R. Why do we faint? *Muscle Nerve* 2001;**24**:981–3.

44 Mouta H, Nishida Y, Motochigawa H, *et al.* Opiate receptor-mediated decrease in renal nerve activity during hypotensive hemorrhage in conscious rats. *Circ Res* 1988;**63**:165–72.

45 Evans RG, Ludbrook J, Potonick SJ. Intracisternal naloxone and cardiac nerve blockade prevent vasodilation during simulated haemorrhage in awake rabbits. *J Physiol (Lond)* 1989;**409**:1–14.

46 Ferguson DW. Naloxone potentiates cardiopulmonary baroreflex sympathetic control in normal humans. *Circ Res* 1992;**70**:172–83.

47 Perna GP, Ficola U, Salvatori P, *et al.* Increase of plasma β-endorphins in vasodepressor syncope. *Am J Cardiol* 1990;**65**:929–30.

48 Wallbridge DR, MacIntyre HE, Gray CE, *et al.* Increase in plasma β-endorphins precedes vasodepressor syncope. *Br Heart J* 1994;**71**:446–8.

49 Foldager N, Bonde-Petersen F. Human cardiovascular reactions to simulated hypovolemia, modified by the opiate antagonist naloxone. *Eur J Appl Physiol* 1988; **57**:507–13.

50 Smith ML, Carlson MD, Sheehan HM, *et al.* Naloxone does not prevent vasovagal syncope during simulated orthostasis in humans. *Physiologist* 1991;**34**:238–9.

51 Grubb BP, Kosinski D. Serotonin and syncope: an emerging connection? *Eur J Cardiac Pacing Electrophysiol* 1996;**5**:306–14.

52 Kuhn D, Wolfe W, Loyenburg W. Review of the central serotonergic neuronal system in blood pressure regulation. *Hypertension* 1980;**2**:243–55.

53 Baum T, Shropshire AT. Inhibition of efferent sympathetic nerve activity by 5-hydroxytryptophan in centrally administered 5-hydroxytryphamine. *Neuropharmacology* 1975;**14**:227–33.

54 Tadepelli A, Mills E, Schanberg S. Central depression of carotid baroreceptor pressor response, arterial pressure, and heart rate by 5-hydroxytryptophan: influence of the supramolecular areas of the brain. *J Pharmacol Exp Ther* 1977;**202**:310–9.

55 Abboud FM. Neurocardiogenic syncope. *N Engl J Med* 1993;**328**:1117–9.

56 Bauer K, Dietersdorfer F, Kaik G. Assessment of β-adrenergic receptor blockade after isamoltane, a 5HT1 receptor active compound in healthy volunteers. *Clin Pharmacol Ther* 1993;**53**(6):675–83.

57 Elam RF, Bergman F, Feverstein G. The use of antiserotonergic agents for the treatment of acute hemorrhagic shock in cats. *Eur J Pharmacol* 1985;**107**:275–8.

58 Hasser E, Schadt J, Grove K. Serotonergic and opioid interactions during acute hemorrhagic hypotension in the conscious rabbit (Abstract). *FASEB J* 1989;**3**:A1014.

59 Morgan DA, Thoren P, Wilczynski E, *et al.* Serotonergic mechanisms mediate renal sympatho-inhibition during severe hemorrhage in rats. *Am J Physiol* 1988;**255**:H496–502.

60 Theodorakis G, Markianos M, Sourlas N, *et al.* Central serotonergic and adrenergic activity in patients with vasovagal syncope (Abstact). *Circulation* 1995;**92**:414.

61 Matzen S, Secher NH, Knigge U, *et al.* Effect of serotonin receptor blockade on endocrine and cardiovascular responses to upright tilt in humans. *Acta Physiol Scand* 1993;**149**:163–76.

62 Samoil D, Grubb BP. Neurally mediated syncope and serotonin reuptake inhibitors. *Clin Auton Res* 1995;**5**:251–5.

63 Grubb BP, Karas BJ. The potential role of serotonin in the pathogenesis of neurocardiogenic syncope and related autonomic disturbances. *J Interv Card Electrophysiol* 1998;**2**:325–32.

64 DiGirolamo E, DiIorio C, Sabatini O, *et al.* Effects of paroxetine hydrochloride, a selective serotonin reuptake inhibitor, on refractory vasovagal syncope: a randomized, double blind placebo controlled study. *J Am Coll Cardiol* 1999;**33**:1227–30.

65 Goldstein D, Spanarkel M, Pitterman A, *et al.* Circulatory control mechanisms in neurocardiogenic syncope. *Am Heart J* 1982;**104**:1071–5.

66 Riegger CA, Wagner A. Excessive secretion of vasopressin during vasovagal reaction. *Am Heart J* 1991;**121**:602–3.

67 Kaufmann H, Oribe E, Oliver JA. Plasma endothelin during upright tilt: relevance for orthostatic hypotension? *Lancet* 1991;**338**:1542–5.

68 Sakuma J, Togashi H, Yoshioka M, *et al.* N-methyl-L-arginine, an inhibitor of L-arginine-derived nitric oxide synthesis, stimulates renal sympathetic nerve activity *in vivo*: a role for nitric oxide in the central regulation of autonomic tone. *Circ Res* 1992;**70**:607–11.

69 Grubb BP, Gerard G, Roush K, *et al.* Cerebral vasoconstriction during head upright tilt-induced vasovagal syncope: a paradoxic and unexpected response. *Circulation* 1991;**84**:1157–64.

70 Janasik D, Gomez C, Njemanze P, *et al.* Abnormalities in cerebral blood flow autoregulation during tilt-induced syncope (Abstract). *Pacing Clin Electrophysiol* 1992;**15**:542.

71 Gomez CR, Janosik DL, Lewis ML. Transcranial Doppler in the evaluation of global cerebral ischemia: syncope and cardiac arrest. In: Babikian VL, Wechsler LR, eds. *Transcranial Doppler Ultrasonography.* St. Louis: Mosby Year Book, 1993: 141–9.

72 Njemanze P. Cerebral circulation dysfunction and hemodynamic abnormalities in syncope during upright tilt test. *Can J Cardiol* 1993;**9**:238–42.

73 Kaminer S, Truemper E, Fisher A. Recurrent syncope in children: intracranial hemodynamics (Abstract). *Pacing Clin Electrophysiol* 1993;**1**:532.

74 Lagi A, Cencetti M, Corsoni M, *et al.* Cerebral vasoconstriction in vasovagal syncope: any link with symptoms? A transcranial Doppler study. *Circulation* 2001;**104**:2649–98.

75 Carey BJ, Manktelow B, Panerai R, Potter J. Cerebral autoregulatory responses to head up tilt in normal subjects and patients with recurrent vasovagal syncope. *Circulation* 2001;**104**:898–902.

76 Daffertshafer M, Hemmerici M. Cardiovascular regulation and vasoneural coupling. *J Clin Ultrasound* 1995;**23**:125–8.

77 Friedman CS, Bierman KM, Patel V, *et al.* Transcranial Doppler ultrasonography during head upright tilt table testing. *Ann Intern Med* 1995;**123**:848–9.

78 Obara C, Kobayashi Y, Ueda H, *et al.* Possible syncopal attack without hypotension during head up tilt table testing: an assessment of middle cerebral blood flow velocity. *PACE* 1996;**19**:711.

79 Grubb BP, Samoil D, Kosinski D, *et al.* Cerebral syncope: loss of consciousness associated with cerebral vasoconstriction in the absence of systemic hypotension. *PACE* 1998;**21**:652–8.

80 Asensio LE, Oseguera M. Reactive hypoglycemia and neurocardiogenic syncope. *Rev Invest Clin* 2000;**52**:596–7.

81 Hoeldtke RD, Boden G. Epinephrine secretion, hypoglycemia unawareness and diabetic autonomic neuropathy. *Ann Intern Med* 1984;**120**:512–7.

82 Folkow B, Neil E. *Circulation.* New York: Oxford University Press, 1971.

83 Linzer M, Felder A, Hackel A, *et al.* Psychiatric syncope. *Psychosomatics* 1990;**31**:181–8.

84 Wayne HH. Syncope: physiologic considerations and an analysis of the clinical characteristics in 510 patients. *Am J Med* 1961;**30**:418–38.

85 Luft NC, Nowell WK. Manifestations of brief instantaneous anoxia in men. *J Appl Physiol* 1956;**8**:444–54.

86 Duvoisin RC. Convulsive syncope induced by the Weber maneuver. *Arch Neurol* 1962;**7**:219–26.

87 Grubb BP, Gerard G, Roush K, et al. Differentiation of convulsive syncope and epilepsy with head up tilt table testing. *Ann Intern Med* 1991;**115**:871–6.

88 Passman R, Horvath G, Thomas J, et al. Clinical spectrum of and prevalence of neurologic events provoked by tilt table testing. *Arch Intern Med* 2003;**163**:1945–8.

89 Zaidi A, Clough P, Cooper P, Scheepers B, Fitzpatrick AP. Misdiagnosis of epilepsy. *J Am Coll Cardiol* 2000; **36**:181–4.

90 Grubb BP, Rubin AM, Wolfe D, et al. Head upright tilt table testing: a useful tool in the evaluation and management of recurrent vertigo of unknown origin associated with syncope or near syncope. *Otolaryngol Head Neck Surg* 1992;**107**:570–5.

91 Grubb BP, Samoil D, Temesy-Armos P, et al. Episodic periods of neurally mediated hypotension and bradycardia mimicking transient ischemic attacks in the elderly. *Cardiol Elderly* 1993;**1**(3):221–6.

92 Sutton R. Vasovagal syndrome: could it be malignant? *Eur J Cardiac Pacing Electrophysiol* 1992;**2**:89.

93 Grubb BP, Temesy-Armos P, Moore J, et al. Head upright tilt table testing in the evaluation and management of the malignant vasovagal syndrome. *Am J Cardiol* 1992;**69**:904–8.

94 Gatzoulis KA, Mamarelis I, Apostolopoulos T, et al. Polymorphic ventricular tachycardia induced during tilt table testing in a patient with syncope and probable dysfunction of the sinus node. *Pacing Clin Electrophysiol* 1995;**18**:1075–9.

95 Kosinski DJ, Grubb BP, Elliott L, Dubois B. Treatment of malignant neurocardiogenic syncope with dual chamber cardiac pacing and fluoxetine hydrochloride. *Pacing Clin Electrophysiol* 1995;**18**:1455–7.

96 Engle GL. Psychologic stress, vasodepressor (vasovagal) syncope and sudden death. *Ann Intern Med* 1978;**89**:403–12.

97 Linzer M, Varia I, Pontinen M, et al. Medically unexplained syncope: relationship to psychiatric illness. *Am J Med* 1992;**92**:185–255.

98 Bou-Holaigh I, Rowe P, Kan J, Calkins H. The relationship between neurally mediated hypotension and the chronic fatigue syndrome. *JAMA* 1995;**274**:961–7.

99 Stevens H, Fazekas J. Experimentally induced hypotension. *Arch Neurol Psych* 1955;**73**:416–24.

100 Milstein S, Reyes W, Benditt D. Upright body tilt for evaluation of patients with recurrent syncope. *Pacing Clin Electrophysiol* 1989;**12**:117–24.

101 Fitzpatrick AP, Theodorakis G, Vardas P, Sutton R. Methodology of head up tilt table testing in patients with unexplained syncope. *J Am Coll Cardiol* 1991; **17**:125–30.

102 Shvartz E. Reliability of quantifiable tilt table data. *Aerospace Med* 1968;**39**:1094–6.

103 Shvartz E, Meyerstein N. Tilt tolerance of young men and women. *Aerospace Med* 1970;**41**:253–5.

104 Vogt FB. Tilt table and volume changes with short term deconditioning experiments. *Aerospace Med* 1967; **38**:564–8.

105 Sutton R, Peterson M. The clinical spectrum of neurocardiogenic syncope. *J Cardiovasc Electrophysiol* 1995; **6**:569–76.

106 Strasberg B, Rechavia E, Sagie A, et al. Usefulness of head up tilt table test in evaluating patients with syncope of unknown origin. *Am Heart J* 1989;**118**:923–7.

107 Raviele A, Gasparini G, DePede F, et al. Usefulness of head up tilt table test in evaluating syncope of unknown origin and negative electrophysiologic study. *Am J Cardiol* 1990;**65**:1322–7.

108 Abi-Samra F, Maloney J, Foulad FM, Castbe L. Usefulness of head up tilt testing and hemodynamic investigations in the workup of syncope of unknown origin. *Pacing Clin Electrophysiol* 1987;**10**:406–10.

109 Almquist A, Goldenburg I, Milstein S, et al. Provocation of bradycardia and hypotension by isoproterenol and upright posture in patients with unexplained syncope. *N Engl J Med* 1989;**320**:346–51.

110 Grubb BP, Temesy-Armos P, Hahn H, Elliott L. Utility of upright tilt table testing in the evaluation and management of syncope of unknown origin. *Am J Med* 1991;**96**:6–10.

111 Pongiglione G, Fish FA, Strasberger JF, Benson DW. Heart rate and blood pressure response to upright tilt in young patients with unexplained syncope. *J Am Coll Cardiol* 1990;**16**:165–70.

112 Sheldon R, Killam S. Methodology of isoproterenol tilt table testing in patients with syncope. *J Am Coll Cardiol* 1992;**19**:773–9.

113 Kapoor WN, Brant N. Evaluation of syncope by upright tilt testing with isoproterenol. *Ann Intern Med* 1992; **116**:358–63.

114 Morillo CA, Klein G, Zandri S, Yee R. Diagnostic accuracy of a low dose isoproterenol head up tilt protocol. *Am Heart J* 1995;**129**:901–6.

115 Natale A, Akhtar M, Jazayeri M, et al. Provocation of hypotension during head up tilt testing in subjects with no history of syncope or presyncope. *Circulation* 1995;**92**:54–8.

116 Grubb BP, Kosinski D, Temesy-Armos P, Brewster P. Responses of normal subjects during head upright tilt table testing with and without low dose isoproterenol infusion. *Pacing Clin Electrophysiol* 1997;**20**:2019–23.

117 Hackel A, Linzer M, Anderson N, Williams R. Cardiovascular and catecholamine responses to head-up tilt in the diagnosis of recurrent unexplained syncope in elderly patients. *J Am Geriatr Soc* 1991;**39**:663–9.

118 Grubb BP, Kosinski D. Tilt table testing: concepts and limitations 1997;**20**(8):781–7.

119 Grubb BP, Wolfe D, Gerard G, *et al*. Syncope and seizures of psychogenic origin: identification with upright tilt table testing. *Clin Cardiol* 1992;**15**:839–42.

120 Grubb BP, Kosinski D, Boehm K, Kip K. The postural orthostatic tachycardia syndrome: a neurocardiogenic variant identified during head up tilt table testing. *Pacing Clin Electrophysiol* 1997;**20**:2205–12.

121 Streeten DH. Abnormal orthostatic changes in blood pressure and heart rate in subjects with intact sympathetic nervous function: evidence for excessive venous pooling. *J Lab Clin Med* 1988;**111**:326–35.

122 Sutton R, Peterson M, Brignole M, *et al*. Proposed classification for tilt-induced vasovagal syncope. *Eur J Cardiac Pacing Electrophysiol* 1992;**2**:180–3.

123 Blanc JJ, Mansourati J, Maheu B, *et al*. Reproducibility of a positive passive upright tilt test at a seven day interval in patients with syncope. *Am J Cardiol* 1993;**72**:469–71.

124 Fish FA, Strasburger JF, Benson W. Reproducibility of a symptomatic response to upright tilt in young patients with unexplained syncope. *Am J Cardiol* 1992;**70**:605–9.

125 Chen XC, Chen MY, Remole S, *et al*. Reproducibility of head up tilt table testing for eliciting susceptibility to neurally mediated syncope in patients without structural heart disease. *Am J Cardiol* 1992;**69**:755–60.

126 Grubb BP, Wolfe D, Temesy-Armos P, *et al*. Reproducibility of head upright tilt table test results in patients with syncope. *Pacing Clin Electrophysiol* 1992;**15**:1477–81.

127 Kerdiet CTP, van Dijk N, Linzer M, *et al*. Management of vasovagal syncope: controlling or aborting faints by leg crossing and muscle tensing. *Circulation* 2002;**106**:1684–9.

128 Jordan J, Shannon JR, Black B, *et al*. The pressor response to water drinking in humans: a sympathetic response? *Circulation* 2000;**101**:504–9.

129 El-Sayed H, Hainsworth R. Salt supplement increases plasma volume and orthostatic tolerance in patients with unexplained syncope. *Heart* 1996;**75**:134–40.

130 Reybrouck T, Heidbuchel H, Van De Werf F, Ector H. Long term follow-up results of tilt training therapy in patients with recurrent neurocardiogenic syncope. *PACE* 2002;**25**:1441–6.

131 Calkins H. Pharmacologic approaches to therapy for vasovagal syncope. *Am J Cardiol* 1999;**84**:20Q–5Q.

132 Grubb BP, Temesy-Armos P, Moor J, *et al*. The use of tilt table testing in the evaluation and management of syncope in children and adolescents. *PACE* 1992;**15**:742–8.

133 Scott WA, Pongiglione G, Bromberg I, *et al*. Randomized comparison of atenolol and fludrocortisone acetate in the treatment of pediatric neurally mediated syncope. *Am J Cardiol* 1995;**76**:400–2.

134 Cox MM, Perlman B, Mayor MR, *et al*. Acute and long-term β-adrenergic blockade for patients with neurocardiogenic syncope. *J Am Coll Cardiol* 1995;**26**:1293–8.

135 Mahananda N, Bhuripanyo K, Kangkagate C, *et al*. Randomized placebo-controlled trial of oral atenolol in patients with unexplained syncope and positive upright tilt table test results. *Am Heart J* 1995;**130**:1250–3.

136 Hjorth S, Sharp T. *In vivo* microdialysis evidence for central serotonin 1A and 1B autoreceptor of the β-receptor antagonist penbutolol. *J Pharmacol Exp Ther* 1993;**265**:707–12.

137 Hjorth S. Penbutolol as a blocker of central 5HT1A receptor-mediated responses. *Eur J Pharmacol* 1992;**222**:121–7.

138 Jhamb DK, Singh B, Sharda B, *et al*. Comparative study of the efficacy of metoprolol and verapamil in patients with syncope and positive head-up tilt test response. *Am Heart J* 1996;**132**:608–11.

139 Biffi M, Boriani G, Sabbatini P, *et al*. Malignant vasovagal syncope: a randomized trial of metoprolol and clonidine. *Heart* 1997;**77**:268–72.

140 Cohen MB, Snow JS, Grasso V, *et al*. Efficacy of pindolol for treatment of vasovagal syncope. *Am Heart J* 1995;**130**:786–90.

141 Iskos D, Dutton J, Scheinman MM, Lurie KG. Usefulness of pindolol in neurocardiogenic syncope. *Am J Cardiol* 1998;**82**:1121–4.

142 Muller G, Deal B, Strasburger JF, Benson DW Jr. Usefulness of metoprolol for unexplained syncope and positive response to tilt testing in young persons. *Am J Cardiol* 1993;**71**:592–5.

143 Brignole M, Menozzi C, Gianfranchi L, Lolli G, Bottoni N, Oddone D. A controlled trial of acute and long-term medical therapy in tilt-induced neurally mediated syncope. *Am J Cardiol* 1992;**70**:339–42.

144 Sheldon R, Rose S, Flanagan P, Koshman L, Killam S. Effects of beta isoproterenol tilt table test. *Am J Cardiol* 1996;**278**:536–9.

145 Di Girolamo E, DiIorio C, Sabatini P, Leonzio L, Barsotti A. Effects of different treatments vs. no treatment on neurocardiogenic syncope. *Cardiologia* 1998;**43**:833–7.

146 Madrid A, Ortega I, Rebollo GJ, *et al*. Lack of efficacy of atenolol for the prevention of neurally mediated syncope in highly symptomatic population: a prospective double-bind, randomized and placebo-controlled study. *J Am Coll Cardiol* 2001;**37**:554–7.

147 Ventura R, Maas R, Zeidler D, *et al*. A randomized and controlled pilot trial of β-blockers for the treatment of recurrent syncope in patients with a positive or negative

response to head-up tilt test. *Pacing Clin Electrophysiol* 2002;**25**:816–21.

148 Flevari P, Livanis E, Theodorakis G, Zarvalis E, Mesiskli T, Kremastinos DT. Vasovagal syncope: a prospective, randomized, cross-over evaluation of the effects of propranolol, nadolol and placebo on syncope recurrence and patients' well-being. *J Am Coll Cardiol* 2002;**40**: 499–504.

149 Fitzpatrick AP, Ahmed R, Williams S, Sutton R. A randomized trial of medical therapy in malignant vasovagal syndrome or neurally mediated bradycardia/hypotension syndrome. *Eur J Card Pacing Electrophysiol* 1991; **1**:191–202.

150 Davgovian M, Jarardilla R, Frumin H. Prolonged asystole during head upright tilt table testing after β-blockade. *Pacing Clin Electrophysiol* 1992;**15**:14–6.

151 Sheldon R. The Prevention of Syncope Trial (POST) Results: Oral Presentation. Heart Rhythm Society Meeting, San Francisco, CA, May 22, 2004.

152 Natale A, Sra J, Dhala A, *et al.* Efficacy of different treatment strategies for neurocardiogenic syncope. *PACE* 1995;**130**:1250–3.

153 Lee TM, Su SF, Chen MF, *et al.* Usefulness of transdermal scopolamine for vasovagal syncope. *Am J Cardiol* 1996;**78**:480–2.

154 Cadman CS. Medical therapy of neurocardiogenic syncope. *Cardiol Clin* 2001;**19**:1–18.

155 Milstein S, Buetikofer J, Durmigan A, *et al.* Usefulness of disopyramide for prevention of upright tilt-induced hypotension bradycardia. *Am J Cardiol* 1990;**65**:1334–44.

156 Morillo CA, Leitch JW, Yee R, Klein GJ. A placebo-controlled trial of disopyramide for neurally mediated syncope induced by head up tilt. *J Am Coll Cardiol* 1993;**22**:1843–8.

157 Kelly PA, Mann DE, Alder SW, *et al.* Low dose disopyramide often fails to prevent neurocardiogenic syncope. *PACE* 1994;**17**:573–6.

158 Strieper MJ, Campbell RM. Efficacy of alpha adrenergic agonist therapy for prevention of pediatric neurocardiogenic syncope. *J Am Coll Cardiol* 1993;**22**:594–7.

159 Janosik D, Holt D, Fredman C, *et al.* Efficacy of oral ephedrine sulfate in preventing neurocardiogenic syncope. *Circulation* 1991;**84**(II):234.

160 Susmano A, Volgman A, Buckingham T. Beneficial effects of dextroamphetamine in the treatment of vasodepressor syncope. *Pacing Clin Electrophysiol* 1993;**16**: 1235–8.

161 Grubb BP, Kosinski D, Kip K. Utility of methylphenidate in the therapy of refractory neurocardiogenic syncope. *Pacing Clin Electrophysiol* 1996;**19**:836–40.

162 Sra J, Maglio C, Biehl M, *et al.* Efficacy of midodrine hydrochloride in neurocardiogenic syncope refractory

to standard therapy. *J Cardiovasc Electrophysiol* 1997; **8**:42–6.

163 Grubb BP, Karas B, Kosinski D, Boehm K. Preliminary observations on the use of midodrine hydrochloride in the treatment of refractory neurocardiogenic syncope. *J Interv Card Electrophysiol* 1999;**3**:139–43.

164 Ward CR, Gray JC, Gilroy JJ, *et al.* Midodrine: a role in the management of neurocardiogenic syncope. *Heart* 1998;**79**:45–9.

165 Perez-Lugones A, Schweikert R, Pavia S, *et al.* Usefulness of midodrine in patients with severely symptomatic neurocardiogenic syncope: a randomized control study. *J Cardiovasc Electrophysiol* 2001;**12**:935–8.

166 Moya A, Permanycr-Miralda G, Sagrista-Sauleda J, *et al.* Limitations of head up tilt test for evaluating the efficacy of therapeutic interventions in patients with vasovagal syncope: results of a controlled study of etilefrine versus placebo. *J Am Coll Cardiol* 1995;**25**:65–9.

167 Raviele A, Brignole M, Sutton R, *et al.* Effect of etilefrine in preventing syncopal recurrence in patients with vasovagal syncope: a double-blind, randomized, placebo-controlled trial. The Vasovagal Syncope International Study. *Circulation* 1999;**99**:1452–7.

168 Biffi M, Boriani G, Sabbatini P, *et al.* Malignant vasovagal syncope: a randomized trial of metoprolol and clonidine. *Heart* 1997;**77**:268–72.

169 Zeng C, Zhu Z, Liu G, Hu W. Randomized double blind placebo controlled trial of oral enalapril in patients with neurally mediated syncope. *Am Heart J* 1998; **135**:852–8.

170 Grubb BP, Wolfe D, Samoil D, *et al.* Usefulness of fluoxetine hydrochloride for prevention of resistant upright tilt-induced syncope. *Pacing Clin Electrophysiol* 1993;**16**:458–64.

171 Grubb BP, Samoil D, Kosinski D, *et al.* The use of sertraline hydrochloride in the treatment of refractory neurocardiogenic syncope in children and adolescents. *J Am Coll Cardiol* 1994;**24**:490–4.

172 McGrady A, Bernal G. Relaxation-based treatment of stress-induced syncope. *J Behav Ther Exp Psychiatry* 1986;**17**:23–7.

173 McGrady AV, Bush EG, Grubb BP. Outcome of biofeedback-assisted relaxation for neurocardiogenic syncope and headache: a clinical replication series. *Appl Psychophysiol Biofeedback* 1997;**22**:63–72.

174 Fitzpatrick AP, Travill CM, Yardas PE, *et al.* Recurrent symptoms after ventricular pacing in unexplained syncope. *Pacing Clin Electrophysiol* 1990;**13**:619–24.

175 Fitzpatrick A, Sutton R. Tilting toward a diagnosis in recurrent unexplained syncope. *Lancet* 1989;**1**:658–60.

176 Fitzpatrick A, Theodorakis G, Ahmed R. Dual chamber pacing aborts vasovagal syncope induced by head up 60° tilt. *Pacing Clin Electrophysiol* 1991;**14**:13–9.

177 McGuinn P, Moore S, Edel T, *et al.* Temporary dual chamber pacing during tilt table testing for vasovagal syncope: predictor of therapeutic success (Abstract). *Pacing Clin Electrophysiol* 1991;**14**:734.

178 Samoil D, Grubb BP, Brewster P, *et al.* Comparison of single and dual chamber pacing techniques in the prevention of upright tilt-induced vasovagal syncope. *Eur J Card Pacing Electrophysiol* 1993;**3**:36–41.

179 Petersen ME, Chamberlain-Weber R, Fitzpatrick A, *et al.* Permanent pacing for prevention of recurrent vasovagal syncope. *Br Heart J* 1994;**71**:274–81.

180 Benditt D, Petersen ME, Lurie K, *et al.* Cardiac pacing for prevention of recurrent vasovagal syncope. *Ann Intern Med* 1995;**122**:204–9.

181 Connolly SJ, Sheldon R, Roberts RS, Gent M. The North American vasovagal pacemaker study (VPS): a randomized trial of permanent cardiac pacing for the prevention of vasovagal syncope. *J Am Coll Cardiol* 1999;**33**:16–20.

182 Sutton R, Brignole M, Menozzi C, *et al.* Dual chamber pacing in the treatment of neurally mediated tilt positive cardioinhibitory syncope. Pacemaker vs. no therapy: multicenter randomized study. *Circulation* 2000;**102**:294–9.

183 Ammirati F, Colivicchi F, Toscano S, *et al.* DDP packing with rate-drop function versus DDI with rate hysteresis pacing for cardioinhibitory vasovagal syncope. *PACE* 1998;**21**:2178–81.

184 Ammirati F, Colivicchi F, Santini M. Permanent cardiac pacing versus medical treatment for the prevention of recurrent vasovagal syncope: a multicentre, randomized controlled trial. *Circulation* 2001;**104**:52–7.

185 Connolly S, Sheldon R, Thorpe K, *et al.* Pacemaker therapy for prevention of syncope in patients with recurrent severe vasovagal syncope. Second vasovagal pacemaker study (VPSII): a randomized trial. *JAMA* 2003;**289**:2224–9.

186 Giada F, Raviele A, Menozzi C, *et al.* The vasovagal syncope and pacing trial (SYNPACE): a randomized placebo controlled study of permanent cardiac pacing for treatment of recurrent vasovagal syncope. *PACE* 2003;**26**:1016.

187 Sutton R. Has cardiac pacing a role in vasovagal syncope? *J Interv Card Electrophysiol* 2003;**9**:145–9.

188 Sra JS. Can we assess the efficacy of therapy in neurocardiogenic syncope? *J Am Coll Cardiol* 2001;**37**: 560–1.

189 Bloomfield DM, Sheldon R, Grubb BP, Calkins H, Sutton R. Putting it together: a new treatment algorithm for vasovagal syncope and related disorders. *Am J Cardiol* 1999;**84**:33Q–9Q.

CHAPTER 3

Dysautonomic (orthostatic) syncope

Blair P. Grubb, MD

Introduction

One of the truly defining moments in the long process of human evolution was the adoption of upright posture. Although it greatly enhanced mobility, upright posture placed a new burden on a blood pressure control system that had evolved principally to meet the needs of an animal in the dorsal position. Thus, humans demonstrate an enhanced susceptibility to the effects of gravity on circulation. Indeed, the very organ that defines our humanity – the brain – is in the most precarious of locations in regard to vascular perfusion. The greatest challenge imposed on the body by upright posture is the downward shift of blood to a level below the heart. Via the sympathetic efferent pathways, the autonomic nervous system is the principal source of both short- and medium-term responses to these positional changes. Although other mechanisms such as the renin-angiotensin-aldosterone system also contribute, their responses are seen over a much longer period. Thus, disturbances in autonomic function resulting in sympathetic failure can result in orthostatic (or positional) hypotension, which may be of a degree sufficient to lead to cerebral hypoperfusion and ultimately to loss of consciousness (syncope).

This chapter focuses on autonomic dysfunction as a cause of orthostatic hypotension leading to syncope. It reviews the physiological and biochemical abnormalities associated with these disorders, as well as the signs and symptoms commonly associated with them. It also provides an outline of both neurogenic and non-neurogenic causes of orthostatic hypotension, a suggested plan of evaluation, and potential treatment options that are available.

Historical aspects

The concept of a sympathetic nervous system whose role is the regulation of the body's multiple functions seems to have been first proposed by the Roman physician Galen in the second century of the current era [1]. Galen described a nerve trunk lying along the posterior ribs and observed that they were connected by fibers to the spinal cord. He thought that the nerves were hollow tubes that served to distribute "animal spirits" throughout the body, thereby leading to "sympathy" or "concert" between various body parts. Centuries later (in 1552) the Renaissance physician Eustachius made detailed descriptions of the sympathetic chain as well as the adrenal glands [2]. Jacobus Winslow (1732) expanded on these ideas and thought that the ganglia served as "small brains" and described the chain as the "great sympathetic nerve" [3].

By the middle of the 19th century much more elaborate anatomical as well as functional studies were being performed. In 1878, Benard first reported on the vasodilatory effects of sympathetic nerve sectioning, whereas Brown-Sequard produced vasoconstriction by stimulating the cut ends of sympathetic nerves [1]. Shortly thereafter Gaskell divided the system (both morphologically and functionally) into two divisions: the thoracolumbar (sympathetic) and craniosacral (parasympathetic) [4]. By 1895 Oliver and Schäfer [5] discovered the cardio-stimulatory effects of adrenal gland extracts. Shortly thereafter Abel and Takamine isolated the active substance from the adrenal glands: epinephrine (also referred to as adrenalin in Europe). The term *autonomic nervous system* (ANS) was first introduced by Langley [6] in 1898 to describe the part of the nervous system that controlled the involuntary or vegetative functions of the organs (as opposed to those involved in the voluntary control of the skeletal muscles). Langley later coined the term *parasympathetic* nervous system to describe the craniosacral portion of the ANS so as to distinguish it from sympathetic nerves that came from the thoracolumbar ganglia.

By the early part of the 20th century the noted physiologist Walter Cannon [7] proposed that the adrenal glands and the sympathetic nerves constituted a single functional unit, which he termed the "sympathico-adrenal system." He further proposed that the sympathetic system principally served to function during emergent situations (fight or flight) while the parasympathetic would serve to run processes such as digestion, during periods of quiescence (rest and digest). To describe the state of balance between these two opposing systems Cannon [8] coined the term *homeostasis*, citing it as an example of "the Wisdom of the Body." Later investigations found evidence that norepinephrine was the principal neurotransmitter of the sympathetic nervous system and acetylcholine that of the parasympathetic system. However, by the 1960s it had become evident that many autonomic nerve fibers were neither adrenergic nor cholinergic [1]. During this period, Burnstock found non-adrenergic, non-cholinergic autonomic neurons in the myenteric plexus of the intestine, thus establishing evidence for what has come to be known as the *enteric nervous system*. Shortly thereafter, adenosine triphosphate (ATP) was identified as a neurotransmitter for these nerves. In 1976, Burnstock [9] found that autonomic nerve cells may actually release more than one neurotransmitter. The amount of the coexistence and co-release of neurotransmitters (referred to as chemical coding) has promoted detailed investigations into the effects of various illnesses on the autonomic neuroeffector junction.

The idea that altered autonomic nervous system function could produce a disease state is a relatively recent one, dating from Bradbury and Eggleston's classic paper in 1925 [10]. Since that time there has been a tremendous growth in our knowledge of autonomic function as well as a greater appreciation of illnesses produced when any aspect of the system fails.

Maintenance of postural normotension

In the normal human subject, approximately 25–30% of the circulating blood volume is in the thorax [11]. Assumption of the upright posture results in the gravity-mediated displacement of approximately 300–800 mL of blood (or 6–8 mL/kg) to the abdomen and lower extremities. This represents a volume drop of 26–30%, with up to 50% of this fall occurring within seconds of standing. This rapid fall in central blood volume results in a drop in venous return to the heart [12]. Because the heart cannot pump out what it does not receive, there is a reduction in stroke volume of approximately 40% resulting from the decrease in cardiac filling pressure [13]. This brings about a decrease in intravascular pressure above, and an increase in intravascular pressure below, what is referred to as the venous hydrostatic indifference point (HIP) [11]. The HIP represents the site in the vascular tree where pressure is independent of posture. In humans, the venous HIP is at roughly the diaphragmatic level, while the arterial HIP is around the level of the left ventricle. Because the level of the venous HIP is to a large extent dependent on venous compliance, it can be affected by muscular activity [14]. During standing, leg muscle contractions combined with the venous valve system actively drive blood back to the heart, moving the HIP upward toward the right atrium. Respiratory activity also contributes to an increase in venous return. During deep inspiration there is a reduction in thoracic pressure favoring inward flow, while at the same time the intra-abdominal pressure increases, reducing retrograde flow because of compression of the iliac and femoral veins [15].

In addition to these changes, upright posture also results in a large increase in the transmural capillary pressure in the dependent regions of the body, resulting in a net increase in fluid filtration into the tissue spaces. Equilibration of this transcapillary fluid shift occurs after approximately 30 min upright, during which there can be a net fall in plasma volume of up to 10% [12].

In order for standing to occur successfully, a series of cardiovascular regulating mechanisms are brought into play, all aimed at preserving a constant level of arterial pressure and cerebral perfusion despite the effects of gravity. In normal subjects, orthostatic stabilization is achieved in 1 min or less [11]. Interestingly, recent investigations have disclosed differences between the initial circulatory responses elicited by standing (active change) and those brought on by head-up tilt (passive change) [16]. Wieling *et al.* [17] and Wieling and van Lieshot [18] have divided the orthostatic response into three phases:

1 initial response (the first 30 s);
2 the early "steady state" circulatory adjustment (after 1–2 min upright);
3 prolonged orthostasis (at least 5 min upright).

These responses seem to differ somewhat according to whether the orthostatic stress is passive (tilt) or active (standing).

Immediately following head-up tilt, cardiac stroke volume remains normal for about six beats, despite a fall in venous return (largely brought about by the blood in the pulmonary circulation). Next there is a gradual decline in both cardiac filling and arterial pressure [13,18]. These changes activate two groups of pressure receptors: high-pressure sites in the carotid sinus and the aortic arch, and low-pressure sites in the cardiac and pulmonary areas. In regard to the latter, mechanoreceptors subserved by unmyelinated vagal afferents are present in all four cardiac chambers. These mechanoreceptors produce a tonic inhibitory effect on the cardiovascular centers of the medulla (in particular the nucleus tractus solitarii) [11]. The reduction in venous return and filling pressure that results from the assumption of upright posture unloads these receptors, decreasing their firing rates thereby eliciting a reflex increase in sympathetic outflow with a resultant increase in vascular constriction in both the systemic resistance vessels and the splanchnic capacitance vessels [13,19]. A second local axon reflex, called the venoarteriolar axon reflex, also constricts arterial flow to muscle, skin, and adipose tissue [20]. This reflex can account for up to half of the increase in limb vascular resistance seen during standing.

Head-up tilt also seems to activate high-pressure receptors located in the carotid sinus. The initial increase in heart rate seen during tilt appears to be modulated by a fall in carotid arterial pressure. The gradual increase in diastolic pressure seen during tilt appears more closely related to an increase in peripheral vascular resistance [21].

The initial circulatory response to standing is somewhat different [18]. The more active process of standing causes contraction of muscles in the legs and abdomen, resulting in the compression of both the capacitance and resistance vessels and an increase in peripheral vascular resistance. This actually results in a mild transient elevation in right atrial pressure and cardiac output that causes activation of low-pressure cardiac receptors [21]. This increase in neural traffic to the brainstem causes a sudden decrease in peripheral vascular resistance that may drop by as much as 40% [14]. This in turn can allow for a fall in mean arterial blood pressure of up to 20 mmHg that will last for up to 6–8 s. This drop is then addressed by the aforementioned mechanisms.

The early steady state period during upright posture is characterized by a steady increase in diastolic pressure of approximately 10%, with little or no change in systolic blood pressure. There is also an increase in heart rate of approximately 10 b min^{-1}. Compared with supine position, there is 30% less blood in the thorax, the cardiac output is 30% less, and the heart rate goes up by 10–15 b min^{-1} [16,21].

Prolonged upright posture also brings neurohumoral mechanisms into play. The exact extent to which these mechanisms are activated depends, to a large extent, on the volume status of the patient. The greater the degree of volume depletion, the greater the degree of activation by the renin-angiotensin-aldosterone system, as well as that of vasopressin [22]. However, the principal mechanism by which prolonged upright posture is compensated for lies in the arterial baroreceptor (especially carotid sinus) influence on peripheral vascular resistance [11]. Failure of any component in these complex responses can lead to a failure of normal compensation to postural change, which can lead to hypotension and resultant syncope. In a broad sense, the term dysautonomia indicates a state in which a disturbance in autonomic nervous system function adversely affects health [23]. These conditions range from relatively benign transient periods of autonomic tone in otherwise normal individuals to potentially lethal neurodegenerative disorders.

Disturbances in orthostatic regulation

Over the last several decades several disturbances in orthostatic regulation have been identified [13]. Although they share many characteristics, each is nevertheless unique. A basic system of classification is presented in Fig. 3.1. In constructing any classification system it should be remembered that when we observe nature we see what we want to see according to what we believe we know about it at the time. In order to make some sense of the apparent chaos of nature, we try to classify it into a coherent system that conforms to our observations and expectations. Thus, any system of classification is in some ways arbitrary and open to revision over time. The system presented here (Fig. 3.1) has proven to be clinically useful and follows the basic guidelines established by the American Autonomic Society (AAS) and the American Academy of Neurology (AAN) in 1996 [24,25]. The reflex syncopes representing disorders such as neurocardiogenic syncope and carotid sinus hypersensitivity are discussed in separate chapters (as are the postural tachycardia syndromes). Some investigators have tended to classify the etiology of these disorders into primary and secondary causes (Table 3.1). The primary forms are, at present, idiopathic in nature and can be further subdivided into acute and chronic forms. The secondary forms are those that are seen in association with other disease processes (such as diabetes, multiple myeloma and amyloidosis), exposure to toxic compounds (alcohol and heavy metals), or medications (antineoplastic drugs, amiodarone, antihypertensive and antidepressant agents). Indeed, orthostatic hypotension may accompany any condition that causes a significant reduction in blood or extracellular fluid volume, or which results in being bedridden for an extended period of time. None the less, orthostatic hypotension is the principal expression of autonomic neurocirculatory dysfunction, and in the absence of any identifiable cause is referred to as autonomic failure (which may either be acute or chronic in presentation) [3].

Chronic autonomic failure
Primary syndromes
The first reports of chronic autonomic failure were made by Bradbury and Eggleston in 1925 [10].

They used the term "idiopathic orthostatic hypotension" to describe an "extensive and peculiar disturbance in the functional activity of the vegetative nervous system" resulting from its lack of coexisting overt neurologic defects. However, the term "idiopathic orthostatic hypotension" has been felt to be inadequate as it fails to express the fact that these patients tend to have a generalized state of autonomic failure that is associated with disturbed bladder, bowel, sudomotor, and sexual function (with a lack of somatic nerve involvement). At present, the term pure autonomic failure (PAF) is used to describe this condition [24]. The terms and definitions employed here are based on those outlined in the joint AAS–AAN consensus statement [25].

Symptoms of PAF usually begin in middle age, with the majority of cases being diagnosed between ages 50 and 70 years [26]. The disorder is more frequent in men than women, with a reported 2 : 1 ratio [27]. The symptoms of PAF are often slow and insidious in onset, with mild symptoms that are concealed for years because of autonomic or other compensatory mechanisms. Orthostatic hypotension is usually the most debilitating symptom of PAF and, while it may not be the first symptom experienced, it is usually the one that prompts patients to seek medical attention. Patients often relate initial vague symptoms of orthostatic weakness, dizziness, and presyncope that are frequently dismissed by physicians as insignificant (which may result in a referral to a psychiatrist). Presyncope and syncope (often in the morning, after meals, exercise, hot baths, or in hot weather) are some of the symptoms that lead patients to seek medical advice. As opposed to neurocardiogenic (vasovagal) syncope, patients with advanced PAF do not relate having nausea, vomiting, diaphoresis, or pallor in association with loss of consciousness [28]. More often, patients will describe their syncope as a gradual fading of consciousness. However, because many patients experience a kind of amnesia to events around the syncopal episode, they may report it as a "drop attack." Other orthostatic complaints include weakness, fatigue, gait disturbance, neck pain, and visual blurring. Supine hypertension is not uncommon in many patients, the etiology of which is still unclear. The full syndrome is characterized by pronounced orthostatic hypotension

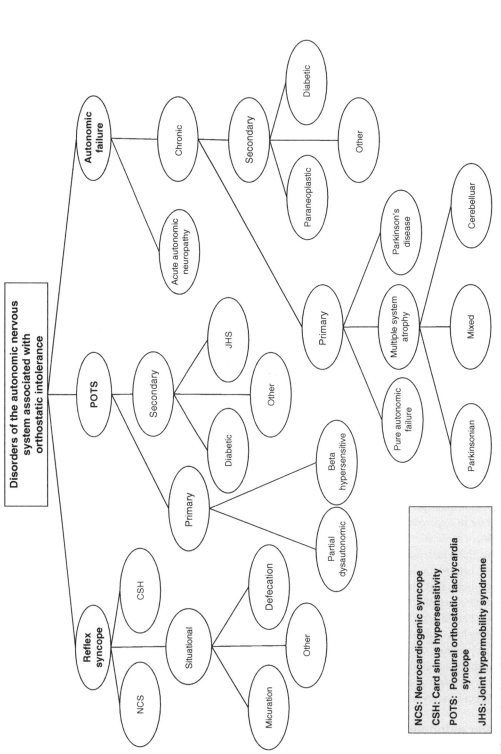

Fig. 3.1 Disorders of the autonomic nervous system associated with orthostatic intolerance.

Table 3.1 Autonomic disorders associated with orthostatic intolerance.

Primary autonomic disorders

Acute pandysautonomia

Pure autonomic failure

Multiple system atrophy

Parkinsonism

Pyramidal/cerebellar

Mixed

Reflex syncopes

Neurocardiogenic syncope

Carotid sinus hypersensitivity

Secondary autonomic failure

Central origin

Cerebral cancer

Multiple sclerosis

Age-related

Syringobulbia

Peripheral forms

Afferent

  Guillain–Barré syndrome

  tabes dorsalis

  Holmes–Adie syndrome

Efferent

  diabetes mellitus

  nerve growth factor deficiency

  dopamine β-hydroxylase deficiency

Afferent/efferent

  familial dysautonomia

Spinal origin

  transverse myelitis

  syringomyelia

  spinal tumors

Other causes

  renal failure

  paraneoplastic syndromes

  autoimmune/collagen vascular disease

  human immunodeficiency virus infection

  amyloidosis

(with presyncope and syncope), constipation, early satiety, abdominal pain (resulting from poor bowel motility), lack of ability to sweat, temperature intolerance, urinary retention, and dry mouth [29]. In men, impotence and loss of libido are often the first symptoms, whereas women usually first complain of urinary retention and incontinence.

While PAF may lead to severe (potentially disabling) functional impairment, it rarely leads to death [30].

A very different situation occurs when primary autonomic failure is associated with other idiopathic somatic neurologic defects, a condition first described by Shy and Drager in 1960 [31,32,]. More recently, the term multisystem atrophy (MSA) has been used to describe this condition (as the term Shy–Drager syndrome was never well defined and led to increasing confusion) [24]. There is little that can match the eloquence of the initial report:

> The full syndrome consists of the following features; orthostatic hypotension, urinary and rectal incontinence, loss of sweating, iris atrophy, external ocular palsies, rigidity, tremor, loss of associated movements, impotence, the findings of an atonic bladder, and loss of rectal sphincter tone, fasciculations, wasting of distal muscles, evidence of a neuropathic lesion in the electromyogram that suggests involvement of the anterior horn cells, and the finding of a neuropathic lesion in the muscle biopsy. The date of onset is usually in the 5th to 7th decade of life [31].

Men are affected by MSA about twice as often as women [27]. While patients may present with initial signs and symptoms that suggest PAF, they slowly begin to develop disturbances in somatic nervous system functions. As in PAF, presyncope and syncope are the symptoms most likely to cause a patient to seek medical attention [28].

MSA is classified into three major subgroups according to the somatic nerve system involved [24,27]. Unlike PAF, in MSA there is significant central nervous system (CNS) involvement. The first subgroup consists of those patients who, in addition to autonomic failure, develop features suggestive of Parkinson's disease (some investigators employ the term striatonigral degeneration to describe this group, others use the designation MSA-P) [33]. These patients may exhibit stiffness, clumsiness, or a change in handwriting early in the course of their illness. As opposed to classic Parkinson's disease, in parkinsonian MSA, there is a predominance of rigidity without much tremor that is associated with a progressive loss of facial expression and limb akinesia [29]. While the parkinsonian MSA patient may develop limb rigidity, they lack the classic "cogwheel" or "lead pipe" rigidity that is typical in true Parkinson's disease. None the less, it may be quite difficult to distinguish the parkinsonian form of MSA from Parkinson's disease [34]. Recent studies have found that between 7% and 22% of patients thought to have Parkinson's disease while alive were, at autopsy, found to exhibit neuropathologic features consistent with MSA [35].

A second group of MSA patients are distinguished by manifesting cerebellar and/or pyramidal features (a condition referred to as "cerebellar" MSA-C or "olivopontocerebellar" atrophy) [36]. In this group of MSA patients there is a prominent disturbance of gait with an associated truncal ataxia that can be severe enough to prevent the patient from standing without support. Slurring of speech is often present as is a progressive loss of diction. A mild to moderate intention tremor often affects the arms and legs. Lastly, there are patients who appear to have a mixed form of the disorder who display both cerebellar and parkinsonian features (some investigators use the term MSA-A [autonomic] to describe these individuals when autonomic dysfunction is the principal clinical manifestation) [37]. The natural history of MSA is one of relentless progression. The majority of patients with MSA die within 5–8 years of onset (although rare cases have survived up to 20 years) [30]. Aspiration, apnea, and ultimately respiratory failure are the principal final events.

Over the last several years it has become evident that true Parkinson's disease itself may be a cause of orthostatic hypotension. Parkinson's disease is an idiopathic neurodegenerative disorder resulting from a loss of pigmented dopanergic cells within the brain's substantia nigra which project to the striatum (involving both the putamen and caudate regions) [38]. Affecting an estimated 1% of the population over the age of 65 years, it causes tremor, bradykinesia, rigidity, and the loss of postural reflexes. Until relatively recently, the presence of orthostatic hypotension in Parkinson's disease was felt to occur mainly as a result of either medications or inactivity. Most of the dopaminergic drugs used to treat Parkinson's disease can cause orthostatic hypotension. However, it is now thought that Parkinson's disease itself may lead to orthostatic hypotension as well as other symptoms of autonomic failure [39]. In Parkinson's disease, extrapyramidal motor problems are the presenting symptoms. Only later in the disease process do patients develop significant autonomic failure, at which point it becomes difficult to distinguish between Parkinson's disease and MSA.

Using neuroimaging techniques applied to the heart, Goldstein et al. [40] have been able to distinguish between different forms of autonomic failure. Sympathetic nerves in the heart absorb both ^{123}I-metaiodobezylguanidine (^{123}I-MIBG) and 6-[^{18}F] fluorodopamine which then radiolabel the vesicles in these sympathetic nerve terminals. This permits the visualization of the sympathetic innervation of the heart by utilizing either single-photon emission computed tomography after administration of ^{123}I-MIBG or by using positron emission tomography (PET) after administration of 6-[^{18}F] fluorodopamine [3]. The visualization occurs independent of adrenoreceptor binding because it depends mainly upon active transport of the labeled tracer by the uptake process, which is followed by its sequestration in the vesicles.

These studies have demonstrated that patients suffering from MSA (of any subtype) have relatively intact cardiac sympathetic innervation and a marked decrease in blood pressure following ganglionic blockade with trimetaphan. Conversely, patients with either PAF or Parkinson's disease have virtually no detectable amounts of the aforementioned tracer substances in the left ventricular myocardium and a very modest decrease in blood pressure in response to trimetaphan. Patients with PAF and Parkinson's disease also display extremely reduced (or absent) cardiac spillover of norepinephrine, levodopa, and dihydroxyphenylglycol (DHPG), all of which indicate a tremendous loss of sympathetic nerve terminal innervation in the heart [3].

These contrasting findings suggest the existence of a preganglionic lesion in MSA and a postganglionic lesion in both PAF and in Parkinson's disease. This later finding has demonstrated that, at least in some instances, Parkinson's disease may have extensive peripheral as well as central involvement. Kaufman [37] has suggested that the same neurodegenerative process is at work in MSA, Parkinson's disease and PAF, because in each of these disorders α-synuclein accumulates in neuronal cytoplasmic inclusions. A gene that codes for alpha-synuclein (a neuronal protein of unknown function) is mutated in the autosomal dominant form of Parkinson's disease. It was recently reported that the cytoplasmic inclusions found in the neural cells of MSA patients stain positive for alpha-synuclein. At the same time, the Lewy bodies found in neural cells of patients with PAF will also stain strongly positive for α-synuclein. Kaufman proposed that abnormalities in the expression or structure of alpha-synuclein or related proteins may result in degeneration of catecholamine-containing neurons, raising the possibility that the chronic primary autonomic failure syndromes are actually three different presentations of one disease. Further studies are underway to evaluate this hypothesis.

Acute autonomic failure

Acute panautonomic neuropathy, causing orthostatic hypotension and syncope, is uncommon but often dramatic in its presentation [41]. The principal features that characterize acute panautonomic neuropathy (also called pandysautonomia) are elaborated by Low and McLeod [42] and consist of:
1 acute or subacute onset;
2 widespread and severe sympathetic and parasympathetic failure;
3 relative or total sparing of somatic nerve fibers.
In almost every case, this acute onset of sympathetic and parasympathetic failure occurs in relatively young people who were previously quite healthy. Malfunction of the sympathetic nervous system results in severe orthostatic hypotension of such a degree that patients are unable to sit upright in bed without losing consciousness. There is often a loss of sweating. Failure of the parasympathetic system results in dry mouth and eyes and a disruption in both bladder and bowel function. The latter is manifested by abdominal pain, bloating, nausea, vomiting, and severe constipation that may occasionally alternate with profuse diarrhea [43]. One of the most prominent features of the disorder is that patients often have a fixed heart rate of approximately 40–55 b min^{-1} with complete chronotropic incompetence. Many patients will also have fixed dilated pupils. Occasionally, acute autonomic fail-

ure is accompanied by acute and inexorable neuropathic pain that may be truly agonizing to the patient [42].

The rapidness of the onset of symptoms is often quite dramatic, and many of our patients have been able to relate the exact moment the illness began. Many patients complain of an antecedent febrile illness (presumed to be a viral infection), suggesting that the illness may be immune mediated. Indeed, Verino et al. [44] have demonstrated high levels of ganglionic acetylcholine receptor (ACLR) autoantibodies in these patients, usually ≥ 1.00 nmol/L. The level of these autoantibodies seems to correlate well with the severity and progression of the illness.

On physical examination these patients display profound orthostatic hypotension, a fixed heart rate, and fixed dilated pupils. Patients often suffer from urinary retention as well as dry, flaky skin. Gross motor strength and sensory perception are usually normal, although occasional patients experience abnormal pain and temperature perception. There has been little systematic evaluation of the course and long-term prognosis of patients with an acute autonomic neuropathy. Although some patients make remarkable recoveries, for others the disease follows a chronic, debilitating course that leaves significant residual defects in its wake [45].

Secondary causes

Secondary autonomic failure (or dysfunction) is said to occur where the exact lesion has been identified or where there is a clear association with a known disease (e.g., diabetes mellitus or a spinal cord injury). As outlined in Table 3.1, there are a large variety of disorders that may be accompanied by autonomic dysfunction.

An acute or chronic autonomic neuropathy may be seen as an effect of a malignancy (most often small cell carcinoma of the lung) [46]. Paraneoplastic autonomic neuropathy may cause a progressive panautonomic neuropathy or may result in gastro-intestinal dysmotility (such as gastroparesis or intestinal pseudo-obstruction). Malignancy-related autonomic dysfunction may also occur in conjunction with other paraneoplastic neurological disturbances (myelopathy, limbic encephalitis, or ataxia). Paraneoplastic autonomic neuropathy has been linked to the production of autoantibodies, in particular autoneuronal nuclear antibody type 1 (ANNA-1 or anti-Hu) [47]. Sometimes, autoantibodies are extremely specific for a particular malignancy. For example, small cell cancer of the lung was found to exist in 80% of patients who were seropositive for ANNA-1. A variety of other malignancy-specific autoantibodies have been isolated and can be effectively identified during serologic screening (see Chapter 9). In a patient with a suspected malignancy-related dysautonomia, screening for all known cancer-related antibodies should be performed, and if found should prompt a rigorous search for the presence of a malignancy.

Diabetic autonomic neuropathy is a common, stealthy complication of diabetes that occurs over prolonged periods of time, affecting virtually any organ of the body from skin to gastrointestinal control [48]. In the peripheral nerves, autonomic unmyelinated fibers are found together with unmyelinated somatic fibers as well as large sensory and motor myelinated fibers. The reported incidence of diabetic autonomic neuropathy varies greatly, with reported ranges from 50 to 100%. While clinical symptoms usually do not appear for years after the onset of diabetes, subclinical neuropathy can be seen with laboratory testing within 1 year of diagnosis in type 2 diabetes and within 2 years in patients with type 1 disease. Orthostatic hypotension often indicates advanced generalized autonomic failure, the frequency of which is reported to be from 17 to 43% [49]. In diabetic patients with symptomatic autonomic dysfunction, approximately 25–50% die within 5–10 years of diagnosis. The 5-year mortality of diabetic patients with autonomic neuropathy is three times higher than for those patients without autonomic involvement, most often because of increased rates of cardiovascular and renal disease. Lack of heart rate variability during exercise or deep breathing is an ominous sign of autonomic neuropathy and is associated with a high risk of coronary artery disease.

Amyloidosis, either as primary disorder or in association with multiple myeloma, often results in a peripheral neuropathy with autonomic failure [50]. Neuropathic symptoms usually begin with distal sensory loss as well as increased temperature thresholds. Autonomic symptoms are common and syncope and near syncope are also quite common. Diffuse anhidrosis with compensatory sweat-

ing of unaffected areas is common. Macroglossia and weight loss can be useful clues to accurate diagnosis. The diagnosis is confirmed by finding amyloid deposits in biopsies of fat, sural nerve, and rectal tissue. Cardiac involvement carries a particularly poor prognosis. Death usually occurs resulting from renal failure or cardiac arrhythmias.

Recent investigations have revealed that orthostatic hypotension may occur as a result of a single enzyme abnormality. An example of this is β-hydroxylase (DβH) deficiency, a syndrome characterized by sympathetic noradrenergic denervation and adrenomedullary failure, with intact vagal and sympathetic cholinergic function [51]. A five- to tenfold increase in normal serum dopamine levels with virtually undetectable levels of serum epinephrine and norepinephrine is diagnostic for the disorder. Another condition that can cause orthostatic hypotension is nerve growth factor deficiency (which may actually cause DβH deficiency) as well as dopa decarboxylase deficiency and reductions in certain sensory neuropeptides. Orthostatic hypotension may also be seen as a complication of neurologic disorders that affect other neuronal systems (such as the thalamus or from prion-mediated disorders such as fatal familial dysautonomia. Orthostatic hypotension may also accompany conditions such as chronic renal failure and the acquired immune deficiency syndrome (AIDS).

Pharmacologic agents that affect the sympathetic nervous system may either cause or exacerbate orthostatic hypotension (Table 3.2). Drugs with central activity include reserpine, barbiturates, methyldopa, clonidine, and tricyclic antidepressants. Peripherally acting agents include prazosin, phenoxybenzamine, guanethidine, angiotensin-converting enzyme inhibitors, and beta-blocking agents. Indeed, virtually any vasodilatory agent may exacerbate on otherwise mild tendency toward orthostatic hypotension.

A variety of other agents have also been implicated in producing orthostatic hypotension [47]. Principal among these have been the chemotherapeutic agents such as cis-platinum and the vinca alkaloids (vinblastine, vincristine, and vindesine). Amiodarone has been associated with a neuropathic syndrome consisting of orthostatic hypotension along with a mixed sensory motor neuropathy associated with a myopathy. Luckily, amiodarone neuropathy

Table 3.2 Pharmacologic agents that may cause or worsen orthostatic intolerance.

Angiotensin-converting enzyme inhibitors
α-Receptor blockers
Calcium-channel blockers
Beta-blockers
Phenothiazines
Tricyclic antidepressants
Bromocriptine
Ethanol
Opiates
Diuretics
Hydralazine
Ganglionic-blocking agents
Nitrates
Sildenafil citrate
Vardenafil HCl
MAO inhibitors

MAO, monoamine oxidase.

usually subsides after the drug is discontinued. Perhexiline maleate is a calcium-channel blocker used in the treatment of angina. Chronic use of the agent has been associated with a mixed sensory motor neuropathy, orthostatic hypotension, weight loss, and liver toxicity. Disturbances in autonomic function have been seen following prolonged exposure to a variety of organic solvents that principally contain aliphatic, aromatic, and other hydrocarbons, alcohols, ketones, esters, and ethers. Carbon disulfide and toluene have also been implicated. Hexacarbon neuropathy may occur from occupational exposure or by intentional inhalation (glue sniffing). A rapidly progressive polyneuropathy associated with orthostatic hypotension, impotence, vasomotor instability, and either excessive or impaired sweating. Indeed, it should be kept in mind that occasional patients may be covertly using illicit drugs (unbeknown to family and friends) that result in orthostatic intolerance. In addition, a patient may be secretly using an agent to produce a fictitious illness (Munchausen syndrome) so as to simulate orthostatic hypotension.

Clinical features

The principal finding in all of the aforementioned disorders is of an impairment of normal cardio-vascular regulation that produces orthostatic (or postural) hypotension. Orthostatic hypotension is usually considered as a fall of > 20 mmHg systolic blood pressure within 2–3 min of standing [24]. However, this definition is somewhat arbitrary, and it is important to realize that a more modest drop in blood pressure associated with symptoms may be just as important. It also should be remembered that some patients will demonstrate a gradual but progressive fall in blood pressure over a longer time frame (such as 10–15 min) that will be associated with symptoms. Symptom provocation is dependent not only on the absolute fall in blood pressure, but also the rate of change and the ability of the cerebral vasculature to auto-regulate sufficiently to maintain perfusion despite systemic hypotension. It is also important to remember that orthostatic hypotension is often only one aspect of a more general disturbance in cardiovascular regulation. Patients may also experience supine hypertension or erratic swings in blood pressure and may exhibit excessive blood pressure responses to a variety of physiologic or pharmacologic challenges.

The syncopal episodes that accompany orthostatic hypotension will, on occasion, be reported as "drop attacks" which occur with little or no warning. More commonly, there is a gradual loss of consciousness over half a minute or so while the patient is standing or walking (and on occasion while sitting). Many patients will describe a neck ache that radiates to the occipital region of the skull and to the shoulders (sometimes called a "coat hanger" distribution) which occurs prior to loss of consciousness. The mechanism of this frequent and virtually unique symptom of orthostatic hypotension is unclear (although some have postulated it to be caused by ischemia in continuously contracting postural muscles) [29]. The neck ache may be associated with a progressive anterior cervical flexion of the neck (anterocollis). Muscle ischemia has also been implicated in other symptoms in autonomic failure. Some patients describe typical symptoms of exertional angina while others describe symptoms of claudication. Blurred vision may also occur as a result of a fall in blood delivery to the retina (the eye is not buffered against blood pressure changes as the brain and brainstem are by the pressure-stabilizing effects of cerebrospinal fluid), as may

Table 3.3 Distinguishing features among pure autonomic failure, autonomic neuropathy, and multiple system atrophy (adapted from Low and Bannister [27]).

Factor	PAF	Autonomic neuropathy	MSA
Onset	Slow	Acute	Slow
Primary symptom	Orthostatic hypotension	Diverse symptoms	Orthostatic hypotension Genitourinary problems
Gastrointestinal problems	Rare (except constipation)	Common	Uncommon
CNS disturbance	Absent	Absent	Present
Somatic neuropathy	Absent	Mild	Occurring in 15–25%
Pain	Absent	Common	Absent
Progression	Slowly progressive	Usually not progressive	Progressive
Principal lesion site	Principally postganglionic	Postganglionic Some somatic	Mainly preganglionic and central
Supine plasma norepinephrine	Low	Low	Normal
Prognosis	Fair to good	Fair to good	Poor

CNS, central nervous system; MSA, multiple system atrophy; PAF, pure autonomic failure.

tunnel vision, scotoma, and hallucinations [52]. Unlike classic vasovagal syncope, there is no associated diaphoresis and the episodes are not accompanied by bradycardia. Often, the symptoms occur within minutes upon standing or walking, when the patient may stumble, fall, or sink to their knees as consciousness is lost. Recovery and loss of most symptoms usually occur within several minutes after becoming supine (although on occasion they may last longer). Most patients report that symptoms are far worse in the morning, in hot weather, after exercise, and following meals (particularly if accompanied by alcohol consumption), all of which result in a redistribution of blood volume to peripheral or mesenteric areas.

Many patients with autonomic failure experience an impairment in temperature regulation which is exacerbated by an inability to sweat properly. This leads them to be prone to overheating during periods of high ambient temperatures. Impotence is common among male patients and may be the first symptom that patients encounter. Bloating and constipation are common, and difficulty swallowing and rectal incontinence may occur in the late stages of MSA [27]. A severe disturbance of bowel function with severe diarrhea and fecal incontinence suggest the possibility of amyloidosis. A relatively common complaint is that of nocturnal polyuria. This is thought to occur when pooled peripheral blood is redistributed to

the central areas during prolonged supine posture (similar to the mechanism causing paroxysmal nocturnal dyspnea). Some patients may lose up to 1 L of urine during a single evening, greatly exacerbating the tendency toward morning hypotension.

The patient with MSA may exhibit progressive muscle wasting, although not to the extent seen in the motor neuron disorders such as amyotrophic lateral sclerosis. In PAF and MSA there is no increased tendency towards dementia, whereas intellectual impairment is a not infrequent feature of Parkinson's disease [29].

Postprandial hypotension can pose a significant problem for patients with autonomic failure. Glucose is the principal component of food responsible for the fall in pressure. Lipids have a somewhat slower hypotensive effect, while protein causes only minimal changes. Insulin has been implicated in the production of hypotension, as it has a blood pressure lowering effect that appears to occur independently of hypoglycemia. Insulin has also been shown to increase arteriovenous shunts controlled by peripheral nerves.

Patients with MSA often develop both obstructive and central sleep apnea, manifested by loud snoring as well as involuntary inspiratory gasps. MSA patients may die suddenly during sleep. Table 3.3 outlines some of the clinical features that can help distinguish PAF from MSA and acute autonomic neuropathy.

Evaluation

As in all of clinical medicine, the first and most important step is a detailed history and physical examination. Laboratory testing is then ordered based on the history and physical examination, and information from all these sources is used to arrive at a diagnosis and outline a reasonable and comprehensive plan of management.

The first and foremost goal is to determine whether an autonomic disorder is present, and if so to ascertain the nature of the involvement. The physician should look for specific patterns that tend to point to one disorder as opposed to another, while at the same time seeking to determine whether autonomic involvement may be occurring secondary to another disorder. Finally, it is important to determine what effects the autonomic disturbance is having on the patient and their family.

Outlining all of the various patterns of autonomic dysfunction that may be present is beyond the scope of this chapter and the interested reader is directed to several excellent texts of autonomic disorders [53,54]. However, several important examples of specific patterns are briefly outlined. Autonomic dysfunction brought about by amyloid polyneuropathy is diffuse in nature, with a selective loss of pain and temperature sensation, orthostatic hypotension, and weight loss. Amyloid infiltration can be demonstrated in the subcutaneous fat, rectal tissue, and nerves. In patients with diabetic neuropathy, not only is there obvious hyperglycemia, there are also signs and symptoms of diffuse autonomic failure involving the cardiovagal, postganglionic sympathetic, sudomotor, and adrenergic systems. It is particularly important to identify any drugs the patient may be taking that could result in orthostatic hypotension (such as antihypertensive agents). In young people with severe autonomic dysfunction it is important to consider the possibility of street drugs (such as cocaine, amphetamines, crack, or phencyclidine) as well as alcohol as contributing factors. Other potentially treatable problems are autonomic dysfunction associated with thallium or arsenic neuropathy.

In the patient's history, the physician should endeavor to identify any cyclic or fluctuating nature to his or her symptoms. Orthostatic hypotension may exhibit spontaneous variations throughout the course of the day, and may vary in respect to medication, meals, and with the menstrual cycle in women. Knowledge of these variations can be quite useful in planning a therapeutic program.

The anatomic location of the preganglionic autonomic nervous system makes it relatively inaccessible to direct physiological assessment. Therefore, tests used to evaluate the adequacy of autonomic function are not direct assessments, rather they measure end-organ responses to various physiological and pharmacological challenges. In addition, it is possible to determine the levels of both autonomic neurotransmitters and neuromodulators in the plasma, urine, and cerebrospinal fluid. Quantification of autonomic receptor density and affinity can also be performed.

The first and simplest test is to test blood pressure in the supine, sitting, and standing positions. The fall in blood pressure that is regarded as significant is somewhat variable between laboratories, but is generally felt to be 20–30 mmHg systolic and 10–15 mmHg diastolic. Care should be taken to measure blood pressure when standing with the arm extended horizontally to prevent the hydrostatic effects of a fluid column in the dependent arm (which could potentially result in a falsely elevated reading). Because the nature of the orthostatic response to active standing differs from that of passive tilting, we often perform tilt table testing on these subjects. Tilting also provides a stable setting for the measurement of other determinants of autonomic function, and it seems to provide an adequate degree of reproducibility [55]. Currently, we perform head-upright tilt table testing while the patient is fasting. A standard tilt table with a footboard made for weight bearing is used and a standard sphygmomanometer is used for blood pressure measurements. Patients are also connected to a standard cardiographic monitor for continuous elevation of heart rate and rhythm. The tilt table is then inclined at an angle 70° from horizontal for a period of 45 min, with blood pressure measured every 3 min until hypotension begins. At this time, measurements are made every 30 s. In some patients we also measure cerebral blood flow during tilt by means of transcranial Doppler ultrasonography. In addition to measuring blood pressure, heart rate responses are also determined at rest and in response to standing and head-up tilt, to deep respiration, and to Valsalva maneuver. Resting heart rate is principally determined by vagal tone, which normally declines upon standing, resulting in an increase in heart rate of between 10 and 30 b min^{-1}. The normal maximum heart rate response to standing occurs after 15 beats, then slows to a stable rate by the 30th beat [56]. This response depends on a normal parasympathetic innervation of the heart.

Other tests include assessment of thermoregulatory sweating by raising the body temperature using an external heat source. The sweat response is then measured by the degree of color change of an indicator substance (which is spread over the body) such as iodine with starch, quinizarin, or alizarin red. Cutaneous bioelectric recordings that measure the degree of skin conductance, skin resistance, or the sympathetic skin potential are also used as another method of ascertaining sudomotor function.

The serum levels of norepinephrine and the way they change between the supine and head-up tilt positions can also be used to determine the nature of suspected autonomic failure [57]. In patients with deficits in the postganglionic sympathetic vasomotor fibers, the supine plasma norepinephrine levels can be abnormally low, whereas in patients with MSA, supine plasma levels are usually normal. With both disorders, however, the expected increase in plasma norepinephrine levels during tilt may either be blunted or absent, indicating a sympathetic outflow dysfunction. Plasma vasopressin levels may also be measured in order to determine the function of the afferent limb of the baroreflex. Failure of vasopressin to increase during hypotension in a patient documented to have a normal response to an infusion of hypertonic saline can be because of lesions affecting the baroreceptor afferents in the vagus nerve or their central connections to the paraventricular hypothalamic nuclei.

The response of the body to pharmacologic challenges with a number of different agents has also been used. These agents include epinephrine, norepinephrine, isoproterenol, clonidine, and atropine. Each is used to determine the sensitivity of different groups of receptors as well as the functional status of the cardiac vagus and sympathetic nerve terminals. The interested reader is directed to several excellent references on these tests [53,54,56].

Discriminating between PAF, MSA and Parkinson's disease can present a particular challenge. Three major differences are present that help determine the presence of MSA as opposed to Parkinson's disease. First are the atypical nature of the Parkinsonian features, the degree to which the extrapyramidal system is affected, and the distinctive autonomic features of each. In regards to the extrapyramidal symptoms in MSA, rigidity, bradykinesia, and ataxia are common whereas tremor is often minimal or absent altogether. Responses to treatment with levodopa are modest at best and usually transient, and there is an absence of the on–off pattern seen in Parkinson's disease. In addition, several tests may be useful in distinguishing PAF, MSA, and Parkinson's disease. An example is that the release of vasopressin in response to hypotension and growth hormone secretions to clonidine are diminished in MSA but are normal in PAF and in Parkinson's disease (MSA alone affects the brainstem-hypothalamic-pituitary pathway) [58,59]. Supine plasma norepinephrine concentration is low in PAF but normal in MSA because in the latter postganglionic neurons are normal. Magnetic resonance imaging of the brain is abnormal only in MSA, where degenerative changes can be seen in the putamen [60].

Goldstein *et al.*'s [3,40] brilliant work in measuring cardiac sympathetic activity with labeled tracers raises the exciting possibility of someday having an accurate, practical, diagnostic modality that will distinguish between Parkinson's disease and MSA.

In selected patients, exercise stress testing may be useful in identifying patients with chronotrophic incompetence or exercise-induced hypotension. Ambulatory blood pressure monitoring is sometimes helpful in determining the range of blood pressure changes over the course of the day.

Therapeutic measures

The first step in the treatment of the patient with orthostatic hypotension is to identify and correct any potentially reversible problems. For example, anemia, dehydration and drug-induced hypotension all represent treatable causes. When no reversible cause is apparent, therapies aimed at reducing symptoms are started.

Foremost in treatment is the education of the patient and family as to the nature of the disorder. Potential aggravating factors such as extreme heat and dehydration should be identified and avoided. Patients are normally encouraged to increase their fluid and salt intake. As large meals may provide a large amount of blood shunting into the mesenteric vasculature and thereby aggravate symptoms, patients should be encouraged to eat smaller and more frequent meals, principally of a protein content. Because of its vasodilatory and diuretic effects, alcohol should be avoided.

Patients and families need to remember that these disorders tend to be chronic in nature and that treatments are palliative rather than curative, and may require periodic alterations to meet the patient's changing needs. Many patients and their families benefit from psychological counseling to help them deal with the stresses and hardships brought about by chronic illness.

Sleeping with the head of the bed elevated is useful, as it appears to lessen the sudden pooling of blood that can occur upon arising in the morning and may also reduce the degree of nocturnal diuresis and supine hypertension. If a hospital bed is used, a 45° head-up angle is used. Alternatively, the back posts of the bed can be elevated by 10–15 cm (4–6 in) (placing a brick under each of the back bedposts is an easy way to accomplish this); however, a footboard may be needed to keep the patient from sliding off the bed. Upon arising in the morning, patients should sit on the edge of the bed for several minutes before slowly standing.

Custom-fitted elastic support hose are often helpful in producing a type of counter-gradient effect in the lower extremities of the body in order to minimize venous pooling. At least 30–40 mmHg ankle counter pressure, extending from the metatarsals to the costal margin is needed to be truly effective. We recommend that the hose be made with an open crotch to make urination easier. While helpful, they may be difficult to put on and uncomfortable when the weather is hot.

Physical measures that can increase pressure include crossing the legs and pushing them against each other and rocking up on the toes [61]. Each of these activate the skeletal muscle pump and can briefly elevate pressure enough to allow the patient to get to a convenient place to sit or lie down. Resistance training to improve the strength of the skeletal muscle pump can also be useful, as may tilt training.

A variety of different pharmacological agents have been used to treat orthostatic hypotension (Table 3.4). One of the most commonly used agents is fludrocortisone, a mineral corticoid that acts on the distal renal tubule to promote the reabsorption of sodium in exchange for a loss of potassium and hydrogen ions [62]. This retention of sodium also promotes retention of water, thereby expanding the total blood volume. In addition, fludrocortisone seems to increase the sensitivity of blood vessels to the effects of circulating norepinephrine, causing an increase in vascular resistance. Some authors have reported that it also appears to increase the number of α-receptors in the peripheral vasculature. The usual starting dosage is 0.1 mg once or twice daily. We usually do not exceed dosages of 0.4 mg/day p.o. The drug may cause hyperkalemia or hypomagnesemia, and the patient should be periodically monitored for these. The agent DDAVP is sometimes a useful volume-expanding agent [63]. Tablets of 0.1–0.2 mg can be given at bedtime and may be useful in preventing nocturnal polyuria.

A second form of therapy is to use sympathetic stimulation to augment peripheral vascular resistance. An example of this is the α_2-receptor antagonist yohimbine [64]. Central α_2-stimulation inhibits sympathetic activity. Therefore, by blocking this, yohimbine increases sympathetic outflow. The agent produces a modest yet significant increase in plasma norepinephrine as well as an increase in blood pressure. Usual therapeutic dosages are in the range of 8–10 mg p.o. 2–3 times daily, with the principal side-effects being nervousness, anxiety, and diarrhea.

Several sympathetic agents have been used in testing patients with orthostatic hypotension. These agents have their actions by either direct or indirect stimulation of α-adrenergic receptors, thereby causing both arteriolar and venous vasoconstriction. Remember that some patients with orthostatic hypotension are quite sensitive to the effects of these agents and they may cause significant supine hypertension. The amphetamine class agents, such as methylphenidate, can control postural hypotension, but its CNS stimulant effects and small potential for dependence limit its widespread use

Table 3.4 Treatment options.

Therapy	Method or dose	Common problems
Head-up tilt of bed	45° head-up tilt of bed (often will need footboard)	Hypotension, sliding off bed, leg cramps
Elastic support hose	Require at least 30–40 mmHg ankle counterpressure, work best if waist high	Uncomfortable, hot, difficult to get on
Diet	Fluid intake of 2–2.5 L/day NA+ intake of 150–250 mEq/day	Supine hypertension. Peripheral edema
Exercise	Aerobic exercise (mild) may aid venous return. Water exercise particularly helpful	May lower blood pressure if done too vigorously
Fludrocortisone	Begin at 0.1–0.2 mg/day may work up to doses not exceeding 1.0 mg/day	Hypokalemia, hypomagnesemia, peripheral edema, weight gain, congestive heart failure
Methylphenidate	5–10 mg p.o. t.i.d. given with meals, give last dose before 6 pm	Agitation, tremor, insomnia, supine hypertension
Midodrine	2.5–10 mg every 2–4 h. May use up to 40 mg/day	Nausea, supine hypertension
Clonidine	0.1–0.3 mg p.o. b.i.d. or patches placed 1/week	Dry mouth, bradycardia, hypotension
Yohimbine	8 mg p.o. b.i.d.–t.i.d.	Diarrhea, anxiety, nervousness
Ephedrine sulfate	12.5–25 mg p.o. t.i.d.	Tachycardia, tremor, supine hypertension
Fluoxetine	10–20 mg p.o. q.d. (requires 4–6 weeks of therapy)	Nausea, anorexia, diarrhea
Venlafaxine	75 mg XR form p.o. q.d. or b.i.d.	Nausea, anorexia, hypertension
Erythropoietin	10,000 IU^2 once weekly	Requires injections, burning of site, increase hematocrit, CVA
Pindolol	2.5–5.0 mg p.o. b.i.d.–t.i.d.	Hypotension, congestive heart failure, bradycardia
Desmopressin	An analog of vasopressin used as a nasal spray or pill at 0.2 mg p.o. q.h.s.	Hyponatremia
Octreotide	25 µg^2 b.i.d., may titrate to 100–200 µg t.i.d.	Nausea, abdominal pain, muscle cramps, hypertension
Pyridostigmine	60 mg p.o. b.i.d.	Nausea, abdominal cramping, diarrhea, diaphoresis

B.i.d., twice daily; CVA, cardiovascular accident; p.o., by mouth; q.d., every day; q.h.s., each evening; t.i.d., three times a day; XR, extended release.

[65]. Another agent, midodrine, is also useful in preventing orthostatic hypotension. Midodrine is a prodrug that is metabolized to an active form, desglymidodrine, which acts on α_1-adrenoreceptors to cause constriction of arterial resistance and venous capacitance vessels [66]. It has a fairly rapid absorption, with peak concentration occurring within 20–40 min, and a short half-life of approximately 30 min [67]. It is given in regimens of 2.5–10 mg, 3–4 times daily. The side-effects include nausea, "goose bumps" of the skin (cutis anserina), tingling of the scalp, and supine hypertension. A number of studies have demonstrated its utility in the treatment of orthostatic hypotension [67,68].

Surprisingly, the drug clonidine, an α_2-adrenoreceptor agonist, can prove extremely useful as a therapy for orthostatic hypotension that occurs as a result of significant postganglionic sympathetic lesions [69]. Postjunctional α_2-receptors are widespread throughout the vasculature (especially in veins) and may become hypersensitive in autonomic failure [70]. While the drug's central activity causes a reduction in sympathetic outflow in normal subjects (thus lowering blood pressure), patients with autonomic failure who have very little remaining sympathetic activity (mainly PAF and spinal cord lesions) will principally experience the peripheral effects of the agent, with an increase in heart rate and blood pressure. Clonidine is also useful in lessening the degree of supine hypertension that some patients experience.

Beta-adrenoceptor blocking agents have been used with the idea that, despite the presence of an α-adrenoceptor defect, these agents could augment peripheral vascular resistance or at least prevent vasodilation [71]. These drugs may also act on pre-synaptic β-adrenoceptors and slow the release of norepinephrine [72]. In our experience, these agents have not proven as useful as others, other than blunting supine hypertension. Beta-blockers with intrinsic sympathetic activity have been reported to be more effective than those without.

The use of serotonin reuptake inhibitors (SSRIs) may prove useful in the management of selected patients. A substantial body of literature has demonstrated that serotonin has a major role in the regulation of blood pressure by the CNS [73]. Several studies have demonstrated that the SSRIs can be an effective means of preventing the sudden hypotension seen in neurocardiogenic syncope. Similar studies have shown that fluoxetine and venlafaxine may be useful in the treatment of orthostatic hypotension [74,75].

Another promising therapy is erythropoietin. Erythropoietin is a polypeptide that is produced mainly in the kidney, and seems to stimulate red blood cell production. Erythropoietin is produced in response to factors such as hypoxic hemorrhage or anemia. While the role of the autonomic nervous system in erythropoietin production is unclear, many patients with autonomic failure are anemic, with a lower than anticipated serum erythropoietin response. A series of studies have demonstrated that erythropoietin can be a remarkable therapy for orthostatic hypotension [76–78]. Interestingly, this effect is independent of its red cell augmentation and appears to be caused by direct construction of the peripheral vasculature [78]. The drawbacks of the agent are that it must be administered subcutaneously and that the red blood cell counts must be monitored on a regular basis to make sure they do not get too high, (we normally do not let the hematocrit rise above 50). The somatostatin analogue octreotide is sometimes useful in refractory patients with orthostatic hypotension. It must be administered at 25 µg subcutaneously twice daily and may be titrated up to 100–200 mg three times daily. The drug may cause nausea and muscle cramping. In the acute autonomic neuropathies there have been reports of immunoglobin therapy and immunosuppressive agents being effective, but large-scale experience is lacking.

Based on the observation that many of the acute (and probably many of the chronic) autonomic neuropathies are caused by the effects of autoantibodies to ganglionic nicotinic acetylcholine receptors, Singer *et al.* [79] have explored the possibility that the acetylcholinesterase inhibitor pyridostigmine would be an effective therapy for orthostatic hypotension. In a pilot study in patients with MSA, Parkinson's disease, amyloid neuropathy, diabetic neuropathy, and idiopathic autonomic neuropathy they found that pyridostigmine caused only a modest non-significant increase in supine blood pressure while at the same time significantly increasing orthostatic blood pressure and reducing the fall in blood pressure during head-up tilt. This may be a particularly useful agent in treating patients with orthostatic hypotension who also have supine hypertension.

The synthetic catecholamino acid L-threo-3,4-dihydroxyphenylserine (L-DOPS) has also been demonstrated to increase upright blood pressure and to decrease orthostatic hypotension [29]. The drug is converted to norepinephrine that is released from sympathetic nerves. Further studies with this unique and promising agent are ongoing.

Finally, a novel approach to the treatment of refractory orthostatic hypotension in patients with severe autonomic failure has been reported. Oldenburg *et al.* [80] have used an ambulatory patient-controlled norepinephrine infusion pump in six patients with refractory orthostatic hypotension. Four patients suffered from PAF, and two suffered from MSA (age range 57–75 years). Ambulatory epinephrine was infused intravenously in individually adjusted dosages through an indwelling infusion system and portable continuous infusion pump. Four patients have enjoyed a dramatic reduction in symptoms of orthostatic hypotension and have not experienced any untoward effects. Two patients demonstrated a beneficial effect initially but died from causes unrelated to their norepinephrine therapy. This therapy should only be considered in the most refractory of cases. It should be noted that of the abovementioned agents, only midodrine is approved by the US Food and Drug Administration for the treatment of orthostatic hypotension. The remaining agents are used "off label." It should also be remembered that the therapies elaborated here are principally aimed at controlling orthostatic hypotension, and that the patient suffering from autonomic failure will have other problems that these agents will not completely address. Both patient and physician should keep in mind that autonomic disorders may be progressive in nature and any treatment program may require modification over time.

An often neglected, but nevertheless important, aspect of these disorders is the tremendous social and emotional toll they take on the patients and their families. The attitude of the physician can have a profound impact on the patient with any chronic autonomic disorder. Some physicians and patients tend to view these disorders as untreatable and both descend into a state of hopelessness. Such a view is unwarranted as the majority, through diligent and patient effort, can be helped. A positive (yet at the same time realistic) approach by a sympathetic and knowledgeable physician not only improves the patient's sense of well-being, but may impact on the course of the disease as well. Hope is a potent medicine and should be encouraged [81]. The secondary problems produced by severe autonomic disorders cause a wide range of personal and social issues that encompass occupational, marital, psychosexual, legal, and financial difficulties. Many physicians are ill prepared (and uncomfortable) to deal with these problems, yet it is in this very area that some patients benefit most. The physician should be aware of the community resources available and should be able to refer to psychologists, counselors, social workers, rehabilitation specialists, and lawyers who can help address their concerns [82]. A patient support organization, the National Dysautonomic Research Foundation (www.ndrf.org) is an excellent source of information for adult patients and their families and now has a number of local support groups. A support group for children and adolescents is the Dysautonomia Youth Network of America (www.dynakids.org).

Conclusions

Orthostatic hypotension is a surprisingly common condition with a diverse number of causes. Recognition of the cause is important in establishing prognosis and a reasonable plan of treatment. A wide variety of different treatments exist that can significantly improve a patient's symptoms and help to restore their quality of life. Additional investigation is needed to better understand and establish treatments for this debilitating and poorly understood group of disorders.

References

1 Tansey EM. Historical perspectives on the autonomic nervous system. In: Mathias CM, Bannister R, eds. *Autonomic Failure: A Textbook of Clinical Disorders of the Autonomic Nervous System*. Oxford, UK: Oxford University Press, 1999: xxiii–xxix.

2 Ackerknecht EH. The history of the discovery of the vegetative nervous system. *Med Hist* 1974;**18**:2–8.

3 Goldstein DS, Robertson D, Esler M, Straus S, Eisenhofer G. Dysautonomias: clinical disorders of the autonomic nervous system. *Ann Intern Med* 2002;**137**:753–63.

4 Gaskell WH. On the structure, distribution, and function of the nerves which innervate the viseral and vascular systems. *J Physiol* 1886;**7**:1–80.

5 Sheehan D. The autonomic nervous system prior to Gaskell. *N Engl J Med* 1941;**224**:457–60.

6 Langley JN. On the union of cranial autonomic (visceral) fibers with the nerve cells of the superior cervical ganglion. *J Physiol* 1898;**23**:240–70.

7 Cannon WB, Rosenblueth A. *Autonomic Neuroeffector Systems*. New York, NY: Macmillan, 1937.

8 Cannon WB. *The Wisdom of the Body*. New York, NY: W.W. Norton, 1939.

9 Burnstock G. Do some nerve cells release more than one neurotransmitter? *Neuroscience* 1976;**1**:239–48.

10 Bradbury S, Eggleston C. Postural hypotension: a report of three cases. *Am Heart J* 1925;**1**:73–86.

11 Joyner M, Shepherd T. Autonomic regulation of the circulation. In: Low P, ed. *Clinical Autonomic Disorders*, 2nd edn. Philadelphia, PA: Lippincott-Raven, 1997: 61–71.

12 Thompson WO, Thompson PK, Dailey ME. The effect of upright posture on the composition and volume of the blood in man. *J Clin Invest* 1988;**5**:573–609.

13 Shepherd R, Shepherd JT. Control of the blood pressure and circulation in man. In: Mathias C, Bannister R, eds. *Autonomic Failure: A Textbook of Clinical Disorders of the Autonomic Nervous System*, 4th edn. Oxford, UK: Oxford University Press, 1999: 72–5.

14 Blomquist CG, Stone HL. Cardiovascular adjustments to gravitational stress. In: Shepherd JJ, Abboud FM, eds. *Handbook of Physiology*, Section 2: *The Cardiovascular System*. Bethesda: American Physiological Society, 1983: 1025–63.

15 Rowell LB. *Human Circulation Regulation During Physical Stress*. Oxford, UK: Oxford University Press, 1986.

16 Streeten DHP. *Orthostatic Disorders of the Circulation: Mechanisms, Manifestations and Treatment.* New York, NY: Plenum Publishing, 1957.

17 Wieling W, TenHarkel A, van Lieshout JJ. Classification of orthostatic disorders based on the short-term circulatory response upon standing. *Clin Sci* 1991;**99**:241–8.

18 Wieling W, van Lieshot JJ. Circulatory adaptation upon standing. In: Yoshikawa M, ed. *New Trends in Autonomic Nervous System Research.* Amsterdam, the Netherlands: Excerpt 2 Medica, 1991: 200–4.

19 Angell-James JE, Daily MB. Comparison of the reflex vasomotor responses to separate and combined stimulation of the carotid sinus and aortic arch baroreceptors by pulsatile and nonpulsatile pressures in the dog. *J Physiol (Lond)* 1970;**209**:257–93.

20 Henriksen O, Sejrsen P. Local reflex in microcirculation in human skeletal muscle. *Acta Physiol Scand* 1977; **99**:19–26.

21 Appenzeller O, Oribe E. Neurogenic control of the circulation, syncope and hypertension. In: Appenzeller O, Oribe E, eds. *The Autonomic Nervous System: An Introduction to Basic and Clinical Concepts,* 5th edn. Amsterdam, Netherlands: Elsevier Science, 1997: 65–182.

22 Sancho J. The role of the renin-angiotensen-aldosterone system in cardiovascular homeostasis in normal human subjects. *Circulation* 1976;**53**:400–5.

23 Grubb BP, Karas B. Clinical disorders of the autonomic nervous system associated with orthostatic intolerance: an overview of classification, clinical evaluation and management. *PACE* 1999;**22**:798–810.

24 Consensus Committee of the American Autonomic Society and the American Academy of Neurology. Consensus statement on the definition of orthostatic hypotension, pure autonomic failure and multiple system atrophy. *Neurology* 1996;**46**:1470–1.

25 Mathias CJ. The classification and nomenclature of autonomic disorders: ending chaos, resolving chaos and hopefully achieving clarity. *Clin Auton Res* 1995;**5**:307–10.

26 Freeman R. Pure autonomic failure. In: Robertson D, Biaggiani I, eds. *Disorders of the Autonomic Nervous System.* Amsterdam, the Netherlands: Harwood Academic, 1995: 61–82.

27 Low P, Bannister R. Multiple system atrophy and pure autonomic failure. In Low P, ed. *Clinical Autonomic Disorders.* Philadelphia, PA: Lippincott-Raven, 1997: 555–75.

28 Schatz IT. Pure autonomic failure. In Robertson D, Low PA, Polinsky RJ, eds. *Primer on the Autonomic Nervous System.* San Diego, CA: Academic Press, 1996: 239–41.

29 Mathias C, Bannister R. Clinical features and evaluation of the primary chronic autonomic failure syndromes. In: Mathias C, Bannister R, eds. *Autonomic Failure: A Textbook of Clinical Disorders of the Autonomic Nervous System,* 4th edn. Oxford, UK: Oxford University Press, 1999: 307–20.

30 Appenzeller O, Oribe E. Progressive autonomic failures. In: Appenzeller O, Oribe E, eds. *The Autonomic Nervous System: An Introduction to Basic and Clinical Concepts,* 5th edn. Amsterdam, the Netherlands: Elsevier Science, 1997: 567–606.

31 Shy GM, Drager GA. A neurologic syndrome associated with orthostatic hypotension. *Arch Neurol* 1960;**3**:511–27.

32 Polinsky RT. Multiple system atrophy and Shy–Drager syndrome. In: Robertson D, Low PA, Polinsky RT, eds. *Primer on the Autonomic Nervous System.* San Diego, CA: Academic Press, 1996: 222–6.

33 Fearnley TM, Less AT. Striatonigral degeneration: a clinico-pathologic study. *Brain* 1990;**113**:1823–42.

34 Tellinger K. Pathology of Parkinson's disease: changes other than the nigrostratal pathway. *Mol Chem Neuropathol* 1991;**14**:153–97.

35 Hughes AJ, Daniel DE, Kilford L, *et al.* Accuracy of clinical diagnosis of idiopathic Parkinson's disease: a clinico-pathologic study of 100 cases. *J Neurol Neurosurg Psychiatry* 1992;**55**:181–4.

36 Gilman S, Quinn NP. The relationship of multiple system atrophy to sporadic olivopontocerebellar atrophy and other forms of late onset cerebellar atrophy. *Neurology* 1996;**46**:1197–9.

37 Kaufman H. Primary autonomic failure: three clinical presentations of one disease? *Ann Intern Med* 2000; **133**:382–4.

38 Goldstein D. Dysautonomia in Parkinson's disease: neurocardiologic abnormalities. *Lancet Neurol* 2003;**2**:669–76.

39 van Dijk JG, Haan J, Zwinderman K, *et al.* Autonomic nervous system dysfunction in Parkinson's disease: relationship with age, medication, duration and severity. *J Neurol Neurosurg Psychiatry* 1993;**56**:1090–5.

40 Goldstein DS, Holmes C, Cannon RO, *et al.* Sympathetic cardioneuropathy in dysautonomias. *N Engl J Med* 1997;**336**:696–702.

41 Grubb BP, Kosinski DJ. Acute pandysautonomic syncope. *Eur J Card Pacing Electrophysiol* 1997;**7**:10–4.

42 Low P, McLeod T. Autonomic neuropathies. In: Low P, ed. *Clinical Autonomic Disorders.* Philadelphia, PA: Lippincott-Raven, 1997: 464–86.

43 Yaki MD, Fronera AT. Acute autonomic neuropathy. *Arch Neurol* 1975;**32**:132–3.

44 Verino S, Low P, Fealy R, *et al.* Autoantibodies to ganglionic acetylcholine receptors in autoimmune autonomic neuropathies. *N Engl J Med* 2000;**343**:347–55.

45 Klein CM, Verino S, Lennon V, *et al.* The spectrum of autoimmune autonomic neuropathies. *Ann Neurol* 2003; **53**:752–8.

46 Khurana RK. Paraneoplastic autonomic dysfunction. In: Robertson D, Low P, Polinsky P, eds. *Primer on the Autonomic Nervous System.* San Diego, CA: Academic Press, 1996: 266–8.

47 Low PA, Verino S, Suarez G. Autonomic dysfunction in peripheral nerve disease. *Muscle Nerve* 2003;**27**:646–61.

48 Vinik A, Erbas T. Recognizing and treating diabetic autonomic neuropathy. *Cleve Clin J Med* 2001;**68**:928–44.

49 Ziegler D. Cardiovascular autonomic neuropathy: clinical manifestations and measurement. *Diabetes Rev* 1999; **7**:342–57.

50 Shaibani AT, Harati Y. Amyloidotic autonomic failure. In: Robertson D, Low P, Polinsky P, eds. *Primer on the Autonomic Nervous System*. San Diego, CA: Academic Press, 1996: 255–9.

51 Mathias CJ, Bannister R. Dopamine β-hydroxylase deficiency: with a note on other genetically determined causes of autonomic failure. In: Mathias C, Bannister R, eds. *Autonomic Failure: A Textbook of Clinical Disorders of the Autonomic Nervous System*, 4th edn. Oxford, UK: Oxford University Press, 1999: 307–20.

52 Wieling W, Gert van Dijk, Lieshout J, Benditt D. Pathophysiology and clinical presentation. In: Benditt D, Blanc JJ, Brignole M, Sutton R, eds. *The Evaluation and Treatment of Syncope*. Elmsford, NY: Futura-Blackwell Publishing, 2003: 20–6.

53 Low P. *Clinical Autonomic Disorders*, 2nd edn. Philadelphia, PA: Lippincott-Raven, 1997.

54 Mathias C, Bannister R. *Autonomic Failure: A Textbook of Clinical Disorders of the Autonomic Nervous System*. 4th edn. Oxford, UK: Oxford University Press, 1999.

55 Grubb BP, Kosinski D. Tilt table testing: concepts and limitations. *PACE* 1997;**20**:781–7.

56 Malik M. *Clinical Guide to Cardiac Autonomic Tests*. Dordrecht, the Netherlands: Kluwer Academic, 1998.

57 Goldstein DS, Polinsky RT, Garty M, *et al*. Patterns of plasma levels of catecholamines in neurogenic orthostatic hypotension. *Ann Neurol* 1989;**26**:558–63.

58 Kaufman H, Oribe E, Miller M, *et al*. Hypotension-induced vasopressin release distinguishes between pure autonomic failure and multiple system atrophy with autonomic failure. *Neurology* 1992;**42**:590–3.

59 Kimber JR, Watson L, Mathias CT. Distinction of idiopathic Parkinson's disease from multiple system atrophy by stimulation of growth hormone release with clonidine. *Lancet* 1997;**349**:1877–81.

60 Konagaya M, Konagaya Y, Honda H, *et al*. A clinico-MRI study of extrapyramidal symptoms in multiple system atrophy: linear hyperintensity in the outer margin of the putamen. *No To Shinkei* 1993;**45**:509–13.

61 Kredict CTP, van Dijk N, Linzer M, *et al*. Management of vasovagal syncope: controlling or aborting faints by leg crossing and muscle tensing. *Circulation* 2002;**106**:1684–9.

62 Hickler RB, Thompson GR, Fox LM, *et al*. Successful treatment of orthostatic hypotension with 9-X-fluohydrodortisone. *N Engl J Med* 1959;**261**:788–91.

63 Mathias CJ, Fosbraey P, de Costa DS, *et al*. Desmopressin reduces nocturnal polyuria, reverses overnight weight loss, and improves morning postural hypotension in autonomic failure. *BMJ* 1986;**293**:353–4.

64 Goldberg MR, Hollister AS, Robertson D. Influence of yohimbine on blood pressure, autonomic reflexes and plasma catecholamines in humans. *Hypertension* 1983; **5**:772–8.

65 Grubb BP, Kosinski D, Kip K. Utility of methylphenidate in the therapy of refractory neurocardiogenic syncope. *PACE* 1996;**19**:836–40.

66 McTavish D, Goa KL. Midodrine: a review of its pharmacologic properties and therapeutic use in orthostatic hypotension and secondary hypotensive disorders. *Drugs* 1989;**38**:757–77.

67 Tankovic T, Gilden JL, Hiner BC, *et al*. Neurocardiogenic orthostatic hypotension: a double blind placebo controlled study with midodrine. *Am J Med* 1993;**95**:38–48.

68 Law P, Gilden TL, Freeman R, *et al*. Efficacy of midodrine versus placebo in neurogenic orthostatic hypotension: a randomized, double-blind multi-center study. *JAMA* 1997;**277**:1046–51.

69 Robertson D, Goldberg MR, Hollister AS, *et al*. Clonidine raises blood pressure in idiopathic orthostatic hypotension. *Am J Med* 1983;**74**:193–9.

70 Onrot T, Goldberg MR, Biaggioni I, *et al*. Post junctional vascular smooth muscle X2-adrenoreceptors in human autonomic failure. *Clin Invest Med* 1987;**10**:20–31.

71 Chobanian AY, Volicer L, Liang DS, *et al*. Use of propranolol in the treatment of idiopathic orthostatic hypotension. *Trans Am Physicians* 1977;**90**:324–34.

72 Man in't, Yeld AJ, Schaekamp MA. Prandolol acts as a beta adrenoreceptors agonist in orthostatic hypotension: therapeutic implications. *BMJ* 1981;**282**:929–31.

73 Grubb BP, Karaa BJ. The potential role of serotonin in the pathogenesis of neurocardiogenic syncope and related autonomic disturbances. *J Interv Card Electrophysiol* 1998;**2**:325–32.

74 Grubb BP, Samoil D, Kosinski D, *et al*. Fluoxetine hydrochloride for the treatment of severe refractory orthostatic hypotension. *Am J Med* 1994;**97**:366–8.

75 Grubb BP, Kosinski D. Preliminary observations on the use of venlafaxine hydrochloride in refractory orthostatic hypotension. *J Serotonin Res* 1996;**6**:89–94.

76 Hoedktke RD, Streeten DH. Treatment of orthostatic hypotension with erythropoietin. *N Engl J Med* 1993; **329**:611–5.

77 Biaggioni S, Robertson D. Krantz S, *et al*. The anemia of primary aoutonomic failure and its reversal with recombinant erythropoietin. *Ann Intern Med* 1994;**121**:181–6.

78 Grubb BP, Lachant N, Kosinski D. Erythropoietin as a therapy for severe refractory orthostatic hypotension. *Clin Auton Res* 1994; **4**:212.

79 Singer W, Opfer-Gehrking TL, McPhee BR, Hiltz MJ, Bharucha AE, Low PA. Acetylcholinesterase inhibition: a novel approach in the treatment of orthostatic hypotension. *J Neurol Neurosurg Psychiatry* 2003;**74**:1294–8.

80 Oldenburg O, Mitchell A, Nurmberger T, *et al.* Ambulatory norepinephrine treatment of severe autonomic orthostatic hypotension. *J Am Coll Cardiol* 2001;**37**:219–23.

81 Li J. Hope and the medical encounter. *Mayo Clin Proc* 2000;**75**:765–7.

82 Li J. The physician as advocate. *Mayo Clin Proc* 1998;**73**:1022–4.

CHAPTER 4

Bradyarrhythmias and syncope

David G. Benditt, MD, *& Richard Sutton,* DScMed

Introduction

The recognition of excessively slow heart rates as a potential cause of syncope long antedates availability of electrocardiographic recordings; careful physical examination yielded the necessary clues. In this regard, description of dissociated "a" and "cv" waves during examination of the neck veins, such as that reported by Stokes in the mid-1800s [1], provided the earliest documentation of AV block as a possible cause of syncope. Somewhat later, Sir James Mackenzie in reviewing his considerable clinical experience in 1913 [2] wrote, "I have made observations and tracings of several patients during syncopal attacks, and have found a variety of conditions.... The most common has been a slowing of the heart rate, with great weakness of the pulse, so that only a slight tracing was obtained by the sphygmograph."

Despite the relative ease with which electrocardiograms (ECGs) can now be recorded, even in free-living individuals, the detection of symptomatic events remains a challenge. Thus, the relationship between a recorded bradycardia and susceptibility to syncope should not be assumed unless the recorded event is associated with symptoms. Not infrequently, marked bradycardia may be recorded (e.g., in healthy individuals during sleep) yet have no bearing on the cause of syncope in that individual. Further, in some of these patients the presence of underlying heart disease may result in susceptibility to any of a number of other symptomatic arrhythmias (e.g., ventricular tachycardia, atrial fibrillation with very rapid ventricular response), which may be the real culprits. In others, even severe symptomatic bradycardia may be of neural reflex origin, and concomitant

vasodilation may have an important role in eliciting symptomatic hypotension. In the latter instance, treatment of bradycardia alone (e.g., cardiac pacing) may not completely resolve the problem.

Overview of bradyarrhythmic causes of syncope

Bradyarrhythmias may be a primary cause of syncope by diminishing cardiac output and cerebrovascular blood flow to a degree sufficient enough to result in transient global impairment of cerebral function. Alternatively, bradyarrhythmias may act in concert with other factors such as inappropriate vasodilation (e.g., vasovagal syncope, carotid sinus syndrome) or inadequate vasoconstriction (e.g., certain dysautonomias) to diminish cerebral perfusion.

Symptomatic bradyarrhythmias imply a disturbance of sinoatrial function, AV conduction, or both. These disturbances may be the result of:
1 intrinsic disturbances of sinus node and/or AV conduction usually associated with congenital or acquired structural cardiac disease;
2 extrinsic conduction system disturbances (most commonly occurring in the presence of some structural abnormality) initiated by or exacerbated by drug effects and occasionally autonomic disturbances; or
3 neurally mediated reflex functional disturbances usually occurring in the absence of structural conduction system disease.

The bradyarrhythmias accompanying neurally mediated reflex phenomena and, perhaps to a lesser extent, intrinsic disturbances of sinus node function, have been importantly associated with concomitant peripheral vascular phenomena, such as inappropriate vasodilation or inadequate vasoconstriction [3–5]. These vascular contributors can have a key role in eliciting systemic hypotension, and as such may be critical to the basis of the faint.

Intrinsic disturbances of sinus node or AV conduction disease

Disturbances of sinus node function and AV conduction may be of either congenital or acquired origin [3]. In this regard, acquired sinus node dysfunction is thought to be a relatively frequent cause of transient neurological symptoms (Table 4.1), and currently accounts for more than half of the

Table 4.1 Causes of sinus node dysfunction.

Intrinsic sinus node dysfunction
Idiopathic degenerative disease (probably most common)
Ischemic
   chronic coronary artery disease occasionally involving
     sinus node artery
   during acute myocardial infarction (particularly inferior
     wall, see "extrinsic" also)
Infiltrative disorders: amyloidosis, hemochromatosis,
   tumors
Inflammatory or postinflammatory: pericarditis,
   myocarditis
Musculoskeletal disorders: Duchenne's or myotonic
   dystrophy, Friedreich's ataxia
Collagen-vascular disease: lupus erythematosus,
   scleroderma
Postoperative: Mustard procedure, atrial septal defect
   repair

Extrinsic sinus node dysfunction
Drug effects (see Table 4.8)
Electrolyte disturbances: particularly hyperkalemia
Endocrine conditions: hypothyroidism or, less commonly,
   hyperthyroidism
Myocardial infarction, acute inferior wall (neural reflex
   effects)
Neurally mediated bradycardia – hypotension syndromes
   carotid sinus syndrome
   vasovagal syncope
   postmicturition syncope
   cough, sneeze syncope
   others
Miscellaneous
   intracranial hypertension
   obstructive jaundice

permanent pacemakers implanted in most Western countries. Similarly, acquired AV conduction system disease is ubiquitous, especially in an aging society. However, given the propensity for the latter to be associated with ventricular dysfunction, the importance of ventricular tachyarrhythmias as a cause of syncope in these same patients requires consideration.

Extrinsic functional disturbances (particularly drug-induced bradycardia)

Drug-induced disturbances of sinus node function have been well described [3,6]. Sympatholytic antihypertensive agents were among the earliest agents to be incriminated. However, as most of these latter agents (e.g., guanethidine, bethanidine, α-methyldopa) are of diminishing clinical importance, the β-adrenergic blockers, calcium-channel blockers, cardiac glycosides, and "membrane-active" antiarrhythmic drugs have become proportionally of greater concern. In regard to drug-induced disturbances of AV conduction, antiarrhythmic agents offer the greatest potential for harm. The risk is greatest in the setting of a pre-existing conduction disturbance (e.g., underlying bundle branch block). In such cases, transient high-grade AV block may cause syncope. However, bradycardia (particularly in the setting of antiarrhythmic drugs, which prolong the QT interval) may also enhance susceptibility to certain bradycardia-dependent tachyarrhythmias (torsade de pointes).

Bradyarrhythmias in this category also comprise those associated with episodic or sustained disturbances of autonomic control of the conduction system (excluding reflex activity, discussed separately). Examples in this group may include marked hypervagatonia in physically fit individuals, or bradyarrhythmias induced as a result of other organ disease (e.g., head trauma).

Neurally mediated reflex disturbances

The neurally mediated reflex syncopal syndromes are the most common causes of syncope [7–16] (Table 4.2). An up-to-date classification of these conditions, as well as an effective approach to their diagnosis and treatment, is provided within the European Society of Cardiology Guidelines on the evaluation and treatment of syncope published in 2001 [17].

Table 4.2 Neurally mediated syncopal syndromes.

Vasovagal faint
Carotid sinus syncope
Gastrointestinal stimulation
  swallow syncope
  defecation syncope
Postmicturition syncope
Cough syncope
Laugh syncope
Sneeze syncope
Glossopyharyngeal neuralgia
Airway stimulation
Raised intrathoracic pressure
  brass wind instrument playing
  weight-lifting

Table 4.3 Carotid sinus massage (CSM), carotid sinus hypersensitivity (CSH), and carotid sinus syndrome (CSS).

Methodology for carotid sinus massage
Site: carotid arterial pulse just below thyroid cartilage
Right side followed by left, pause between
Massage, NOT occlusion
Duration: 5–10 s
Posture: supine and erect

Outcomes
Carotid sinus hypersensitivity
Abnormal response to CSM (> 3 s asystole and/or
  > 50 mmHg fall in systolic blood pressure)
Absence of symptoms attributable to CSS
CSH reported frequent in "fallers" [17]

Carotid sinus syndrome
> 3 s asystole and/or 50 mmHg fall in systolic blood pressure
  with reproduction of symptoms

Contraindications/risks of CSM
Carotid bruit
Known significant carotid arterial disease
Previous CVA
Myocardial infarction in last 3 months
Risk: approximately 1 in 5000 CSM complicated by TIA

CVA, cerebrovascular accident; TIA, transient ischemic attack.

Within the category of neurally mediated reflex faints, the so-called vasovagal or "common" faint is by far the most important condition. However, carotid sinus syndrome (CSS) is now believed to be more frequent than previously appreciated, and has become more widely recognized as an important factor in previously unexplained faints and falls in the elderly [17,18]. In this regard, the clinical laboratory recognition of CSS (Table 4.3) has improved with the more frequent application of carotid sinus massage with the patient in the upright posture (usually making use of a tilt table for undertaking this procedure safely).

The various conditions comprising the neurally mediated syncopal syndromes appear to exhibit many common pathophysiologic elements, but the "trigger factors" differ (e.g., pain, carotid sinus stimulation, cough, micturition). In regard to these triggers, afferent neural signals that initiate the neural reflex may originate from within the central nervous system (CNS) directly (e.g., syncope associated with fear or anxiety), or from any of a variety of peripheral "receptors." The peripheral "receptors" respond to various triggers such as mechanical or chemical stimuli, or pain (e.g., carotid sinus syncope, postmicturition syncope). For reasons alluded to earlier, the subsequent electrophysiologic and hemodynamic picture may be quite variable. Certain patients exhibit a predominantly "cardioinhibitory" picture, with an extended period of bradycardia (or asystole) being the apparent cause of the faint. However, most present a mixed "vasodepressor" and "cardioinhibitory" response [16–24]. Only on rare occasions does a pure "vasodepressor" syndrome occur.

A detailed classification of neurally mediated hypotensive responses, as observed during tilt table testing, has been provided (and subsequently revised) by a multicenter European working group (Vasovagal International Study, VASIS) [22,23]. This classification has merit in terms of our better understanding the various possible clinical presentations. However, as pointed out recently as a result of the ISSUE trial [24], findings during tilt testing may not predict outcomes in the same patient during spontaneous syncope events.

Overview of diagnostic techniques

Electrocardiographic recordings

Given the overwhelming contribution of cardiac rhythm disturbances to the causes of syncope, electrocardiographic documentation during a spontaneous symptomatic episode would be of obvious diagnostic value in the assessment of the basis of syncope. The concomitant documentation of ambulatory blood pressure would also be of substantial additional value.

As a rule, if ambulatory electrocardiographic monitoring is successful in providing a symptom–arrhythmia correlation, the need for additional diagnostic testing may be substantially diminished (differentiating neurally mediated bradycardia with a concomitant vasodepressor element from other forms of bradycardia remains a consideration). However, outpatient monitoring necessitates exposing patients to recurrence of potentially serious arrhythmias.

Obtaining ECG documentation of symptomatic arrhythmia causing syncope is difficult, because syncopal symptoms tend to be infrequent and unpredictable [25]. The 12-lead ECG, being only a brief sample of the cardiac rhythm (approximately 12 s) is unlikely to "capture" a syncopal event, and consequently rarely provides specific findings in the patient with syncope. Certain 12-lead ECG observations may, however, provide indirect clues leading to further investigation. For instance, the presence of ventricular pre-excitation (e.g., Wolff–Parkinson–White syndrome), QT interval prolongation, or evidence of acute cardiac injury (e.g., evolving myocardial infarction) may suggest a basis for syncope. Conversely, relatively common findings such as sinus bradycardia, right or left bundle branch block, or bifascicular conduction system disease, are more often than not non-specific findings.

Longer term ambulatory ECG recording systems are widely available and would seem, in theory, to be an effective tool for evaluating arrhythmias as a cause of syncope. Guidelines on the use of ambulatory ECG recording systems have recently been summarized in an ACC/AHA/NASPE statement [26]. However, apart from implanted loop recorders (ILRs), ambulatory ECG monitoring has proved relatively inefficient as a diagnostic tool for the patient with syncope. Even ECG "event" recorders, which can be used in a continuous-loop mode for patients whose symptoms preclude responding appropriately when the episode begins, have proved disappointing. In a review of the effectiveness of ambulatory ECG recordings in the evaluation of syncope, an ACC/AHA Task Force reported that among 2,612 patients, only 19% reported symptoms [26]. Further, only 4% of all patients had an arrhythmia in association with their symptoms.

Several reports have attested to the value of ILRs in evaluating syncope patients [27–29]. In a relatively recent, randomized study, Krahn *et al.* [29] followed outcomes in 60 patients with syncope of unknown etiology. Patients were randomized to either ILR (27 patients) or conventional testing incorporating a standard external loop recorder, tilt testing, and electrophysiologic testing (30 patients). A diagnosis was obtained in 52% of the ILR group versus 20% of the conventional group ($P = 0.012$). Thereafter, undiagnosed patients were offered crossover to the other diagnostic modality. In these cases, diagnoses were made in eight of 13 patients who accepted ILRs, compared with only one of six patients who went to the conventional arm. Thus, prolonged ILR monitoring was relatively effective. Further, bradyarrhythmias were the largest single diagnostic category accounting for syncope (Fig. 4.1). Consequently, ILR monitoring systems will likely become of increasing importance in the evaluation of difficult syncope cases. Further, as the Internet becomes increasingly used for medical monitoring, wireless ILR transmission might be expected to further enhance the speed with which diagnostic endpoints are achieved.

Exercise testing

Exercise testing is not typically very productive in the evaluation of the patient with syncope, and is best reserved for patients with exercise-induced symptoms or those in whom myocardial ischemia is suspected. In terms of bradyarrhythmias associated with syncope, certain exercise test observations may be pertinent in the management of individual cases. For example, exercise testing may identify severe degrees of chronoscopic incompetence [3], excessively rapid heart rate deceleration after exercise, tachycardia-related AV block, or the exercise-associated variant of neurally mediated syncope [30]. Similarly, ECG rarely provides a definitive basis for syncope, but may be highly suggestive in patients with hypertrophic obstructive cardiomyopathy (HOCM) or severe valvular aortic stenosis.

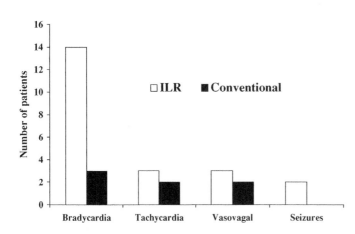

Fig. 4.1 Bar graph illustrating the relative frequency of various syncope diagnosis categories identified in the Randomized Assessment of Syncope Trial [29]. In this group of patients in whom a thorough initial clinical evaluation failed to reveal a basis for syncope, the patients were randomized to receive an implanted loop recorder (ILR) or to continue conventional evaluation. Subsequently, if a diagnosis was not made, crossover was offered. In brief, ILRs appeared to provide more diagnoses than did the conventional approach. Further, as illustrated here, bradyarrhythmias ultimately appeared to be more common than tachyarrhythmias as a cause of syncope.

Electrophysiologic testing

In general, invasive electrophysiologic testing has not proved particularly helpful in defining brady-cardic causes of syncope. Apart from exceedingly prolonged sinus node recovery times (SNRT) or HV intervals well in excess of 100 ms, the diagnostic value of such testing has proved disappointing. Not unexpectedly then, electrophysiologic studies have tended to have their greatest (albeit limited) impact in very selected clinical settings, specifically individuals with underlying structural heart disease. On the other hand, such testing has proved far less useful among patients without apparent structural substrate for arrhythmia [13,17,31–34]. For example, in the review by Camm and Lau [13], electrophysiologic testing was deemed to have provided a diagnosis in 56% of all patients. However, the testing was clearly more successful in patients with evident structural cardiac disease (71%) than in patients without (36%).

As with any test, care must be taken in interpreting findings of invasive electrophysiologic studies, as "false-positive" findings are frequent. For example, in one study, in which bradyarrhythmias were known to be the cause of syncope (21 syncopal patients with known symptomatic AV block or sinus pauses [33]), electrophysiologic testing only correctly identified three of eight patients with documented sinus pauses (sensitivity 37.5%) and two of 13 patients with documented AV block (sensitivity 15.4%). On the other hand, other abnormalities, not known to have occurred spontaneously in these individuals, were often induced during electrophysiologic study. Potentially, tilt table testing may have proved helpful in these patients, and may have permitted placing the apparently "false-positive" electrophysiologic findings in perspective.

Head-up tilt table testing and carotid sinus massage

Among all causes of syncope, the neurally mediated syncopal syndromes are the most frequent (especially the "common" or vasovagal faint). These conditions and their evaluation are discussed in more detail in Chapter 2 and pp. 110–12. However, with respect to identifying susceptibility to the vasovagal faint, head-up tilt testing has become a particularly important diagnostic technique [34,35]. In order to obtain a detailed discussion of tilt table testing protocols, test reproducibility, and estimated specificity and sensitivity, the reader is referred to the ACC Expert Consensus Report [34] and the recent guidelines document from the European Society of Cardiology [17].

The addition of tilt table testing to electrophysiologic testing appears to have markedly enhanced diagnostic capabilities in syncope patients. For example, Sra et al. [31] reported results of electrophysiologic testing in conjunction with head-up tilt testing in 86 consecutive patients referred for evaluation of unexplained syncope. Electrophysiologic testing was abnormal in 29 (34%) of patients; with the majority of these (21 patients) having inducible sustained monomorphic ventricular tachycardia.

The remainder comprised patients with inducible supraventricular tachycardias (five patients), sinoatrial dysfunction (one patient), and conduction system disease (two patients). Among the remaining patients, head-up tilt testing proved positive in 34 cases (40%) while 23 patients (26%) remained undiagnosed. In general, patients exhibiting positive electrophysiologic findings were older, more frequently male, and exhibited lower ventricular ejection fractions and higher frequency of evident heart disease than was the case in patients with positive head-up tilt tests or patients in whom no diagnosis was determined. During follow-up, syncope recurrence occurred in approximately 13% of patients. Importantly, however, syncope recurrence in patients in whom treatment was directed by electrophysiologic testing or tilt table testing seemed to be highly associated with discontinuation of recommended therapies.

A further evaluation of the combined use of electrophysiologic testing and head-up tilt testing in the assessment of syncope is provided in the report by Fitzpatrick *et al.* [36]. Among 322 syncope patients evaluated between 1984 and 1988, conventional electrophysiologic testing provided a basis for syncope in 229 of 322 cases (71%), with 93 patients having a normal electrophysiologic study. Among the patients with abnormal electrophysiologic findings, AV conduction disease was diagnosed in 34%, sinus node dysfunction in 21%, carotid sinus syndrome in 10%, and an inducible sustained tachyarrhythmia in 6%. In the 93 patients with normal conventional electrophysiologic studies, tilt table testing was undertaken in 71 cases, and reproduced syncope, consistent with a vasovagal mechanism, in 53 of 71 patients (75%). Overall, a diagnosis of neurally mediated vasovagal syncope was made in 16% of the entire patient population. This percentage likely reflects the selected nature of the study population, and is lower than is expected in a broader range of syncope patients (e.g., those presenting to emergency rooms or general medical clinics).

Syncope caused by bradyarrhythmias in the setting of intrinsic sinus node or AV conduction system disease

Sinus node dysfunction

Sinus node dysfunction (also termed "sick sinus syndrome" or sinoatrial disease) encompasses an array of sinus node and/or atrial arrhythmias that result in persistent or intermittent periods of inappropriate slow or fast heart beating (Figs 4.2 and 4.3) [3]. Clinical manifestations of sinus node dysfunction vary from seemingly asymptomatic electrocardiographic findings to a wide range of complaints including syncope, lightheadedness, dizziness, shortness of breath, palpitations, fatigue, lethargy, and dementia. In the patient experiencing syncope, the cause may be a transient severe bradyarrhythmia, or tachyarrhythmia, or both. On occasion, and particularly in the setting of patients being treated with antiarrhythmic drugs, atrial bradycardia may be associated with development of symptomatic ventricular tachyarrhythmias (Fig. 4.4).

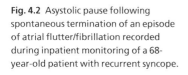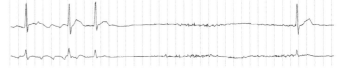

Fig. 4.2 Asystolic pause following spontaneous termination of an episode of atrial flutter/fibrillation recorded during inpatient monitoring of a 68-year-old patient with recurrent syncope.

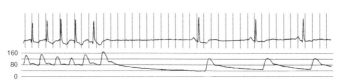

Fig. 4.3 Prolonged pause following termination of atrial tachycardia in a patient with recurrent dizziness. Symptoms of palpitation were associated with the tachyarrhythmias, but bradycardia following termination was accompanied by near-syncope. Note the tendency for post-pause blood pressure to be lower than baseline. This finding suggests a possible reflex vasodilatory component to the event.

II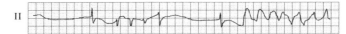

Fig. 4.4 Recording from an 80-year-old patient with recent onset of recurrent syncope. The individual had been being taking a type 1A antiarrhythmic agent for control of paroxysmal atrial fibrillation. ECG monitor reveals junctional bradycardia, marked QT interval prolongation, and polymorphous ventricular tachycardia (torsade de pointes). Syncopal symptoms in this case were caused by the bradycardia-dependent tachycardia. The bradycardia could be attributed to the adverse antiarrhythmic drug action on native cardiac pacemaker function in a patient in whom sinus node dysfunction presented initially as paroxysmal atrial fibrillation.

Most often though, it is believed that the arrhythmias associated with syncope in sinus node dysfunction patients are those producing relatively long periods (in the range of 10–15 s) of severe bradycardia with consequent inadequate cerebral blood flow (i.e., sinus pauses and sinoatrial block).

Brady- or tachyarrhythmias may also be the cause of presyncopal symptoms, which are often variously described by patients as "lightheadedness," "dizziness," "wooziness," or other relatively nonspecific complaints. For example, atrial fibrillation with a slow ventricular response or chronotropic incompetence (inadequate heart rate responsiveness during physical exertion or emotional stress) may play a part. However, these same complaints (especially "dizziness" and "lightheadedness") are relatively common in many patients, (especially in the elderly, who comprise a large proportion of the sinus node dysfunction population), and their causes are often difficult to pinpoint. Although arrhythmic etiologies are perhaps among the easiest possibilities to evaluate, establishing an unequivocal relation between symptoms and arrhythmia is often difficult.

Etiology of intrinsic sinus node dysfunction

Although congenital or familial disorders of sinus node function occur (Fig. 4.5), most clinically important disturbances of sinus node dysfunction are acquired as a result of the aging process or concomitant disease (see Table 4.1). Degenerative and/or fibrotic changes within the sinoatrial node region often accompany aging. However, such changes also result from commonly occurring disease states such as hypertension, atherosclerotic cardiovascular disease, cardiomyopathy, and inflammation (e.g., pericardial disease, myocarditis, collagen vascular diseases). Surgical trauma (particularly well known to occur after the Mustard procedure for transposition of the great arteries, and with closure of atrial septal defects, especially of the sinus venous type) is also an important contributor. The role of ischemic heart disease is difficult to ascertain. The significance of finding a close association between sinus node dysfunction and coronary artery disease is uncertain because both conditions are inherently more common in older individuals, especially in Western countries. Overall, it is believed that in only approximately one-third of adult patients with sinus node disease does ischemia caused by sinus node artery disease appear to account for the disturbance [3]. In some additional patients, however, the consequences of previous myocardial infarction may be relevant, especially if myocardial damage was extensive and complicated by congestive heart failure or hypotension. Additional factors

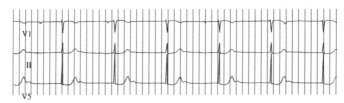

Fig. 4.5 ECG recording from an asymptomatic male, aged 48 years, who presented with a first episode of atrial fibrillation. Following cardioversion, the patient exhibited severe atrial bradycardia (note regular but very slow atrial rate) and absence of antegrade AV conduction. Cardiac evaluation was normal apart from the ECG findings. Family history was positive for the patient's mother having had a pacemaker implanted at a relatively young age for reasons that are not fully known.

Table 4.4 Syncope in sinus node dysfunction.

Reference	All patients (age range in years)	Syncope/ dizziness	Brady-induced*
Easley & Goldstein [157]	13 (63–82)	12 (92%)	13 (100%)†
Rubenstein et al. [37]	56 (26–92)	40 (71%)	32/40 (80%)
Wan et al. [158]	15 (20–85)	6 (40%)	5/6 (83%)
Kulbertus [159]	13 (57–95)	12 (92%)	12 (100%)
Obel et al. [160]	34 (25–82)	26 (78%)	NA
Hartel & Talvensaari [161]	90 (22–86)	49 (54%)	32/49 (65%)
Strauss et al. [162]	20 (32–87)	12 (60%)	NA
Sauerwein et al. [163]	30 (53–81)	22 (73%)	22/22 (100%)
Scheinman et al. [164]‡	28 (24–80)	23 (82%)	23 (100%)
Sutton et al. [165]§	37 (36–89)	22 (59%)	NA

* Differentiation of syncope etiology (bradycardia versus tachycardia) was not always clear; best estimate provided here.
† Syncope resulting from bradycardia alone in six patients, and resulting from post-tachy bradyarrhythmia in seven patients.
‡ Patients were selected based on the presence of sinus pauses or sinoatrial exit block.
§ Only patients with syncope included from this study.

such as cardioactive drugs or autonomic influences are considered separately later.

Orthotopic cardiac transplantation has provided an important new group of patients with an apparently high propensity for exhibiting disturbance of sinus node function in the early postoperative period. Fortunately, however, despite the combination of surgical trauma, ischemic time, rejection, and drug effects, only a small proportion of transplant patients develop sufficiently severe bradycardia to require implantation of cardiac pacemakers. The frequency of pacemaker implantation in heart transplant patients is approximately 2% in the University of Minnesota experience. In the majority of these cases the indication is chronotropic incompetence. Syncope caused by sinus node dysfunction appears to be rare in this setting.

Syncope in sinus node dysfunction
Prevalence
It is generally agreed that intrinsic sinus node dysfunction is an important cause of bradycardia-related syncope. However, the frequency with which this occurs in free-living individuals is unknown. Among those selected symptomatic sinus node dysfunction patients referred to centers that have taken an interest in reporting their clinical experience, syncope and dizziness are relatively common presenting features (range 40–92%; Table 4.4). In part, this apparently high frequency may be caused both by being more readily recognized by patients and physicians than some of the other symptoms associated with sinus node dysfunction, and because they are often considered among the most worrisome of all symptoms. Thus, among 56 patients with either severe bradyarrhythmias or bradycardia-tachycardia syndrome described by Rubenstein et al. [37], 25 (45%) presented with syncope and an additional 15 (27%) reported various presyncopal symptoms. In the vast majority of these cases (80%), bradyarrhythmias were considered to be the principal responsible rhythm disturbance. Similarly, among 22 patients with sinus node dysfunction and syncope, Sutton and Perrins [38] reported resolution of symptoms with prevention of bradycardia by cardiac pacing in 16 cases (73%). Of the patients with residual symptoms, treatment failure because of pacing system dysfunction occurred in one case, while symptomatic tachyarrhythmias were ultimately uncovered in several others.

Electrocardiographic observations
The electrocardiographic manifestations of sinus node dysfunction may include both bradyarrhythmias (most importantly, sinus bradycardia, sinus

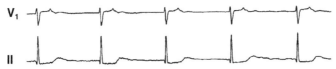

Fig. 4.6 ECG recording depicting junctional rhythm with retrograde atrial activation (P-waves superimposed on the T-waves) in a patient with "fluttering in the chest, weakness and lightheadedness." In cases such as this, atrial contraction against a closed AV valve can be expected to cause a clinical picture comparable with that associated with "pacemaker syndrome" (i.e., pseudo-pacemaker syndrome). Symptoms in this setting are multifactorial in origin, including regurgitation of blood into systemic and pulmonary veins, diminished contribution of atrial systole to cardiac output, and neurohumoral effects presumably triggered by atrial wall stretch.

pauses, sinoatrial exit block, inexcitable atrium, chronotropic incompetence) and tachyarrhythmias (principally paroxysmal or persistent atrial fibrillation or atrial flutter). Although bradyarrhythmias have been more often associated with syncope in published reports of patients classified as having sinus node dysfunction, every effort should be made to keep an open mind in the assessment of such patients and identify the specific arrhythmia(s) responsible. Of concern is the fact that patients with sinus node dysfunction tend to be in an age group in which other cardiac disease is also present, and therefore susceptibility to ventricular tachyarrhythmias or AV conduction disturbances must be considered.

Sinus bradycardia, even if relatively severe, is rarely a cause of syncope. However, presyncopal symptoms may be expected, especially during periods of physical exertion. While such symptoms are probably primarily the result of inadequate cerebral nutrient flow because of bradycardia, the presence of junctional rhythm with retrograde atrial capture or rhythmic AV dissociation may be an exacerbating factor (Fig. 4.6). In the latter circumstances, the basis for symptomatology may be both because of diminished cardiac output (i.e., loss of atrial contribution) and neurohumoral factors (including release of atrial peptides). In essence, the mechanism is comparable with that associated with "pacemaker syndrome" [39,40].

A sinus pause or sinus arrest implies failure of normal pacemaker discharge with consequent lack of an expected atrial activation of sinus node origin. The duration necessary to qualify as a "sinus pause" or "sinus arrest" remains difficult to define, and in a given individual depends in part on the magnitude of underlying sinus arrhythmia (i.e., the degree with which that individual's sinus rate varies on a regular basis). As a rule, however, asymptomatic sinus pauses of up to 3 s in duration are relatively common and without clear-cut adverse prognostic implications [26]. Pauses in excess of 3 s are rare during ambulatory monitoring (2.4 and 0.8% of patients, respectively [41,42]) and, although the clinical significance may vary, they warrant careful assessment to detect symptomatic correlations. Thus, in patients presenting with syncope or dizziness, the identification of pauses greater than 3 s suggests (but does not prove) a basis for the symptoms. The same general rules may be applied to sinoatrial exit block.

Coexistence in the same patient of periods of bradyarrhythmias and atrial tachycardias (usually atrial fibrillation, but possibly atrial flutter or other primary atrial tachycardias) is a common manifestation of sinus node dysfunction often termed bradycardia-tachycardia syndrome [3,43–45]. Symptoms may result from either excessively rapid heart beating, bradycardia, or both. A prolonged pause following termination of a tachycardia episode is one of the most frequent causes of syncope and dizziness in patients with sinus node dysfunction (see Figs 4.2 and 4.3). Such pauses may be aggravated by antiarrhythmic drug therapy initiated to suppress tachycardia susceptibility. Finally, it should be borne in mind that bradyarrhythmias may increase susceptibility to tachycardia, and that the tachyarrhythmia may be responsible for symptoms. A common example is the tendency for atrial fibrillation to occur in the setting of excessive atrial bradycardia. However, symptomatic ventricular ectopy (Fig. 4.7) and ventricular tachyarrhythmias (especially torsade de pointes; see Fig. 4.4) may also become a problem in bradycardic patients, especially if the patient is being treated with antiarrhythmic drugs.

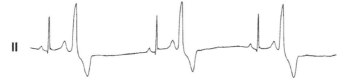

Fig. 4.7 Rhythm strip obtained during a symptomatic period in an elderly male who presented with near-syncope associated with modest exertion. In this case, chronotropic incompetence further complicated by ventricular bigeminy resulted in an inappropriately low "effective" heart rate. Atrial rate-adaptive pacing in conjunction with antiarrhythmic drug therapy proved beneficial.

Persistent atrial fibrillation, particularly in association with a very slow ventricular response (unrelated to drugs), is considered part of the spectrum of sinus node dysfunction. Unless the ventricular rate is exceedingly slow, syncope or dizziness is unlikely. Nevertheless, intermittently very long R-R intervals may occur, thereby causing bradycardia-related symptoms. In the case of individuals with such slow ventricular rates, concomitant AV conduction system disease may be part of the problem. However, although diffuse conduction system disease may occur as part of the sinus node dysfunction picture, the predilection for development of clinically worrisome AV block has probably been overemphasized. In fact, many patients with sinus node dysfunction manifest surprisingly rapid ventricular responses during atrial tachycardias.

AV block in sinus node dysfunction
Concomitant disturbances of AV conduction in patients with sinus node dysfunction is a well-recognized and important, although poorly understood, phenomenon. Its importance becomes most apparent when subsidiary pacemaker sites (i.e., junctional or ventricular) fail to provide expected "back-up" in the setting of an inadequate sinus rate. Additionally, a propensity to AV conduction failure has substantial implications with respect to the choice of cardiac pacing mode for symptomatic patients. Sutton and Kenny [45] have provided a succinct assessment of this issue. In their review of published reports encompassing 1808 patients, 300 (16.6%) manifested conduction system disease at the time sinus node dysfunction was diagnosed. However, more severe degrees of AV block (e.g., high-grade AV block) were uncommon (5–10% of cases). In studies for which follow-up was available, only 117 of 1395 patients (8.4%) developed conduction system disturbances over a mean follow-up time of 34.2 months (i.e., approximately 2.7% per year). Furthermore, for the most part these new conduction disturbances were of relatively minor forms (e.g., first-degree AV block, Wenckebach block at slower heart rates than before). Finally, in an important, prospective study of atrial versus ventricular pacing, Andersen et al. [46,47] estimated the annual risk of AV block to be approximately 0.6%.

In regard to the likelihood of the development of syncope, the acuteness with which new AV conduction system disturbances develop is a crucial factor. This aspect cannot be assessed from the Sutton and Kenny report [45]. However, findings such as those reported by Rosenqvist et al. [48], Stangl et al. [49], and Sutton and Bourgeois [50] suggest that the rate of progression is typically slow and should be detectable by careful periodic clinical and electrocardiographic follow-up. For example, in the Rosenqvist report [48], only one of 30 patients experienced high-grade AV block during a 5-year follow-up (i.e., less than 1% incidence of progression per year), and that patient had marked HV interval prolongation on entry into the study. Similarly, in the experience reported by Stangl et al. [49], only six of 110 patients observed over a period of 52 ± 28 months exhibited conduction disease progression, and in most cases the progression was minor (third-degree AV block, none; Mobitz II second-degree AV block, 1; first-degree AV block, 5).

It appears that susceptibility to subsequent conduction system involvement or aggravation of existing conduction system disease in patients with sinus node dysfunction is largely unrelated to the nature of the presenting electrocardiographic abnormalities [51]. Among 17 patients with bradycardia followed for 36 months, high-grade AV block developed in one (approximately 2% per year) compared with three instances among 22 patients with bradycardia-tachycardia syndrome followed for 53 months (approximately 3.1% per year). However, iatrogenic influences may be important. For example, van Mechelen et al. [52] used serial electrophysiologic measurements to assess AV conduction properties in 24 patients with sinus node dysfunction followed over a 3-year period. The investigators found that deterioration of AV conduction system performance (as assessed by serial estimation of the atrial paced rate at which type I second-degree AV block was observed) appeared to correlate more closely with the use of antiarrhythmic drugs than with conduction system degeneration itself. Santini et al. [53] made a similar observation. Thus, careful control of patient exposure to antiarrhythmic drugs may be among the most important factors for diminishing risk of developing clinically significant conduction system disease in patients with sinus node dysfunction.

Comorbidities

Patients with sinus node dysfunction, in large measure because of their age and tendency to harbor coexisting diseases (especially cardiovascular disorders), are also susceptible to "loss of consciousness" spells that may not be caused by a primary arrhythmia. Thromboembolic complications, myocardial ischemia, or new-onset seizure disturbances are important considerations. The first of these, thromboembolism, is primarily responsible for the excess morbidity and mortality associated with sinus node disease [3,45,54,55]. As a rule, medical history, physical examination, and relatively straightforward testing permit these conditions to be distinguished from syncope of arrhythmic origin.

Many aspects of sinus node dysfunction remain poorly understood. Among the more curious of these is the relationship between sinus node disease and apparent dysfunction of subsidiary pacemaker sites leading to risk of prolonged symptomatic asystole. Whether a common disease process is responsible for both remains to be clarified. Potentially, autonomic disturbances may be contributory. In this regard, Brignole et al. [56] have proposed that sinus node dysfunction incorporates (and perhaps in some patients may be considered a variant of)

the autonomic dysfunction associated with carotid sinus syndrome and vasovagal syncope. Conceivably, in such circumstances, neural influences may explain the diffuse nature of native pacemaker dysfunction.

Treatment

Appropriate treatment of the patient with symptomatic bradycardia resulting from sinus node dysfunction and syncope necessitates consideration of the underlying electrophysiologic and arrhythmic disturbance, the effects of drugs on sinus node function, current indications for and available modes of cardiac pacing, and the role of anticoagulation [3]. In addition, although less pertinent to bradycardia control, the evolving role of transcatheter or surgical ablation for arrhythmia control also warrants examination.

In general, cardiac pacemaker therapy has proved highly effective in patients with sinus node dysfunction when bradyarrhythmia has been demonstrated to account for symptoms (Table 4.5). For the most part, when economic circumstances permit, modern pacing practice has moved away from use of single-chamber ventricular pacing (VVI, VVIR modes) in sinus node dysfunction patients, unless intractable atrial fibrillation or other atrial disease (e.g., atrial inexcitability) precludes use of an atrial-based pacing mode. Pacing techniques that endeavor to maintain a normal AV relationship offer not only better hemodynamic responses, but also eliminate symptoms commonly associated with "pacemaker syndrome," and tend to diminish the likelihood of later development of atrial fibrillation and its consequent risk of thromboembolism [45–48,57]. Finally, because a diagnosis of sinus node dysfunction is inherently associated with an

Table 4.5 Indications for pacing in sinus node dysfunction.

Class I: Indicated
Documented bradycardia-related symptoms

Class II: Possibly indicated
Symptomatic sinus node dysfunction in which a relationship between symptoms and bradycardia has been sought but not established

Class III: Not indicated
Asymptomatic sinus node dysfunction

inappropriate chronotropic response, the use of rate-adaptive pacing (i.e., implantable devices incorporating one or more physiologic sensors) is usually warranted for purposes of optimizing exertional tolerance.

Although theophylline has been reported to be helpful in a few cases (predominantly autonomically mediated bradyarrhythmias), drug therapy is now only rarely used to treat bradyarrhythmias in patients with sinus node dysfunction. On the other hand, by virtue of their age and associated disease processes, patients with sinus node dysfunction are often exposed to a wide range of drugs. These agents may inadvertently exacerbate or unmask underlying susceptibility to bradycardia. This problem is considered in more detail later in this chapter (see p. 109).

Thromboembolic complications (probably primarily associated with atrial fibrillation) are an important contributing factor to excess mortality and morbidity in patients with sinus node dysfunction. While these complications do not cause "true syncope," they do cause neurologic disturbances that may be interpreted as dizziness or syncope. Consequently, stroke risk reduction by anticoagulation is an important element in the treatment of individuals with sinus node dysfunction, particularly those with paroxysmal or persistent atrial fibrillation. The reader is referred to a review of the major anticoagulation trials [58]. In this regard, there is solid evidence supporting the use of warfarin therapy, and while the merits of full dose (325 mg) aspirin therapy remain to be resolved, warfarin is clearly superior to "mini-dose" aspirin (75 mg). In brief, long-term oral anticoagulant therapy should be considered for all patients older than 65 years, and for younger patients with the following risk factors: a previous transient ischemic attack (TIA) or stroke, hypertension, heart failure, diabetes, clinical coronary artery disease, mitral stenosis, prosthetic heart valve, or thyrotoxicosis. Additionally, although the reported clinical experience is sparse and largely anecdotal, early anticoagulation may be warranted in the setting of the inexcitable and/or quiescent atrium. These individuals appear to have an increased thromboembolic risk at any age.

Ablation currently has a relatively small role in the treatment of sinus node dysfunction, and has virtually no importance in regard to bradyarrhythmias. His bundle ablation is perhaps the most important technique in this patient population, and is used to facilitate control of ventricular rate in individuals with permanent or intractable atrial tachyarrhythmias [59]. For the most part, these patients become pacemaker dependent (i.e., absence of an adequate supporting native cardiac rhythm), and any pacemaker system failure in this setting may lead to a life-threatening circumstance. Syncope would certainly be expected.

Other forms of ablation may also be relevant in terms of bradycardia susceptibility. Transcatheter ablation for control of atrial flutter (particularly of right atrial origin) has become highly successful. Similarly, techniques are rapidly evolving for transcatheter ablation of certain forms of atrial fibrillation (particularly with the emergence of "focal" ablation in the setting of paroxysmal or persistent atrial fibrillation) [60–63]. Surgical methods for direct treatment of atrial fibrillation (most commonly using some form of compartmentalization technique) has also matured, although still largely restricted to individuals undergoing cardiac surgery for other reasons (e.g., mitral valve replacement) [64,65]. In all of these cases, tendency to symptomatic bradycardia (particularly chronotropic incompetence) may become more apparent after the tachyarrhythmia problem has been successfully suppressed. Prior to undertaking an ablation procedure, consideration must always be given to the part played by the tachyarrhythmia (albeit troublesome) in supporting the circulation, and the subsequent potential need for permanent pacemaker implantation.

Finally, innovative pacing and/or atrial defibrillation techniques may become a part of the treatment strategy in patients with sinus node dysfunction. Multisite atrial pacing has recently been the subject of a multicenter trial to assess the potential for suppressing atrial fibrillation [66,67]. In brief, the findings tended to support its utility in a subset of individuals with relatively frequent paroxysmal atrial fibrillation, but the differences compared with single-site atrial pacing were fewer than had been expected. Potentially, the addition of seemingly effective atrial fibrillation suppression algorithms within newer multisite atrial pacing systems will enhance effectiveness. A multicenter trial to assess this possibility is currently being developed.

Implantable atrial defibrillators have developed beyond clinical trial stage and have received regulatory approval in many countries [68,69]. These devices, used in conjunction with drugs or pacemakers, offer an opportunity to reverse atrial tachyarrhythmia breakthroughs promptly, thereby reducing the need for aggressive antiarrhythmic drug therapy. However, without highly effective, painless treatment algorithms, these devices are likely to be used only infrequently, perhaps in selected patients with symptomatic bradycardia-tachycardia syndrome in whom syncope may occur either because of excessively slow or excessively rapid heart rates.

AV conduction disturbances

Disturbances of AV conduction range from slowing of AV conduction (first-degree AV block), to intermittent failure of impulse transmission (second-degree AV block), and complete conduction failure (third-degree AV block). In terms of clinical importance in the patient with syncope, both the type of block and the site at which block occurs must be considered [70–72]. A complete discussion of these issues is beyond the scope of this chapter. However, by way of example, in both first- and second-degree (type I) AV block, the AV node (prolonged AH interval) is almost always responsible when there is no evidence of underlying cardiac disease and when the QRS morphology is normal. In the presence of a narrow QRS complex, first-degree AV block has been reported to be caused by AV nodal delay in more than 85% of patients, and by delay within the His bundle in only 13% [70]. In the setting of a wide QRS complex, first-degree AV block was AV nodal in origin in only 22% of cases, infranodal in 45%, and as a result of delay in more than one site in approximately 33% of cases. Similarly, in patients with a narrow QRS complex, type I second-degree AV block is AV nodal in origin in approximately 70% of cases, whereas in the presence of a wide QRS complex infranodal conduction delay may account for 60–70% of cases.

Etiology

Table 4.6 summarizes the principal recognized causes of AV block. Progressive idiopathic fibrosis of the cardiac conduction system is the most common cause of acquired conduction system disease

Table 4.6 Causes of AV block.

Atherosclerotic disease (ASD)
Acute myocardial infarction
Healed myocardial infarction

Calcific infiltration
Calcific valvular heart disease

Cardiomyopathy

Collagen-vascular diseases
Ankylosing spondylitis, dermatomyositis, rheumatoid arthritis, scleroderma, systemic lupus erythematosus

Congenital AV block
Associated with congenital heart disease (ostium primum ASD, transposition of the great vessels)
Associated with maternal systemic lupus erythematosus

Drug effects
β-Adrenergic blockers, cardiac glycosides, "membrane-active" antiarrhythmic agents

Idiopathic fibrosis (Lev's disease)

Infiltrative diseases
Amyloidosis, hemochromatosis, sarcoidosis

Inflammatory diseases
Endocarditis
Myocarditis
Bacterial (diphtheria, Lyme disease, rheumatic fever, tuberculosis)
Viral (measles, mumps)
Parasitic (Chagas' disease)

Neurally mediated AV block
Carotid sinus syndrome, other neurally mediated syncopal syndromes (e.g., vasovagal syncope)

Trauma
Catheter trauma/ablation, radiation, cardiac surgery

Tumors
Mesothelioma, rhabdomyoma

[73,74]. In general, this can be considered an aging-related process of sclerosis of the cardiac skeleton and is particularly likely in patients without evidence of significant underlying structural heart disease. Acute myocardial infarction is associated with the various forms of AV block, and is another common cause of acquired, complete AV block. Chronic ischemic heart disease is also commonly associated with various degrees of AV block,

although it is often impossible to be certain of a causal relationship.

Studies examining the association of acute myocardial infarction to development of AV block largely predate the thrombolytic era [75–77]. These reports suggest that in individuals with inferior wall myocardial infarction, complete AV block occurs in 10–15% [75]. Many of these cases occur early following onset of symptoms and over 60% of those who will develop AV block manifest it within the first 24 h. Fortunately, complete AV block in this setting is usually transient, often evolves from less severe degrees of block (first-degree, type I second-degree), is most often at the level of the AV node, and can often be reversed or ameliorated with atropine. The mechanisms eliciting this form of AV block are multiple, including nodal ischemia, adenosine release, and enhanced parasympathetic tone. Approximately 5% of patients with anterior myocardial infarctions develop complete heart block [76,77]. Among these latter patients the site of block tends to be within the specialized cardiac conduction system, and is associated with a poor prognosis because of the magnitude of associated ventricular damage. As a rule, patients who develop transient or fixed AV block during acute myocardial infarction tend to be older, and to have sustained a more severe myocardial infarction.

Current clinical experience suggests that early revascularization procedures (i.e., thrombolytics, acute angioplasty) may have reduced the frequency of clinically significant AV block, particularly in the case of anterior myocardial infarction [78,79]. This benefit probably coincides with diminished severity of myocardial dysfunction. However, the differences in heart block frequency have not been dramatic with inferior infarction in which neural reflex effects are probably more critical.

Other causes of infranodal AV block include certain complications of valvular heart disease, especially aortic stenosis. In many of these cases, extension of calcification or fibrosis into the nearby conducting system is at fault. The specialized cardiac conduction system may also be damaged by infiltrative cardiomyopathies such as amyloidosis, hemochromatosis, and sarcoid, as well as by certain non-infectious inflammatory conditions including ankylosing spondylitis, lupus erythematosus, and scleroderma [80–83]. While abnormalities of car-diac conduction are relatively common in many patients with congestive or hypertrophic cardiomyopathy, the development of clinically significant AV block is unpredictable.

Cardiac surgery is an important cause of acquired AV block [84]. Block most frequently complicates aortic valve replacement but is seldom associated with coronary artery bypass grafting in the absence of an exceedingly prolonged procedure, lengthy ischemic time, or myocardial infarction. Repair of certain forms of congenital heart disease, especially those physically close to the conducting system (e.g., ostium primum atrial septal defects, ventricular septal defects), is frequently complicated by AV block.

Syncope associated with AV conduction

Both congenital and acquired disturbances of AV conduction may be associated with syncope. As a rule, the risk of syncope or life-threatening brady-cardia being associated with the various forms of AV block is dependent on the underlying disease process. Thus, even in the case of high-grade AV block, the long-term outcome may be excellent in terms of survival when the disturbance is caused by neurally mediated hypervagotonia (e.g., carotid sinus syndrome, vasovagal syncope). Conversely, high-grade AV block occurring during the course of an anterior myocardial infarction is associated with a high propensity for syncope and sudden death (the latter largely because of the magnitude of myocardial damage and consequent risk of ventricular arrhythmia).

First-degree AV block
First-degree AV block is generally non-progressive and essentially a benign finding. For example, among almost 4,000 pilots followed for 27 years, this finding was noted in 148 individuals (approximately 3.5%) [85]. Outcomes in the first-degree AV block group did not differ from that observed in the normal population. An exception to the benign nature of first-degree AV block are those cases in which the condition occurs in conjunction with bifascicular block; infranodal conduction disease may contribute directly to the apparent conduction delay [70,71,86]. These latter individuals are susceptible to development of progressively higher degrees of AV block with associated symptoms.

As a solitary finding, first-degree AV block is almost never the cause of syncope. When syncope does occur in this setting, there is usually no direct causal relationship. However, the presence of first-degree AV block, especially in the absence of structural heart disease, may suggest hypervagotonia and thereby raise suspicion of neurally mediated syncope (see p. 110). Rarely, presyncopal symptoms (but only exceptionally "true syncope") may occur if the PR interval is sufficiently prolonged such that atrial systole occurs against a closed AV valve. In this case, the mechanism of symptomatic hypotension is comparable with that in "pacemaker syndrome" [39,40]. Several factors may be involved, including loss of atrial contribution to cardiac output, neurohumoral influences triggered by excessive stretch on the atrial walls, and retrograde ejection of blood into the systemic and pulmonary veins.

Second-degree AV block
Type I second-degree AV block (Wenckebach type) is generally considered to be a relatively innocent conduction disturbance when the QRS complex is narrow and there is no evidence of associated infranodal conduction system involvement. In this setting, bradycardia is rarely of sufficient severity to account for syncope. However, there remains some doubt regarding the supposedly benign nature of Mobitz type I block in older individuals. Shaw *et al.* [87] followed 214 patients with chronic second-degree block prospectively. The 5-year survival was similar in those with Mobitz type I (mean age 69 years; 57% survival), Mobitz type II (mean age 74 years; 61% survival), and patients with 2 : 1 and 3 : 1 block (mean age 75 years; 53% survival). These authors concluded that Mobitz type I and II AV block were associated with similar risks in this older population, that the presence of bundle branch block did not affect their conclusion, and that pacing improved prognosis.

When type I second-degree block occurs in healthy, physically fit individuals, the cause is most often increased vagal tone. In the absence of certain drug toxicities (e.g., cardiac glycosides) there is no clinical concern. Similarly, in the setting of acute inferior wall myocardial infarction this form of AV block tends to resolve without need for permanent pacing. However, when second-degree type I block occurs in the setting of evident infranodal conduction system disease (e.g., wide QRS), the conduction delay is often within the intraventricular specialized conduction system and risk of progression to complete AV block is a concern.

In contrast to type I second-degree AV block, type II AV block is widely agreed to carry a worrisome prognosis (Fig. 4.8). Type II block is most often seen in conjunction with bundle branch block and is indicative of severe disease of the infranodal specialized cardiac conduction system. In this case there is a predilection for Stokes–Adams attacks and the development of higher grades of AV block (Fig. 4.9). Cardiac pacing is indicated.

2 : 1 AV block
Syncope is not typically associated with 2 : 1 AV block, but may occur if higher grade block develops periodically in these patients. As noted above, 2 : 1 AV block may be the result of AV nodal or infranodal disease. In this case, the site(s) of block may be suspected by the presence of other observations occurring in temporal proximity to the 2 : 1 event (e.g., periods of second-degree type I block may suggest an AV nodal site), but only intracardiac recordings can provide positive proof. The natural history of 2 : 1 AV block and its association with syncopal symptoms may be expected to parallel, for comparable sites of disease, the clinical pictures described above for second-degree AV block.

Third-degree AV block
Third-degree AV block may be high grade (in

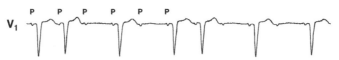

V_1 P   P   P   P   P   P

Fig. 4.8 Mobitz type II AV block in a patient with a history of syncope. Note that the PR interval is unchanging and that there is intermittent absence of a QRS complex. Mobitz type II block is often associated with periods of high-grade AV block and warrants cardiac pacemaker implantation in a setting such as this.

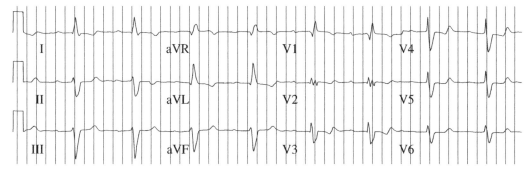

Fig. 4.9 ECG recording in an older patient with infrequent syncopal episodes. Record reveals a wide QRS (right bundle branch block), left axis deviation, and a markedly prolonged PR interval (approximately 320 ms). These findings (sometimes referred to as trifascicular block) are highly suspicious of severe conduction system disease. Although the tracing does not provide an absolute diagnostic basis for syncope, the likelihood of intermittent high-grade AV block is substantial. However, ventricular tachycardia is also of concern in this setting. Electrophysiologic studies is a reasonable recommendation before a therapy choice is made.

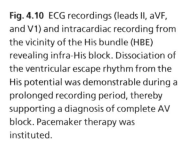

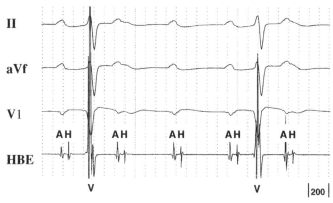

Fig. 4.10 ECG recordings (leads II, aVF, and V1) and intracardiac recording from the vicinity of the His bundle (HBE) revealing infra-His block. Dissociation of the ventricular escape rhythm from the His potential was demonstrable during a prolonged recording period, thereby supporting a diagnosis of complete AV block. Pacemaker therapy was instituted.

which multiple P-waves are blocked; Fig. 4.10) or complete. In either case there is failure of conduction of multiple atrial impulses to the ventricles. The cardiac rhythm then depends on subsidiary pacemakers. These subsidiary sites may be located within either the proximal portions of the specialized cardiac conduction system (i.e., His bundle) resulting in relatively narrow QRS complexes, or within its more distal ramifications resulting in wide QRS complexes at a rate of 40 b min^{-1} or less.

Syncope is common in patients with high grade and complete AV block, having been variously reported to occur in 38–61% of cases [88,89]. In acute anterior myocardial infarction with associated AV block, the prognosis is ultimately related to the magnitude of ventricular damage. By contrast, complete AV block after inferior wall myocardial infarction rarely persists and its occurrence is often preceded by a progression through stages beginning with PR interval prolongation and/or type I second-degree AV block. The site of block in this setting is usually within the AV node and its transient occurrence has no adverse long-term prognostic implication [90].

In general, the risk for syncope or dizziness is greatest at onset of block, prior to establishment of a subsidiary rhythm. Thereafter, the ventricular rhythm often regularizes, and averages 35–40 b min^{-1} in acquired third-degree AV block. In fixed complete AV block, syncope may occur as a result of the unreliability of subsidiary pacemakers, or because of inability of the circulation to provide sufficient cerebral blood flow during periods of exercise or stress. In both cases, the close association with severe underlying heart disease also raises concern regarding tachyarrhythmia-induced syncope (including increased proarrhythmia risk in patients being treated with antiarrhythmic drugs).

Congenital complete heart block occurs with an approximate frequency of 1 in 15,000–25,000 live births (60% female predominance). Unlike most acquired forms of complete AV block, the site of block is typically at the level of the AV node (i.e., His bundle potentials are recorded before each ventricular electrogram). The QRS is narrow in most cases of congenital AV block, and the subsidiary junctional rhythm is relatively rapid and tends to increase in rate with exercise. Nevertheless, the range of available heart rates with exertion is less than normal, and the ventricular rate cannot parallel the atrial rate response (the usual marker of physiologic demand). Consequently, affected individuals exhibit sufficient heart rate excursion to remain physically active in their younger years. Ultimately, however, exertional intolerance often becomes an issue by middle age.

Until recently, congenital complete AV block was considered to have a relatively benign outcome (i.e., is less often accompanied by syncope or life-threatening consequences) than does acquired forms of AV block [91]. However, this view has changed. Syncope and unexpected premature death are now recognized to be more frequent than previously expected [92,93]. In the report from Pordon and Moodie [92], among 14 adult patients in one series who had been followed for 25 years, cardiac pacemakers were deemed necessary in seven individuals. The indications for pacing were syncope in five and dizziness in two. In a substantially larger follow-up study, 102 patients (61 women, 41 men) who had been asymptomatic up to age 15, were followed for an additional 7–30 years [93]. Among these individuals, syncope occurred at least once in 27 instances and was fatal in eight cases. Prolonged QT intervals associated with syncope were noted in seven cases. Thus, current thinking has evolved to favor early application of prophylactic cardiac pacing in adults with isolated congenital complete AV block.

The prognosis associated with congenital complete heart block is also determined by any associated congenital heart disease (e.g., corrected transposition of the great vessels, atrial septal defect). In the absence of concomitant abnormalities, children with congenital AV block tend to display normal growth.

Bundle branch and fascicular blocks
Whether syncope occurs in patients with various forms of bundle branch block and fascicular blocks depends both on the risk of developing high grade or complete AV block, as well as on the risk of occurrence of ventricular tachyarrhythmias. In the Framingham study [94,95], an 18-year follow-up of approximately 5,200 individuals initially believed free of cardiovascular disease revealed a 2.4% incidence of new bundle branch block (0.13% annually). Right bundle branch block was most common (70 of 125 patients) and was unassociated with acute events, but was associated with hypertension and was accompanied by greater incidence of coronary artery disease (2.5 times), congestive heart failure (4 times) and cardiovascular mortality (3 times) than was observed in age-matched controls. By contrast, in almost one-half of patients developing left bundle branch block an acute event was identified. Their subsequent 10-year follow-up was accompanied by a mortality 5 times that of age-matched controls.

In patients with chronic infranodal conduction system disease manifest by bifascicular block, progression to second- or third-degree AV block is usually slow. However, susceptibility increases the longer the HV interval, and appears to be particularly great when the HV interval exceeds 100 ms [96–98]. Evidence of susceptibility to potentially significant infranodal conduction system disease may be uncovered by demonstration of HV prolongation or infranodal block during incremental atrial pacing studies [99], or after parenteral antiarrhythmic drug administration (e.g., procainamide, ajmaline). Indications for undertaking electrophysiologic studies in this setting were summarized in an ACC/AHA guideline published in 1989 [100]. Although rather dated, the guideline recommendations remain reasonable for current use.

Treatment

Apart from the use of atropine in certain forms of transient AV block (e.g., AV block associated with inferior wall myocardial infarction, or occurring during the course of an invasive cardiovascular procedure such as an angiogram), cardiac pacing

Table 4.7 Guidelines for undertaking electrophysiologic study for acquired AV block or chronic intraventricular conduction delay.

Class I: Indicated

1 Syncope or near-syncope in patients with suspected, but not electrocardiographically documented, infranodal block.

2 Patients with a pacemaker for treatment of AV block but in whom symptoms persist and tachyarrhythmias are suspected as the cause.

3 In the setting of bundle branch block, when tachyarrhythmias are a suspected cause of symptoms.

Class II: Possibly indicated

1 AV block or chronic bundle branch block when it is thought that determining site of block is of value for treatment or prognostic purposes.

2 Suspected concealed junctional extrasystoles as cause of AV block.

Class III: Not indicated

1 Symptomatic AV block or intraventricular conduction delay already correlated with electrocardiographic findings.

2 Neurally mediated (vagally mediated) AV block (usually recognized by concomitant sinus slowing).

3 Asymptomatic patients with intraventricular conduction delays.

Table 4.8 Drugs affecting sinus node function.

Antiarrhythmic drugs

Amiodarone: may be associated with *de novo* evidence of sinus node dysfunction

Flecainide, propafenone, sotalol: may be expected to exacerbate sinus node dysfunction

Quinidine, dispoyramide, procainamide: less often worsens sinus node function possibly because of vagolytic properties

Bretylium, lidocaine, mexiletine: rarely a problem

Antihypertensives (sympatholytic)

α-Methyldopa, reserpine, clonidine

β-Adrenergic blocking drugs

Without intrinsic sympathomimetic action (ISA):
   e.g., propranolol, nadolol

With ISA, less severe affects: e.g., pindolol, acebutolol

Calcium-channel blockers

Verapamil and diltiazem more prominently than nifedipine

Cardiac glycosides

Rarely a clinical problem

Miscellaneous

Carbamazepine

Cimetidine

Lithium

Phenytoin

has replaced pharmacologic therapy in the treatment of patients with symptomatic AV block. Syncope, when clearly documented to be associated with bradycardia or when bradycardia is strongly suspected in the setting of AV block (Table 4.7), is a well-defined indication for pacing [101,102].

Extrinsic disturbances of sinus node function and AV conduction

Extrinsic disturbances of sinus function

Conventionally, "extrinsic disturbances" of sinus node function refers to neural influences. However, the impact of drugs and other pharmacologic agents can reasonably be included in this context. This broader definition of "extrinsic disturbances" is used here and elsewhere in the text.

Numerous extrinsic factors can affect sinus node function without inducing structural disturbances. Of these, autonomic nervous system influences, cardioactive drugs, and, less importantly, metabolic

disturbances, are the most common [3,6,103–106]. Drug-induced disorders are dealt with here, while neurally mediated causes are considered separately below.

Cardioactive drugs may initiate or aggravate sinus bradyarrhythmias, or induce chronotropic incompetence (Table 4.8). Cardiac glycosides may aggravate sinus node dysfunction, but this group of agents only rarely cause clinical problems. The drugs most often associated with causing or aggravating bradyarrhythmic aspects of sinus node dysfunction include the now infrequently used (in "developed" countries) sympatholytic anti-hypertensive agents (e.g., α-methyldopa, guanethidine), as well as widely used agents such as β-adrenoceptor blockers, calcium-channel blockers, membrane-active antiarrhythmics (especially amiodarone, sotalol, flecainide, and propafenone) and the anti-epileptic drug carbamazepine (Tegretol®) [3,6]. Less commonly, lithium carbonate, cimetidine, amitriptyline, and the phenothiazines may be responsible [3,6]. Certain antiarrhythmic drugs may result in difficult to recognize proarrhythmic effects in the atrium (i.e., an unexpected increase in the frequency of atrial tachyarrhythmias), as well as ventricular proarrhythmia.

Extrinsic disturbances of AV conduction

The AV nodal region is heavily innervated, and in the normal resting state sympathetic and parasympathetic influences tend to be approximately balanced (in contrast to the sinus node where parasympathetic influences usually dominate). However, in some situations (e.g., well-trained athletes, cardiac glycoside excess, transient hypervagotonia associated with conditions such as carotid sinus syndrome, cough syncope, and vasovagal syncope) parasympathetic control may become predominant [20,21,107–109]; first-degree, second-degree type I, or even paroxysmal high degree of AV block may then occur. In the latter case (i.e., paroxysmal AV block) bradycardia may be sufficiently severe to account for syncope. More often though, syncope in the setting of demonstrable hypervagotonia is the result of neurally mediated reflex activity in which bradycardia is associated with peripheral vascular dilation. Consequently, recurrent syncope in association with extrinsic disturbances of AV conduction may be multifactorial in origin.

Drug effects are a common cause of AV nodal conduction disturbances, and may be the most important factor resulting in deterioration of AV conduction in patients with sinus node dysfunction [3]. In this regard, a variety of cardioactive drugs affect the AV node, either resulting from direct pharmacologic actions (e.g., adenosine, many conventional antiarrhythmic drugs), or indirectly as a result of their actions on the autonomic nervous system (e.g., β-adrenergic blocking drugs), or both. Cardiac glycosides are perhaps the most widely recognized drugs to have such an effect, being well known for inducing first-degree or Mobitz type I second-degree AV block by enhancing the effects of vagal tone at the AV node. Beta-blockers, by diminishing sympathetic effects on the node, are equally important in this regard. Calcium-channel blockers and other antiarrhythmic drugs (e.g., quinidine, sotalol) may act directly, as well as through effects on the autonomic nervous system, to alter conduction in the AV node.

At usual dosage, antiarrhythmic drugs are rarely associated with *de novo* development of complete AV block at the AV nodal level. However, especially in patients with wide QRS morphology indicative of intrinsic infranodal conduction system disease, these drugs may induce symptomatic AV block occurring within the intraventricular specialized conduction system tissues. Furthermore, certain antiarrhythmic drugs, particularly Class 1C agents (e.g., flecainide, propafenone), have the potential to induce sufficient conduction slowing to cause a wide QRS. However, syncope in this setting cannot be assumed to be bradycardic in origin because drug-induced tachycardias (i.e., proarrhythmic effects of antiarrhythmic drugs) are also more common in this situation (see Fig. 4.9).

Syncope of neurally mediated reflex origin

Neurally mediated reflex syncope includes vasovagal syncope, carotid sinus syndrome, and other unusual forms of neurally mediated syncope such as cough, deglutition, and micturition syncope (see Table 4.2). All of these conditions involve both an element of vasodilation as well as the more easily recognized bradycardia (which in some cases may be prolonged asystole). The development of tilt table testing for the clinical investigation of syncope [16,17,19,22,23,110] has greatly increased the capability of confirming the diagnosis of these conditions in symptomatic patients. Optimum treatment, however, remains less well defined.

Clinical presentation

Vasovagal syncope is essentially the "simple" or "common" faint. In young people, this type of faint tends to be easy to diagnose because a clear history of preceding dizziness together with other typical phenomena is obtained (see review by Sutton and Petersen [111]). The patient often reports feelings of lack of air, a change in breathing pattern, detachment from surroundings, sweating, loss of hearing, and nausea prior to total loss of consciousness. Prolonged attacks may be associated with incontinence, usually of urine. Witnesses commonly report that the patient exhibited marked pallor, and may also report the occurrence of muscular jerking. During the recovery phase there is rapid resumption of orientation, but weakness, nausea, and headache may last from minutes to hours. In older subjects, the premonitory symptoms may be very brief and therefore entirely unrecognized, or completely lacking. In such cases, syncope occurs without warning. Such an outcome often results in falls and physical injury, a presentation difficult to distinguish by history alone from syncope complicating conduction disturbances of the heart.

Vasovagal syncope may be triggered by any of a variety of situational factors. Some of the latter include unpleasant sights (e.g., sight of blood), pain, extreme emotion, prolonged standing, stuffy rooms, boredom, and the previous consumption of alcohol. Typical venues for fainting are churches, hospitals, the sports field (usually in association with injury), parties, queues, traveling by air, and restaurants. When prodromal symptoms are lacking, a suspicious venue may be helpful in suggesting the correct diagnosis.

Carotid sinus syndrome usually presents with syncope without warning, but with a slower recovery than is expected in Stokes–Adams attacks. Although rare, a history suggesting that head movements trigger dizziness or syncope supports this diagnosis. As a rule, the condition almost exclusively afflicts older people, with substantial male dominance. These features are in contrast to those of vasovagal syncope; the latter tends to affect the sexes equally and occurs at all ages.

Until recently, bradycardia was considered to be a more prominent feature in carotid sinus syndrome than in vasovagal syncope. However, recent insights obtained from the use of ILRs suggest that spontaneous vasovagal spells are more often associated with bradycardia than had been previously appreciated [17,27–29,112]. Further, with the increasing use of carotid massage with the patient in an upright posture, the importance of vasodilation in carotid sinus syndrome patients has become more evident.

Pathophysiological mechanisms

The efferent reflex pathways (i.e., CNS to major organ systems and peripheral circulation) causing hypotension and bradycardia in the various neurally mediated syncopes are relatively well understood. Essentially, enhanced efferent neural signals in the vagus nerve mediate bradycardia while almost simultaneous diminution of sympathetic neural activity is believed to be primarily responsible for causing dilation of skeletal muscle arterioles [113,114] and splanchnic venules (i.e., the vasodilation component) [115]. However, the "trigger" factors, the afferent neural pathways (i.e., from "trigger" sites to the CNS), and the processing in the vasomotor center are far less clear.

In general, the risk of triggering neurally mediated reflex syncope is accentuated by the loss of central venous volume. This may occur spontaneously as a result of dehydration, hemorrhage, or adoption of the erect posture. The latter has been associated with displacement of 500–1000 mL from the central circulation to dependent regions (higher in patients with inadequate peripheral vascular compensation). Originally, in typical vasovagal syncope, cardiac baroreceptors (particularly those in the left ventricular wall) were implicated as principal sites of inappropriate triggering of the bradycardia-hypotension reflex [108, 116–118]. However, given the documented occurrence of vasovagal syncope in orthotopic heart transplant recipients [119], the focus of interest has shifted toward other residual central mechano- and chemoreceptors (e.g., those baroreceptors that persist in the right atrial remnant in transplanted patients, receptors in the great vessels and pulmonary circulation). These various receptors may be triggered by very low filling pressures known to occur in developing vasovagal syncope [120]. The latter may simply reflect concomitant central volume diminution as a result of the factors noted above. Whether patients particularly susceptible to vasovagal syncope respond in an exaggerated manner to this "stress" is as yet uncertain. In carotid sinus syndrome, the afferent side of the reflex loop is somewhat more clear-cut. In this case, the mode of triggering is neurological arising from stimulation of autonomic receptors in the cervical region [21,121–123], potentially in conjunction with absence of parallel inputs from the sternocleidomastoid muscles [123]. This direct stimulation may account for its rapid onset. If there are central processing abnormalities they are probably similar to those in vasovagal syncope The latter, if they exist, and shared efferent mechanisms may explain the observed clinical overlap between carotid sinus syndrome and vasovagal syncope [124].

The principal afferent neural pathways from central mechano- and chemoreceptors to the medulla in classic vasovagal syncope are generally thought to be via vagal C-fibers. In "susceptible" patients, activity triggered in these pathways initiates a poorly understood series of events within the medullary cardiovascular control areas that result in the efferent response noted above. For other non-vasovagal types of neurally mediated syncope (e.g., carotid sinus syncope, postmicturition syncope), separate afferent neural pathways from the trigger site to the brain have been identified, although central chemo- and mechanoreceptors may also contribute secondarily in these settings [124].

The factors that impart "susceptibility" to neurally mediated syncope in humans remain to be elucidated. It seems that most humans are capable of experiencing vasovagal reactions from time to time, although only a subset (and these often only for a brief period in their lives) seem to exhibit marked susceptibility to recurrent episodes. Potentially, susceptibility may arise from enhanced "trigger site" sensitivity, abnormal medullary response to an otherwise normal afferent signal, an excessive and/or inappropriately balanced efferent neural response, or an undesirable peripheral response (perhaps related to the concept of accentuated antagonism between sympathetic and parasympathetic pathways). Susceptibility may also be characterized by certain neurohumoral responses that have been recorded in fainters but not control subjects. Thus, for example, marked elevation of circulating adrenaline, vasopressin and beta-endorphins [58,125–127] have been reported to precede vasovagal syncope. Whether these are causal, or secondary phenomena is unknown.

Incidence and prognosis

Vasovagal syncope is a condition that can occur in anybody, given sufficiently adverse circumstances. The reported prevalence varies from 15% to 35% of the study population, depending on the group surveyed. For instance, in a recent examination of findings in 641 consecutive patients referred to tertiary care centers for evaluation, Mathias *et al.* [16] concluded that vasovagal syncope accounted for 35%. Fitzpatrick *et al.* [36] estimated that approximately 18% of presentations of two or more syncopal episodes prompting referral for permanent pacing are vasovagal in origin.

Vasovagal syncope is not thought to carry a high risk of fatality. However, the impact of recurrent faints on employment, lifestyle, and susceptibility to physical injury is real. Further, although a more remote concern, sudden asystole is known to be a mode of death [128]. Consequently, the possibility of a rare association between vasovagal syncope and sudden death has been raised [129]. The tendency for vasovagal syncope to occur in young physically fit individuals has raised concern regarding its possible contribution to sports-related syncope with the rare occurrence of physical injury or death as a result of asystole [21].

The incidence of carotid sinus syndrome has been calculated to be 35–40 new patients per million per year [121,122]. As a cause of syncope, carotid sinus syndrome is generally reported to account for approximately 5% of cases [15,16]. However, in clinical practice the condition may be easily overlooked. The reasons for this include:
1 failure to perform carotid sinus massage and tilt table testing routinely in syncope patients;
2 misclassification resulting from failure to record both blood pressure and heart rate response when carotid massage is undertaken (i.e., in the absence of adequate arterial pressure measurements, predominant vasodilatory responses may be overlooked); and
3 failure to perform carotid sinus massage with the patient in the upright posture.

In general, carotid sinus syndrome is not considered to be a life-threatening condition. A 70-year-old patient at presentation is expected to have a 65% 5-year survival. Nevertheless, given the usual effectiveness of appropriately selected pacing therapy, failure to recognize the diagnosis unduly exposes elderly patients (those most often afflicted) to risk of physical injury associated with recurrent syncope and dizzy spells.

Investigation

The most common form of carotid sinus syndrome (i.e., predominant cardioinhibitory form) is diagnosed when carotid sinus massage in the erect position for 5–10 s is associated with symptom reproduction because of the occurrence of asystole or paroxysmal AV block of at least 3 s in duration [17,21,121,122]. The vasodilatory component can be assessed separately by controlling the bradycardia using a temporary dual-chamber pacing system and beat-to-beat arterial pressure monitoring in the erect position. These tests are best performed on a tilt table using digital plethysmography (or, less desirably, an intra-arterial line) to record beat-to-beat arterial pressure changes.

Vasovagal syncope may be suspected as a result of the clinical history, but this is not always possible. Consequently, although protocols have been in a state of evolution in recent years, tilt table testing techniques have proved very valuable [16,17,19,22,23,34]. As a rule, the first step is "passive" head-up tilt at 60–70° during which the patient is supported by a footplate and gently applied body straps for a period not less than 30 min and preferably 45 min [17,34]. Tilt angle of less than 60° and more than 80° leads to loss of sensitivity and specificity. Subsequently, if needed, tilt testing in conjunction with a drug challenge (e.g., isoproterenol, edrophonium, nitroglycerin) may be undertaken either immediately or as a separate procedure [17,34]. The most frequently used drug is isoproterenol, usually given in escalating dosage from 1–3 µg min^{-1} [17,34]. Nitroglycerine intravenously or sublingually has recently gained particular favor in Europe [130].

Tilt testing has a false-positive rate of approximately 10% [34,131]. Acute (i.e., same day or within a few days) test reproducibility in terms of whether syncope is induced or not is approximately 80–90%. Longer term reproducibility (i.e., over more than 1 year) is approximately 60% [132–135]. As there is no "gold standard" for diagnosis of neurally mediated syncope, the sensitivity of tilt testing cannot accurately be estimated. Thus, tilt table testing is an imperfect test. Nevertheless, tilt testing remains the only test that provides the opportunity to precipitate a typical attack under the eyes of the physician. Tilt testing also provides the patient valuable experience that may help them to recognize impending faints and thereby avert future events. Further, its specificity and reproducibility are comparable with many other widely accepted useful diagnostic procedures.

It has been known for some time that tilt testing does not always result in the same hemodynamic picture when repeated in the same patient. Thus, cardioinhibition (i.e., bradycardia) may predominate on one occasion whereas vasodilation with hypotension may occur at another time. Thus, tilt testing may not be optimal for directing treatment strategy. In this regard, the recently published ISSUE study [112] indicates that even when tilt testing indicated a prominent vasodilatory component to the faint, the subsequent recording of spontaneous faints by means of an ILR often revealed bradycardic events. Further study of this phenomenon with devices that can monitor blood pressure (or a surrogate of blood pressure), as well as heart rate, could prove very enlightening.

Treatment

The mainstay in treatment of typical vasovagal syncope is explanation, reassurance, and advice regarding appropriate salt/volume intake. This approach proves most effective when there is a prodrome of sufficient duration to permit the patient to take suitable evasive action. Patients whose symptoms demand more than mere reassurance are those whose attacks have minimal or no prodrome (especially if they have had resulting injury), those who cannot be taught to abort attacks, and those in whom attacks are complicated by seizure-like activity or incontinence. Additionally, patients with "high-risk" occupations or avocations in which syncope might lead to injury to themselves or others present a concern (e.g., pilots, commercial drivers, window-cleaners, swimmers, etc.).

Of greatest recent treatment interest is the concept of "tilt training." In this case, progressively longer periods of forced quiet upright posture are prescribed and carried out over a prolonged period of time [136,137]. Results suggest that this procedure enhances vascular reactivity to gravitational stress and reduces susceptibility to recurrent vasovagal faints. The same technique may also be recommended in orthostatic faints [137].

There exists a vast literature on medication for patients with vasovagal syncope, which is discussed in depth in Chapter 2. Most of the published experience has been based on uncontrolled studies [138]. The few controlled studies that have been reported (atenolol, cafedrine, disopyramide, scopolamine, etilefrine, and midodrine) have tended to be small and of short duration [139–143]. For instance, one β-adrenergic blocker study that demonstrated the benefit of atenolol had only had 1 month's follow-up. Recent, randomized, placebo controlled studies have reported benefit from agents such as midodrine and paroxetine [144,145]. The POST trial, comparing placebo and metoprolol, showed a benefit for those over 42 years of age, but no benefit for those less than 42 years of age (see Chapter 2) [144,145].

Cardiac pacing has proved highly successful in carotid sinus syndrome when bradycardia has been documented [146,147]. Currently, pacing is acknowledged to be the treatment of choice in all but the most mild forms of carotid sinus syndrome. In general, dual-chamber pacing is favored. A rate-drop response diagnostic and rapid pacing rate hysteresis are desirable. The VVI or VVIR pacing mode should only be chosen if there is clear absence of both susceptibility to "ventricular pacing effect" (i.e., a drop in systemic pressure as a result of ventricular pacing alone) and a substantial concomitant vasodepressor element [121,147]. Single-chamber atrial pacing (AAI or AAIR) is contraindicated in carotid sinus syndrome (and other forms of neurally mediated syncope) because of the propensity for these patients to exhibit paroxysmal high-grade AV block during the episodes. Incidentally, the presence of AV block may be "masked" by marked sinus bradycardia or asystole, but becomes immediately evident upon pacing the atrium.

In contrast to carotid sinus syndrome, experience with pacing in other forms of neurally mediated syncope has been much more limited [148–151]. Nevertheless, two important multicenter, controlled trials favor the utility of this strategy. In these two multicenter, randomized trials, the focus was treatment of individuals who appeared to demonstrate predominantly cardioinhibitory faints. In the case of the North American trial [151], there was an actuarial first year rate of recurrent syncope of 18% for pacemaker patients and 60% for controls. The results of the pacing arm of the European VASIS trial [152] were similar but with a longer follow-up in less severely affected (and thus perhaps more typical) patients. A third study has recently been published which further supports the potential for pacing in vasovagal fainters. Ammirati *et al.* [153] reported results in 93 patients (over 55 years of age) who had experienced more than three syncopal events over a 2-year period of time, and who had positive tilt tests with evidence of bradycardia. Patients were randomized to either pacing (DDD mode with rate-drop algorithm, $n = 46$) or β-adrenergic blocker therapy ($n = 47$). Paced patients had two syncope recurrences during a mean follow-up of 390 days; whereas beta-blocker-treated

patients had 12 syncopal recurrences over a mean follow-up of 135 days.

Thus, in vasovagal syncope, pacing may have a useful role when reserved for severe cases in which cardioinhibition appears to be responsible for symptoms. In this setting, only a dual-chamber system is capable of slowing the fall of cardiac output in the face of diminishing venous return.

Two trials have recently been published that may change our approach to pacing in vasovagal syncope. The first of these was the VPS2 trial [154]. After 6 months of follow-up of 100 patients, all of whom received a dual-chamber device either programmed "on" or "off", no significant difference was seen in the time to the first syncope recurrence. The 30% relative risk reduction of the pacing "on" versus pacing "off" may have been demonstrating a trend toward a benefit in the paced group. However, this will never be known as the trial design determined that at 6 months the comparison would be changed to conventional rate of hysteresis versus rate drop response. The investigators made the preliminary conclusion that while the pacemaker treatment effect was not as significant as in the VPS1 trial, the results were nevertheless favorable for pacing in the patients studied. The authors of the study also recommended that pacing for vasovagal syncope should not be considered first-line therapy.

The other trial was the SYNPACE study [155]. Of 29 patients with recurrent syncope receiving pacemakers, there was no significant difference between the pacemaker "on" group versus those with the pacemaker implanted but not activated (OFF). One significant result was that patients with an asystolic tilt table response prior to implant experienced their first syncopal recurrence after pacing at 96 days versus 11 days for those who only demonstrated bradycardia during tilt ($P < 0.03$). These more recent trials tend to cast doubt on the benefit afforded by pacing, and the benefit noted during prior studies attributed to the placebo effect of the surgical procedure required to implant the device. However, it may be too early to conclude that it is all placebo effect as neither of these trials had a sufficiently long follow-up period to make a final judgment (in particular the VPS2 where follow-up ended at 6 months by the trial design).

Thus, dual-chamber pacing with some form of rate hysteresis is effective in tilt-induced and in postimplant follow-up studies of vasovagal syncope. Pacing also appears to have a powerful placebo effect. Careful patient selection of those who are the most symptomatic and have clear cardioinhibitory collapse patterns should be considered for pacing. Pacing should not be considered first-line therapy for vasovagal syncope. Candidates would include those who are older (over 40 years), who have little or no warning prior to syncope, and those who have prolonged attacks complicated by abnormal (epileptiform) movements associated with incontinence [156]. The development of future technologies that will allow for the onset of pacing at an earlier point in a vasovagal attack may provide for a more effective means of therapy.

Conclusions

Bradyarrhythmias resulting from sinus node dysfunction, AV conduction disturbances, and neurally mediated reflex hypotension bradycardia (especially vasovagal syncope) are important causes of syncope. However, establishing the diagnosis in these cases may be challenging. For instance, although bradyarrhythmias may account for symptoms in patients with sinus node and/or AV conduction disturbances, these same symptoms may be caused by tachyarrhythmias. Consequently, identifying the presence of sinus node or AV conduction abnormalities is by itself insufficient to discern the nature of the problem. In the absence of definitive information, it is impossible to develop an effective treatment strategy. Thus, additional careful evaluation is needed to define as precisely as possible the arrhythmia at fault. Similar difficulties arise with respect to the neurally mediated syncopal syndromes. In these cases, the electrocardiographic manifestations encompass a spectrum of possibilities from severe sinus arrest and/or high-grade AV block, to syncope in the absence of overt bradycardia (i.e., systemic hypotension resulting from vasodilation). The first may be interpreted as suggesting the presence of underlying conduction system disease, whereas in the case of pure vasodepressor syncope the diagnosis may be missed entirely if electrocardiographic recordings are obtained in the absence of concomitant blood pressure recordings. Thus, even when electrocardiographic recordings documenting bradycardia during spontaneous symptoms are available, the ultimate basis for syncopal

symptoms may still require further careful diagnostic assessment.

The principal diagnostic step in the syncope patient is differentiation of those individuals with normal cardiovascular status from those with evident structural disease. In the former, assuming that the medical history or physical examination has not identified another system problem, autonomic nervous system studies including carotid sinus massage and tilt table testing should be undertaken. In the latter group, a functional assessment of the suspected structural disturbance (i.e., hemodynamic, angiographic, and electrophysiologic studies as appropriate), and on occasion evaluation of susceptibility to tachy- and bradyarrhythmias by conventional electrophysiologic testing is appropriate. Tilt table testing should follow if the diagnosis remains in doubt. Frequently, long-term monitoring may be necessary to obtain a satisfactory diagnosis. In such cases, ILRs appear to be a particularly promising tool. In only a few instances should special neurologic studies be selected as an initial step. In all cases, the ultimate objective is obtaining a sufficiently strong correlation between the syncopal symptoms and detected abnormalities to permit both an accurate assessment of prognosis and initiation of an appropriate treatment plan.

Acknowledgments

The authors would like to thank Wendy Markuson and Barry L.S. Detloff for assistance in preparation of the manuscript.

References

1 Stokes W. Observations on some cases of permanently slow pulse. *Dublin Q J Med Sci* 1846:**2**;73–85.

2 Mackenzie J. *Diseases of the Heart*. London: Oxford Medical Press, 1913: 48.

3 Benditt DG, Sakaguchi S, Goldstein MA, *et al.* Sinus node dysfunction: pathophysiology, clinical features, evaluation and treatment. In: Zipes DP, Jalife J, eds. *Cardiac Electrophysiology: From Cell to Bedside*, 2nd edn. Philadelphia, PA: W.B. Saunders, 1995: 1215–46.

4 Brignole M, Menozzi C, Gianfranchi L, Oddone D, Lolli G, Bertulla A. Neurally mediated syncope detected by carotid sinus massage and head-up tilt test in sick sinus syndrome. *Am J Cardiol* 1991;**68**:1032–6.

5 Alboni P, Menozzi C, Brignole M, *et al.* An abnormal neural reflex plays a role in causing syncope in sinus bradycardia. *J Am Coll Cardiol* 1993;**22**:1130–4.

6 Benditt DG, Benson DW Jr, Dunnigan A, *et al.* Drug therapy in sinus node dysfunction. In: Rapaport E, ed. *Cardiology Update.* New York, NY: Elsevier, 1984: 79–101.

7 Wayne HH. Syncope: physiological considerations and an analysis of the clinical characteristics in 510 patients. *Am J Med* 1961;**30**:418–38.

8 Day SC, Cook EF, Funkenstein H, *et al.* Evaluation and outcome of emergency room patients with transient loss of consciousness. *Am J Med* 1982;**72**:15–23.

9 Silverstein MD, Singer DE, Mulley AG, *et al.* Patients with syncope admitted to medical intensive care units. *JAMA* 1982;**248**:1185–9.

10 Gendelman HE, Linzer M, Gabelman M, *et al.* Syncope in a general hospital population. *N Y State J Med* 1983; **83**:116–65.

11 Martin GJ, Adams SL, Martin HG, *et al.* Prospective evaluation of syncope. *Ann Emerg Med* 1984;**13**:499–504.

12 Kudenchuk PJ, McAnulty JH. Syncope: evaluation and treatment. *Mod Conc Cardiovasc Dis* 1985;**54**: 25–9.

13 Camm AJ, Lau CP. Syncope of undetermined origin: diagnosis and management. *Prog Cardiol* 1988;**1**:139–56.

14 Ross RT. *Syncope.* London: W.B. Saunders, 1988.

15 Kapoor W. Evaluation and outcome of patients with syncope. *Medicine* 1990;**69**:160–75.

16 Mathias CJ, Deguchi K, Schatz I. Autonomic-function investigations aid in the diagnosis of the cause of syncope and presyncope. *Lancet* 2001;**357**:348–53.

17 Brignole M, Alboni P, Benditt DG, *et al.* Guidelines on management (diagnosis and treatment) of syncope. *Eur Heart J* 2001;**22**:1256–306.

18 Shaw FE, Kenny RA. Overlap between syncope and falls in the elderly. *Postgrad Med J* 1997;**73**:635–9.

19 Benditt DG, Fahy GJ, Lurie GF, Sakaguchi S, Fabian W, Samniah N. Pharmacotherapy of neurally mediated syncope. *Circulation* 1999;**100**(11):1242–8.

20 Chen M-Y, Goldenberg IF, Milstein S, *et al.* Cardiac electrophysiologic and hemodynamic correlates of neurally mediated syncope. *Am J Cardiol* 1989;**63**:66–72.

21 Almquist A, Gornick CC, Benson DW Jr, *et al.* Carotid sinus hypersensitivity: evaluation of the vasodepressor component. *Circulation* 1985;**67**:927–36.

22 Sutton R, Petersen M, Brignole M, *et al.* Proposed classification for tilt induced vasovagal syncope. *Eur J Card Pacing Electrophysiol* 1992;**2**:180–3.

23 Brignole M, Menozzi C, Del Rosso A, *et al.* New classification of haemodynamics of vasovagal syncope: beyond the VASIS classification. Analysis of the pre-syncopal phase of the tilt test without and with nitroglycerin challenge. Vasovagal Syncope International Study. *Europace* 2000;**2**:66–76.

24 Moya A, Brignole M, Menozzi C, *et al.* and ISSUE Investigators. Mechanism of syncope in patients with isolated syncope and in patients with tilt-positive syncope. *Circulation* 2001;**104**:1261–7.

25 Gibson JC, Heitzman MR. Diagnostic efficacy of 24 hour electrocardiographic monitoring for syncope. *Am J Cardiol* 1984;**53**:1013–7.

26 Crawford MH, Bernstein SJ, Deedwania PC, *et al.* ACC/AHA Guidelines for Ambulatory Electrocardiography. *J Am Coll Cardiol* 1999;**34**:912–48. (Executive summary and recommendations. *Circulation* 1999;**100**:886–93.)

27 Krahn AD, Klein GJ, Norris C, *et al.* The etiology of syncope in patients with negative tilt table and electrophysiologic testing. *Circulation* 1995;**92**:1819–24.

28 Krahn A, Klein GJ, Yee R, Takle-Newhouse T, Norris C. Use of an extended monitoring strategy in patients with problematic syncope. Reveal Investigators. *Circulation* 1999;**99**:406–10.

29 Krahn A, Klein GJ, Yee R, Skanes AC. Randomized assessment of syncope trial: conventional diagnostic testing versus a prolonged monitoring strategy. *Circulation* 2001;**104**:46–51.

30 Sakaguchi S, Shultz J, Remole S, *et al.* Syncope associated with exercise, a manifestation of neurally mediated syncope. *Am J Cardiol* 1995;**75**:476–81.

31 Sra JS, Anderson AJ, Sheikh SH, *et al.* Unexplained syncope evaluated by electrophysiologic studies and head-up tilt testing. *Ann Intern Med* 1991;**114**:1013–9.

32 DiMarco JB, Garan H, Hawthorne WJ, *et al.* Intracardiac electrophysiologic techniques in recurrent syncope of unknown cause. *Ann Intern Med* 1981;**95**:542–8.

33 Fujimura O, Yee R, Klein GJ, *et al.* The diagnostic sensitivity of electrophysiologic testing in patients with syncope caused by bradycardia. *N Engl J Med* 1989;**321**: 1703–7.

34 Benditt DG, Ferguson DW, Grubb BP, *et al.* Tilt-table testing for assessing syncope: an American College of Cardiology expert consensus document. *J Am Coll Cardiol* 1996;**28**(1):263–75.

35 Benditt DG. Head-up tilt table testing: rationale, methodology, and applications. In: Zipes DP, Jalife J, eds. *Cardiac Electrophysiology: From Cell to Bedside*, 3rd edn. Philadelphia, PA: W.B. Saunders, 2000: 746–53.

36 Fitzpatrick A, Theodorakis G, Vardas P, *et al.* Methodology of head-up tilt testing in patients with unexplained syncope. *J Am Coll Cardiol* 1991;**17**:125–30.

37 Rubenstein JJ, Schulman CL, Yurchak PM, *et al.* Clinical spectrum of the sick sinus syndrome. *Circulation* 1972;**46**:5–13.

38 Sutton R, Perrins EJ. Neurological manifestations of the sick sinus syndrome. In: Busse EW, ed. *Cerebral Manifestations of Episodic Cardiac Dysrhythmias.* Amsterdam, the Netherlands: Excerpta Medica, 1979: 174–81.

39 Ausubel K, Furman S. The pacemaker syndrome. *Ann Intern Med* 1985;**103**:420–9.

40 Ellenbogen KA, Wood MA, Stambler B. Pacemaker syndrome: clinical, hemodynamic, and neurohumoral features. In: Barold SS, Mugica J, eds. *New Perspectives in Cardiac Pacing 3.* Mt. Kisco, NY: Futura, 1993: 85–112.

41 Ector H, Rolies L, De Geest H. Dynamic electrocardiography and ventricular pauses of 3 seconds and more: etiology and therapeutic implications. *PACE* 1983;**6**:548–51.

42 Hilgard J, Ezri MD, Denes P. Significance of ventricular pauses of three seconds or more detected on 24 hour Holter recordings. *Am J Cardiol* 1985;**55**:1005–8.

43 Ferrer MI. The sick sinus syndrome in atrial disease. *JAMA* 1968;**206**:645.

44 Kaplan BM, Langendorf R, Lev M, Pick A. Tachycardia-bradycardia syndrome (so-called "sick sinus syndrome"). *Am J Cardiol* 1973;**26**:497–508.

45 Sutton R, Kenny R-A. The natural history of sick sinus syndrome. *PACE* 1986;**9**:1110–4.

46 Andersen HR, Thuesen L, Bagger JP, Vesterlund T, Thomsen PEB. Prospective randomised trial of atrial versus ventricular pacing in sick-sinus syndrome. *Lancet* 1994;**344**:1523–8.

47 Andersen HR, Nielsen JC, Thomsen PE, *et al.* Long-term follow-up of patients from a randomised trial of atrial versus ventricular pacing for sick-sinus syndrome. *Lancet* 1997;**350**:1210–6.

48 Rosenqvist M, Brandt J, Schuller H. Atrial versus ventricular pacing in sinus node disease: a treatment comparison study. *Am Heart J* 1986;**111**:292–7.

49 Stangl K, Wirtzfeld A, Seitz K, *et al.* Atrial stimulation (AAI): long-term follow-up of 110 patients. In: Belhassen B, Feldman S, Copperman Y, eds. *Cardiac Pacing and Electrophysiology. Proceedings of the VIIIth World Symposium on Cardiac Pacing and Electrophysiology.* Jerusalem: R & L Creative Communications, 1987: 283–5.

50 Sutton R, Bourgeois I. *The Foundations of Cardiac Pacing. Part 1.* Mt Kisco, NY: Futura Publishing, 1991: 131.

51 Gijs Mast E, Van Hemel NM, Bakea L, *et al.* Is chronic atrial stimulation a reliable method for single chamber pacing in sick sinus syndrome? *PACE* 1986;**9**:1127–30.

52 van Mechelen R, Segers A, Hagemeijer F. Serial electrophysiologic studies after single chamber atrial pacemaker implantation in patients with symptomatic sinus node dysfunction. *Eur Heart J* 1984;**5**:628–36.

53 Santini M, Alexidou G, Ansalone G, *et al.* Relation of prognosis in sick sinus syndrome at age, conduction defects and modes of permanent cardiac pacing. *Am J Cardiol* 1990;**565**:729–35.

54 Skagen K, Hansen JF. The long-term prognosis for patients with sinoatrial block treated with permanent pacemaker. *Acta Med Scand* 1975;**199**:13–5.

55 Sasaki Y, Shimotori M, Akahane K, *et al.* Long-term follow-up of patients with sick sinus syndrome: a comparison of clinical aspects among unpaced, ventricular inhibited paced, and physiologically paced groups. *Pacing Clin Electrophysiol* 1988;**11**:1575–83.

56 Brignole M, Menozzi C, Gianfranchi L, *et al.* Neurally mediated syncope detected by carotid sinus massage and head-up tilt test in sick sinus syndrome. *Am J Cardiol* 1991;**68**: 1032–6.

57 Rosenqvist M, Brandt J, Schuller H. Long-term pacing in sick sinus node disease: effects of stimulation mode on cardiovascular morbidity and mortality. *Am Heart J* 1988;**116**:16–22.

58 Laupacis A, Albers G, Dalen J, *et al.* Antithrombotic therapy in atrial fibrillation. *Chest* 1995;**108**:352S–9S.

59 Scheinman MM, Evans-Bell T, and the Executive Committee of the Percutaneous Cardiac Mapping and Ablation Registry. Catheter ablation of the atrioventricular junction: a report of the percutaneous mapping and ablation registry. *Circulation* 1984;**70**:1024–9.

60 Haissaguerre M, Gencel L, Fischer B, *et al.* Successful catheter ablation of atrial fibrillation. *J Cardiovasc Electrophysiol* 1994;**5**:1045–52.

61 Gaita F, Riccardi R, Calo L, *et al.* Atrial mapping and radiofrequency catheter ablation in patients with idiopathic atrial fibrillation: electrophysiological findings and ablation results. *Circulation* 1998;**97**:2136–45.

62 Haissaguerre M, Jais P, Shah D, *et al.* Spontaneous initiation of atrial fibrillation by ectopic beats originating in the pulmonary veins. *N Engl J Med* 1998; **339**:659–66.

63 Oral H, Knight BP, Tada H, *et al.* Pulmonary vein isolation for paroxysmal and persistent atrial fibrillation. *Circulation* 2002;**105**:1077–81.

64 Cox JL. The surgical treatment of atrial fibrillation. IV. Surgical technique. *J Thorac Cardiovasc Surg* 1991; **101**:5884–92.

65 Cox JL, Boineau JP, Schuessler RB, *et al.* Modifications of the MAZE procedure for atrial flutter and atrial fibrillation. I. Rationale and surgical results. *J Thorac Cardiovasc Surg* 1995;**110**:473–84.

66 Saksena S, Prakash A, Hill M, *et al.* Prevention of recurrent atrial fibrillation with chronic dual site right atrial pacing. *J Am Coll Cardiol* 1996;**28**:687–94.

67 Prakash A, Delfaut P, Krol RB, Saksena S. Regional right and left atrial activation patterns during single and dual site atrial pacing in patients with atrial fibrillation. *Am J Cardiol* 1998;**82**(10):1197–204.

68 Murgatroyd FD, Johnson EE, Cooper RA, *et al.* Safety of low energy atrial defibrillation: world experience (Abstract). *Circulation* 1994;**99**(Suppl. I):14.

69 Wellens HJJ, Lau C-P, Luderitz B, *et al.* for the METRIX Investigators. Atrioverter: an implantable device for the treatment of atrial fibrillation. *Circulation* 1998;**98**:1651–6.

70 Puech P, Grolleau R, Guimond C. Incidence of different types of AV block and their localization by His bundle recordings. In: Wellens HJJ, Lie KI, Janse MJ, eds. *The Conduction System of the Heart.* Leiden, the Netherlands: Stenfert Kroese, 1976: 467–84.

71 Rosen KM, Rahimtoola SH, Chuquimia R, *et al.* Electrophysiological significance of first degree atrioventricular block with intraventricular conduction disturbance. *Circulation* 1971;**43**:491–502.

72 Narula OS, Scherlag BJ, Javier RP, *et al.* Analysis of the A-V conduction defect in complete heart block utilizing His bundle electrograms. *Circulation* 1970;**41**:437–48.

73 Lev M. The pathology of atrioventricular block. *Cardiovasc Clin* 1972;**4**:159–86.

74 Lev M, Bharati S. Atrioventricular and intraventricular conduction system disease. *Arch Intern Med* 1975; **135**:405–10.

75 Rotman M, Wagner GS, Wallace AG. Bradyarrhythmias in acute myocardial infarction. *Circulation* 1973;**45**:703–22.

76 Sutton R, Davies M. The conduction system in acute myocardial infarction complicated by heart block. *Circulation* 1968;**38**:987–92.

77 Rosen KM, Loeb HS, Chuquimia R, *et al.* Site of heart block in acute myocardial infarction. *Circulation* 1970; **42**:925–33.

78 Berger PB, Ruocco NA Jr, Ryan TJ, *et al.* Incidence and prognostic implications of heart block complicating inferior myocardial infarction treated with thrombolytic therapy: results from the TIMI II. *J Am Coll Cardiol* 1992;**20**:533–40.

79 Rathore SS, Gersh BJ, Berger PB, *et al.* Acute myocardial infarction complicated by heart block in the elderly: prevalence and outcomes. *Am Heart J* 2001;**141**(47):47–54.

80 Vigorita VJ, Hutchins GM. Cardiac conduction system in hemochromatosis: clinical and pathological features in six patients. *Am J Cardiol* 1979;**44**:418–23.

81 Bharati S, Lev M, Denes P, Modlinger J, *et al.* Infiltrative cardiomyopathy with conduction disease and ventricular arrhythmia: electrophysiologic and pathologic correlations. *Am J Cardiol* 1980;**45**:163–73.

82 Bharati S, de la Fuente DJ, Kallen RJ, *et al.* Conduction system in systemic lupus erythematosus with atrioventricular block. *Am J Cardiol* 1975;**35**:299–304.

83 Hassel D, Heinsimer J, Califf RM, *et al.* Complete heart block in Reiter's syndrome. *Am J Cardiol* 1984;**53**:967–8.

84 Kastor JA. Atrioventricular block. In: Kastor JA, ed. *Arrhythmias.* Philadelphia, PA: W.B. Saunders, 1994: 150.

85 Mathewson FA, Rabkin SW, Hsu PH. Atrioventricular heart block: 27 year follow-up experience. *Trans Assoc Life Ins Med Dir Am* 1976;**60**:110–30.

86 McAnulty JH, Murphy E, Rahimtoola SH. A prospective evaluation of intraHisian conduction delay. *Circulation* 1979;**59**:1035–9.

87 Shaw DB, Kekwick CA, Veale D, Gowers J, Whistance T. Survival in second degree atrioventricular block. *Br Heart J* 1985;**53**:587–93.

88 Rowe JC, White PD. Complete heart block: a follow-up study. *Ann Intern Med* 1958;**49**:260–70.

89 Penton GB, Miller H, Levine SA. Some clinical features of complete heart block. *Circulation* 1956;**13**:801–24.

90 Berger PR, Roucco NA Jr, Ryan TJ, *et al.* Incidence and prognostic implications of heart block complicating inferior myocardial infarction treated with thrombolytic therapy: results from TIMI II. *J Am Coll Cardiol* 1992;**20**:533–40.

91 Michaelsson M, Engle MA. Congenital complete heart block: an international study of the natural history. *Cardiovasc Clin* 1972;**4**:86–101.

92 Pordon CM, Moodie DJ. Adults with congenital complete heart block: 25-year follow-up. *Cleve Clin J Med* 1992;**59**:587–90.

93 Michaelsson M, Jonzon A, Riesenfeld T. Isolated congenital complete atrioventricular block in adult life. *Circulation* 1995;**92**:442–9.

94 Schneider JF, Thomas HE Jr, Kreger BE, *et al.* New acquired left bundle branch block: the Framingham Study. *Ann Intern Med* 1979;**90**:303–10.

95 Schneider JF, Thomas HE Jr, Kreger BE, *et al.* Newly acquired right bundle-branch block: the Framingham Study. *Ann Intern Med* 1980;**92**:37–44.

96 Dhingra RC, Denes P, Wu D, *et al.* Syncope in patients with chronic bifascicular block. *Ann Intern Med* 1974; **81**:302–6.

97 Scheinman MM, Peters RW, Sauve MJ, *et al.* Value of H-Q interval in patients with bundle branch block and the role of prophylactic permanent pacing. *Am J Cardiol* 1982;**50**:1316–22.

98 Dhingra RC, Amat y Leon F, Pouget M, *et al.* Infranodal block: diagnosis, clinical significance and management. *Med Clin North Am* 1976;**60**:175–92.

99 Dhingra RC, Wyndham CRC, Bauernfiend RA, *et al.* Significance of bundle branch block distal to the His bundle induced by atrial pacing in patients with chronic bifascicular block. *Circulation* 1979;**60**:1455–64.

100 Fisch C, DeSanctis RW, Dodge HT, *et al.* Guidelines for intracardiac electrophysiologic studies: a report of the American College of Cardiology/American Heart Association Task Force on Assessment of Diagnostic and Therapeutic Cardiovascular Procedures. *Circulation* 1989;**80**:1925–39.

101 Gregoratos G, Cheitlin MD, Conill A, *et al.* ACC/AHA guidelines for implantation of cardiac pacemakers and antiarrhythmia devices: executive summary. A report of the American College of Cardiology/American Heart Association Task Force on Practice Guidelines (Committee on Pacemaker Implantation). *Circulation* 1998; **97**;1325–35.

102 Rattes MF, Klein GJ, Sharma AD, *et al.* Efficacy of empirical cardiac pacing in syncope of unknown cause. *CMAJ* 1989;**140**:381–5.

103 Jordan JL, Yamaguchi I, Mandel WJ. Studies on the mechanism of sinus node dysfunction in the sick sinus syndrome. *Circulation* 1978;**57**:217–23.

104 Scheinman MM, Strauss HC, Evans GT, Ryan C, Massie B, Wallace A. Adverse effects of sympatholytic agents in patients with hypertension and sinus node dysfunction. *Am J Med* 1978;**64**:1013–20.

105 Seipel L, Both A, Breithardt G, *et al.* Action of antiarrhythmic drugs on His bundle electrogram and sinus node function. *Acta Cardiol (Brux)* 1974;**18** (Suppl):251–67.

106 Linker NJ, Camm AJ. Drug effects on the sinus node: a clinical perspective. *Cardiovasc Drugs Ther* 1988;**2**:165–70.

107 Lieshout JJV, Wieling W, Karemaker JM, *et al.* The vasovagal response. *Clin Sci* 1991;**81**:575–86.

108 Almquist A, Goldenberg IF, Milstein S, *et al.* Provocation of bradycardia and hypotension by isoproterenol and upright posture in patients with unexplained syncope. *N Engl J Med* 1989;**320**:346–51.

109 Smith ML, Carlson MD, Thames MD. Reflex control of the heart and circulation: implications for cardiovascular electrophysiology. *J Cardiovasc Electrophysiol* 1991;**2**: 441–9.

110 Kenny RA, Ingram A, Bayliss J, *et al.* Head-up tilt: a useful test for investigating unexplained syncope. *Lancet* 1986;**2**:1352–4.

111 Sutton R, Petersen MEV. The clinical spectrum of neurocardiogenic syncope. *J Cardiovasc Electrophysiol* 1995;**6**:569–76.

112 Moya A, Brignole M, Menozzi C, *et al.* and ISSUE Investigators. Mechanism of syncope in patients with isolated syncope and in patients with tilt-positive syncope. *Circulation* 2001;**104**:1261–7.

113 Barcroft H, Edholm OG. On the vasodilatation in human skeletal muscle during posthaemorrhagic fainting. *J Physiol* 1945;**104**:161–75.

114 Vallin BG, Sundlof G. Sympathetic outflow to muscles during vasovagal syncope. *J Auton Nerv Syst* 1982;**6**: 287–91.

115 Bearn AG, Billing B, Edholm OG, Sherlock S. Hepatic blood flow and carbohydrate changes in man during fainting. *J Physiol* 1951;**115**:442–5.

116 Sharpey-Schafer EP, Hayter CJ, Barlow ED, *et al.* Mechanism of acute hypotension from fear and nausea. *Br Med J* 1958;**46**: 878–80.

117 Thoren P. Role of cardiac C fibres in cardiovascular control. *Rev Physiol Biochem Pharmacol* 1979;**86**:1–94.

118 Oberg B, Thoren P. Increased activity in left ventricular receptors during hemorrhage or occlusion of caval veins in the cat: a possible cause of the vaso-vagal reaction. *Acta Physiol Scand* 1972;**85**:164–73.

119 Fitzpatrick AP, Banner N, Cheng A, *et al.* Vasovagal syncope may occur after orthotopic heart transplantation. *J Am Coll Cardiol* 1993;**21**:1132–7.

120 Dickinson CJ. Fainting precipitated by collapse firing of venous baroreceptors. *Lancet* 1993;**342**:970–2.

121 Morley CA, Sutton R. Carotid sinus syncope. *Int J Cardiol* 1984;**6**:287–93.

122 Benditt DG, Sakaguchi S, Lurie KG, *et al.* Pathophysiology of neurally mediated syncope. In: Saksena S, Luderitz B, eds. *Interventional Electrophysiology: A Textbook*, 2nd edn. Armonk, NY: Futura Publishing, 1996.

123 Tea SH, Mansourati J, L'Heveder G, Mabin D, Blanc J-J. New insights into the pathophysiology of carotid sinus syndrome. *Circulation* 1996;**93**:1411–6.

124 Benditt DG, Goldstein MA, Adler S, *et al.* Neurally mediated syncopal syndromes: pathophysiology and clinical evaluation. In: Mandel WJ, ed. *Cardiac Arrhythmias*, 3rd edn. Philadelphia, PA: J.B. Lippincott, 1995: 879–906.

125 Sander-Jensen K, Secher NH, Astrup A, *et al.* Hypotension induced by passive head-up tilt: endocrine and circulatory mechanisms. *Am J Physiol* 1986;**251**:R743–9.

126 Wallbridge DR, MacIntyre HE, Gray CE, *et al.* Increase in plasma beta-endorphins precedes vasodepressor syncope. *Br Heart J* 1994;**71**:446–8.

127 Jardine DL, Melton I, Crozier IG, Bennett SI, Donald RA, Ikram H. Neurohumoral response to head-up tilt and its role in vasovagal syncope. *Am J Cardiol* 1997; **79**:1302–6.

128 Pepine C, Morganroth J, McDonald J, *et al.* Sudden death during ambulatory electrocardiographic monitoring. *Am J Cardiol* 1991;**68**:785–8.

129 Milstein S, Buetikofer J, Lesser J, *et al.* Cardiac asystole: a manifestation of neurally mediated hypotension bradycardia. *J Am Coll Cardiol* 1989;**14**:1626–32.

130 Raviele A, Menozzi C, Brignole M, *et al.* Value of head-up tilt testing potentiated with sublingual nitroglycerin to assess the origin of unexplained syncope. *Am J Cardiol* 1995;**76**:267–72.

131 Natale A, Akhtar M, Jazayeri M, *et al.* Provocation of hypotension during head-up tilt testing in subjects with no history of syncope or presyncope. *Circulation* 1995; **92**:54–8.

132 Chen XC, Chen MY, Remole S, *et al.* Reproducibility of head-up tilt-table testing for eliciting susceptibility to neurally mediated syncope in patients without structural heart disease. *Am J Cardiol* 1992;**69**:755–60.

133 Grubb BP, Wolfe DA, Temesy-Armos PN, *et al.* Reproducibility of head upright tilt table test results in patients with syncope. *PACE* 1992;**15**:1477–81.

134 Sheldon R, Splawinski J, Killam S. Reproducibility of isoproterenol tilt-table tests in patients with syncope. *Am J Cardiol* 1992;**69**:1300–5.

135 Petersen MEV, Price D, Williams T, *et al.* Short AV delay VDD pacing does not prevent vasovagal syncope in patients with cardioinhibitory vasovagal syndrome. *PACE* 1994;**17**:882–91.

136 Ector H, Reybrouck T, Heidbuchel H, Gewillig M, Van de Werf F. Tilt training: a new treatment for recurrent neurocardiogenic syncope or severe orthostatic intolerance. *PACE* 1998;**21**:193–6.

137 Di Girolamo E, Di Iorio C, Leonzio L, Sabatini P, Barsotti A. Usefulness of a tilt training program for prevention of refractory neurocardiogenic syncope in adolescents: a controlled study. *Circulation* 1999;**100**: 1798–801.

138 Sutton R. Therapy of vasovagal syncope: is there a role for drugs today? In: Raviele R, ed. *Arrhythmias*. Milan, Italy: Springer, 2001: 75–82.

139 Fitzpatrick AP, Ahmed R, Williams S, *et al*. A randomized trial of medical therapy in malignant vasovagal syndrome or neurally mediated bradycardia/hypotension syndrome. *Eur J Card Pacing Electrophysiol* 1991;**1**:91–202.

140 Brignole M, Menozzi C, Gianfranchi L, *et al*. A controlled trial of acute and long-term medical therapy in tilt-induced neurally mediated syncope. *Am J Cardiol* 1992;**70**(3):339–42.

141 Morillo CA, Leitch JU, Yee R, *et al*. A placebo-controlled trial of intravenous and oral disopyramide for prevention of neurally mediated syncope induced by head-up tilt. *J Am Coll Cardiol* 1993;**22**:1843–8.

142 Moya A, Permanyer-Miralda G, Sagrista-Sauleda J, *et al*. Limitations of head-up tilt test for evaluating the efficacy of therapeutic interventions in patients with vasovagal syncope: results of a controlled study of etilefrine versus placebo. *J Am Coll Cardiol* 1995;**25**:65–9.

143 Mahanonda N, Bhuripanyo K, Kangkagate C, *et al*. Randomized double-blind placebo-controlled trial of oral atenolol in patients with unexplained syncope and positive upright tilt table results. *Am Heart J* 1995;**130**:1250–3.

144 Samniah N, Sakaguchi S, Lurie KG, Iskos D, Benditt DG. Efficacy and safety of midodrine hydrochloride in patients with refractory vasovagal syncope. *Am J Cardiol* 2001;**88**(1):80–3.

145 Perez-Lugones A, Schweikert R, Pavia S, *et al*. Usefulness of midodrine in patients with severely symptomatic neurocardiogenic syncope: a randomized control study. *J Cardiovasc Electrophysiol* 2001;**12**:935–8.

146 Brignole M, Menozzi C, Lolli G, *et al*. Long-term outcome of paced and nonpaced patients with severe carotid sinus syndrome *Am J Cardiol* 1992;**69**:1039–43.

147 Benditt DG, Remole S, Asso A, *et al*. Cardiac pacing for carotid sinus syndrome and vasovagal syncope. In: Barold SS, Mugica J, eds. *New Perspectives in Cardiac Pacing*, 3rd edn. Mount Kisco, NY: Futura Publishing, 1993: 15–28.

148 Benditt DG, Sutton R, Gammage M, *et al*. Clinical experience with Thera DR rate-drop response pacing algorithm in carotid sinus syndrome and vasovagal syncope. *PACE* 1997;**20**(Suppl. II):832–9.

149 Benditt DG, Peterson M, Lurie K, *et al*. Cardiac pacing for prevention of recurrent vasovagal syncope. *Ann Intern Med* 1995;**122**:204–9.

150 Petersen MEV, Chamberlain-Webber R, Fitzpatrick AP, *et al*. Permanent pacing for cardioinhibitory malignant vasovagal syndrome. *Br Heart J* 1994;**71**:274–81.

151 Connolly SJ, Sheldon R, Roberts RS, Gent M. The North American Vasovagal Pacemaker Study (VPS): a randomized trial of permanent cardiac pacing for the prevention of vasovagal syncope. *J Am Coll Cardiol* 1999;**33**:16–20.

152 Sutton R, Brignole M, Menozzi C, *et al*. for the VASIS investigators. Dual-chamber pacing is efficacious in treatment of neurally mediated tilt-positive cardioinhibitory syncope. Pacemaker versus no therapy: a multicentre randomized study. *Circulation* 2000;**102**: 294–9.

153 Ammirati F, Colivicchi F, Santini M, *et al*. Permanent cardiac pacing versus medical treatment for the prevention of recurrent vasovagal syncope: a multicenter, randomized, controlled trial. *Circulation* 2001;**104**(1): 52–6.

154 Connolly SJ, Sheldon R, Thorpe KE, *et al*. for the VPS investigators. Pacemaker therapy for prevention of syncope in patients with recurrent severe vasovagal syncope. Second vasovagal pacemaker study (VPS-2): a randomized trial. *JAMA* 2003;**209**:2224–9.

155 Giodo F, Raviele A, Monozzi C, *et al*. The vasovagal syncope and pacing trial (SYNPACE): a randomized placebo controlled study of permanent pacing for treatment of recurrent vasovagal syncope. *Pacing Clin Electrophysiol* 2003;**26**:1016.

156 Sutton R. Has cardiac pacing a role in vasovagal syncope? *J Interv Card Electrophysiol* 2003;**9**:145–9.

157 Easley RM Jr, Goldstein S. Sino-atrial syncope. *Am J Med* 1971;**50**:166–7.

158 Wan SH, Lee GS, Toh CC. The sick sinus syndrome. A study of 15 cases. *Br Heart J* 1972; **34**:942–52.

159 Kulbertus HE. The magnitude of risk of developing complete heart block in patients with LAD-RBBB. *Am Heart J* 1973;**86**:278–80.

160 Obel IW, Cohen E, Millar RN. Chronic symptomatic sinoatrial block: a review of 34 patients and their treatment. *Chest* 1974;**65**:397–402.

161 Hartel G, Talvensaari T. Treatment of sinoatrial syndrome with permanent cardiac pacing in 90 patients. *Acta Med Scand* 1975;**198**:341–7.

162 Strauss HC, Bigger JT, Saroff AL, Giardina EG. Electrophysiologic evaluation of sinus node function in patients with sinus node dysfunction. *Circulation* 1976;**53**:763–76.

163 Sauerwein HP, Roos JC, Becker AE, Dunning AJ. The sick sinus syndrome. *Acta Med Scand* 1976;**199**:467–73.

164 Scheinman MM, Strauss HC, Abbott JA, *et al*. Electrophysiologic testing in patients with sinus pauses and/or sinoatrial exit block. *Eur J Cardiol* 1978;**8**:51–60.

165 Sutton R, Perrins J, Citron P. Physiological cardiac pacing. *Pacing Clin Electrophysiol* 1980;**3**:207–19.

CHAPTER 5

Tachyarrhythmias as a cause of syncope

Frank Pelosi, Jr., MD, *& Fred Morady,* MD

Introduction

Approximately 25% of syncope cases are caused by tachyarrhythmias. Of these, ventricular tachycardia accounts for 85% of cases and 15% result from supraventricular tachycardia [1]. Syncope in the presence of ventricular tachycardia can be an ominous predictor of future mortality in the presence of structural heart disease. In contrast, syncope associated with many supraventricular tachycardias is less concerning and treatment can be directed at the underlying arrhythmia. Depending on the tachycardia mechanism, syncope can result in either direct mechanical disruptions, autonomic maladjustments, or both. Therefore, a clinical evaluation based on identification of the causative arrhythmia and those cardiac conditions that can predict future adverse events is critical to developing a sound therapeutic strategy. The proper approach to these patients involves distinguishing the features of ventricular from supraventricular arrhythmias contributing to syncope.

Syncope-related tachyarrhythmias

Ventricular arrhythmias

Ventricular arrhythmias account for 21% of all patients presenting with otherwise unexplained syncope [1]. In patients with sustained ventricular tachycardia, 30% experience syncope or near-syncope [2]. Along with syncope, patients with ventricular arrhythmias commonly experience palpitations and lightheadedness. Ventricular tachycardia is most commonly associated with structural heart disease. In a study of 88 patients referred for electrophysiologic testing, 75% of patients presenting

with ventricular tachycardia had structural heart disease and, of the nine patients who died during the study's follow-up period, eight had left ventricular ejection fraction of less than 0.30 [3].

Idiopathic ventricular tachycardia arises from the right ventricular outflow tract in 75–90% of cases and can be treated with pharmacologic agents or radiofrequency ablation [4]. The long QT syndrome has an incidence of 1 in 7000 and is associated with increased mortality in the presence of syncope [5]. Syncope is often the initial presentation with the long QT syndrome, occurring in approximately 5% per year with an overall annual mortality of approximately 1% per year [6]. The presence of syncope in this syndrome, along with aborted sudden death in the patient or close relative, may be predictive of an increased risk of sudden death where defibrillator implantation should be considered [7]. Arrhythmogenic right ventricular dysplasia is characterized by fatty infiltration of the right ventricle, which can present with either monomorphic or polymorphic ventricular tachycardia. In patients with disorders of sodium channel known as the Brugada syndrome, the presence of sudden syncope and characteristic atypical right bundle branch block pattern is associated with a sixfold increase in sudden cardiac death [8].

Supraventricular arrhythmias

Supraventricular tachycardia encompasses approximately 12 different arrhythmia mechanisms and can be present in 3% of the population. Syncope is unusual with these arrhythmias and prognosis is generally favorable, so treatment can be directed at eliminating the underlying arrhythmia.

Supraventricular tachycardia originating primarily in the atrium includes atrial fibrillation, flutter, and tachycardia. Atrial fibrillation is the most common cardiac arrhythmia requiring hospitalization in the USA, but is an unusual cause of syncope. One important exception is atrial fibrillation in the presence of a rapidly conducting extranodal accessory pathway. Lacking the usual decremental properties of the atrioventricular node, atrial depolarizations are capable of triggering ventricular fibrillation as they conduct directly to the ventricles via the accessory pathway. Atrial flutter cycle lengths can be as rapid as 220 ms, but usually conduct to the ventricles in a 2 : 1 or 3 : 1 ratio. Patients can experience presyncope or syncope when atrial flutter conducts to the ventricles with a 1 : 1 relationship.

Supraventricular tachycardias involving the atrioventricular node as part of the re-entrant circuit encompass one of the most common cardiac rhythms seen in electrophysiology laboratories for intervention. Atrioventricular nodal reentrant tachycardia involves a re-entrant rhythm involving the atrioventricular bundle with ventricular rates approaching 230 b min^{-1}. Atrioventricular tachycardias utilizing extranodal accessory pathways involve two major types. Orthodromic re-entrant tachycardia is where antegrade conduction from the atria to the ventricles takes place over the atrioventricular node and His–Purkinje system. This results in a tachycardia with a usually normal QRS duration. Antidromic re-entrant tachycardia occurs when antegrade conduction occurs over the extranodal pathway, leading to a tachycardia with a wide QRS morphology. Although not typically thought of as an arrhythmia associated with syncope, some reports cite a history of syncope in as many as 20% of patients [9]. Elimination of accessory pathway conduction with radiofrequency ablation has emerged as a first-line therapy for these arrhythmias.

Pathophysiology of tachyarrhythmia-induced syncope

Ventricular tachycardia

The onset of ventricular tachycardia causes uncoordinated ventricular contraction with severe regurgitation of the atrioventricular valves. Accelerated rates decrease diastolic filling times and ultimately lead to decreased diastolic filling and diastolic dimension. Hamer *et al.* [10] studied 40 patients undergoing electrophysiologic study and observed that patients both with and without syncope had drops in mean arterial blood pressure to approximately 40 mmHg at the onset of ventricular tachycardia. Patients who did *not* experience syncope experienced recovery of mean arterial pressure to at least 50 mmHg within 1 min. Those who experienced syncope did not demonstrate such a recovery. In this same report, patients who developed syncope had ventricular tachycardia mean rates of 253 b min^{-1} versus 193 b min^{-1} in those without syncope. Interestingly, there was no association between left ventricular ejection fraction or ventricular tachycardia morphology and the development of syncope. Calkins *et al.* [11] evaluated the effect of quinidine and amiodarone on blood pressure during rapid ventricular pacing. Blood pressure decreased at baseline with pacing cycle lengths of less than 350 ms. In the presence of amiodarone and quinidine, blood pressure did not decrease significantly except at pacing cycle lengths of 350 and 280 ms. If extrapolated to spontaneous ventricular tachycardia, these findings suggest tachycardia cycle length is an important determinant in the hemodynamic stability of ventricular tachycardia.

Autonomic factors also have a role in the development of syncope during ventricular tachycardia. In an animal model, Feldman *et al.* [12] studied the hemodynamic effects of ventricular tachycardia under different autonomic challenges. At baseline, left ventricular systolic pressure drops recovered within 1 min. Sinus cycle length decreased as ventricular tachycardia duration increased. In the presence of β-adrenergic blockade, recovery of left ventricular systolic pressure and sinus cycle length changes were blunted. In the presence of α-adrenergic blockade, left ventricular pressure remained persistently low and sinus cycle length demonstrated a pattern similar to the pattern at baseline. Complete ganglionic blockade produced a combination of features similar to those seen with α- and β-adrenergic blockade. These data show that autonomic influences play an important part in the recovery of blood pressure and thus the hemodynamic stability of ventricular tachycardia. Smith *et al.* [13] evaluated the correlation of sympathetic nerve activity and ventricular tachycardia in patents undergoing electrophysiologic testing and found a surge in sympathetic activity after the onset of ventricular tachycardia, then a gradual decrease while still remaining above baseline levels. In patients undergoing electrophysiologic study, ventricular tachycardia associated with sustained drops in blood pressure was associated with drops in the sinus rate; however, in ventricular tachycardia that is otherwise well tolerated, the sinus rate increased [14]. This suggests that sympathetic withdrawal or augmented vagal tone may contribute to hemodynamic changes in unstable ventricular tachycardia. It has been observed that patients with left ventricular dysfunction have abnormal control of peripheral circulation during stimulated orthostatic stress, perhaps a result of impairment of cardiopulmonary and arterial baroreflexes.

Supraventricular tachycardia

With the onset of supraventricular tachycardia, ventricular filling is diminished because of decreased diastolic filling times [15]. Arterial pressure drops dramatically as a result of reduced ventricular filling and attenuated left atrial pressure. This leads to presyncope and cerebral hypoperfusion. A compensatory increase in systemic vascular resistance at least partially relieves the initial hypotension of the supraventricular tachycardia. It has also been suggested that alterations of atrioventricular conduction during supraventricular tachycardia result in atrial contraction against a closed atrioventricular valve. This lack of effective atrial contraction further contributes to decrease left ventricular filling.

The relationship between supraventricular tachycardia cycle length and syncope is less clear. Some investigators have suggested that a supraventricular tachycardia rates greater than 170 b min^{-1} are associated with higher rates of syncope [9]. Others have suggested that autonomic influences similar to vasodepressor syndrome contribute to syncope in supraventricular tachycardia. Leitch et al. [16] performed electrophysiologic studies in 23 patients with supraventricular tachycardia, in both the supine and upright positions. Shorter tachycardia cycle lengths did not correlate with an increase risk of syncope when induced in the upright position. In the supine position, a correlation between tachycardia cycle length and syncope was found. In addition, vasodepressor changes induced during

passive upright tilt table testing were predictive of syncope in the upright position during supraventricular tachycardia. It is believed that diminished left ventricular filling and increased contractility causes activation of cardiac mechanreceptors, triggering a response similarly to vasodepressor syndrome.

Cerebral hypoperfusion is the hallmark of syncope; therefore, abnormalities in cerebral autoregulation have been suggested as a critical component in the development of syncope. Paradoxical cerebral vasoconstriction has been observed with transcranial Doppler studies during upright tilt table testing in patients with ventricular tachycardia and fibrillation [17]. Others have shown a reduction of 69% in middle cerebral artery flow velocity during electrophysiology testing for supraventricular and ventricular tachycardia in patients with syncope [18]. What is unclear is whether these changes represent a critical dysfunction of cerebral autoregulation or simply a response to decreased blood flow as a result of diminished cardiac output. In studies in patients with vasodepressor syncope, changes in cerebral autoregulation have been observed shortly before syncope, while others report that this is a response to hypocapnia which occurs long after the onset of presyncope [19,20]. The role of cerebral autoregulation in the development of syncope associated with supraventricular tachycardia remains unclear and is the subject of future investigation.

Evaluation and management of tachyarrhythmia-related syncope

The evaluation of a patient with syncope where tachyarrhythmia is suspected should be focused on identification of the responsible arrhythmia and those cardiac disorders that may predict future adverse events. A baseline 12-lead electrocardiogram can identify patients with long QT syndrome, Brugada syndrome, and sometimes arrhythmogenic right ventricular dysplasia. It is important to note that these abnormal electrocardiographic findings can be intermittent, so a normal electrocardiogram does not rule out these disorders. Evaluation of left ventricular function and morphologic evaluation of cardiac structure can be obtained with two-dimensional echocardiography. If ischemia is suspected, exercise testing or cardiac catheterization should be considered. Abnormalities of the right ventricle found in arrhythmogenic right ventricular dysplasia can be evaluated with contrast right ventriculography, and gated cardiac magnetic resonance imaging or gated blood-pool imaging of right ventricular function.

Ambulatory monitoring is usually the first step to identify tachyarrhythmias responsible for syncope. Selecting the appropriate monitor is based on the nature and frequency of symptoms. Continuous 24- or 48-h Holter monitoring can be used for patients where symptoms are expected to occur during the recording period. In a study of various methods of arrhythmia evaluation, 24-h Holter monitoring had a diagnostic yield of 21% [21]. Patient-activated loop event recorder can be used for longer periods of time and have been shown to be effective in identifying responsible arrhythmias. In a prospective comparison of patient-activated loop recorders and Holter monitors, external loop recorders had a diagnostic yield of 56% versus 22% for Holter monitors [22]. Their usefulness is limited in patients who have little or no prodrome before syncope or for those who cannot activate the recording device. Implantable loop recorders can be used to identify arrhythmias in those with less frequent symptoms. These devices have a battery longevity of approximately 1 year and can detect arrhythmias in both automated and patient-activated modes [23].

The role of electrophysiologic testing in identifying the causative arrhythmia for patients has been studied by several investigators. In one study, 53 patients with syncope, 54% of whom had structural heart disease, sustained or non-sustained ventricular tachycardia was induced in approximately 45% of cases [24]. Of these patients, the absence of structural heart disease was predictive of a normal electrophysiology study. In a separate study of 100 patients with unexplained syncope and non-diagnostic or normal electrophysiologic tests, 2% subsequently died suddenly and 20% had recurring syncope [25]. Of these 19 patients, a cause of syncope could not be identified except for four who had high-degree atrioventricular block and sinus node dysfunction.

Once the responsible arrhythmia and underlying substrate have been determined, treatment is directed to preventing sudden death and alleviating symptoms. Patients with severe left ventricular dysfunction and syncope attributed to ventricular tachycardia should be considered for defibrillator implantation [26]. In a study by Knight et al. [27], patients with non-ischemic cardiomyopathy and unexplained syncope who received implantable defibrillators had similar rates of appropriate defibrillator therapies as those receiving an implantable defibrillator for cardiac arrest, a finding validated by other investigators [27,28]. Implantable defibrillators are suitable for patients without structural heart disease and syncope secondary to ventricular tachycardia that is refractory to other treatments. Patients with syncope who have conditions that place them at risk for sudden cardiac death, such as long QT syndrome, Brugada syndrome, or arrhythmogenic right ventricular dysplasia should be considered for defibrillator implantation, especially if the syncope is attributed to ventricular arrhythmias.

For patients with supraventricular tachycardia causing syncope, treatment should be focused on treating the underlying arrhythmia. Catheter-based ablation has eclipsed the use of antiarrhythmic drugs for a wide variety of cardiac arrhythmias. Syncope caused by supraventricular arrhythmias has been effectively cured when the responsible arrhythmia has been successfully ablated [29,30].

References

1 Krol RB, Morady F, Flaker GC, et al. Electrophysiologic testing in patients with unexplained syncope: clinical and non-invasive predictors of outcome. J Am Coll Cardiol 1987;**10**:358–63.

2 Morady F, Shen EN, Bhandari A, Schwartz AB, Scheinman MM. Clinical symptoms in patients with sustained ventricular tachycardia. West J Med 1985;**142**: 341–4.

3 Middlekauff HR, Stevenson WG, Saxon LA. Prognosis after syncope: impact of left ventricular function. Am Heart J 1993;**125**:121–7.

4 Lerman BB, Stein KM, Markowitz SM, Mittal S, Slotwiner DJ. Ventricular arrhythmias in normal hearts. Cardiol Clin 2000;**18**:265–91, vii.

5 Vincent GM. Long QT syndrome. Cardiol Clin 2000; **18**:309–25.

6 Moss AJ, Schwartz PJ, Crampton RS, et al. The long QT syndrome: prospective longitudinal study of 328 families. Circulation 1991;**84**:1136–44.

7 Zareba W, Moss AJ, Daubert JP, Hall WJ, Robinson JL, Andrews M. Implantable cardioverter defibrillator in high-risk long QT syndrome patients. *J Cardiovasc Electrophysiol* 2003;**14**:337–41.

8 Priori SG, Napolitano C, Gasparini M, *et al.* Natural history of Brugada syndrome: insights for risk stratification and management. *Circulation* 2002;**105**:1342–7.

9 Wood KA, Drew BJ, Scheinman MM. Frequency of disabling symptoms in supraventricular tachycardia. *Am J Cardiol* 1997;**79**:145–9.

10 Hamer AW, Rubin SA, Peter T, Mandel WJ. Factors that predict syncope during ventricular tachycardia in patients. *Am Heart J* 1984;**107**:997–1005.

11 Calkins H, Shyr Y, Schork A, Kadish A, Morady F. Effects of quinidine and amiodarone on blood pressure during rapid ventricular pacing in coronary artery disease. *Am J Cardiol* 1992;**70**:1206–9.

12 Feldman T, Carroll JD, Munkenbeck F, *et al.* Hemodynamic recovery during simulated ventricular tachycardia: role of adrenergic receptor activation. *Am Heart J* 1988;**115**:576–87.

13 Smith ML, Ellenbogen KA, Beightol LA, Eckberg DL. Sympathetic neural responses to induced ventricular tachycardia. *J Am Coll Cardiol* 1991;**18**:1015–24.

14 Huikuri HV, Zaman L, Castellanos A, *et al.* Changes in spontaneous sinus node rate as an estimate of cardiac autonomic tone during stable and unstable ventricular tachycardia. *J Am Coll Cardiol* 1989;**13**:646–52.

15 Goldreyer BN, Kastor JA, Kershbaum KL. The hemodynamic effects of induced supraventricular tachycardia in man. *Circulation* 1976;**54**:783–9.

16 Leitch JW, Klein GJ, Yee R, Leather RA, Kim YH. Syncope associated with supraventricular tachycardia: an expression of tachycardia rate or vasomotor response? *Circulation* 1992;**85**:1064–71.

17 Grubb BP, Durzinsky D, Brewster P, Gbur C, Collins B. Sudden cerebral vasoconstriction during induced polymorphic ventricular tachycardia and fibrillation: further observations of a paradoxic response [see comment]. *Pacing Clin Electrophysiol* 1997;**20**:1667–72.

18 Zunker P, Haase C, Borggrefe M, Georgiadis D, Georgiadis A, Ringelstein EB. Cerebral hemodynamics during induced tachycardia in routine electrophysiologic studies: a transcranial Doppler study. *Neurol Res* 1998;**20**:504–8.

19 Carey BJ, Manktelow BN, Panerai RB, Potter JF. Cerebral autoregulatory responses to head-up tilt in normal subjects and patients with recurrent vasovagal syncope. *Circulation* 2001;**104**:898–902.

20 Lagi A, Cencetti S, Corsoni V, Georgiadis D, Bacalli S. Cerebral vasoconstriction in vasovagal syncope: any link with symptoms? A transcranial Doppler study [see comment]. *Circulation* 2001;**104**:2694–8.

21 Lacroix D, Dubuc M, Kus T, Savard P, Shenasa M, Nadeau R. Evaluation of arrhythmic causes of syncope: correlation between Holter monitoring, electrophysiologic testing, and body surface potential mapping. *Am Heart J* 1991;**122**:1346–54.

22 Sivakumaran S, Krahn AD, Klein GJ, *et al.* A prospective randomized comparison of loop recorders versus Holter monitors in patients with syncope or presyncope [see comment]. *Am J Med* 2003;**115**:1–5.

23 Ashby DT, Cehic DA, Disney PJ, Mahar LJ, Young GD. A retrospective case study to assess the value of the implantable loop recorder for the investigation of undiagnosed syncope. *Pacing Clin Electrophysiol* 2002;**25**:1200–5.

24 Morady F, Shen E, Schwartz A, *et al.* Long-term follow-up of patients with recurrent unexplained syncope evaluated by electrophysiologic testing. *J Am Coll Cardiol* 1983;**2**:1053–9.

25 Kushner JA, Kou WH, Kadish AH, Morady F. Natural history of patients with unexplained syncope and a nondiagnostic electrophysiologic study. *J Am Coll Cardiol* 1989;**14**:391–6.

26 Gregoratos G, Abrams J, Epstein AE, *et al.* ACC/AHA/NASPE 2002 guideline update for implantation of cardiac pacemakers and antiarrhythmia devices: summary article. A report of the American College of Cardiology/American Heart Association Task Force on Practice Guidelines (ACC/AHA/NASPE Committee to Update the 1998 Pacemaker Guidelines). *J Cardiovasc Electrophysiol* 2002;**13**:1183–99.

27 Knight BP, Goyal R, Pelosi F, *et al.* Outcome of patients with non-ischemic dilated cardiomyopathy and unexplained syncope treated with an implantable defibrillator [see comment]. *J Am Coll Cardiol* 1999;**33**:1964–70.

28 Andrews NP, Fogel RI, Pelargonio G, Evans JJ, Prystowsky EN. Implantable defibrillator event rates in patients with unexplained syncope and inducible sustained ventricular tachyarrhythmias: a comparison with patients known to have sustained ventricular tachycardia. *J Am Coll Cardiol* 1999;**34**:2023–30.

29 Antz M, Weiss C, Volkmer M, *et al.* Risk of sudden death after successful accessory atrioventricular pathway ablation in resuscitated patients with Wolff–Parkinson–White syndrome. *J Cardiovasc Electrophysiol* 2002;**13**:231–6.

30 Brembilla-Perrot B, Beurrier D, Houriez P, Claudon O, Wertheimer J. Incidence and mechanism of presyncope and/or syncope associated with paroxysmal junctional tachycardia. *Am J Cardiol* 2001;**88**:134–8.

CHAPTER 6

Use of electrophysiology studies in syncope: practical aspects for diagnosis and treatment

Edward A. Telfer, MD, *& Brian Olshansky,* MD

Introduction

The cause of syncope can be difficult to determine with certainty. Despite a careful history and physical examination, and even with properly directed non-invasive testing, the etiology can remain unidentified in almost 50% of syncope patients [1]. The prognosis for the majority of patients can be favorable [2–6], but varies widely depending on underlying (and causative), or concomitant, diagnoses, specifically, cardiac causes [7–11].

Cardiac arrhythmias, often a suspected and serious cause for syncope, are generally transient and difficult to record and diagnose. They can represent a potentially life-threatening situation. Underlying structural cardiac disease is not always a prerequisite for arrhythmic syncope. Even for patients with cardiac disease in whom an arrhythmia is suspected as the cause for syncope, the etiology can be difficult to diagnose with absolute certainty unless electrocardiographic (ECG) assessment, hemodynamic monitoring, and direct observation are all present at the time of syncope. Clinical variability in presentation further confounds the diagnosis. Empiric therapy directed against the suspected or potential arrhythmic cause for syncope can worsen the prognosis, ironically, without necessarily treating either the arrhythmia or syncope effectively.

Syncope, undiagnosed, despite an extensive non-invasive evaluation, is problematic. It often requires more than diagnostic acumen to determine that the cause is self-limited and benign, and clearly is not always associated with a good outcome. The mortality may approach 20–30% in the first year after presentation if syncope resulted from a cardiovascular cause, such as ventricular tachycardia, and structural heart disease is present [1,6–12].

This chapter focuses on the practical use of electrophysiology (EP) studies to evaluate and treat patients with otherwise undiagnosed syncope; illustrative case examples are included.

Background

Several abnormalities could potentially be diagnosed from an EP study. These include bradycardias caused by sinus node dysfunction and AV/His–Purkinje conduction problems as well as supraventricular and ventricular tachycardias (Table 6.1).

Beginning in the 1960s, endocardial catheters were placed in the heart and used to record, pace, and deliver premature extrastimuli from the atria and the ventricles ("EP studies"). Initial application of this technique was used to assess conduction through the heart [13,14]. Later, the EP study was used in patients with known tachycardias to reproduce re-entrant supraventricular tachycardias (SVTs) [14–16] (excluding, perhaps, atrial flutter and fibrillation, for which the technique has questionable efficacy) and ventricular tachycardia [15–17]. For ventricular tachycardia, EP studies were found particularly sensitive (90–95%) to initiate "clinical" (spontaneous) sustained monomorphic ventricular tachycardia in patients with coronary artery disease. Sustained monomorphic ventricular

Table 6.1 Data acquired during an electrophysiology study.

Sinus node function
AV nodal function
His–Purkinje conduction properties
Induction of supraventricular tachycardia
Induction of ventricular tachycardia

tachycardia was rarely induced at EP study in patients without spontaneous, sustained ventricular tachycardia. Vanderpol *et al.* [17] showed that the test was less sensitive (appproximately 50%) in reproducing non-sustained ventricular tachycardia in patients who had spontaneous non-sustained ventricular tachycardia. This is important because non-sustained ventricular tachycardia could cause syncope.

Electrophysiology studies were used as a method to evaluate conduction, pathologic and normal, through the AV node and His–Purkinje system [14,18–20]. Sinus node function was also assessed at EP study in patients with known sinus node dysfunction [21–28]. Several techniques were described.

By the 1970s, the use of EP studies expanded to assess the *potential* risk of arrhythmia in patients with suspected, but not clinically documented, arrhythmias [29]. This application included attempting to identify arrhythmias in patients with syncope of unknown origin [30–45]. In these early investigations, the patient population enrolled in the studies comprised those with undiagnosed syncope as the only criterion for study. Patients were not specifically selected or targeted with any specific diagnoses in mind. Various types of arrhythmias, including non-sustained and sustained ventricular tachycardia, ventricular fibrillation, polymorphic ventricular tachycardia, and supraventricular arrhythmias were induced and correlated to syncope. It was recognized that abnormalities discovered at EP study did not convincingly reproduce the patient's clinical syncopal episodes. It was hypothesized, however, that the observed abnormalities of conduction and induced tachycardias were related to the patient's syncope.

Induction techniques and the specificity of the EP study were assessed further in the mid-1980s to determine the potential clinical significance of the arrhythmias initiated [45–54]. Techniques to perform EP studies were also assessed in greater detail. Stimulation protocols, patient recruitment, even the definitions of abnormal responses, were highly variable, making comparison between different investigations difficult. As experience with EP studies in syncope patients grew, a consensus emerged concerning reasonable stimulation protocols and definitions of induced arrhythmia abnormalities [14]. Investigators became more sophisticated in the interpretation of EP study results. Also, an attempt to correlate the prognosis to EP study results was undertaken [45,55–58]. Treatment based upon the EP study results was evaluated to assess if the test had utility in directing therapy. Several reports showed that treatment of abnormalities observed at EP study resulted in a better prognosis and/or a reduction in the rate of recurrent syncope [45,55–61].

Teichman *et al.* [62] popularized the notion of quantifying the severity of abnormalities observed from normal to minor ("borderline"), to "clearly abnormal" findings. The diagnostic yield of EP studies was 36% if only "clearly abnormal" results were considered, but by combining "borderline" abnormalities with "clearly abnormal" results the diagnostic yield rose to 75%.

The diagnostic yield of arrhythmia abnormalities found at EP study varied tremendously between investigations. This was likely related to patient selection, stimulation protocols, and definition of EP abnormalities. Despite these issues, the most common abnormality of clinical significance noted was induction of sustained monomorphic ventricular tachycardia. This finding suggested a potential cause for syncope and provided predictive data regarding the risk of cardiac death.

Some patient subgroups clearly did not benefit from an EP study, meaning that the EP results were non-diagnostic. Identification of these patients became important so that the risk and expense of EP study could be avoided. Krol *et al.* [63] found that the predictors of an abnormal study (ventricular tachycardia in 71%) included: left ventricular ejection fraction (LVEF) ≤ 40%; bundle branch block; presence of coronary artery disease; history of remote myocardial infarction; use of class I antiarrhythmic drugs; injury related to loss of consciousness; and male sex. Predictors of non-diagnostic study included: left ventricular ejection fraction ≥ 40%; absence of structural heart disease; a normal 12-lead ECG; and normal 24-h ambulatory monitoring. The probability of a normal EP study increased with the number and duration of the syncopal episodes. While these predictors are generally accurate:

1 Not all reports show the same results (e.g., injury that does not clearly predict a poor prognosis or an arrhythmic etiology of syncope, but this point is controversial [63,64]).

2 A positive study could still occur without any of above predictors. If fact, 35% of all positive EP studies occurred in patients with LVEF ≥ 0.40.

Krol *et al.* [63] had restrictive definitions of an abnormal EP study:

1 sinus node recovery time ≥ 3 s;
2 HV interval ≥ 100 ms;
3 infra-Hisian block during atrial pacing;
4 monomorphic ventricular tachycardia;
5 SVT associated with hypotension.

The "clearly abnormal" EP study results have remained the accepted standard [64].

Kushner *et al.* found that patients with normal or less serious and specific abnormalities than defined by Krol *et al.* had a good prognosis independent of the frequency of recurrent syncope [56,65]. Some investigators have even suggested that there is a reduction in syncope recurrence even if the EP study is non-diagnostic (a "placebo" effect of the EP study, perhaps; M.M. Scheinman, personal communication). The non-diagnostic EP study has other important implications: a patient with coronary artery disease with impaired left ventricular function and syncope who has a negative EP study has a good long-term prognosis.

Other investigators identified a high incidence of inducible ventricular tachycardia in syncope patients with bundle branch block [32,36]. The expected cause for syncope (in this example, infra-Hisian block) may be instead only a predictor for other potentially life-threatening arrhythmic problems including ventricular tachycardia.

EP studies have continued to emerge over the past decade as a common diagnostic tool for syncope patients. In the 1990s, at Loyola University Medical Center, approximately 20% of primary EP studies were performed to assess patients with otherwise undiagnosed syncope.

According to recent ACC/AHA guidelines, syncope in association with suspected heart disease and no other apparent cause is considered a "class I" indication for EP study [66]. The study may help to provide a potential cause for syncope in this group.

Electrophysiology study protocols

The EP study is an invasive, but relatively low risk procedure requiring placement of venous sheaths through which electrode catheters are placed to determine sinus node function and conduction properties through the heart as well as the presence of inducible supraventricular and ventricular arrhythmias [67]. The procedure takes approximately 1–3 h. Each EP study protocol has been well tested for its sensitivity and specificity in specific pathologic conditions and in normal subjects. A consensus on a "standard" EP test for syncope has now been reached [66,68].

After catheters are placed in the heart, conduction intervals are measured. Then sinus node recovery time is measured by rapid pacing of the atria followed by abrupt termination and measurement of the time for the sinus node to "recover." AV conduction is determined by progressively shorter fixed rate and by ramp pacing to assess AV nodal and His–Purkinje conduction. The presence of conduction block below the His bundle is distinctly abnormal and indicative of the need for a pacemaker.

Single extrastimuli are then introduced at two or more cycle lengths in the high right atrium. Then single, double, and triple premature extrastimuli are introduced at two or more paced cycle lengths in the ventricular at two sites (generally at the apex and outflow tract of the right ventricle). There are several acceptable, well-tested protocols to attempt to induce tachycardias. Isoproterenol can be given and may be helpful to attempt to induce both SVT and ventricular tachycardia but should be reserved for patients for whom EP studies without isoproterenol infusion are non-diagnostic and there is little risk of exacerbating severe ischemia [69]. The sensitivity and specificity of isoproterenol in this setting is unknown. Some arrhythmias, such as right ventricular outflow tract ventricular tachycardia, may actually be more inducible with isoproterenol than with pacing maneuvers. Epinephrine (and isoproterenol) has been used to uncover subtle forms of the long QT syndrome [70,71]. Procainamide infusion, up to 15 mg kg^{-1}, can be used as a conduction "stress test" in patients suspected of having infra-Hisian block (those with bundle branch block, bifasicular block, or a prolonged HV interval). Procainamide can further impair conduction though the His–Purkinje system. Patients who show infra-Hisian block become pacemaker dependant in short order and do not tend to have recurrent syncope after pacemaker implantation [72]. Procainamide can also be used to facilitate induction of bundle branch re-entry ventricular tachycardia when it is suspected but cannot be induced with extrastimuli alone (including long–short coupling interval). More recently, intravenous: amjaline (1 mg kg^{-1}; 10 mg min^{-1}), flecanide (2 mg kg^{-1}, max 150 mg; in 10 min), and procainamide (10 mg kg^{-1}; 100 mg min^{-1}) have been shown to provoke, or exacerbate, the ECG changes associated with Brugada syndrome [73,74]. In the USA, intravenous amjaline and flecanide are not available. Drugs including atropine, adenosine, and beta-blockers may also have utility in conjunction with pacing maneuvers.

Expected yield of electrophysiology studies

The expected yield from an EP study is variable, dependent upon anticipated abnormalities and patient risk factors [75,76]. Some findings, such as severe sinus node disease, are generally independent of left ventricular function, but can be anticipated by non-invasive monitoring. Unequivocally abnormal findings (symptomatic sinus node recovery time ≥ 3 s) are quite specific for serious sinus node dysfunction, but are rare findings in syncope patients (see Fig. 2.4). While the EP study techniques are specific to reproduce serious sinus node dysfunction, the technique is unreliable in syncope patients to detect sinus node dysfunction as cause for syncope [77–79].

Fujimura *et al.* [77] described an alarmingly high incidence of "missed" conduction and sinus node disease in syncope patients using EP studies. In this study, they identified 21 patients with intermittent AV block (13 patients) or sinus pauses (eight pati-

ents) associated with syncope, who then underwent EP study prior to the implantation of a permanent pacemaker. For the patients with documented sinus node disease, only three of eight (sensitivity = 37.5%) had evidence of sinus node disease at EP study. Three of these same eight patients with documented sinus node disease as a cause for syncope demonstrated other abnormalities at EP study, including dual AV nodal physiology, atrial flutter, and sustained monomorphic ventricular tachycardia. Only two of 13 patients with documented intermittent AV block demonstrated evidence of AV block at EP study (sensitivity = 15.4%). These same 13 patients displayed other abnormalities including inducible atrial fibrillation with rapid ventricular response associated with hypotension.

Similarly, Krahn *et al.* [78] found a high incidence of intermittent sinus arrest and AV block in recurrent syncope patients who had previously undergone a negative tilt table test and a non-diagnostic EP study using implanted long-term ambulatory monitors. In this study, five of 16 patients demonstrated sinus arrest associated with syncope and two of 16 patients demonstrated AV block associated with syncope. Interestingly, no patient suffered any complications or sequelae from the time of the initial non-diagnostic EP study to the time that the diagnosis was established by the subcutaneous long-term ambulatory monitor.

Severe conduction system disease is most commonly found in patients with some type of advanced conduction delay on non-invasive monitoring and 12-lead ECG. Severe infra-Hisian conduction delay or block is rare in patients without a wide QRS (QRS duration ≥ 120 ms) or AV block (first degree or higher). Syncope patients with bifasicular block have been described as having a high incidence of sustained monomorphic ventricular tachycardia, making the EP study as useful for excluding co-existing ventricular tachycardia as for confirming infra-Hisian block in this group [32].

Patients with a history of SVT, who later develop syncope, should, in general, undergo EP studies. The same holds true for patients with documented or suspected pre-excitation on a 12-lead ECG [45]. The situation is less clear-cut for patients with atrial fibrillation or atrial flutter discovered on non-invasive monitoring, if a direct association with syncope is lacking. Atrial fibrillation can rarely cause syncope because of alterations in ventricular response, but the yield of the EP study tends to be low, unless there is another coexisting reason to perform it. Reproduction of a suspected tachycardia-bradycardia syndrome is sometimes accomplished in patients with atrial flutter, given that atrial flutter is often terminated with pacing maneuvers. Once in sinus rhythm, an assessment of underlying sinus node function and AV nodal conduction properties is possible. Termination of atrial fibrillation is occasionally successful with antiarrhythmic drug infusion, but generally requires electrical cardioversion. However, the pause, occurring occasionally after electrical cardioversion, provides almost no diagnostic information. Both atrial fibrillation and atrial flutter are associated with an increased risk of thromboembolic events, especially around the time of cardioversion (by whatever means). The risk of thromboembolic events must weigh in the decision to perform an EP study, especially if either atrial fibrillation or atrial flutter is the only reason that the study is performed. Because atrial flutter can also be "cured" with current radiofrequency ablation techniques (without concurrent need for a permanent pacemaker), the yield of the EP study is perhaps higher for atrial flutter than for atrial fibrillation.

The yield of EP study for sustained monomorphic ventricular tachycardia, is most dependent on ventricular function and the type of underlying heart disease (see Table 6.5). For patients with ventricular dysfunction, the etiology of heart disease is vital in determining the expected yield of EP studies [15–17,79–84]. The yield is highest for patients who have a history of distant myocardial infarction associated with left ventricular dysfunction (LVEF ≤ 0.35) [63]. Patients with a history of distant myocardial infarction but with preserved left ventricular function (LVEF ≥ 0.40) associated with late potentials on a signal-averaged ECG (SAECG) may also have a high incidence of inducible sustained monomorphic ventricular tachycardia [85–87]. The diagnostic yield of ventricular stimulation protocols is lower (but not zero) in patients with left ventricular dysfunction because of dilated or non-ischemic cardiomyopathy than those with a history of distant myocardial infarction. The potential for inducible sustained monomorphic ventricular tachycardia cannot be dismissed in patients with non-ischemic or dilated cardiomyopathy [88]. However,

an EP study may be negative in a patient with dilated cardiomyopathy and syncope but the risk of death and recurrent syncope resulting from a ventricular arrhythmia can remain high [89]. Sustained monomorphic ventricular tachycardia is the most specific induced arrhythmia, but other responses may be important prognostically. Link *et al.* [90] showed that syncope patients with inducible ventricular arrhythmias treated with an implanted cardioverter defibrillator (ICD) "appropriate" ICD shocks. Kaplan Meier estimated that 50% would have a shock in 3 years. This included patients with inducible non-sustained ventricular tachycardia and ventricular fibrillation [90].

In patients without ventricular dysfunction, ventricular stimulation has an extraordinarily low yield and in general should not be performed unless there is some specific reason to expect that syncope is caused by ventricular tachycardia. Examples include patients with syncope in whom right ventricular dysplasia [91,92], Brugada syndrome [93,94], right ventricular outflow tract ventricular tachycardia, idiopathic left ventricular tachycardia ("narrow" right bundle branch block [RBBB]/left anterior fascicular block [LAFB] morphology), or sarcoid-associated cardiomyopathy are *strongly* suspected [95].

Interpretation of electrophysiology study results

Goals

Several important questions arise in patients with syncope who undergo EP study and in whom an arrhythmia is found.

1 Is the arrhythmia clinically relevant?

2 Is the arrhythmia the cause for syncope?

3 How can the arrhythmia be treated? Will treatment prevent recurrent syncope?

4 What is the implication of multiple arrhythmia abnormalities at testing?

5 Is a well-tolerated, but abnormal, arrhythmia the cause for syncope?

6 What are the prognostic implications of abnormal results?

While there are no tacit answers to these questions, clinical acumen in light of the test results is always the key to proper and effective long-term treatment. The next several sections attempt to clarify and answer these questions.

The level of uncertainty

Clinical correlation between an arrhythmia induced at EP study can be difficult to correlate with symptoms in syncope. Abnormal results must be interpreted in the context of the individual patient. In patients with a history of left ventricular dysfunction, particularly associated with previous myocardial infarction, the induction of sustained monomorphic ventricular tachycardia has been historically the most specific and prognostic induced arrhythmia. Inducible ventricular fibrillation may be an appropriate endpoint in some, but not all or even most patients.

For the MADIT I study of patients with non-sustained ventricular tachycardia, LVEF < 0.36, and coronary artery disease (but no syncope), ventricular fibrillation induction at EP testing was considered an endpoint for prophylactic ICD implantation, if induced with two or less ventricular extrastimuli [96]. This study also opened the way for consideration of prophylactic ICD implantation in a larger population of patients at risk for sudden death even if syncope was not present.

Link et al. [90] showed that appropriate shocks occur in patients with syncope. Actuarial probability of appropriate shocks was 22% and 50% at 1 and 3 years, respectively. In this report, most patients had sustained monomorphic ventricular tachycardia induced. However, five patients had inducible non-sustained ventricular tachycardia and 10 patients had inducible ventricular fibrillation. In Link et al.'s report, these latter patients received appropriate ICD shocks with a similar frequency as the former patients and at a similar frequency to those patients in the MADIT I trial. These data suggest that induced ventricular fibrillation may be specific enough to warrant treatment in some syncope patients, particularly in those patients with severe left ventricular dysfunction.

Link et al. [97] expanded their experience in a subsequent study of 274 coronary artery patients with syncope or presyncope who underwent EP studies. Ventricular fibrillation was induced in 23 of 274 patients (8%), ventricular flutter in 24 of 274 (9%), and non-sustained ventricular tachycardia in 42 of 274 (15%). At follow-up, clinically apparent ventricular arrhythmias occurred in three of 23 (13%) patients with inducible ventricular fibrillation, seven of 24 (30%) of those with induced ventricular flutter, and had a higher incidence (seven of 42 [17%]) in those with inducible non-sustained ventricular tachycardia.

In a small, retrospective case–control study, Andrews et al. [98] examined the rate of ICD therapies in syncope patients compared with a group of patients with similar characteristics who presented with ventricular tachycardia. This high-risk cohort had structural heart disease and inducible sustained monomorphic ventricular tachycardia and were all treated with ICDs. There was no difference in the subsequent number of ICD therapies at follow-up, with both groups receiving frequent therapies.

Mittal et al. [12] found a high incidence of subsequent significant arrhythmias but less impact on long-term mortality in syncope patients with coronary artery disease. The low (45%) 2-year survival rate observed in those with inducible sustained monomorphic ventricular tachycardia despite ICD therapy was surprising.

The conundrum of what to do with the syncope patient who has impaired left ventricular function and coronary artery disease may be solved, in part, by results from the MADIT I and II trials [96,99]. These studies indicated that patients with impaired ventricular function and coronary artery disease might benefit from an ICD regardless of the presence of syncope or, in MADIT II, inducible ventricular tachycardia. The MADIT II trial of patients with left ventricular ejection fractions < 0.30 and coronary artery disease indicated an improved survival with an ICD even if there was no specific clinical scenario such as syncope or sustained ventricular tachycardia present.

Alternatively, while an ICD may be indicated in a syncope patient based on other clinical criteria, the diagnostic information to help plan subsequent therapeutic interventions cannot be underestimated. An ICD may not solve the problem as to why a patient with a poor ejection fraction passed out. EP testing may help in specific circumstances.

However, EP testing is not always helpful. Induced ventricular fibrillation has long been observed in patients with hypertrophic cardiomyopathy and syncope [100]. Unfortunately, it has been harder to show that induced arrhythmias predict subsequent outcome, or that a normal EP study is associated with a better prognosis. Reasons for this may include selection bias, heterogeneous populations at risk, and variable risk associated with specific gene mutations.

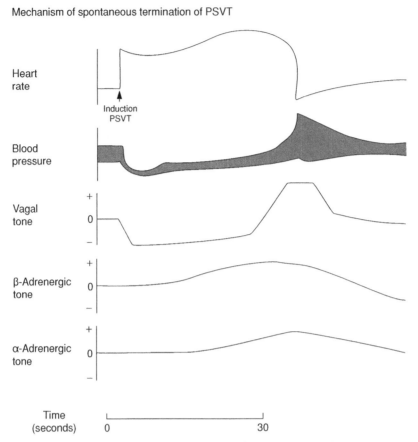

Mechanism of spontaneous termination of PSVT

Fig. 6.1 The effects of autonomic tone associated with the initiation of supraventricular tachycardia. (Reprinted with permission from Waxman *et al.* [103].) PSVT, paroxysmal supraventricular tachycardia.

Induced ventricular fibrillation is a very specific response in patients with Brugada syndrome [10,11]. Furthermore, a negative study, used as one of several variables, may be associated with a better prognosis.

Leitch *et al.* [101] examined the changes in vasomotor tone imposed by inducing SVT in patients while on a tilt table in the supine and the passive head-up positions. Seven of 22 patients developed syncope in the head-up position. The mean SVT rate was identical to the 15 patients who did not develop syncope. It was hypothesized that syncope was related to inadequate compensation of "vasomotor factors" rather than tachycardia rate. Waxman *et al.* [102,103] described the autonomic responses imposed by an abrupt increase in heart rate brought about by the initiation of SVT (Fig. 6.1). From these data, it is clear that body position,

autonomic tone, and vasoregulatory factors, all of which are patient dependent, can precipitate syncope when syncope is present. Because the vast majority of EP studies are performed in sedated and supine patients, reproduction of syncope cannot be used as a confirmatory marker that the observed or induced abnormality is clinically relevant. Intuitively, the absence of syncope during an induced monomorphic tachycardia is not an appropriate reason to dismiss the tachycardia as clinically irrelevant.

There is no reason to suspect that any evaluation, including EP study, should completely clarify causes for syncope in all instances [75]. Regarding EP testing, the endpoints of the test are not always clear and vary depending on the patient and the disease process. For example, what is the significance of reproducibly inducible non-sustained monomorphic ventricular tachycardia? Some non-sustained monomorphic ventricular tachycardia can be self-terminating and still result in hemodynamic intolerance and syncope. Such a response to ventricular stimulation may be labeled "non-specific" in the EP laboratory [48–50]. The prognostic implications of inducible non-sustained monomorphic ventricular tachycardia are unknown and will likely remain so [12,90,97]. Alternatively, induced sustained monomorphic ventricular tachycardia may not be the cause for syncope, but the weight of available data suggest that its induction, in general, is associated with a poorer prognosis [9,12,104–107]. The ultimate prognostic implications of inducible sustained monomorphic ventricular tachycardia are also intertwined with other factors such as left ventricular function and the nature of the structural heart disease (if any). Aggressive EP testing protocols open the way for a potential increase in non-specific responses [45,50,52]. Non-sustained polymorphic ventricular tachycardia is not uncommon during EP study of syncope patients but probably has much less significance than non-sustained monomorphic ventricular tachycardia; however, sustained polymorphic ventricular tachycardia, a potentially abnormal response to stimulation, may have clinical significance [90,96,97]. Polymorphic ventricular tachycardia is most common with short coupling intervals for premature extrastimuli and is most likely to occur with triple extrastimuli at intervals close to the ventricular refractory period. Polymorphic ventricular tachycardia can be an ominous marker if it is sustained, and if it occurs with two or less ventricular extrastimuli. Polymorphic ventricular tachycardia induced with two ventricular extrastimuli was an inclusion arrhythmia in MADIT I [96].

One possible way to enhance the specificity of EP study in patients with induced polymorphic ventricular tachycardia is to repeat the stimulation protocol after procainamide infusion. If a slower monomorphic ventricular tachycardia is then induced, the specificity of the abnormal response is likely to be more relevant clinically [104]. Ventricular fibrillation induction is a non-specific EP study finding in a syncope patient because it causes death, not syncope, unless promptly electrically defibrillated. Alternatively, in syncope patients, inducible ventricular fibrillation may be a moder-

ately specific marker of subsequent ICD shocks [90,97]. Only rarely has ventricular fibrillation been found to be a direct cause for syncope [108].

If ventricular tachycardia or SVT is initiated, it is obviously abnormal, but is it the cause for syncope? SVT can be autonomically mediated with respect to rate and hemodynamic response [102–104]. The induction of SVT occurs in approximately 13% of syncope patients referred for EP study, but the induction of SVT is highly unlikely in a general patient population without symptoms. SVT is more likely the cause for syncope if the rate is fast or if the tachycardia is poorly tolerated. Simultaneous atrial and ventricular activation can further worsen hemodynamic tolerance of a tachycardia even at slower rates. SVT is population dependent but is a very likely cause for syncope if no other abnormality is found.

EP studies can provide the diagnosis for an arrhythmic cause that may have been associated with hypotension and collapse in a clinical setting, independent of whether or not syncope is precipitated during the procedure. Sympathetic tone and postural position affect the ability of patients to compensate for alterations in cardiac output that are associated with an arrhythmia. Most EP studies are performed in the supine position, while most arrhythmic syncope occurs while non-supine.

The abrupt change in heart rate at initiation of a tachycardia is associated with hypotension, with release of parasympathetic tone and gradual increase in sympathetic tone as time progresses (Fig. 6.1). Overshoot in sympathetic tone can lead to an increase in parasympathetic tone and accentuated antagonism, stopping the tachycardia [103,104]. This is one way that SVT can cause syncope but stop spontaneously. An abrupt change in heart rate in hypotension can be enhanced by orthostatic positional change.

Even a non-sustained ventricular tachycardia, not associated with syncope in the EP laboratory, may result in syncope clinically. The EP study is not focused on recreating syncope in the EP laboratory but instead on trying to diagnose a potential arrhythmic cause for syncope. Non-invasive data (telemetry, ECG, echocardiogram, signal-averaged ECG, and loop recorders) help the electrophysiologist to interpret the EP study more accurately [109–113]. The use of newer non-invasive tests, such as T wave alternans, heart rate variability, and QT dispersion, are emerging. At this time, these additional non-invasive tests cannot be incorporated effectively into algorithms to evaluate syncope.

Prognostic implications

EP abnormalities have been identified in 12–70% of patients with otherwise unexplained syncope, with sustained monomorphic ventricular tachycardia the most common abnormality (see Chapter 2). Studies are performed in the hope of not only identificating abnormalities, leading to therapy to prevent recurrent syncope, but also to determine prognosis. Therapy directed at treating the underlying abnormality (most commonly sustained monomorphic ventricular tachycardia) has been associated with a reduction in the risk of death and recurrent syncope in some, but not all, studies [45,55,56,58]. In high-risk patients, treatment may alter the course, but no randomized prospective trials have been performed.

Analysis of the ESVEM trial (in the context of syncope) is illustrative [114]. Based on retrospective analysis of this prospective study, no statistically significant difference was found in the incidence of arrhythmic death and cardiac arrest between the four defined subgroups. In other words, patients who presented with a diagnosis of syncope, but without documented tachycardia, and who met the inclusion criteria (≥ 10 PVCs h^{-1} and induced sustained monomorphic ventricular tachycardia), carried a prognosis similar to patients with documented ventricular tachycardia (with or without syncope) or ventricular fibrillation/cardiac arrest. The incidence of arrhythmic death in the syncope-alone group at 1 year was 24%, and not significantly different from the 20% mortality found in those patients who had survived a prior cardiac arrest. By the fourth year, the mortality in the syncope group was 37%. It is not clear that syncope imparts an excess risk of death, but patients with sustained monomorphic ventricular tachycardia, premature ventricular contractions (PVCs), a decreased LVEF, and syncope are a particularly high-risk group.

The finding that syncope alone in patients with inducible ventricular tachycardia and frequent ventricular ectopy on Holter monitoring carries a mortality comparable to cardiac arrest survivors is not only interesting but of substantial clinical

importance. Based on these results, it appears that syncope in the face of organic heart disease and inducible ventricular tachycardia, in association with frequent ectopy , is associated with a substantial mortality. Until more data are available, an aggressive approach to treat the underlying ventricular arrhythmias appears to be warranted in syncope patients who fulfill ESVEM inclusion criteria.

Based on a consensus of the present data, it appears that patients with unexplained syncope found to have inducible ventricular tachycardia at EP study appear to have a poorer prognosis compared with those without inducible ventricular tachycardia [105–107].

Treatment guided by EP study diagnoses in syncope patient is associated with an improved prognosis in several small, uncontrolled trials, but no prospective controlled trials are currently available. A normal or non-diagnostic study carries a favorable prognosis. Alternatively, syncope has been associated with a poor prognosis independent of etiology or results of EP studies in some groups; severe cardiomyopathy, particularly in those with non-ischemic cardiomyopathy.

Data conflict on these issues. It is very possible that patients with advanced heart disease can develop syncope from profound, but transient, hemodynamic collapse. This may be related to autonomic failure, aggressive vasodilator therapy, or even temporary electromechanical dissociation without even the presence of an arrhythmia. Death in these patients may be by a non-arrhythmic mechanism that would not be expected to be diagnosed at EP testing.

Using the electrophysiology study to direct therapy

The EP study can be used to assess the prognostic implications of syncope and can help to direct therapy. Studies such as Olshansky *et al.* [45], Krol and Kushner *et al.* [63,65] are most useful in defining the EP-related results for which treatment is indicated. Thus, certain abnormalities found at EP study may require treatment independent of whether they caused syncope. If findings are definitive, and indicate high risk for arrhythmic death, treatment should be offered to prevent syncope *and* to prevent arrhythmic cardiac death, independent of the true cause of syncope (Table 6.2).

Table 6.2 Definite abnormality (treatment indicated).

Sustained monomorphic ventricular tachycardia with hypotension

Rapid supraventricular tachycardia with marked hypotension

AV block in the His–Purkinje system (intra- or infra-His) at an atrial cycle length < 320 ms (not pseudo infra-Hisian block) ± procainamide infusion

Symptomatic sinus node recovery time (> 3 s)

Table 6.3 Borderline abnormality (treatment may be needed).

Non-sustained monomorphic ventricular tachycardia with hypotension

AV nodal refractory period > 600 ms

HV > 100 ms (very rare) ± procainamide infusion

Supraventricular tachycardia rate > 180 b min^{-1} without hypotension

Sinus node recovery time > 2 s without symptoms

There are "borderline" abnormalities found at EP study that *may* require treatment, but experience (and the literature) suggests that it is safe to withhold treatment until the situation is better clarified [56,65]. In other words, borderline abnormalities may reflect the true cause of syncope but have less prognostic meaning; immediate treatment is less pressing (Table 6.3). Further diagnostic tests or a period of observation may be indicated. Normal or non-diagnostic test results suggest that an arrhythmic cause of syncope is unlikely.

The use of the EP study results, in order to guide therapy, is disease and stimulation protocol specific. For example, the absence of inducible sustained monomorphic ventricular tachycardia has little meaning in patients with dilated cardiomyopathy or long QT interval syndrome (Tables 6.3– 6.5).

It is clear that interpretation of the EP study requires thorough understanding of the technique, its strengths, and limitations. The answers to questions raised in interpreting abnormal responses are *specific* only to each particular patient subgroup. While limited, the strategy of using the results of the EP study to guide therapy provides a necessary framework to further care for the individual patient.

Table 6.4 Non-diagnostic findings (treatment generally not needed).

Polymorphic ventricular tachycardia without other supportive history

Sinus node recovery time < 2 s without symptoms

No induced tachycardia

Several clinical examples below illustrate the complexity of interpreting EP study results in syncope patients. The cases are chosen deliberately for their complexity and may not necessarily be indicative of the routine syncope patient. However, the EP study can always raise more questions than it answers.

Case 1

A 55-year-old male truck driver with non-ischemic cardiomyopathy presented to an emergency room with one episode of syncope. He had an intermittent "unusual feeling" (Fig. 6.2a). Lidocaine was given and the "unusual feeling" resolved. At EP study, no ventricular tachycardia was induced with up to three ventricular extrastimuli at two sites. Isoproterenol infusion, with rapid pacing, precipitated prolonged episodes of ventricular tachycardia lasting up to 16 s associated with hypotension (Fig. 6.2b). Radiofrequency ablation successfully treated the ventricular tachycardia originating from the right ventricular outflow tract. He was discharged off all antiarrhythmic therapy and has not had any recurrent symptoms.

Comments. The 12-lead ECG during symptoms provided the diagnosis of right ventricular outflow tract ventricular tachycardia. Had that information not been available, the diagnosis may have been missed at EP study because isoproterenol may not have been given, or the result dismissed as non-specific.

Syncope in patients with left ventricular dysfunction has been associated with a poor prognosis. Given the low sensitivity and specificity of EP studies for patients with dilated cardiomyopathy, the patient may have been offered an empiric therapy such as an ICD. Fortunately, during his study, he had very long runs of ventricular tachycardia observed before and during EP study.

Table 6.5 Utility of specific protocols within an electrophysiology study.

Atrial stimulation likely to very useful
1 Chronotropic incompetence proven or suspected
2 Tachycardia-bradycardia syndrome suspected by monitoring
3 Bundle branch block on ECG
4 Supraventricular tachycardia suspected by history or on monitoring
5 Second-degree heart block or higher

Atrial stimulation protocols may be useful
1 Asymptomatic sinus pauses
2 To assess coexisting sinus node or conduction system disease in patients with impaired ventricular function and suspected ventricular tachycardia

Atrial stimulation protocols are unlikely to be useful
1 As part of routine protocol to replace the role of non-invasive monitoring
2 Chronic atrial fibrillation (except for measurement of HV interval)

Ventricular stimulation protocols are likely to be very useful
1 Structural heart disease, LVEF > 0.4, and an abnormal SAECG
2 LVEF < 0.40, coronary artery disease but no acute myocardial infarction
3 Bundle branch block and suspected structural heart disease
4 Idiopathic ventricular tachycardia suspected by monomorphic ectopy on monitoring
5 Recurrent syncope in a patient already treated for ventricular tachycardia
6 Right ventricular dysplasia is strongly suspected

Ventricular stimulation protocols may be useful
1 Long QT (to assess response to epinephrine and monophasic action potentials)
2 Dilated cardiomyopathy
3 Palpitations with syncope early after cardiac surgery and myocardial infarction
4 Syncope associated with use of antiarrhythmic drugs
5 Recurrent, undiagnosed syncope
6 Sarcoid cardiomyopathy
7 Suspected Brugada syndrome

Ventricular stimulation protocols not useful and may be counterproductive
1 Hypertrophic cardiomyopathy without documented arrhythmia
2 Structurally normal heart when specific, occult cardiac disease is not strongly suspected

Ventricular stimulation protocols should be deferred or are contraindicated
1 Severe, uncorrected electrolyte disorders
2 Atrial fibrillation without previous adequate anticoagulation, or with known cardiac thrombus
3 Critical valvular stenosis
4 Known critical coronary artery stenosis with active ischemia, prior to revascularization
5 Severely decompensated heart failure (Class IV)

ECG, electrocardiogram; LVEF, left ventricular ejection fraction; SAECG, signal-averaged ECG.

Case 2
A 70-year-old man with a history of myocardial infarction and impaired left ventricular function developed recurrent, otherwise unexplained, syncope. An EP study was positive for sustained monomorphic ventricular tachycardia. An ICD was implanted and programmed appropriately. He had received apparently "appropriate" ICD shocks, associated with near-syncope. Subsequently, he developed atrial fibrillation, was admitted to the hospital, and placed on amiodarone. He underwent a non-invasive EP study through his defibrillator, along with defibrillation threshold testing, prior to discharge on amiodarone.

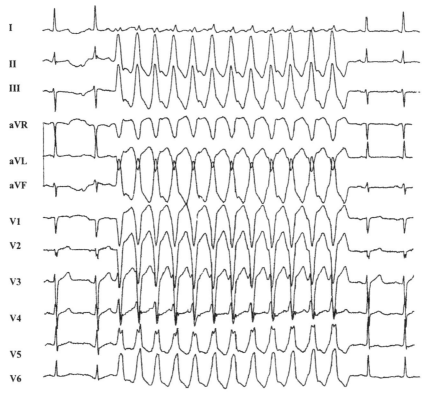

Fig. 6.2a A 12-lead ECG for a patient with syncope who experienced similar but more intense symptoms of palpitations prior to syncope. The morphology is consistent with right ventricular outflow tract ventricular tachycardia.

Two years later, he developed recurrent syncope. An EP study was again performed non-invasively via the ICD. Sustained monomorphic ventricular tachycardia was induced below the programmed rate cut-off of the ICD (Fig. 6.3). Since the ICD was reconfigured to detect and treat the slower, but recurrent, poorly tolerated, ventricular tachycardia, he has not had recurrent syncope.

Comments. Several points are apparent:
1 An ICD can treat induced arrhythmias in syncope patients, and abort syncope.
2 EP studies can be performed without catheters, directly via the ICD.
3 Subsequent syncopal episodes in patients who appear to have been effectively treated in the past need further evaluation. The cause for recurrent syncope may represent a failure of the previously effective therapy, or the patient may have developed syncope from a different etiology.

4 Ventricular tachycardia can result in hemodynamic collapse and syncope, independent of the rate.
5 ICDs may also prevent death in such patients independent of the ability to prevent recurrent syncope.

Case 3
A 74-year-old man with a recent history of chest discomfort developed palpitations associated with "near-syncope" and syncope. The ECG was normal. There was normal systolic function on an echocardiogram. Less intense palpitations occurred without other symptoms during a 12-lead ECG (Fig. 6.4a). A cardiac catheterization demonstrated a critical lesion in a large ramus intermedius branch for which he underwent angioplasty associated with dissection and stent placement but the artery remained patent. He continued to have near-incessant, non-sustained ventricular tachycardia similar to Fig. 6.4a with near-syncope. Beta-blockers

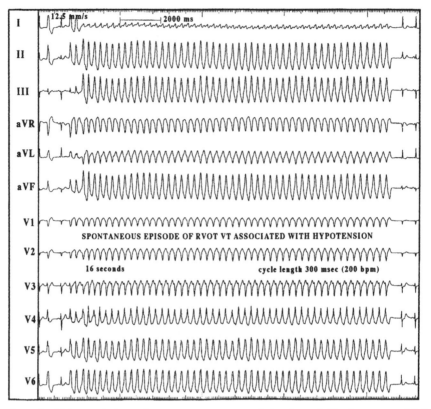

Fig. 6.2b A diagnosis of right ventricular outflow tract ventricular tachycardia is confirmed at electrophysiology study. Salvos of prolonged but self-terminating ventricular tachycardia are associated with hypotension but not syncope during the study. The tissue responsible for tachycardias is successfully ablated using radiofrequency ablation techniques.

suppressed the ventricular tachycardia but rendered him temporary pacemaker-dependent. An EP study of beta-blockers was negative for sinus node dysfunction and sustained ventricular tachycardia but reproduced the clinical arrhythmia (non-sustained ventricular tachycardia). Fig. 6.4b demonstrates the effect of spontaneous non-sustained ventricular tachycardia on his arterial pressure.

Comments. This case illustrates several points:
1 The EP study could reproduce the clinical arrhythmia even though sustained ventricular tachycardia could not be induced.
2 Non-sustained ventricular tachycardia can result in syncope.
3 While ablation of the tachycardia origin was possible, the EP study was inadequate to guide medical therapy.

4 Prognosis, based upon left ventricular function, is good.
5 An ICD would not prevent recurrent symptoms and in this patient's circumstances may result in multiple shocks resulting from non-sustained ventricular tachycardia.

Case 4
A 63-year-old man had a history of angina. He had one episode of syncope and was found to have atrial flutter with a left bundle branch block (LBBB) and a controlled ventricular response. The duration of the atrial flutter and LBBB were unknown. He had a witnessed, but undocumented, cardiac arrest (requiring electrical cardioversion of ventricular fibrillation) while in the hospital, not associated with chest pain. During resuscitation, he converted to sinus rhythm with a first-degree block and a

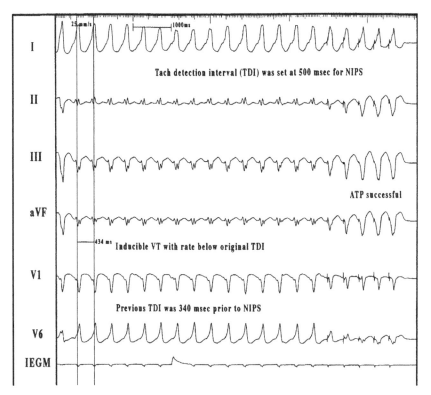

Fig. 6.3 Induction of ventricular tachycardia in a patient who had been previously successfully treated for ventricular tachycardia associated with syncope with an implantable defibrillator. After presenting with recurrent syncope, he is found to have a slower morphology of ventricular tachycardia with a rate that is below the previous cut-off for the device.

LBBB. He was found to have critical three-vessel coronary artery disease and left ventricular dysfunction and therefore underwent coronary artery bypass graft surgery. At EP study, the baseline HV interval was 67 ms (Fig. 6.5a). He developed infra-Hisian block with atrial pacing at 460 ms, (Fig. 6.5b). He had inducible atrial flutter, which was associated with prolonged infra-Hisian block lasting several seconds (Figs 6.5c & 6.5d). Sustained ventricular tachycardia could not be induced.

Comments. This patient had several potential etiologies for syncope. Infra-Hisian block precipitated by paroxysmal atrial flutter was most likely. Alternatively, the patient may have had a self-limited, ischemia-mediated episode of ventricular tachycardia. It is not unusual for cardiac arrest to be predated by one or more episodes of syncope. He was treated with a combination of amiodarone and a dual-chamber pacemaker with mode-switching capabilities. In several months of follow-up he has done well, without cardiac arrest or recurrent syncope. In addition, this patient underwent cardiac catheterization after the cardiac arrest. Syncope without cardiac arrest is a very poor indication for cardiac catheterization unless the diagnosis of critical aortic stenosis is confirmed.

Case 5
A 37-year-old man with treated non-Hodgkin's lymphoma complicated by pericarditis had unexplained syncope. On admission, he was in atrial flutter with a controlled ventricular response at rest, raising suspicion that a rapid response to atrial flutter may have precipitated syncope. Despite a normal two-dimensional echocardiogram, an EP study was performed to treat his atrial flutter and assess other arrhythmic causes. Atrial flutter terminated during radio frequency ablation (Fig. 6.6a). He had a 6.3-s pause prior to the first junctional

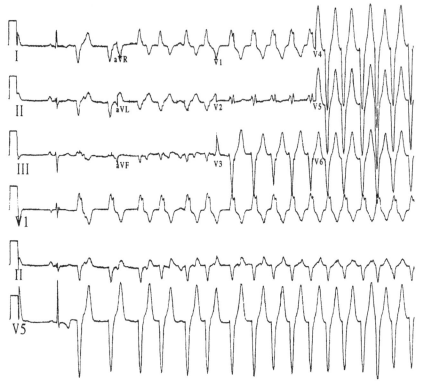

Fig. 6.4a A 12-lead ECG of a man who presents with recent onset syncope and near syncope.

beat and a 39-s sinus node recovery time. The sinus node recovery time and the corrected sinus node recovery time were both abnormal (Fig. 6.6b). The patient was treated with a rate responsive, dual-chamber permanent pacemaker, with mode-switching capabilities. He has not had recurrent syncope.

Comments. This patient probably had syncope resulting from the tachycardia-bradycardia syndrome. In this example, EP study was very useful even though the heart was grossly normal by echocardiographic criteria. At study, the abnormal sinus node recovery time did not mimic the duration of the pause that occurred at the termination of atrial flutter. If the patient had presented in sinus rhythm, it is conceivable that a diagnosis of atrial flutter associated with the tachycardia-bradycardia syndrome may not have been considered. Because his heart was "normal," EP study may not have been considered or the sinus node abnormality may have been considered borderline. Non-invasive monitor-

ing may have been similarly able to demonstrate sinus node dysfunction but perhaps at the cost of recurrent syncope.

Case 6

A 77-year-old man had syncope while driving, and drove his car into a river. Although he had no cardiac history, he did have hypertension and diabetes mellitus. Telemetry revealed non-sustained ventricular tachycardia (Fig. 6.7a). He was found to have significant coronary artery disease and moderate left ventricular dysfunction at cardiac catheterization. Both his referring cardiologist and the patient wished to avoid coronary artery bypass graft surgery, so he was treated medically for ischemia. At EP study, the HV interval was 70 ms (Fig. 6.7b). With the infusion of procainamide 15 mg kg^{-1}, his HV interval prolonged to 100 ms (Fig. 6.7c). Atrial pacing after procainamide induced 2 : 1 infra-Hisian block (Fig. 6.7d). He did not have monomorphic ventricular tachycardia induced. A permanent pacemaker was placed. He

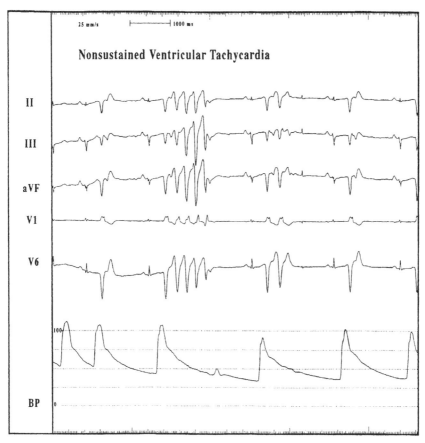

Fig. 6.4b Non-sustained ventricular tachycardia associated with a fall in perfusion pressure in a syncope patient. Blood pressure (BP) is measured from a radial artery catheter.

has remained asymptomatic, although he has become pacemaker dependent.

Comments. Atrioventricular block was shown conclusively on telemetry. The arterial pressure showed an immediate drop in blood pressure after the first dropped QRS complex. The referring physician performed cardiac catheterization prior to consulting us. We would not have automatically performed cardiac catheterization, but we used the information. Because he had left ventricular dysfunction associated with non-sustained ventricular tachycardia in the setting of coronary artery disease, coexisting ventricular tachycardia needed to be excluded. The EP study revealed a baseline HV of 70 ms. The HV lengthened to 100 ms on procainamide. Infra-Hisian block was demonstrable only with procainamide. Despite the non-invasive

evidence of AV block, it took a provocative maneuver (procainamide) to demonstrate infra-Hisian block. In the current era, it is quite likely this patient would have been offered a dual-chamber ICD, despite disappointing battery longevity of the units to date.

Case 7
A 69-year-old man with a history of a non-ischemic cardiomyopathy was admitted with syncope. At EP study, multiple morphologies of sustained monomorphic ventricular tachycardia were reproducibly induced. An arterial sheath had been placed with the hopes of finding a well-tolerated, predominant morphology suitable for ablation. Fig. 6.8a reveals a beat-to-beat alteration in arterial blood pressure associated with a "slow" ventricular tachycardia. The tachycardia terminated spontaneously with an

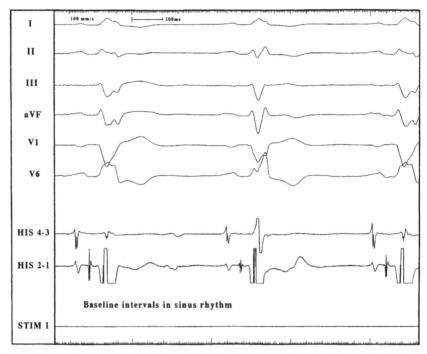

Fig. 6.5a Baseline His bundle electrogram (His 4–3 and His 2–1) during sinus rhythm. The HV interval is slightly abnormal at 67 ms.

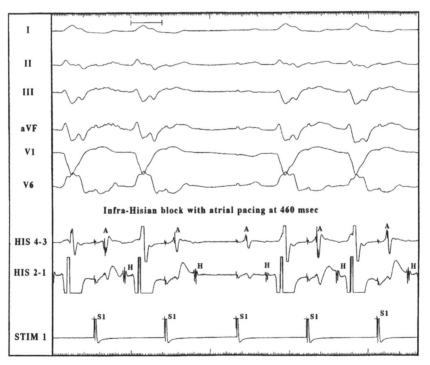

Fig. 6.5b Atrial pacing (STIM 1) at 460 ms induces block below the level of the His bundle.

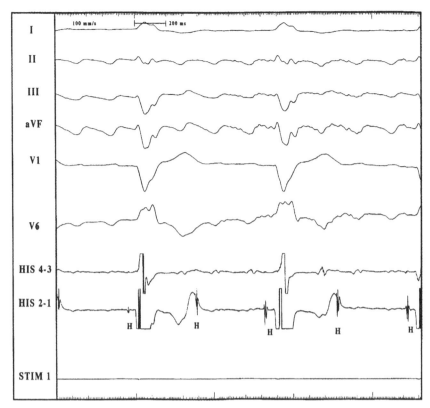

Fig. 6.5c Atrial flutter is induced with rapid atrial pacing. This is associated with 2 : 1 infra-Hisian block. There are two His bundle electrograms (see HIS 4–3 and HIS 2–1) for every conducted QRS complex.

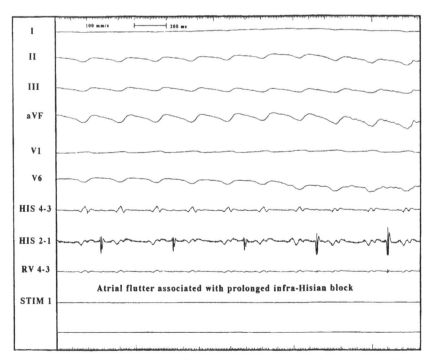

Fig. 6.5d Subsequently, the patient develops ventricular asystole associated with complete infra-Hisian block (see HIS 2–1). The rhythm is atrial flutter with complete AV block. Ventricular pacing is instituted within a matter of seconds.

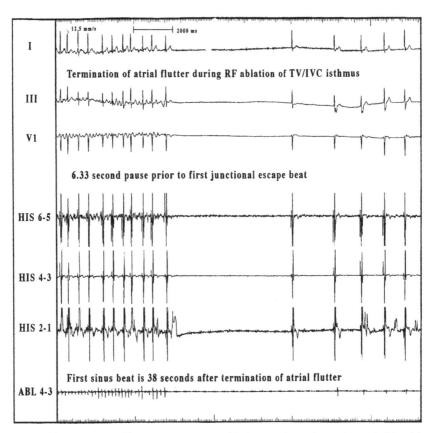

Fig. 6.6a A 37-year-old man presents with new onset syncope and is found to be in atrial flutter associated with a controlled ventricular response. After successful termination of atrial flutter during radiofrequency ablation, a prolonged pause is noted with a delay of 6.3 s prior to the first junctional beat. Analysis suggests that the first sinus depolarization occurred 38 s after the termination of atrial flutter.

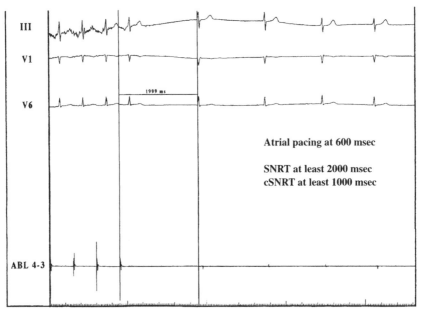

Fig. 6.6b Sinus node recovery times are clearly abnormal but not to the degree seen after the termination of atrial flutter. Sinus node recovery time is at least 2000 ms. The corrected sinus node recovery time (cSNRT) is at least 1000 ms. The upper limit of normal for the cSNRT is 545 ms.

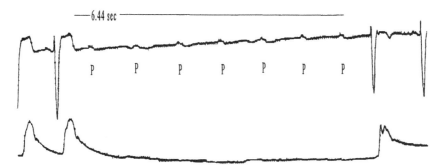

Fig. 6.7a High-degree heart block (top tracing) associated with a decrease in the arterial blod pressure (lower tracing) in a man who presents with new onset syncope. He also demonstrates non-sustained ventricular tachycardia on telemetry.

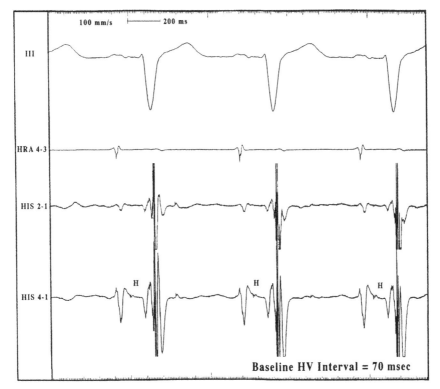

Fig. 6.7b Baseline HV interval in sinus rhythm is 70 ms in a patient who presents with syncope and is found to have the telemetry findings shown in Fig. 6.7a. Atrial pacing is associated with block above the level of the His bundle. HIS, His bundle position; HRA; high right atrial position.

immediate improvement in blood pressure (Fig. 6.8b). A second, faster ventricular tachycardia was associated with electromechanical dissociation (Fig. 6.8c). He was treated with amiodarone and an ICD.

Comments. Even though this patient had a non-ischemic cardiomyopathy, he had inducible sustained monomorphic ventricular tachycardia.

Although bundle branch re-entry can occur commonly in this population, it was not present here. While it is less common to be able to induce sustained monomorphic ventricular tachycardia in these patients, the response is still very specific.

Case 8
The patient is a 54-year-old male with recurrent syncope. It was determined that he had deglutition

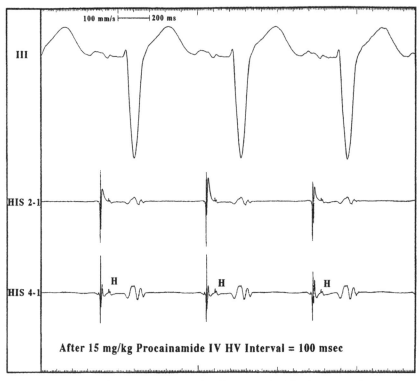

Fig. 6.7c This tracing represents conduction seen in the His bundle catheter (HIS) for the same patient shown in Figs 6.7a and 6.7b. The HV interval prolongs to 100 ms after the infusion of 15 mg kg⁻¹ of procainamide.

syncope when he drank excessively cold liquids. He also had carotid hypersensitivity. An EP study was performed to assess the benefits of dual- and single-chamber pacing to prevent hemodynamic collapse (Fig. 6.9a). During carotid massage in the EP laboratory, the patient became asystolic (Fig. 6.9b). With ventricular pacing he remained hypotensive (Fig. 6.9c), but with AV sequential pacing his systolic blood pressure remained intact (Fig. 6.9d). He underwent the implantation of a DDD pacemaker. Subsequently to this, he remains asymptomatic with no recurrent syncope on carotid massage or drinking cold liquids.

Case 9

A 34-year-old man presented with recent onset syncope without prodrome and postsyncopal diaphoresis. Past medical history and family history were unremarkable. Physical examination was normal. ECG results consistent with Brugada syndrome were obtained (Fig. 6.10). Two-

dimensional echocardiogram was normal. At EP study, he was inducible for ventricular fibrillation with single and double ventricular extrastimuli. The rest of the study was normal. He was treated with a single-chamber ICD, and given a rate cut-off of 300 ms.

Subsequently, he had recurrent syncope. However, the ICD was interrogated and found to be functional without any episodes being detected. A monitor zone was programmed. Because the EP study had been otherwise normal, he also underwent early tilt table testing. This test reproduced his symptoms and was positive for vasodepressor syncope.

Comments. The patient's presentation was atypical for vasodepressor syncope given the rare episodes and lack of prodrome. It is reasonable to assume that the diagnosis of Brugada syndrome was made incidentally. It does not follow that ICD implant was neither indicated nor wise. As with many other

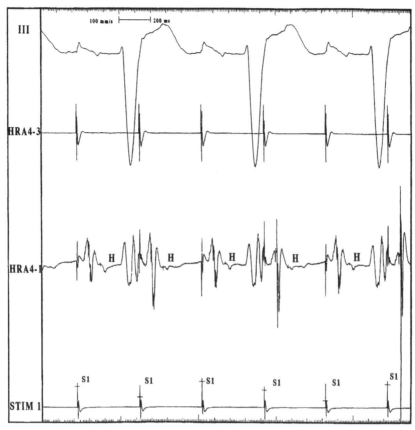

Fig. 6.7d In the same patient shown in Figs 6.7a, 6.7b and 6.7c, atrial pacing results in 2 : 1 infra-Hisian block after infusion of 15 mg kg^{-1} of procainamide.

pathophysiologic conditions, sudden death prophylaxis and treatment of syncope are linked, but not necessarily the same thing. While syncope is associated with a worse prognosis in Brugada syndrome, it is unclear what the role of coexisting vasodepressor syncope is.

Also, because an EP had been performed, once the patient was found to have recurrent syncope not caused by ventricular fibrillation, secondary evaluation shifted immediately away from arrhythmias with a high level of confidence that a slower VT or SVT was not the culprit. A monitor zone was programmed only for insurance.

Case 10

An 83-year-old woman with a history of rheumatic heart disease and coronary artery disease and previous mitral commissurotomy and bypass surgery presents with syncope and was found to be in atrial fibrillation. She had previously been in sinus rhythm but has symptoms in atrial fibrillation. ECG revealed atrial fibrillation with a non-specific intraventricular conduction delay. A transesophageal echocardiogram (TEE) revealed a left atrial thrombus with smoke and moderate left ventricular dysfunction with segmental wall motion abnormalities. The patient was treated with a dual-chamber, high-output ICD without defibrillation threshold testing. The rate cut-off was set for 200 b min^{-1}. She was anticoagulated with heparin and coumarin for several weeks. Repeat TEE revealed resolution of clot. She then underwent non-invasive programmed stimulation which revealed sustained monomorphic ventricular tachycardia at 170 b min^{-1} associated with near-syncope. A single defibrillator shock terminated the ventricular tachycardia and

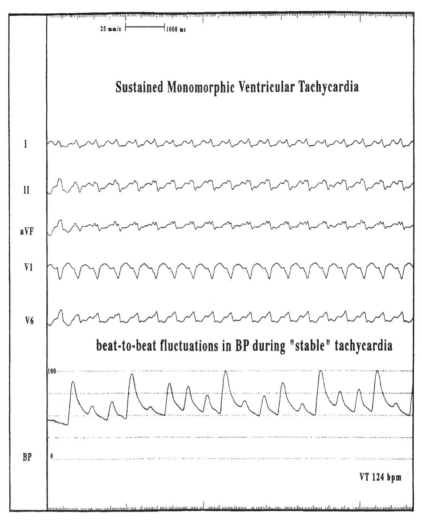

Fig. 6.8a Despite a stable rate of "slow" ventricular tachycardia, there is a fluctuation of the arterial blood pressure and therefore hemodynamic impairment in a patient with syncope that had been presumed to be secondary to this ventricular tachycardia.

she reverted to sinus rhythm. She has subsequently been treated with amiodarone (successfully) for recurrent atrial fibrillation and ventricular tachycardia and is doing well.

Comments. This case illustrates potential pitfalls in the evaluation of complex patients with syncope. On one hand, she may be at risk for sudden death, but either the diagnostic evaluation or treatment may predictably result in serious morbidity (in this case stroke). In this instance, the ICD was chosen, but immediate programming was focused upon termination of ventricular fibrillation until it

was safer to proceed with a complete diagnostic evaluation.

The role of the electrophysiology study in frequent recurrent syncope

In the 50% of patients in whom no obvious cause for syncope is found, syncope itself appears to be self-limited and often benign. Many patients appear to have spontaneous resolution of syncope. For others, non-invasive monitoring can help to identify patients in whom the EP study will provide a high yield. Several variables have been identified that are

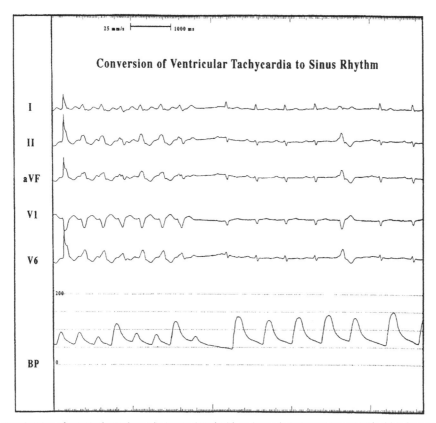

Fig. 6.8b Termination of ventricular tachycardia is associated with an immediate improvement in the blood pressure. The fluctuations in beat-to-beat arterial pressure also improve.

Table 6.6 Variables associated with an abnormal electrophysiology study.

Presence of structural heart disease
Previous myocardial infarction
Late potentials present on signal-averaged ECG
Bifasicular block present on 12-lead ECG
Pre-excitaition present on 12-lead ECG
Waxing/waning atypical right bundle brunch block
  (Brugada syndrome) on 12-lead ECG
Non-invasive monitoring suggestive of sinus node
  dysfunction
Non-invasive monitoring suggestive of fixed AV block
Older age
History of supraventricular tachycardia
Fatty infiltration of the right/left ventricle on cardiac MRI

ECG, electrocardiogram; MRI, magnetic resonance imaging.

associated with a positive EP test (Table 6.6). In this group, the EP study should be performed early in the work-up. However, there is a group of patients who have frequent, recurrent episodes of syncope, for whom all non-invasive parameters are normal and who have undergone repeated non-invasive evaluations. In this small group, an EP study can be offered later into a diagnostic work-up. Data from Krol *et al.* [63] and Krahn *et al.* [78] suggest that the EP study will occasionally find surprising and possibly clinically important abnormalities even in "low yield" patients. However, when performing and interpreting results in "low yield" patients, one should be extremely careful to ensure that any abnormality discovered is clinically relevant. Recommendations for when to consider an EP study in a patient with syncope are listed in Table 6.7.

Unusual indications for electrophysiology studies in syncope

There are other unusual reasons to consider EP studies. Ventricular stimulation protocols may occa-

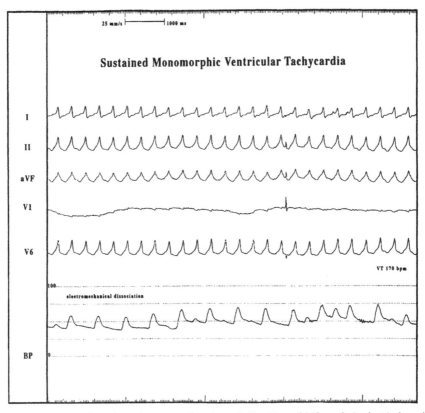

Fig. 6.8c A faster ventricular tachycardia in the same patient shown in Figs 6.8a and 6.8b results in electrical–mechanical dissociation without alterations in the rate of the ventricular tachycardia.

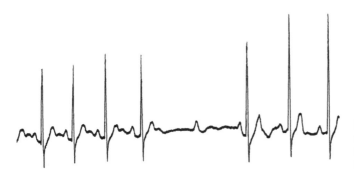

Fig. 6.9a In a patient who presents with recurrent syncope, after swallowing cold water, slowing of the sinus rate precedes AV block.

sionally be useful in conjunction with the infusion of epinephrine in patients who are suspected of having the long QT interval syndrome, to assess the effects of pacing rate and epinephrine dose on the QT_C interval [115].

An emerging indication for EP studies is to determine risk in patients with known or suspected Brugada syndrome associated with syncope. The role of EP studies for first-degree relatives is still unclear, but drug provocation of typical ECG changes seems to a more prudent screening tool.

Patients with hypertrophic cardiomyopathy can develop syncope as part of their clinical syndrome, of which sustained monomorphic ventricular tachycardia is an occasional cause [100]. In the past, there have been many attempts to assess the

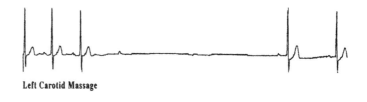

Left Carotid Massage

Right Carotid Massage

Fig. 6.9b Carotid sinus massage is associated with long sinus pauses. Atrial pacing demonstrates concurrent high-degree block in the AV node.

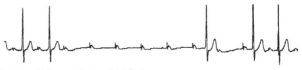
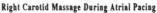

Right Carotid Massage During Atrial Pacing

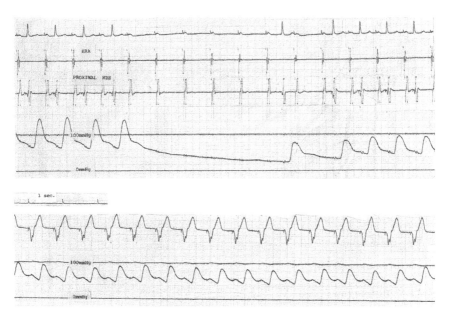

Fig. 6.9c The effects of atrial and ventricular pacing on the blood pressure with carotid sinus massage. Top, carotid massage with atrial pacing. Bottom, carotid massage with ventricular pacing.

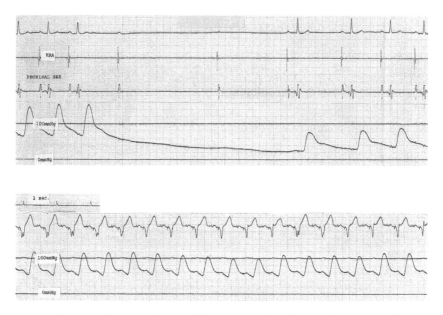

Fig. 6.9d Temporary AV sequential pacing during carotid sinus massage virtually normalizes the arterial blood pressure. This effect is more pronounced than the effect of ventricular pacing as shown in Fig. 6.9c. Top, carotid massage. Bottom, carotid massage with AV sequential pacing.

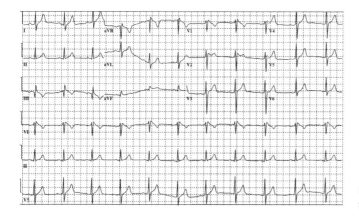

Fig. 6.10 ECG consistent with Brugada syndrome.

utility of programmed stimulation in patients with hypertrophic cardiomyopathy and syncope. While it is clear that syncope is associated with an increased risk in some patients with hypertrophic cardiomyopathy, the results of programmed stimulation have had disappointingly little impact on predicting outcome. Currently, there is a limited role for the routine use of EP studies to deter-

mine which hypertrophic cardiomyopathy patients should receive an ICD [11].

EP studies are counterproductive and possibly dangerous in some patients, such as those with uncorrected critical valvular (generally aortic) stenosis or coronary artery disease. Syncope patients who are found to have these pathological conditions should undergo operative or intervention

Table 6.7 Indications for electrophysiology (EP) study in syncope patients.

Strong indications for EP study in syncope patients
(High utility*)

Previous myocardial infarction associated with left
ventricular dysfunction

Bundle branch block including bifasicular block on 12-lead
ECG

Pre-excitation on 12-lead ECG

Late potentials present on signal-averaged ECG

Fatty infiltration of the right/left ventricle on cardiac MRI†

Previous history of supraventricular tachycardia

Non-invasive monitoring suggests but does not
convincingly demonstrate sinus node dysfunction

Non-invasive monitoring suggests but does not
convincingly demonstrate AV block

To exclude coexisting ventricular tachycardia

To reassess previously effective antiarrhythmic therapy

Other indications for EP study in syncope patients
(Variable utility‡)

Frequent recurrent syncope in low yield patients

Long QT interval syndrome†

Dilated cardiomyopathy†

Hypertrophic cardiomyopathy†

---

* The EP study is generally indicated, with results
influencing therapy.

† The EP study should not be used to guide the
appropriateness of ICD therapy.

‡ The EP study may be useful in some circumstances, but
should be interpreted with caution.

ECG, electrocardiogram; MRI, magnetic resonance imaging;
ICD, implantable cardioverter defibrillator.

correction prior to EP studies. Severe electrolyte abnormalities and/or decompensated heart failure should be stabilized prior to study (see Table 6.5).

Patients with unrecognized atrial fibrillation without previous adequate anticoagulation should undergo pre-procedure TEE to exclude pre-existing left atrial thrombus and EP studies should be performed with anticoagulation. Even clinically irrelevant ventricular arrhythmias may prompt electrical cardioversion and reversion to sinus rhythm. If left atrial or mural thrombus *is* found, then treatment based upon presumed diagnosis should be strongly considered in combination with anticoagulation (see Case 10).

Occasionally, EP studies are performed for "pol-itical" reasons. This tends to occur in situations when syncope or near-syncope episodes occur in patients who are at low risk, non-invasive work-up is inconclusive, and the patient is at low risk for either injury or recurrence, but said patients have an agenda to find or exclude a diagnosis at all costs. Examples include patients with high-risk professions (pilots, bus drivers, certain construction workers) or activities (competitive athletes, deep sea divers).

In patients with syncope and relative bradycardia, the hemodynamic effects of AV sequential pacing can be assessed to see if the patient would benefit from a dual-chamber pacemaker. In other patients with paroxysmal bradycardia, it may not be clear if the cause for the sinus node dysfunction is a result of intrinsic sinus node disease or a reflex neurocardiogenic cause. In these cases, the EP study may help differentiate one cause from the other. Some investigators have advocated a role for dual-chamber pacing for some patients with neurocardiogenic syncope [116,117]. The placement of temporary atrial and ventricular pacing wires during a tilt table test may provide insight into the utility of dual-chamber pacing as therapy in selected patients.

The role of catheter ablation in the treatment of syncope

For over a decade, catheter ablation has become the standard of care for the treatment of syncopal SVT resulting from the Wolff–Parkinson–White syndrome, atrioventricular nodal re-entry, sinoatrial re-entry, atrial flutter, and many atrial tachycardias (Table 6.8). The latter three tachycardias are often associated with sinus node dysfunction, with the termination of the tachycardia resulting in a long sinus pause. While it is standard practice to assess sinus nodal and atrioventricular conduction properties after catheter ablation, particular attention should be paid to the possibility of pre-existing sinus nodal dysfunction as a contributing factor for syncope in patients with sinoatrial re-entry, atrial flutter, and atrial tachycardia (see Case 5).

Catheter ablation of atrial fibrillation is evolving and will likely have a pivotal role in the management of atrial fibrillation in the future. However, atrial fibrillation with associated rapid ventricular

Table 6.8 Potential ablation targets in syncope patients.

Atrial/supraventricular tachycardia
Sinoatrial re-entry*
Atrial tachycardia*
Atrial fibrillation*
Atrial flutter*
Atrioventricular nodal re-entry
SVT associated with pre-excitation syndromes
Ventricular/ventricular tachycardia associated with normal function
Right ventricular outflow tract ventricular tachycardia (LBBB/inferior axis)
Idiopathic left ventricular tachycardia ("narrow" RBBB/left axis) morphology
Ventricular/ventricular tachycardia associated with abnormal function†
Bundle branch re-entry
Scar-mediated ventricular tachycardia associated with chronic coronary disease
Re-entry ventricular tachycardia associated with arrhythmogenic RV dysplasia

LBBB, left bundle branch block; RBBB, right bundle branch block; RV, right ventricular; SVT, supraventricular tachycardia.

* Consider concurrent sinus nodal dysfunction.

† Additional treatment for sudden cardiac death prophylaxis is generally appropriate.

response is rarely a direct cause of syncope. Patients with atrial fibrillation who present with syncope are *much* more likely to have coexisting sinus nodal or atrioventricular conduction abnormalities as the etiology of the syncope. Therefore, the role of catheter ablation of atrial fibrillation for the treatment syncope needs to be clarified.

Syncope resulting from ventricular tachycardia is a common presentation in patients with ventricular tachycardia. In those patients with normal cardiac function, catheter ablation of the ventricular tachycardia is the only necessary treatment, and their subsequent prognosis is excellent. Other patients, with left or right ventricular dysfunction, may also benefit from catheter ablation of the clinical ventricular tachycardia but may still have a poor or uncertain prognosis. In patients with left or right ventricular dysfunction resulting from a variety of causes, consideration of other treatments

options in addition to catheter ablation, such as the implantation of an ICD, is necessary.

Conclusions

There is a clearly role for EP studies to manage patients with syncope. Use of EP studies, guided by information collected during the history, physical examination, and non-invasive testing, provides supportive information not easily available in any other way. While the EP study is a potent method to diagnose arrhythmias and help to guide therapy, it has several important limitations. In essence, the EP study provides additional supportive data regarding the diagnostic cause for syncope. It is useful only in this regard.

The greatest yield of the EP study is in patients with impaired left ventricular function, structural heart disease, and other suggestive findings or history of serious arrhythmia problems. For this population, the EP study can help to direct further appropriate arrhythmia management decisions to reduce the risk of recurrent syncope and to reduce the risk of death.

References

1 Kapoor WN, Karpf M, Wienand S, Peterson JR, Levey GS. A prospective evaluation and follow-up of patients with syncope. *N Engl J Med* 1983;**309**:197–204.

2 Silverstein MD, Singer DE, Mulley AG, *et al.* Patients with syncope admitted to medical intensive care units. *JAMA* 1982;**248**:1185–9.

3 Savage DD, Corwin L, McGee DL, *et al.* Epidemiologic features of isolated syncope: the Framingham study. *Stroke* 1985;**16**:626–9.

4 Kapoor WN, Hanusa BH. Is syncope a risk factor for poor outcomes? Comparison of patients with and without syncope. *Am J Med* 1996;**100**:646–55.

5 Eagle KA, Block HR, Cook EF, *et al.* Evaluation of prognostic classifications for patients for patients with syncope. *Am J Med* 1985;**79**:455–60.

6 Kapoor, WN. Evaluation and outcome of patients with syncope. *Medicine (Baltimore)* 1990;**69**: 160–75.

7 The Antiarrhythmics versus Implantable Defibrillators (AVID) Investigators. A comparison of antiarrhythmic drug therapy with implantable defibrillators in patients resuscitated from near-fatal ventricular arrhythmias. *N Engl J Med* 1997;**337**:1576–83.

8 Anderson JL, Hallstrom AP, Epstein AE, *et al.* Design and results of the antiarrhythmics vs implantable

defibrillators (AVID) registry. *Circulation* 1999;**99**: 1692–9.

9 Steinberg JS, Beckman K, Greene HL, *et al.* Follow-up of patients with unexplained syncope and inducible ventricular tachyarrhythmias: analysis of the AVID registry and an AVID substudy. *J Cardiovasc Electrophysiol* 2001;**12**:996–1001.

10 Brugada P, Brugada R, Brugada P. Determinants of sudden cardiac death in individuals with the electrocardiographic pattern of Brugada syndrome and no previous cardiac arrest. *Circulation* 2003;**108**:3092–6.

11 Maron BJ, Estes NA, Maron MS, *et al.* Primary prevention of sudden death as a novel treatment strategy in hypertrophic cardiomyopathy. *Circulation* 2003; **107**:2872–5.

12 Mittal S, Iwai S, Stein K, *et al.* Long-term outcome of patients with unexplained syncope treated with an electrophysiologic-guided approach in the implantable cardioverter-defibrillatior era. *J Am Coll Cardiol* 1999;**34**:1082–9.

13 Scherlag BJ, Lau SH, Helfant RH, *et al.* Catheter technique for recording His bundle activity in man. *Circulation* 1969;**39**:13–8.

14 Rosen K, Mehta A, Miller RA. Demonstration of dual atrioventricular nodal pathways in man. *Am J Cardiol* 1974; **33**:291–4.

15 Josephson ME. *Clinical Cardiac Electrophysiology: Techniques and Interpretations*, 2nd edn. Philadelphia, PA: Lea & Febiger, 1993.

16 Fisher JD. Role of electrophysiologic testing in the diagnosis and treatment of patients with known and suspected bradycardias and tachycardias. *Prog Cardiovasc Dis* 1981;**24**:25–90.

17 Vanderpol CJ, Farshidi A, Spielman S, *et al.* Incidence and clinical significance of induced ventricular tachycardia. *Am J Cardiol* 1980;**45**:725–31.

18 Dhingra RC, Wyndham C, Bauernfeind R, *et al.* Significance of block distal to the His bundle induced by atrial pacing in patients with chronic bundle branch block. *Circulation* 1979;**60**:1455–64.

19 Dhingra RC, Palileo E, Strasberg B, *et al.* Significance of the HV interval in 517 patients with chronic bifasicular block. *Circulation* 1981;**64**:1265–71.

20 McAnulty JH, Rahimtoola SH. Bundle branch block. *Prog Cardiovasc Dis* 1983;**26**:333–54.

21 Narula O, Samet P, Javier R. Significance of the sinusnode recovery time. *Circulation* 1972;**45**:40–58.

22 Mandel W, Hayakawa H, Danzig R, *et al.* Evaluation of sino-atrial node function in man by overdrive suppression. *Circulation* 1971;**44**:59–66.

23 Rosen KM, Loeb HS, Sinno MZ, *et al.* Cardiac conduction in patients with symptomatic sinus node disease. *Circulation* 1971;**43**:835–44.

24 Scheinman MM, Strauss HC, Abbott JA, *et al.* Electrophysiologic testing in patients with sinus pauses and/or sinoatrial exit block. *Eur J Cardiol* 1978;**8**:51–60.

25 Gupta PK, Lichstein E, Chadda KD, *et al.* Appraisal of sinus nodal recovery time in patients with sick sinus syndrome. *Am J Cardiol* 1974;**34**:265–70.

26 Strauss HC, Bigger JT, Saroff AL, *et al.* Electrophysiologic evaluation of sinus node function in patients with sinus node dysfunction. *Circulation* 1976;**53**:763–76.

27 Gang ES, Reiffel JA, Livelli FD Jr. Sinus node recovery times following the spontaneous termination of supraventricular tachycardia and following atrial overdrive pacing: a comparison. *Am Heart J* 1983;**105**:210–5.

28 Breithardt G, Seipel L, Loogen F. Sinus node recovery time and calculated sinoatrial conduction time in normal subjects and patients with sinus node dysfunction. *Circulation* 1977;**56**:43–50.

29 Gann D, Tolentino A, Samet P. Electrophysiologic evaluation of elderly patients with sinus bradycardia: a long-term follow-up study. *Ann Intern Med* 1979;**9**:24–9.

30 DiMarco JP, Garan H, Harthorne JW, *et al.* Intracardiac electrophysiologic techniques in recurrent syncope of unknown origin. *Ann Intern Med* 1981;**95**:542–8.

31 Hess DS, Morady F, Scheinman MM. Electrophysiologic testing in the evaluation of patients with syncope of undetermined origin. *Am J Cardiol* 1982;**50**:1309–15.

32 Ezri M, Lerman BB, Marchlinski FE, *et al.* Electrophysiologic evaluation of syncope in patients with bifasicular block. *Am Heart J* 1983;**106**:693–7.

33 Akhtar M, Shenasa M, Denker S, Gilbert CJ, Rizwi N. Role of cardiac electrophysiologic studies in patients with unexplained recurrent syncope. *Pacing Clin Electrophysiol* 1983;**6**:192–201.

34 Morady F, Shen E, Schwartz A, *et al.* Long-tem follow-up of patients with recurrent unexplained syncope evaluated by electrophysiologic testing. *J Am Coll Cardiol* 1983;**2**:1053–9.

35 Scharma AD, Klein GJ, Milstein S. Diagnostic assessment of recurrent syncope. *PACE* 1984;**7**:749–59.

36 Morady F, Higgins J, Peters RW, *et al.* Electrophysiologic testing in bundle branch block and unexplained syncope. *Am J Cardiol* 1984;**54**:587–91.

37 Morady F. The evaluation of syncope with electrophysiologic studies. *Cardiol Clin* 1986;**4**:515–26.

38 DiMarco JP. Electrophysiologic studies in patients with unexplained syncope. *Circulation* 1987;**75** (Suppl. 3): 140–3.

39 McAnulty JH. Syncope of unknown origin: the role of electrophysiologic studies. *Circulation* 1987;**75** (Suppl. 3);144–5.

40 Click RL, Gersh BJ, Sugrue DD, *et al.* Role of invasive electrophysiologic testing in patients with symptomatic bundle branch block. *Am J Cardiol* 1987;**59**:817–23.

41 Nelson SD, Kou WH, de Buitleir M, *et al.* Value of programmed ventricular stimulation in presumed carotid sinus syndrome. *Am J Cardiol* 1987;**60**:1073–7.

42 Winters SL, Deshmukh P, Gomes JA. Role of electrophysiologic testing in syncope of unknown origin. *Cardiovasc Rev Rep* 1988;**9**:49–55.

43 Kapoor WN, Hammill SC, Gersh BJ. Diagnosis and natural history of syncope and the role of invasive electrophysiologic testing. *Am J Cardiol* 1989;**63**:730–4.

44 Paul T, Guccione P, Garson A. Relation of syncope in young patients with Wolff–Parkinson–White syndrome to rapid ventricular response during atrial fibrillation. *Am J Cardiol* 1990;**65**:318–21.

45 Olshansky B, Mazuz M, Martins JB. Significance of inducible tachycardia in patients with syncope of unknown origin: a long-term follow-up. *J Am Coll Cardiol* 1985;**5**:216–23.

46 Platia EV, Greene HL, Vlay SC, Werner JA, Gross B, Reid PR. Sensitivity of various extrastimulus techniques in patients with serious ventricular arrhythmias. *Am Heart J* 1983;**106**:698–703.

47 Brugada P, Abdollah H, Heddle B, *et al.* Results of a ventricular stimulation protocol using a maximum of four premature stimuli in patients without documented or suspected ventricular arrhythmias. *Am J Cardiol* 1983;**52**:1214–8.

48 DiCarlo LA, Morady F, Schwartz AB, *et al.* Clinical significance of ventricular fibrillation-flutter induced by ventricular programmed stimulation. *Am Heart J* 1985;**109**:959–63.

49 Platia EV, Reid PR. Non-sustained ventricular tachycardia during programmed stimulation: criteria for a positive test. *Am J Cardiol* 1985;**56**:79–83.

50 Wellens HJ, Brugada P, Stevenson WG. Programmed electrical stimulation of the heart in patients with life-threatening ventricular arrhythmias: what is the significance of induced arrhythmias and what is the correct stimulation protocol? *Circulation* 1985;**72**:216–27.

51 Morady F, DiCarlo L, Winston S, *et al.* A prospective comparison of triple extrastimuli and left ventricular stimulation in studies of ventricular tachycardia induction. *Circulation* 1984;**70**:52–7.

52 Kou WH, de Buitleir M, Kadish AH, Morady F. Sequelae of non-sustained polymorphic ventricular tachycardia induced during programmed ventricular stimulation. *Am J Cardiol* 1989;**64**:1148–51.

53 Morady F, Shapiro W, Shen W, *et al.* Programmed ventricular stimulation in patients without spontaneous ventricular tachycardia. *Am Heart J* 1984;**107**:875–82.

54 Meinertz T, Treese N, Kasper W, *et al.* Determinants of prognosis in idiopathic dilated cardiomyopathy as determined by programmed electrical stimulation. *Am J Cardiol* 1985;**56**:337–41.

55 Bass EB, Elson JJ, Fogoros RN, *et al.* Long-term prognosis of patients undergoing electrophysiologic studies for syncope of unknown origin. *Am J Cardiol* 1988;**62**:1186–91.

56 Doherty JU, Pembrook-Rogers D, Grogan EW, Falcone RA, *et al.* Electrophysiologic evaluation and follow-up characteristics of patients with recurrent unexplained syncope and presyncope. *Am J Cardiol* 1985;**55**:703–8.

57 Moazez F, Peter T, Simonson J, *et al.* Syncope of unknown origin: clinical, noninvasive, and electrophysiologic determinants of arrhythmia induction and symptom recurrence during long-term follow-up. *Am Heart J* 1991;**121**:81–8.

58 Kall JG, Olshansky B, Wilber DJ. Sudden death and recurrent syncope in patients presenting with syncope of unknown origin: predictive value of electrophysiologic testing [Abstract]. *PACE* 1991;**14**:714.

59 Sra JS, Anderson AJ, Sheikh SH, *et al.* Unexplained syncope evaluated by electrophysiologic studies and head-up tilt testing. *Ann Intern Med* 1991;**114**:1013–9.

60 Muller T, Roy D, Talajic M, *et al.* Electrophysiologic evaluation and outcome of patients with syncope of unknown origin. *Eur Soc Cardiol* 1991;**20**:139–43.

61 Englund A, Bergfeldt L, Rehnqvist N, *et al.* Diagnostic value of programmed ventricular stimulation in patients with bifasicular block: a prospective study of patients with and without syncope. *J Am Coll Cardiol* 1995;**26**:1508–15.

62 Teichman SL, Felder SD, Matos JA, *et al.* The value of electrophysiologic studies in syncope of undetermined origin: report of 150 cases. *Am Heart J* 1985;**110**:469–79.

63 Krol RB, Morady F, Flaker GC, *et al.* Electrophysiologic testing in patients with unexplained syncope: clinical and non-invasive predictors of outcome. *J Am Coll Cardiol* 1987;**10**:358–63.

64 Day SC, Cook EF, Funkenstein H, Goldman L. Evaluation and outcome of emergency room patients with transient loss of consciousness. *Am J Med* 1982;**73**:15–23.

65 Kushner JA, Kou WH, Kadish AH, Morady F. Natural history of patients with unexplained syncope and a non-diagnostic electrophysiology study. *J Am Coll Cardiol* 1989;**14**:391–6.

66 Zipes DP, DiMarco JP, Gillette PC, *et al.* Task force on practice guidelines (Committee on clinical intracardiac electrophysiologic and catheter ablation procedures). *J Am Coll Cardiol* 1995;**26**:555–73.

67 Horowitz LN, Kay HR, Kutalek SP, *et al.* Risks and complications of clinical electrophysiologic studies: a prospective analysis of 1,000 consecutive patients. *J Am Coll Cardiol* 1987;**9**:1261–8.

68 Brooks R, Garan H, Ruskin JN. Evaluation of the patient with unexplained syncope. In: Zipes DP, ed. *Cardiac*

Electrophysiology: From Cell to Bedside. Philadelphia, PA: Saunders, 1990: 646–66.

69 Olshansky B, Martins JB. Isoproterenol facilitation of ventricular tachycardia induction during extrastimulus testing predicts effective chronic therapy with beta-adrenergic blockade. *Am J Cardiol* 1987;**59**:573–7.

70 Jackman WM, Friday KJ, Anderson JL, *et al.* The long QT syndromes: a critical review, new clinical observations and a unifying hypothesis. *Prog Cardiovasc Dis* 1988;**31**:115–72.

71 Shimizu W, Noda T, Takaki H, *et al.* Epinephrine unmasks latent mutation carriers with LQT1 form of congenital long QT syndrome. *J Am Coll Cardiol* 2003;**41**:633–42.

72 Wilber DW, Kall J, Olshansky B, Scanlon P. Pacing induced infra-His block in patients with syncope of unknown origin: incidence and clinical significance. *PACE* 1990;**13**:562A.

73 Wilde AA, Antzelevitch C, Borggrefe M, *et al.* For the Study Group on the molecular basis of arrhythmias of the European Society of Cardiology. Proposed diagnostic criteria for the Brugada syndrome: consensus report. *Circulation* 2002;**106**:2514–9.

74 Chinushi M, Washizuka T, Okumura H, Aizawa Y. Intravenous administration of class I antiarrhythmic drugs induced T wave alternans in a patient with Brugada syndrome. *J Cardiovasc Electrophysiol* 2001;**12**: 493–5.

75 Klein GJ, Gersh BJ, Yee R. Electrophysiological testing: the court of final appeal for the diagnosis of syncope? *Circulation* 1995;**92**:1332–5.

76 Bachinsky WB, Linzer M, Weld L, Estes NA, 3rd. Usefulness of clinical characteristics in predicting the outcome of electrophysiologic studies in unexplained syncope. *Am J Cardiol* 1992;**69**(12):1044–9.

77 Fujimura O, Yee R, Klein GJ, *et al.* The diagnostic sensitivity of electrophysiologic testing in patients with syncope caused by transient bradycardia. *N Engl J Med* 1989; **3321**:1703–7.

78 Krahn AD, Klein GJ, Norris C, *et al.* The etiology of syncope in patients with negative tilt table and electrophysiologic testing. *Circulation* 1995;**92**:1819–24.

79 Brignole M, Menozzi C, Bottoni N, *et al.* Mechanisms of syncope caused by transient bradycardia and the diagnostic value of electrophysiologic testing and cardiovascular reflexivity maneuvers. *Am J Cardiol* 1995;**76**(4):273–8.

80 Middlekauff H, Stevenson W, Stevenson L, *et al.* Syncope in advanced heart failure: high risk of sudden death regardless of origin of syncope. *J Am Coll Cardiol* 1993;**21**:110–6.

81 Middlekauff HR, Stevenson WG, Saxon LA. Prognosis after syncope: impact of left ventricular function. *Am Heart J* 1993;**125**:121–7.

82 Brembilla-Perrot B, Donetti J, Terrier de la Chaise A, *et al.* Diagnostic value of ventricular stimulation in patients with idiopathic dilated cardiomyopathy. *Am Heart J* 1991;**121**:1124–31.

83 Olhausen KV, Stienen U, Schwarz F, *et al.* Long-term prognostic significance of ventricular arrhythmias in idiopathic dilated cardiomyopathy. *Am J Cardiol* 1988; **61**:146–51.

84 Poll DS, Marchlinski FE, Buxton AE, *et al.* Usefulness of programmed stimulation in idiopathic dilated cardiomyopathy. *Am J Cardiol* 1986;**112**:992–7.

85 Gang ES, Peter T, Rosenthal PT, *et al.* Detection of late potentials on the surface electrocardiogram in unexplained syncope. *Am J Cardiol* 1986;**58**:1014–20.

86 Winters SL, Stewart D, Targonski A, *et al.* Signal averaging of the surface QRS complex predicts inducibility of ventricular tachycardia in patients with syncope of unknown origin: a prospective study. *J Am Coll Cardiol* 1987;**10**:775–81.

87 Kuchar DL, Thornburn CW, Sammel NL. Signal averaged electrocardiogram for evaluation or recurrent syncope. *Am J Cardiol* 1986;**58**:949–53.

88 Hsia HH, Marchlinski FE. Electrophysiology studies in patients with dilated cardiomyopathies. *Card Electrophysiol Rev* 2002;**6**:472–81.

89 Tchou P, Krebs AC, Sra J, *et al.* Syncope: a warning sign of sudden death in idiopathic dilated cardiomyopathy patients. *J Am Coll Cardiol* 1991;**17**:196A.

90 Link MS, Costeas XF, Griffith JL, *et al.* High incidence of appropriate implantable cardiovertor–defibrillator therapy in patients with syncope of unknown etiology and inducible ventricular arrhythmias. *J Am Coll Cardiol* 1997;**29**:370–5.

91 Thiene G, Nava A, Corrado D, *et al.* Right ventricular cardiomyopathy and sudden death in young people. *N Engl J Med* 1988;**318**:129–33.

92 Ricci C, Longo R, Pagnan L, *et al.* Magnetic resonance imaging in right ventriclar dysplasia. *Am J Cardiol* 1992;**70**:1589–95.

93 Brugada P, Geelen P, Brugada R, *et al.* Prognostic value of electrophysiologic investigations in Brugada syndrome. *J Cardiovasc Electrophysiol* 2001;**12**:1004–7.

94 Paydak H, Telfer EA, Kehoe RF, *et al.* Brugada syndrome: an unusual cause of convulsive syncope. *Arch Intern Med* 2002;**162**:1416–9.

95 Goldschlager N, Epstein AE, Grubb BP, *et al.* Etiologic considerations in patients with syncope and an apparently normal heart. *Arch Intern Med* 2003;**163**:151–62.

96 Moss AJ, Hall WJ, Cannom DS, *et al.* Improved survival with an implanted defibrillator in patients with coronary artery disease at high risk for ventricular arrhythmia. Multicenter Automatic Defibrillator Implantation Trial Investigators. *N Engl J Med* 1996;**335**:1933–40.

97 Link MS, Saeed M, Gupta N, *et al.* Inducible ventricular flutter and fibrillation predict for arrhythmia occurrence in coronary artery disease patients presenting with syncope of unknown origin. *J Cardiovasc Electrophysiol* 2002;**13**:1103–8.

98 Andrews NP, Fogel RI, Pelargonio G, Evans JJ, Prystowsky EN. Implantable defibrillator event rates in patients with unexplained syncope and inducible sustained ventricular tachyarrhythmias: a comparison with patients known to have sustained ventricular tachycardia. *J Am Coll Cardiol* 1999;**34**:2023–30.

99 Moss AJ, Zareba W, Hall WJ, *et al.* Prophylactic implantation of a defibrillator in patients with myocardial infarction and reduced ejection fraction. *N Engl J Med* 2002;**346**:877–83.

100 Fananapazir L, Chang AC, Epstein SE, McAreavey D. Prognostic determinants in hypertrophic cardiomyopathy: prospective evaluation of a therapeutic strategy based on clinical, Holter, hemodynamic, and electrophysiological findings. *Circulation* 1992;**86**:730–40.

101 Leitch JW, Klein GJ, Yee R, *et al.* Syncope associated with supraventricular tachycardia: an expression of tachycardia rate or vasomotor response? *Circulation* 1992;**85**:1064–71.

102 Waxman MB, Wald RW, Cameron D. Interactions between the autonomic nervous system and tachycardias in man. *Cardiol Clin* 1982;**1**:143–85.

103 Waxman MB, Sharma AD, Cameron DA, Huerta F, Wald RW. Reflex mechanisms responsible for early spontaneous termination of paroxysmal supraventricular tachycardia. *Am J Cardiol* 1982;**49**:259–72.

104 Buxton AE, Josephson ME, Marchlinski FE, *et al.* Polymorphic ventricular tachycardia induced by programmed stimulation: response to procainamide. *J Am Coll Cardiol* 1993;**21**:90–8.

105 Morady F, DiCarlo L, Winston S, *et al.* Clinical features and prognosis of patients with out of hospital cardiac arrest and a normal electrophysiologic study. *J Am Coll Cardiol* 1984;**4**:39–44.

106 Wilber DJ, Garan H, Finkelstein D, *et al.* Out-of-hospital cardiac arrest: use of electrophysiologic testing in the prediction of long-term outcome. *N Engl J Med* 1988;**318**:19–24.

107 Wyndham CR. Role of invasive electrophysiologic testing in the management of life-threatening ventricular arrhythmias. *Am J Cardiol* 1988;**62**:I13–7.

108 Masrani K, Cowley D, Bekheit S, *et al.* Recurrent syncope for over a decade due to idiopathic ventricular fibrillation. *Chest* 1994;**106**:1601–3.

109 Prystowsky EN, Knilans TK, Evans JJ. Diagnostic evaluation and treatment strategies for patients at risk for serious cardiac arrhythmias. Part 1. Syncope of unknown origin. Modern concepts of cardiovascular disease. *Am Heart Assoc* 1991;**60**:49–54.

110 Manolis AS, Linzer M, Salem D, *et al.* Syncope: current diagnostic evaluation and management. *Ann Med* 1990;**112**:850–63.

111 Denes P, Uretz E, Ezri MD, *et al.* Clinical predictors of electrophysiologic findings in patients with syncope of unknown origin. *Arch Intern Med* 1988;**148**:1922–8.

112 Bachinsky WB, Linzer M, Weld L, *et al.* Usefulness of clinical characteristics in predicting the outcome of electrophysiologic studies in unexplained syncope. *Am J Cardiol* 1992;**69**:1044–9.

113 Lacroix D, Dubuc M, Kus T, *et al.* Evaluation of arrhythmic causes of syncope: correlation between Holter monitoring, electrophysiologic testing, and body surface potential mapping. *Am Heart J* 1991;**122**:1346–54.

114 Olshansky B, Hahn E, Hartz V and the ESVEM Investigators. Is syncope in the ESVEM trial a marker of cardiac arrest of all-cause mortality? *Circulation* 1994;**90**:I-456A.

115 Bhandari AK, Shapiro WA, Morady F, *et al.* Electrophysiologic testing in patients with the long QT syndrome. *Circulation* 1985;**71**:63–71.

116 Sra JS, Jazayeri MR, Avitall B, *et al.* Comparison of cardiac pacing with drug therapy in the treatment of neurocardiogenic (vasovagal) syncope with bradycardia or asystole. *N Engl J Med* 1993;**328**:1085–90.

117 Benditt DG, Petersen M, Lurie KG, *et al.* Cardiac pacing for prevention of recurrent vasovagal syncope. *Ann Intern Med* 1995;**122**:204–9.

CHAPTER 7

Tilt table testing

Michele Brignole, MD, FESC

Background

During the act of moving from supine to erect posture there is a large gravitational shift of blood away from the chest to the distensible venous capacitance system below the diaphragm. This shift is estimated to total 0.5–1.0 L of thoracic blood, and the bulk of the total change occurs in the first 10 s. In addition, with prolonged standing, the high capillary transmural pressure in dependent parts of the body causes a filtration of protein-free fluid into the interstitial spaces. It is estimated that this results in an approximate 15–20% (700 mL) decrease in plasma volume in 10 min in healthy humans [1]. As a consequence of this gravitationally induced blood pooling and the superimposed decline in plasma volume, the return of venous blood to the heart is reduced, resulting in a rapid diminution of cardiac filling pressure and thereby in a decrease in stroke volume. Despite decreased cardiac output, a fall in mean arterial pressure is prevented by a compensatory vasoconstriction of the resistance and the capacitance vessels in the splanchnic, musculocutaneous, and renal vascular beds. Vasoconstriction of systemic blood vessels is the key factor in the maintenance of arterial blood pressure in the upright posture. Pronounced heart rate increases are insufficient to maintain cardiac output because the heart cannot pump blood that it does not receive [1]. The rapid, short-term adjustments to orthostatic stress are mediated exclusively by the neural pathways of the autonomic nervous system. During prolonged orthostatic stress, additional adjustments are mediated by the humoral limb of the neuroendocrine system [1]. The main sensory receptors involved in orthostatic neural reflex adjustments are the arterial mechanoreceptors (baroreceptors) located in the aortic arch and carotid sinuses. Mechanoreceptors located in the heart and lungs (cardiopulmonary receptors) are thought to have a minor role. Reflex activation of central sympathetic outflow to the systemic blood vessels can be reinforced by local reflex mechanisms such as the venoarteriolar reflex. The skeletal muscle pump and the respiratory pump play an important adjunctive part in the maintenance of arterial pressure in the upright posture by promoting venous return. The static increase in skeletal muscle tone induced by the upright posture opposes pooling of blood in limb veins even in the absence of movement of the subject [1]. Failure of these compensatory adjustments to orthostatic stress is thought to have a predominant role in a large number of patients with syncope. This forms the basis for the use of tilt testing in the evaluation of patients with syncope.

Vasovagal tilt-induced syncope refers to a reflex that, when triggered, gives rise to vasodilation and bradycardia, although the contribution of both to systemic hypotension and cerebral hypoperfusion may differ considerably. Hypotension is caused by vasodilation in the skeletal muscles brought about by inhibition of sympathetic vasoconstrictive activity [2–6]. Experience from tilt testing showed that a vasovagal reaction lasts on average 3 min before causing loss of consciousness [7]. A decrease in systolic blood pressure to 90 mmHg is associated with symptoms of impending syncope [2,8] and to 60 mmHg is associated with syncope [2,9]. A sudden cessation of cerebral blood flow for 6–8 s has been shown to be sufficient to cause complete loss of consciousness [10]. Prodromal symptoms are present in virtually all cases of tilt-induced vasovagal syncope, which occurs, on average, 1 min after the onset of prodromal symptoms [2,8]. During the prodromal phase, blood pressure falls markedly; this fall usually precedes the decrease in heart rate, which may be absent at least at the beginning of this phase [2,7,8].

Isometric arm and leg exercises are able to activate the specific antagonist mechanisms and to abort the vasovagal reaction induced during tilt test [8,11]. Indeed, these maneuvers increase blood pressure during the phase of impending vasovagal syncope by means of muscle sympathetic nerve discharge and vascular resistance increase and allow the patient to avoid losing consciousness. Isometric counter-pressure maneuvers are proposed as a new, feasible, safe and well-accepted first-line specific treatment for vasovagal syncope.

Tilt test protocols

In 1986, Kenny et al. [12] observed an abnormal response to tilt test in 10 of 15 patients with syncope of unknown origin. This response consisted of hypotension and/or bradycardia. They also performed the test in 10 healthy controls without previous syncope, and an abnormal response was provoked in only one. In this study, the authors used an inclination of 60° during 60 min of tilt duration. Since then, tilt testing has been used extensively by many authors proposing different protocols for diagnostic, investigational, and therapeutic purposes. Tilt testing protocols have varied with respect to many factors including the angle of tilting, time duration, and the use of different provocative drugs.

In 1991, Fitzpatrick et al. [13] showed that the use of a bicycle saddle with the legs hanging free for tilt testing gave a low specificity when compared with footboard support. They also showed that tilting at an angle of less than 60° resulted in a low rate of positive responses. Analyzing the time to positive response, they reported a mean time of 24 ± 10 min and proposed 45 min of passive tilting as an adequate duration for the test because this incorporated the mean duration to syncope plus 2 standard deviations. This method is widely known as the Westminster protocol. They reported a rate of positive response in patients with syncope of unknown origin of 75% and a specificity of 93%.

Almquist et al. [14] and Waxman et al. [15] used intravenous isoproterenol during tilt testing. In the study of Almquist et al. [14], after 10 min of passive tilt test without drugs, patients were returned to the supine position and isoproterenol infusion at an initial dosage of 1 μg min^{-1} was administered. When patients achieved a stable increase in heart rate they were tilted again. This maneuver was repeated at increasing dosage up to 5 μg min^{-1}. With this protocol, nine of 11 patients with syncope of unknown origin and negative electrophysiologic studies showed hypotension and/or bradycardia, whereas such responses were found in two of 18 control subjects. In 1992, Kapoor and Brant [16], using an isoproterenol tilt test at 80°, in which isoproterenol was administered in progressive dosages from 1 to 5 μg min^{-1}, without returning the patient to the supine position before each dose increase, reported a low specificity (between 45 and 65%). In 1995, Morillo et al. [17] and Natale et al. [18] proposed a "shortened" low-dose isoproterenol tilt test in which, after 15–20 min of baseline tilt at 60–70°, incremental doses of isoproterenol designed to increase average heart rate by approximately 20–25% over baseline (usually ≤ 3 μg min^{-1}) were administered without returning the patient to the supine position in one study, or returning to the supine position in the other. With this protocol the rate of positive response was 61%, with a specificity of 92–93% (Table 7.1).

In 1994, Raviele et al. [19] proposed the use of intravenous nitroglycerin infusion. With their protocol, 21 of 40 (53%) patients with syncope of unknown origin had positive responses, with a specificity of 92%. Ten of 40 patients (25%) had progressive hypotension without bradycardia. This response was classified as an exaggerated response consisting of an excessive hypotensive effect of the drug. More recently, Raviele et al. [20] have used sublingual nitroglycerin instead of an intravenous infusion. After 45 min of baseline tilting, 0.3 mg of sublingual nitroglycerin was administered. With this protocol, the overall rate of positive responses in patients with syncope of unknown origin was 51% (25% with baseline tilt test and 26% after nitroglycerin administration), with a specificity of 94%. An exaggerated response was observed in 14% of patients and 15% of controls. The main advantage of sublingual nitroglycerin is that venous cannulation is not needed for the protocol. Oraii et al. [21] and Raviele et al. [22] have compared the

Table 7.1 Recommended tilt test protocols (according to ACC expert consensus document [35] and ESC guidelines [39]).

- Supine pre-tilt phase of at least 5 min when no venous cannulation is performed, and at least 20 mm when cannulation is undertaken
- Tilt angle is 60–70°
- Passive phase of a minimum of 20 mm and a maximum of 45 mm
- Use of either intravenous isoproterenol/isoprenaline or sublingual nitroglycerin for drug provocation if passive phase has been negative. Drug challenge phase duration of 15–20 mm
- For isoproterenol, an incremental infusion rate from 1 up to 3 μg min^{-1} in order to increase average heart rate by approximately 20–25% over baseline, administered without returning the patient to the supine position
- For nitroglycerin, a fixed dose of 400 μg nitroglycerin spray sublingually administered in the upright position
- The endpoint of the test is defined as induction of syncope or completion of the planned duration of tilt including drug provocation. The test is considered positive if syncope occurs

isoproterenol test with the nitroglycerin test, with similar rates of positive response and specificity, but with a lower rate of side-effects with nitroglycerin. The optimal duration of the unmedicated phase before the administration of sublingual nitroglycerin has not been fully established. Bartoletti *et al.* [23] compared the effect of an unmedicated phase of 45 mm with 5 mm on the overall positive rate of the nitroglycerin test. The test with the short passive phase was associated with a significant reduction in the rate of positive response, and they concluded that at least some baseline unmedicated tilt testing is needed. Recently, many authors have used a shortened protocol using 400 mg nitroglycerin spray sublingually after a 20-min baseline phase. Pooled data from three studies using this protocol [24–26], in a total of 304 patients, showed a positive response rate of 69%, which was similar to the positive rate of 62% observed in 163 patients from three other studies [23,26,27] using a passive phase duration of 45 min and 400 mg nitroglycerin spray administration. With this protocol, specificity remained high: 94% in 97 controls [24–26]. Thus, a 20-min passive phase before nitroglycerin

administration appears to be an alternative to the more prolonged 45 min passive phase. This method is known as the Italian protocol (Table 7.1).

Other drugs used as provocative agents during tilt testing include isosorbide dinitrate [28,29], edrophonium [30,31], clomipramine [32], and adenosine [33,34].

Irrespective of the exact protocol, some general measures may be suggested when tilt testing is performed. Many of the following rules were published in 1996 as an expert consensus document [35]. The room where the test is performed should be quiet and with dim lights. The patient should fast for at least 2 h before the test. The patients should be in a supine position 20–45 min before tilting. This time interval was proposed to decrease the likelihood of a vasovagal reaction in response to venous cannulation [36,37]. With the protocols that do not use venous cannulation, time in supine position before tilting can be reduced to 5 min. Continuous beat-to-beat finger arterial blood pressure should be monitored non-invasively [38]. Invasive measurements of arterial blood pressure can affect the specificity of the test, especially in the elderly [36] and in children [37]. Although intermittent measurement of pressure using a sphygmomanometer is less desirable, it is an accepted method of testing and is widely used in clinical practice, especially in children. The tilt table should be able to achieve the upright position smoothly and rapidly and to reset to the supine position quickly (< 10 s) when the test is completed in order to avoid the consequences of prolonged loss of consciousness. Only tilt tables with footboard support are appropriate for syncope evaluation. An experienced nurse or medical technician should be in attendance during the entire procedure. The need for a physician to be present throughout the tilt test procedure is less well established because the risk to patients of such testing is very low. Therefore, it is sufficient that a physician is in close proximity and immediately available should a problem arise.

Responses to the tilt test

In patients without structural heart disease, tilt testing can be considered diagnostic, and no further tests need to be performed when spontaneous syncope is reproduced. In patients with structural heart dis-

Table 7.2 Classification of positive responses to tilt testing.

Type I　Mixed
Heart rate falls at the time of syncope but the ventricular rate does not fall to less than 40 b min⁻¹ or falls to less than 40 b min⁻¹ for less than 10 s with or without asystole of less than 3 s
Blood pressure falls before the heart rate falls

Type 2A　Cardioinhibition without asystole
Heart rate falls to a ventricular rate less than 40 b min⁻¹ for more than 10 s but asystole of more than 3 s does not occur
Blood pressure falls before the heart rate falls

Type 2B　Cardioinhibition with asystole
Asystole occurs for more than 3 s
Blood pressure fall coincides with or occurs before the heart rate falls

Type 3　Vasodepressor
Heart rate does not fall more than 10% from its peak at the time of syncope
- *Exception 1.* Chronotropic incompetence
  No heart rate rise during the tilt testing (i.e., less than 10% from the pre-tilt rate)
- *Exception 2.* Excessive heart rate rise
  An excessive heart rate rise both at the onset of the upright position and throughout its duration before syncope (i.e., greater than 130 b min⁻¹)

ease, arrhythmias or other cardiac causes should be excluded prior to considering positive tilt test results as evidence suggesting neurally mediated syncope [35–39]. The clinical meaning of abnormal responses other than induction of syncope is unclear.

In 1992, Sutton *et al.* [40], using the details of hemodynamic responses to tilt testing, proposed a classification of the positive responses, which has been recently modified [7]. This classification is shown in the Table 7.2. Since the decision to terminate tilting influences the type of response [41], for a correct classification of responses tilting should be interrupted at the precise occurrence of loss of consciousness with simultaneous loss of postural tone [7]. Premature interruption underestimates and delayed interruption overestimates the cardio-inhibitory response and exposes the patient to the consequences of prolonged loss of consciousness. However, a consensus does not exist in this regard

and many physicians consider a steadily falling blood pressure accompanied by symptoms sufficient to stop the test.

Grubb and Karas [42] have analyzed the behaviour of blood pressure and heart rate during the period of upright position that precedes the onset of the vasovagal reaction. Different patterns have been recognized. Their results have been confirmed by others [7]. To summarize, two of these are the most frequent. The typical pattern (Fig. 7.1) is characterized by an initial phase of rapid and full compensatory reflex adaptation to the upright position resulting in a stabilization of blood pressure and heart rate (which suggests normal baroreflex function) to the time of an abrupt onset of the vasovagal reaction. The patients with this pattern are largely those who are young and healthy; they have a long history of several syncopal episodes; in many cases the first syncopal episodes occurred in the teenage years; and secondary trauma is infrequent. This pattern, also called "classic", is felt to represent a "hypersensitive" autonomic system that overresponds to various stimuli. Conversely, a different pattern is frequently observed that is characterized by inability to obtain a steady-state adaptation to the upright position and, therefore, a progressive fall in blood pressure and heart rate occurs until the onset of symptoms (Fig. 7.2). The cause of symptoms in this case seems to be a compromised capability to adapt promptly to some external influences ("hyposensitive" autonomic function). Different subtypes have been described, with slight differences between them. The patients affected are predominantly elderly and many have associated diseases; they have a short history of syncope with few episodes per patient; and syncopal episodes begin late in life, suggesting they are caused by the occurrence of some underlying dysfunction. This pattern resembles that seen in patients with autonomic failure and suggests an overlap between the typical vasovagal syncope and more complex disturbances of the autonomic nervous system. Tilt testing can be useful to discriminate between these two syndromes.

Complications

Head-up tilt testing is a safe procedure and the rate

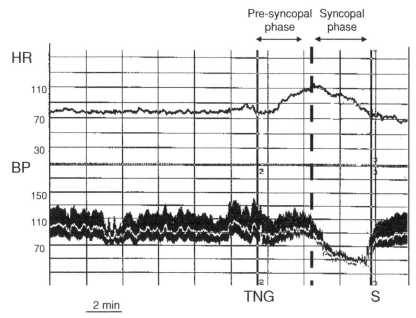

Fig. 7.1 A case of classic (vasovagal) syncope pattern occurring during nitroglycerin challenge. The figure is expanded and the first part of the passive phase of the tilt testing is not shown. The top trace shows the heart rate curve; the bottom trace shows systolic, diastolic, and mean blood pressure curves. Immediately after the administration of 0.4 µg TNG, there is a mild decrease in blood pressure as a consequence of the hemodynamic effect of the drug.

The presyncopal phase lasts approximately 2 min and is characterized by an increase in diastolic blood pressure of 15 mmHg, which indicates a full compensatory reflex adaptation with peripheral vasoconstriction. The heart rate rises approximately 35 b min⁻¹.

The vertical dashed line indicates the time of onset of the vasovagal reaction, which is characterized by a rapid fall in both blood pressure and heart rate that leads to syncope in approximately 3 min. BP, blood pressure; HR, heart rate; S, syncope; TNG, trinitroglycerin.

of complications is very low. Although asystolic pauses as long as 73 s have been reported [43], the presence of such prolonged asystole during a positive response cannot be considered a complication, because this is an endpoint of the test. Rapid return to supine position as soon as syncope occurs is usually all that is needed to prevent or to limit the consequences of prolonged loss of consciousness; brief resuscitation maneuvers are seldom needed. Case reports have documented life-threatening ventricular arrhythmias with isoproterenol in the presence of ischemic heart disease [44] or sick sinus syndrome [45]. No complications have been published with the use of nitroglycerin. Minor side-effects are common and include palpitations with isoproterenol and headache with nitroglycerin. Atrial fibrillation can be induced during or after a positive tilt test and is usually self-limited [46].

Indications

There is general consensus [35–39] that tilt table testing is indicated for diagnostic purposes in the following settings: in case of an unexplained single syncopal episode in high-risk settings (e.g., occurrence of, or potential risk for, physical injury or with occupational implications); recurrent episodes in the absence of organic heart disease; or in the presence of organic heart disease, after cardiac causes of syncope have been excluded, when it will be of clinical value to demonstrate susceptibility to neurally mediated syncope to the patient, their families, and other parties.

Other less common indications may include: differentiating syncope with jerking movements from epilepsy; for evaluating patients with recurrent unexplained falls; and for assessing recurrent presyncope or dizziness.

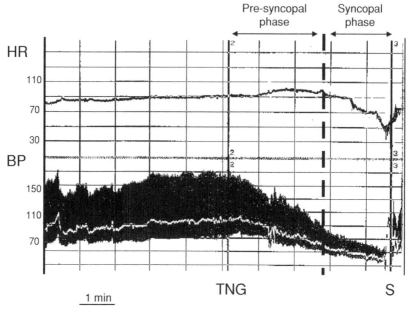

Fig. 7.2 A case of dysautonomic (vasovagal) syncope pattern occurring during nitroglycerin challenge.

The figure is expanded and the first part of the passive phase of tilt testing is not shown. The top trace shows the heart rate curve; the bottom trace shows systolic, diastolic, and mean blood pressure curves. There is an absence of adaptation of blood pressure to the upright position; blood pressure declines slightly and progressively throughout the presyncopal and the syncopal phases without a change in slope; because systolic pressure decreases more than diastolic, pulse pressure also decreases. During the presyncopal phase, heart rate rises but less than in the classic pattern.

The vertical dashed line indicates the time of onset of the vasovagal reaction which, in this case, can be identified only by the decrease in heart rate. BP, blood pressure; HR, heart rate; S, syncope; TNG, trinitroglycerin.

Limitation of tilt table testing in treatment selection for vasovagal syncope

In order to use tilt table testing effectively in the evaluation of the therapeutic options, two conditions are needed: a good reproducibility of the test and responses to tilt testing that are predictive of outcomes at follow-up. The reproducibility of tilt testing has been widely studied [47–51]. The overall reproducibility of an initial negative response (85–94%) is higher than the reproducibility of an initial positive response (31–92%). In addition, data from controlled trials showed that approximately 50% of patients with a baseline positive tilt test became negative when the test was repeated with treatment or with placebo [52–54]. Moreover, acute studies were not predictive of the long-term outcome of pacing therapy [55]. These data show that the use of tilt table testing is limited for assessing the effectiveness of different treatment modalities.

Correlating spontaneous syncopal episodes with tilt table responses

Typically, patients with syncope are asymptomatic at the time of evaluation, and the opportunity to capture a spontaneous event during testing is rare. Because of the episodic nature of syncope, however, correlating spontaneous syncopal episodes with an abnormal finding can be considered as a reference standard. The implantable loop recorder (ILR) has recently become available and has been validated in patients with unexplained syncope [56,57]. Additional information on the ILR can be found in Chapter 19.

In the International Study of Syncope of Uncertain Etiology (ISSUE) [58], an ILR was implanted

Table 7.3 Patient characteristics at enrollment and electrocardiographic findings recorded at the time of syncopal recurrence in patients with isolated syncope and in those with tilt-positive response in the ISSUE study [58]. ECG, electrocardiogram; ILR, implantable loop recorder.

	Syncope	
	Isolated (n = 82)	Tilt-positive (n = 29)
A) Patient characteristics		
Mean age	63 ± 17	64 ± 15
Sex, male	55%	38%
Duration of syncope, years	4 (2–6)	3 (2–10)
Syncopes last 2 years	4 (3–6)	3 (2–10)
Severe trauma	28%	21%
No warning	76%	66%
Structural heart abnormalities	32%	31%
Abnormal ECG	26%	24%
B) ILR-documented syncope		
Follow-up (months)	9 ± 5	10 ± 5
Documented syncope, n (%)	24 (29)	8 (28)
Median time to first episode, days (range)	105 (47–226)	59 (22–98)
Findings at the time of syncope:		
Asystolic pause, n (%)	11 (46)	5 (62)
Maximal duration, sec (range)	15 ± 6 (6–24)	17 ± 9 (3–21)
Sinus arrest (n)	10	5
Atrioventricular block (n)	2	0
Bradycardia < 40 b min^{-1}, n (%)	2 (8)	1 (12)
Normal sinus rhythm, n (%)	9 (37)	2 (25)
Sinus tachycardia, n (%)	1 (4)	0
Atrial tachycardia, n (%)	1 (4)	0

in patients with isolated syncope and in patients with tilt-positive syncope, in order to obtain further information on the mechanism of syncope and to evaluate the natural history of these patients. The isolated syncope group included patients without structural heart disease or with minor heart abnormalities that were considered to be without clinical relevance and not suggestive of a cardiac cause of syncope. The patients had no intraventricular conduction defects, and a comprehensive evaluation (including tilt table testing) revealed no abnormalities. The tilt-positive group was similar to the isolated syncope group except that tilt testing induced isolated syncope. The patients with isolated unexplained syncope and those with an abnormal response to tilt testing had similar clinical characteristics and outcomes (Table 7.3). This finding suggests that the two groups may have been part of the same population. Among the patients in both groups who had a documented recurrence, the most frequent finding was bradycardia at the time of the episode. Typically, these patients had progressive sinus bradycardia, most often followed by ventricular asystole resulting from sinus arrest, or progressive tachycardia followed by progressive bradycardia and ventricular asystole resulting from sinus arrest. Very long asystolic pauses were recorded at the time of syncope in most cases (Fig. 7.3). These findings strongly suggest that, in both groups, syncope was probably neurally mediated and that the most frequent mechanism was a dominant cardioinhibitory reflex with prolonged asystolic pauses. The finding that spontaneous syncope is often associated with long asystolic pauses had never been observed before. In tilt-positive patients, asystolic syncope was also recorded despite a vasodepressor or mixed response to tilt testing. It therefore seems that spontaneous syncope is much more frequently asystolic than was previously appreciated and greater than would be expected on the basis of the results of tilt testing. Thus, while tilt table testing can be used to determine an

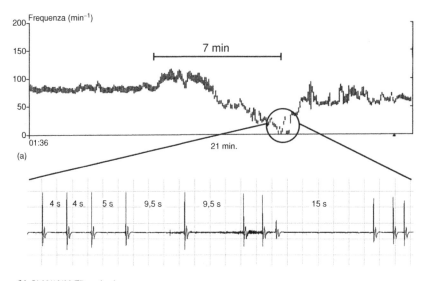

(b) BI 23/12/98 Tilt + mixed

Fig. 7.3 Tilt-positive patient. During the test, the patient had a mixed, "classic" response.

(a) Heart rate trend during 21 min of loop recording. Initially, the heart rate is stable at approximately 80 b min^{-1}; at the beginning of the episode the heart rate increases to 120 b min^{-1}, then progressively decreases to a very low rate.

(b) The expanded electrocardiogram at the time of syncope shows prolonged multiple pauses resulting from sinus arrest. Note the similarity of the heart rate trend with that observed during tilt test in the patient seen in Fig. 7.1. Isolated n = 82. (Adapted from [58].)

individual susceptibility to vasovagal syncope, it cannot always predict the exact type of cardiac response that will occur during a spontaneous event (possibly because tilt table testing employs a relatively modest orthostatic stress that does not fully duplicate the exact type, intensity, or duration of the provocative stimuli encountered in normal life). However, it is important to remember that the study looked only at heart rate changes during spontaneous syncopal events and not the vasodilatory blood pressure changes that are felt to be the more significant factor leading to loss of consciousness.

Consequently, in regard to the electrocardiographic findings documented during spontaneous syncopal events, tilt table testing appears less able to detect some patients with vasovagal syncope (reduced sensitivity) and to yield only a modest correlation between the heart rhythm responses observed during induced and spontaneous episodes. None the less, despite these limitations, tilt table testing remains a useful tool in the evaluation of recurrent unexplained syncope. Further studies

will help to improve its sensitivity and specificity as well as its ability to predict the nature of spontaneous syncopal events.

References

1 Smit AAJ, Halliwill JR, Low PA, Wieling W. Topical review: pathophysiological basis of orthostatic hypotension in autonomic failure. *J Physiol* 1999;**519**:1–10.

2 Alboni P, Dinelli M, Gruppillo P, *et al.* Haemodynamic changes early in prodromal symptoms of vasovagal syncope. *Europace* 2002;**4**:333–8.

3 Mosqueda-Garcia R, Furlan R, Fernandez-Violante R, *et al.* Sympathetic and baroreceptor reflex function in neurally mediated syncope evoked by tilt. *J Clin Invest* 1997;**99**:2736–44.

4 Morillo C, Eckberg D, Ellenbogen K, *et al.* Vagal and sympathetic mechanisms in patients with orthostatic vasovagal syncope. *Circulation* 1997;**96**:2509–13.

5 Lipsitz LW, Mietus J, Moody GB, Goldberger AL. Spectral characteristics of heart rate variability before and during postural tilt. *Circulation* 1990;**81**:1803–10.

6 Van Lieshout JJ, Wieling W, Karemaker JM, Eckberg DL. The vasovagal response. *Clin Sci* 1991;**81**:575–86.

7 Brignole M, Menozzi C, Del Rosso A, *et al.* New classification of haemodynamics of vasovagal syncope: beyond the VASIS classification. Analysis of the pre-syncopal phase of the tilt test without and with nitroglycerin challenge. *Europace* 2000;**2**:66–76.

8 Brignole M, Croci F, Menozzi C, *et al.* Isometric arm counter-pressure maneuvers to abort impending vasovagal syncope. *J Am Coll Cardiol* 2002;**40**:2054–60.

9 Sheldon R, Kiilam S. Methodology of isoproterenol-tilt table testing in patients with syncope. *J Am Coll Cardiol* 1992;**19**:773–9.

10 Rossen R, Kabat H, Anderson JP. Acute arrest of cerebral circulation in man. *Arch Neurol Psychiatr* 1943;**50**:510–28.

11 Krediet P, van Dijk N, Linzer M, Lieshout J, Wieling W. Management of vasovagal syncope: controlling or aborting faints by leg crossing and muscle tensing. *Circulation* 2002;**106**:1684–9.

12 Kenny RA, Ingram A, Bayliss J, Sutton R. Head-up tilt: a useful test for investigating unexplained syncope. *Lancet* 1986;**1**:1352–5.

13 Fitzpatrick AP, Theodorakis G, Vardas P, Sutton R. Methodology of head-up tilt testing in patients with unexplained syncope. *J Am Coll Cardiol* 1991;**17**:125–30.

14 Almquist A, Goldenberg IF, Miistein S, *et al.* Provocation of bradycardia and hypotension by isoproterenol and upright posture in patients with unexplained syncope. *N Engl J Med* 1989;**9**:320, 346–51.

15 Waxman MB, Yao L, Cameron DA, Waid RW, Roseman J. Isoproterenol induction of vasodepressor type reaction in vasodepressor-prone persons. *Am J Cardiol* 1989;**63**:58–65.

16 Kapoor WN, Brant N. Evaluation of syncope by upright tilt testing with isoproterenol: a non-specific test. *Ann Intern Med* 1992;**116**:358–63.

17 Morillo CA, Klein GJ, Zandri 5, Yee R. Diagnostic accuracy of a low-dose isoproterenol head-up tilt protocol. *Am Heart J* 1995;**129**(5):901–6.

18 Natale A, Aktar M, Jazayeri M, *et al.* Provocation of hypotension during head-up tilt testing in subjects with no history of syncope or presyncope. *Circulation* 1995;**92**:54–8.

19 Raviele A, Gasparini G, Di Pede F, *et al.* Nitroglycerin infusion during upright tilt: a new test for the diagnosis of vasovagal syncope. *Am Heart J* 1994;**127**:103–11.

20 Raviele SA, Menozzi C, Brignole M, *et al.* Value of head-up tilt testing potentiated with sublingual nitroglycerin to assess the origin of unexplained syncope. *Am J Cardiol* 1995;**76**:267–72.

21 Oraii S, Maleki M, Minooii M, Kafai I. Comparing two different protocols for tilt table testing: sublingual glyceryl trinitrate versus isoprenaline infusion. *Heart* 1999;**81**:603–5.

22 Raviele A, Giada F, Brignole M, *et al.* Diagnostic accuracy of sublingual nitroglycerin test and low-dose isopro-

terenol test in patients with unexplained syncope: a comparative study. *Am J Cardiol* 2000;**85**:1194–8.

23 Bartoletti A, Gaggioli G, Bottoni N, *et al.* Head-up tilt testing potentiated with oral nitroglycerin: a randomized trial of the contribution of a drug-free phase and a nitroglycerin phase in the diagnosis of neurally mediated syncope. *Europace* 1999;**1**:183–6.

24 Del Rosso A, Bartoli P, Bartoletti A, *et al.* Shortened head-up tilt testing potentiated with sublingual nitroglycerin in patients with unexplained syncope. *Am Heart J* 1998;**135**:564–70.

25 Natale A, Sra J, Akhtar M, *et al.* Use of sublingual nitroglycerin in patients with unexplained syncope. *Am Heart J* 1998;**135**:564–70.

26 Del Rosso A, Bartoletti A, Bartoli P, *et al.* Methodology of head-up tilt testing potentiated with sublingual nutroglycerin in unexplained syncope. *Am J Cardiol* 2000;**85**:1007–11.

27 Foglia Manzillo G, Giada F, Beretta S, Corrado G, Santarone M, Raviele A. Reproducibility of head-up tilt testing potentiated with sublingual nitroglycerin in patients with unexplained syncope. *Am J Cardiol* 1999;**84**:284–8.

28 Zeng C, Zhu Z, Hu W, *et al.* Value of sublingual isosorbide dinitrate before isoproterenol tilt test for diagnosis of neurally mediated syncope. *Am J Cardiol* 1999;**83**:1059–63.

29 Ammirati F, Colivicchi F, Biffi A, Magris B, Pandozi C, Santini M. Head-up tilt testing potentiated with low-dose sublingual isosorbide dinitrate: a simplified time-saving approach for the evaluation of unexplained syncope. *Am Heart J* 1998;**135**:671–6.

30 Voice RA, Lurie KG, Sakaguchi S, Rector TS, Benditt DG. Comparison of tilt angles and provocative agents (edrophonium and isoproterenol) to improve head-upright tilt-table testing. *Am J Cardiol* 1998;**81**:346–51.

31 Fitzpatrick AP, Lee RJ, Epstein LM, Lesh MD, Eisenberg S, Sheinman MM. Effect of patient characteristics on the yield of prolonged baseline head-up tilt testing and the additional yield of drug provocation. *Heart* 1996;**76**:406–11.

32 Theodorakis G, Markianos M, Zarvalis E, *et al.* Provocation of neurocardiogenic syncope by clomipramine administration during the head-up tilt test in vasovagal syncope. *J Am Coll Cardiol* 2000;**36**:174–8.

33 Shen WK, Hammil S, Munger T, *et al.* Adenosine: potential modulator for vasovagal syncope. *J Am Coll Cardiol* 1996;**28**:146–54.

34 Mittal S, Stein K, Markowitz S, Slotwiner D, Rohatgi S, Lerman B. Induction of neurally mediated syncope with adenosine. *Circulation* 1999;**99**:1318–24.

35 Benditt DG, Ferguson DW, Grubb BP, *et al.* Tilt table testing for assessing syncope. ACC expert consensus document. *J Am Coll Cardiol* 1996;**28**:263–75.

36 McIntosh SJ, Lawson J, Kenny RA. Intravenous cannulation alters the specificity of head-up tilt testing for vasovagal syncope in elderly patients. *Age Ageing* 1994;**63**: 58–65.

37 De Jong-de Vos van Steenwijk CCE, Wieling W, Johannes JM, Harms MPM, Kuis W, Wesseling KH. Incidence and hemodynamics of near-fainting in healthy 6–16-year-old subjects. *J Am Coll Cardiol* 1995;**25**:1615–21.

38 Imholz BPM, Wieiing W, van Montfrans GA, Wesseiing KH. Fifteen years' experience with finger arterial pressure monitoring: assessment of the technology. *Cardiovasc Res* 1998;**38**:605–16.

39 Brignole M, Alboni P, Benditt D, *et al.* for the Task Force on Syncope, European Society of Cardiology. Guidelines on management (diagnosis and treatment) of syncope. *Eur Heart J* 2001;**22**:1256.

40 Sutton R, Petersen M, Brignole M, Raviele A, Menozzi C, Giani P. Proposed classification for tilt induced vasovagal syncope. *Eur J Card Pacing Electrophysiol* 1992;**3**:180–3.

41 Wieling W, van Lieshout JJ, ten Harkel ADJ. Dynamics of circulatory adjustments to head-up tilt and tilt back in healthy and sympathetically denervated subjects. *Clin Sci* 1998;**94**:347–52.

42 Grubb BP, Karas B. Diagnosis and management of neurocardiogenic syncope. *Curr Opin Cardiol* l998;**13**:29–35.

43 Maloney J, Jaeger F, Fouad-Tarazi F, Morris H. Malignant vasovagal syncope: prolonged asystole provoked by head-up tilt. *Cleve Clin J Med* 1988;**55**:542–8.

44 Leman RB, Clarke E, Gillette P. Significant complications can occur with ischemic heart disease and tilt table testing. *PACE* 1999;**22**:675–7.

45 Gatzouiis KA, Mamarelis IE, Apostolopoulos T, Dilaveris P, Gialafos J, Toutouzas M. Polymorphic ventricular tachycardia induced during tilt table testing in a patient with syncope and probable dysfunction of the sinus node. *PACE* 1995;**18**:1075–9.

46 Leitch J, Klein G, Yee R, Murdick C, Teo WS. Neurally mediated syncope and atrial fibrillation (Letter). *N Engl J Med* 1991;**324**:495–6.

47 Sheldon R, Splawinski J, Killam S. Reproducibility of isoproterenol tilt-table tests in patients with syncope. *Am J Cardiol* 1992;**69**:1300–5.

48 Grubb BP, Wolfe D, Tenesy Armos P, Hahn H, Elliot L. Reproducibility of head upright tilt-table test in patients with syncope. *PACE* 1992;**15**:1477–81.

49 De Buitler M, Grogan EW Jr, Picone MF, Casteen JA. Immediate reproducibility of the tilt table test in adults with unexplained syncope. *Am J Cardiol* 1993;**71**:304–7.

50 Brooks R, Ruskin JN, Powell AC, Newell J, Garan H, McGovern BA. Prospective evaluation of day-to-day reproducibility of upright tilt-table testing in unexplained syncope. *Am J Cardiol* 1993;**71**:1289–92.

51 Blanc JJ, Mansourati J, Maheu B, Boughaleb D, Genet L. Reproducibility of a positive passive upright tilt test at a 7-day interval in patients with syncope. *Am J Cardiol* 1993;**15**:469–71.

52 Moya A, Permanyer-Miralda G, Sagrista-Sauleda J, *et al.* Limitations of head-up tilt test for evaluating the efficacy of therapeutic interventions in patients with vasovagal syncope: results of a controlled study of etilefrine versus placebo. *J Am Coll Cardiol* 1995;**25**:65–9.

53 Morillo CA, Leitch JW, Yee R, Klein GL. A placebo-controlled trial of intravenous and oral disopyramide for prevention of neurally mediated syncope induced by head-up tilt. *J Am Coll Cardiol* 1993;**22**:1843–8.

54 Raviele A, Brignole M, Sutton R, *et al.* Effect of etilefrine in preventing syncopal recurrence in patients with vasovagal syncope: a double-blind, randomized, placebo-controlled trial. The Vasovagal Syncope International Study. *Circulation* 1999;**99**(11):1452–57.

55 Sutton R, Brignoie M, Menozzi C, *et al.* Dual-chamber pacing in treatment of neurally mediated tilt-positive cardioinhibitory syncope: pacemaker versus no therapy: a multicentre randomized study. *Circulation* 2000;**102**: 294–9.

56 Krahn A, Klein G, Norris C, Yee R. The ethiology of syncope in patients with negative tilt table and electrophysiologic testing. *Circulation* 1995;**92**:1819–26.

57 Krahn AD, Klein GJ, Yee R, Takle-Newhouse T, Norris C. Use of an extended monitoring strategy in patients with problematic syncope. Reveal Investigators. *Circulation* 1999;**26**:406–10.

58 Moya A, Brignole M, Menozzi C, *et al.* Mechanism of syncope in patients with isolated syncope and in patients with tilt-positive syncope. *Circulation* 2001;**104**:1261–7.

CHAPTER 8

Syncope and the implantable cardioverter defibrillator

Brian Olshansky, MD

Introduction

One potential precipitant of syncope is a poorly tolerated, potentially life-threatening, ventricular arrhythmia. The presentation of such a malignant arrhythmia can vary from minimal symptoms to recurrent syncope or even a full-blown cardiac arrest should it recur. This potentially life-threatening cause for syncope can portend future events, including recurrent sustained ventricular tachycardia and, ultimately, death. Indeed, it is often difficult to distinguish a cardiac arrest in its earliest throes from a syncopal event in progress, causing some to remark: "Syncope is the same as sudden death except in one you wake up" [1].

Recent compelling evidence indicates that implantable cardioverter defibrillators (ICDs) can reduce the risk of sudden arrhythmic, cardiac, and total death in populations at high risk for malignant ventricular arrhythmia [2–5]. These devices can rapidly and effectively stop a malignant arrhythmia with an internal shock.

It makes sense therefore that some patients with syncope, who have a malignant ventricular arrhythmia as the root cause, may benefit from an ICD to reduce the risk of death. This chapter focuses on indications for ICD implantation in patients with syncope. It describes disorders that may identify a patient at risk and provides guidelines for which patient with syncope may merit consideration for an ICD.

Methods to identify risk – who is at highest risk of sudden cardiac death?

Those with syncope at highest risk of arrhythmic death include patients with cardiomyopathy, infiltrative cardiac disease, valvular disease, congenital syndromes (long QT interval syndrome, Brugada syndrome, arrhythmogenic right ventricular dysplasia, and hypertrophic cardiomyopathy).

In patients with ischemic and non-ischemic cardiomyopathy, New York Heart Association Functional Class and left ventricular ejection fraction (LVEF) remain the best predictors of sudden cardiac death and total mortality. Other risk factors depend on the underlying medical condition.

Other common, rather non-specific indicators of risk include ongoing ischemia and ventricular arrhythmias. Syncope may portend sudden cardiac death for patients with impaired ventricular function, those with congenital long QT interval syndrome, and other genetic conditions that predispose to arrhythmias.

Risk stratification has been attempted by using non-invasive markers such as heart-rate variability [6], spectral turbulence [7], T-wave alternans [8,9], QT interval measurements and dispersion [10,11], brain natriuretic peptide [11,12], and late potentials measured by signal-averaged electrocardiogram (ECG) [13,14]. No such approach has yet proved to be highly reliable or gained broad acceptance.

Electrophysiology testing has been used with mixed results [15–21] (see Chapter 6). The test can predict outcome and define rhythm disturbances but not for all syncope patients at risk for sudden

Table 8.1 ACC/AHA guidelines for electrophysiology testing in syncope patients. (Adapted from [22].)

Class I (definitely indicated)
Patients with suspected structural heart disease and syncope that remains unexplained after appropriate evaluation

Class II (reasonable to do)
Patients with recurrent unexplained syncope without structural heart disease and a negative head-up tilt test

Class III (contraindicated)
Patients with a known cause of syncope for whom treatment will not be guided by electrophysiology testing

---

cardiac death. Most data apply to those patients who have coronary artery disease. The capability to stratify risk using electrophysiology testing remains unsettled. ACC/AHA guidelines provide some guidance for when an electrophysiology test is appropriate in a syncope patient but these guidelines are now almost 10 years old (Table 8.1 [22]).

One thing appears clear: the electrophysiology test results have little meaning in a vacuum. The results are patient-, symptom-, and disease-specific. Data from recent investigations suggest that electrophysiology testing may not be as effective to predict risk as initially suspected. Nevertheless, this approach has a clear role in the diagnosis of patients with syncope. For patients who have unexplained syncope and have structural heart disease (non-ischemic and ischemic cardiomyopathy), electrophysiology studies continue to have a role (see Chapter 6 and Table 8.1). However, the ideal method to detect long-term risk or recurrent syncope and sudden cardiac death remains obscure.

Is syncope an independent predictor of death?

This question has never been answered with any certainty. It is difficult to design a controlled clinical trial to demonstrate that syncope patients with similar heart conditions have the same or worse outcomes as those patients who do not have syncope. Syncope is not necessarily an independent prognostic indicator in the general population of patients with heart disease [23], in patients in in-

tensive care units [24], in the elderly, in hospitalized patients, in patients with Wolff–Parkinson–White syndrome, and even in patients with hypertrophic cardiomyopathy.

Future studies may indicate whether syncope acts as an independent predictor of death. Patients who have syncope and are matched to those without syncope but with similar underlying serious cardiovascular conditions have a similar outcome [25]. It appears that patients with syncope, structural heart disease, impaired LVEF, and with the same mix of coronary artery disease have as high a risk of sudden death over the next 2–3 years as patients who have already presented with ventricular tachycardia or ventricular fibrillation [26,27].

Patients with dilated cardiomyopathy and syncope may be an extremely high-risk group for sudden cardiac death as well as total mortality [28]. The mechanism for syncope in these patients may not be completely clear. It can be caused by hemodynamic collapse or other causes of syncope (as it may be in any patient who has underlying structural heart disease). Nevertheless, small, non-randomized, uncontrolled studies show benefit from ICD implantation in patients such as those with dilated cardiomyopathy and syncope of undetermined etiology.

Reducing chance of death in syncope patients at risk of sudden and cardiovascular death

Reduction in risk with standard medical therapy

Despite advances in medical therapy and declining death rates resulting from heart disease, sudden death from a cardiovascular cause continues to reign as the number one killer. Several standard drug therapies, when used properly, markedly improve survival from cardiovascular disease. These include beta-blockers, aspirin, angiotensin-converting enzyme inhibitors, anticoagulants (including warfarin and aspirin), and HMG-CoA reductase inhibitors ("statins"). Myocardial revascularization, when obstructive coronary artery disease is causing active ischemia, and valve replacement for aortic stenosis are some approaches shown to reduce risk in selected patients. These therapies, while effective, do not eliminate the risk for death completely.

The risk can remain high for those with underlying cardiovascular disease who have congestive heart failure or ventricular dysfunction.

Antiarrhythmic drugs

Attempts to reduce mortality in those at high risk have included empiric (untested use of) anti-arrhythmic drug therapy, serial-guided antiarrhythmic drug therapy, ventricular tachycardia ablation, and ICDs. Antiarrhythmic drugs, despite theoretical benefits, can worsen survival despite apparent arrhythmia suppression. Ablation can eliminate recurrent ventricular tachycardia but alone has not been shown to reduce the risk of cardiac mortality in patients at high risk of arrhythmic death.

Empiric antiarrhythmic drug therapy, including amiodarone, has failed to show consistent survival benefit [29,30]. Antiarrhythmic drugs have been tested as a primary means to prevent ventricular tachyarrhythmias and death. While they may suppress arrhythmias, little compelling evidence exists that any antiarrhythmic drug lowers the risk for death [31]. Antiarrhythmic drugs, used in the post-myocardial infarction period, and in association with congestive heart failure, provide no apparent benefit; often, harm occurred.

A serial-guided drug therapy approach using Holter monitoring or electrophysiology testing is similarly ineffective [32]. Drugs given based on markers that suggest success also have failed to prevent recurrent arrhythmias (at rates of over 50%) and prevent death. The benefit of antiarrhythmic drugs to prevent recurrent ventricular arrhythmias and also prevent death may only occur in patients with relatively preserved left ventricular ejection function (LVEF > 0.35, no right ventricular abnormalities, and no heart failure symptoms). These patients have a low risk of death from the start and therapy is aimed at reducing the arrhythmia burden to reduce symptoms.

Studies are still performed to assess the benefits of antiarrhythmic drug therapies in high-risk populations but no drug therapy has yet shown consistent and definite risk reduction. Randomized clinical trials with antiarrhythmic medications have failed to demonstrate clear benefit to reduce risk of sudden and all-cause death in any specific patient population.

When drugs are used, they are often stopped because of side-effects. For amiodarone, in regimens used to treat ventricular arrhythmias, the discontinuation rate often exceeds 40%. To treat ventricular arrhythmias, amiodarone is the only antiarrhythmic shown to be at least as safe as placebo in high-risk patients with structural heart disease but it has not been shown to be better than placebo at preventing death. While data conflict, there is ongoing concern about the use of antiarrhythmic drug therapy as the primary means to improve survival in high-risk patients. It appears, for the populations tested, that empiric use of almost any antiarrhythmic drug appears to be of little long-term survival benefit. Further, the "substrate" causing ventricular arrhythmias may change unexpectedly. While therapy may be effective initially, as the substrate changes drug therapy may no longer be beneficial.

For syncope patients with malignant ventricular arrhythmias, the best candidates to consider for antiarrhythmic drug therapy are those who are not candidates for ICD therapy. These include:

1 patients with an otherwise poor prognosis despite treatment of the underlying arrhythmia;

2 patients with intact ventricular function despite structural heart disease (as the prognosis is otherwise good);

3 patients with well-tolerated ventricular tachycardia; and

4 patients with idiopathic ventricular tachycardia.

Ablation of ventricular tachycardia

Radiofrequency catheter ablation has been used to treat ventricular tachycardia. While feasible in patients without structural heart disease, this approach is questionable in patients with structural heart disease for preventing all ventricular tachyarrhythmias and reducing the risk of sudden cardiac death. This approach is really meant to prevent well-tolerated ventricular tachycardia from becoming a clinical problem in these patients, not to prevent death. It may even prevent syncope.

No study shows a survival benefit with ablation of ventricular tachycardia. Patients who have recurrent ventricular tachycardia may benefit. Ablation performed during electrophysiology testing can modify the ventricular tachycardia recurrences that might lead to frequent ICD activation resulting from a specific ventricular tachycardia. No data show that ventricular tachycardia ablation can substitute for the benefits of ICD therapy.

Combination therapy

There is likely a role for combining ablation approaches and/or antiarrhythmic drugs with ICD therapy. The role of the ICD is to reduce the risk of death from a malignant ventricular arrhythmia and prevent symptoms (depending on how it is programmed). It is likely that the ICD may create new symptoms caused by the shocks to treat the arrhythmias and may not prevent the arrhythmia itself. The issue is that there is a distinction between prevention of syncope and prevention of death. The ICD is meant to prevent arrhythmic death but it may not prevent syncope.

Few data (no randomized trials) show that a specific antiarrhythmic therapy is better than no antiarrhythmic therapy in an ICD population. Clinical experience alone dictates that there are benefits when antiarrhythmic drugs are used together with an ICD. Fortunately, even if the patient has a proarrhythmic drug reaction, the ICD can provide back-up defibrillation. Frequently used antiarrhythmic drugs include sotalol and amiodarone. Amiodarone is used in patients with impaired ventricular function and congestive heart failure, a common condition in patients with ICDs. If the patient is stable enough, amiodarone can be started as an outpatient. Drugs may:

1 slow ventricular tachycardia below the programmed rate cut-off;
2 increase energy threshold to defibrillate;
3 have an effect on pace termination of ventricular tachycardia; and
4 be proarrhythmic.

If they are used in conjunction with an ICD, appropriate testing must be carried out.

Based on these possible interactions, it is best to use an antiarrhythmic drug only if necessary. The reason to use an antiarrhythmic drug is if there are frequent episodes of ventricular tachycardia or fibrillation requiring ICD activations. While antitachycardia pacing can generally be well tolerated by most patients, some patients have chest pain and dizziness and an antiarrhythmic drug or an ablation must be considered. For ICD shocks, the problem is almost always worse. Patients who have frequent shocks will require an antiarrhythmic drug.

ICDs

Evidence of benefit

The weight of evidence from observational studies, single-site trials, and multicenter, randomized, controlled trials of ICD therapy suggests that life-threatening ventricular tachyarrhythmias can be prevented from causing death when used in addition to the best medical therapy. Highly effective, the ICD simplifies management, can be cost-effective and shortens hospital stay, while improving patient longevity and quality of life (in many, but not all patients).

Most single-center studies show advantages of the ICD. The risk of sudden arrhythmic death with the ICD implant is generally less than 2% per year. Over time, the majority of patients receive therapy from the ICD. Proving benefit from ICD therapy has challenged the electrophysiology community for over 18 years. Now, a large body of clinical experience and experimental evidence supports these initial reports [2–5]. Several hundred thousand patients have had ICDs implanted. The risk of sudden death remains consistently low in almost all high-risk patients. The skeptics point to the continued risk for total mortality in the studies evaluating patients with ICDs. There are several studies that demonstrate benefits of ICDs in syncope patients [33].

Large, multicenter, clinical trials were designed to determine the survival benefit of the ICD [2]. Now, with good controlled data, the benefits of the ICD are undisputed. Based on these results, guidelines have been created to address which patients benefit most from the ICD [34]. Also not to be underestimated is the now growing acceptance of ICD use by the medical community and the public. There are no large multicenter trials that have addressed the benefits of an ICD specifically in syncope patients.

Technological advances

The ICD has advanced from its early development in the 1970s. The first human ICD implant was in 1980 and the device was FDA approved in 1985. The first programmable ICD was developed in 1988. The first biphasic defibrillation waveform ICD with tiered-therapy device was FDA approved in 1993. A pectoral unipolar lead system was approved in 1995. The first dual-chamber ICD implants were performed in 1997.

The original "AID" (automatic implantable defibrillator) had no cardioversion potential (it could only sense ventricular fibrillation), weighed 250 g and had an 18-month longevity. The AID and other early devices were not programmable and could only deliver a shock. Implantation required general anesthesia. A surgeon was required to perform a sternotomy or thoracotomy. Patches and screw-in sensing leads were placed directly on the heart. The ICD delivered an inefficient waveform shock so that two or three epicardial defibrillation patches were required to ensure adequate defibrillation capabilities (adequate defibrillation thresholds). The devices were placed in the abdomen. Recovery required 5–8 days in hospital. Mortality from the implant itself was 3–4%. The early ICDs were "committed," so that once a rapid rhythm was detected, the ICD would charge and discharge the shock into the patient. It was difficult to assess lead or patch problems and determine the integrity of the ICD system. Despite these and other limitations, the older devices were still shown to be lifesaving. If the patient received a shock, however, there was no way to establish exactly what caused it.

ICDs have become highly advanced technologically. The device has progressed from a bulky, epicardial patch/lead system with an abdominal implant to a sleek, single-chamber, right ventricular "shock box." More recent ICDs have the capability to act as a dual-chamber (DDDR) pacemaker/ICD combination. Now there are AV ICDs that are capable of stopping atrial and ventricular arrhythmias, and biventricular ICDs that can pace the atria and the left and right ventricles as well as stop ventricular arrhythmias. ICDs have the capability of providing effective back-up bradycardia pacing as well as preventing death from ventricular tachycardia and ventricular fibrillation. No specific algorithms have yet been developed to prevent initiation of ventricular tachycardia and ventricular fibrillation (they are on the way), but antiarrhythmic drug therapy and/or ventricular tachycardia ablation used in conjunction with ICD implantation may reduce initiation of ventricular tachycardia and reduce the risk of death from episodes should they occur.

ICDs are capable of performing atrial and ventricular defibrillation, atrial and ventricular pacing, and sensing and biventricular pacing. They can terminate rhythms with low and high energy shocks and can attempt to pace terminate ventricular tachycardia (a potential advantage in the syncope patient). Detection capabilities are enhanced so that modern ICDs can better distinguish nonsustained and sustained arrhythmias. They are more capable of aborting inappropriate or unnecessary activations from atrial arrhythmias and they are not committed to shock for a non-sustained arrhythmia.

There are different tachycardia zones in modern ICDs so that different therapies can be delivered depending on the rhythm. The sensing capabilities have become more sophisticated to detect ventricular arrhythmias with a high degree of sensitivity but not at the expense of specificity.

The ICD is now smaller (< 50 ml and 70 g), is easier to implant, and has longer lasting batteries and capacitors (> 7 years). Device memory capabilities allow for more intense monitoring and detection of sustained and non-sustained tachycardias and amount of ventricular and atrial pacing. They allow for rate-responsive pacing. Present devices have the capability of storing electrogram documentation of episodes of tachycardia and delivered or aborted therapy. Many can also record the template for the normal conducted beat to distinguish it from a ventricular tachycardia beat. The devices can sense and pace in both the atria and ventricles.

The waveform for defibrillation is more efficient, enhanced by the advent of biphasic shocks. The ICD "can" is, typically, "active," helping to minimize the amount of implanted hardware. The lead has the other pole(s). This and the changes in the waveform have allowed the ICD implant to be placed in the upper chest and the ease of implantation is similar to that of a pacemaker.

Several therapy "zones" can be programmed to deliver defibrillation shocks and/or antitachycardia pacing by a multiprogrammable approach. Detection algorithms are more sophisticated to help differentiate supraventricular from ventricular tachycardia. Newer devices can monitor lead impedance and even determine the rhythm disturbance that preceded the ventricular arrhythmia leading to device activation. The devices are now implanted by electrophysiologists using a non-thoracotomy approach, often in < 1 h, using local anesthesia and conscious sedation. Patients now have shorter hospital stays (< 24 h), lower implant mortality (0.5–0.8%), and better quality of life.

ICD indications – the list is growing

Initially, ICDs were used to prevent sudden cardiac death in patients who had already experienced a cardiac arrest (or two) from malignant ventricular arrhythmias that required resuscitation and were not the result of a correctable cause. This population was already identified to be at risk for recurrent episodes of cardiac arrest. It made sense to consider an ICD implant in this population of patients. The multicenter, NIH sponsored, AVID trial demonstrated definitively that patients who had poorly tolerated ventricular tachycardia or ventricular fibrillation benefited more from an ICD than from any specific antiarrhythmic drug therapy (in addition to properly prescribed medications for the underlying cardiac condition) [2].

Subsequent multicenter, prospective, large, randomized, clinical trial data identified other patients who may benefit from an ICD even after the patient is placed on the proper and best medical therapy. These were patients at risk for, but who had not yet had a cardiac arrest. The prophylactic use of ICDs extended to patients who had:

1 LVEF ≤ 0.35, asymptomatic non-sustained ventricular tachycardia, chronic coronary artery disease, and an electrophysiology study positive for inducible sustained, monomorphic, ventricular tachycardia (MADIT).

2 LVEF ≤ 0.30, status postmyocardial infarction, and New York Heart Association (NYHA) Functional Class I–III congestive heart failure compared with best medical therapy alone (MADIT II [3]).

3 LVEF ≤ 0.35, frequent ventricular ectopy, no NYHA Functional Class IV congestive heart failure, ventricular ectopy, dilated non-ischemic cardiomyopathy compared with best medical therapy alone (DEFINITE [5]).

4 LVEF ≤ 0.35, NYHA Functional Class II and III congestive heart failure (and no other specific disease features) compared with amiodarone and placebo in addition to best medical therapy [31].

5 LVEF # 0.30, NYHA Functional Class II–IV heart failure and a wide QRS complex for a biventricular ICD (COMPANION [4]).

Details of inclusion and exclusion criteria can be found elsewhere.

It is likely that other high-risk groups will be identified who may benefit from an ICD. The patients in the above groups benefited from simple, single-chamber ICDs without additional features. Recent advances, however, have led to the development of ICDs that are capable of more than simply shocking ventricular tachycardia or ventricular fibrillation. New devices have the capability of atrial and ventricular sensing and pacing, better algorithms to distinguish supraventricular from ventricular tachycardia, advanced algorithms for pace termination of ventricular tachycardia and, importantly, biventricular pacing.

With biventricular pacing algorithms present in select ICD devices, there is also the possibility of improving quality of life, cardiac output, New York Heart Association Functional Class, and reducing sequelae of congestive heart failure in properly selected patients, including those who have New York Heart Association Functional Class III and IV congestive heart failure and a wide QRS complex (> 0.12 s) [4].

There are other selected high-risk patients for whom no randomized controlled clinical trial has demonstrated benefit of an ICD implant but the preponderance of data indicate that they may benefit from an ICD. These include patients with the long QT interval syndrome, hypertrophic cardiomyopathy, and Brugada syndrome.

It is also important to realize that not all "high-risk" patients who appear to be good candidates benefit from ICD implant. Randomized trials that show no benefit from an ICD include:

1 status postcoronary artery bypass graft surgery who have LVEF < 0.36 and a positive signal-averaged ECG (CABG-PATCH trial [35,36]); and

2 patients with large myocardial infarction early in the throes of the myocardial infarction (DINAMIT [37]).

Circumspect clinical assessment is needed prior to considering an ICD in any patient. To date, no study involving ICDs has looked specifically at a population of syncope patients.

Guidelines for ICD implantation

In 1991, indications for ICD implantation were developed by the North American Society of Pacing and Electrophysiology (NASPE) and separately by an American College of Cardiology and American Heart Association (ACC/AHA) task force. Based on the available data in 1991, the ACC/AHA concurred with the NASPE guidelines in most respects. Based on recent trials and further experience with the ICD, these guidelines for ICD implantation were revised in 1998. In 2002, the guidelines were again revised as new evidence become available [34]. Guidelines specifically relevant to syncope, with additional comments, are listed in Table 8.2 [34]. Revisions from prior 1998 guidelines are listed in Table 8.3 [34].

When to consider an ICD in a syncope patient

The decision to implant an ICD in a patient with syncope is based in part on an accurate diagnosis and identification of risk for preventable arrhythmic death (Table 8.4). This is based on an amalgamation of clinical evidence and on a high level of suspicion. The proper identification of the patient who ultimately may benefit from an ICD is open to scrutiny and divisive opinions. If a life-threatening arrhythmia is a potential cause for syncope, an electrophysiologist may be able to provide an informed decision concerning the risks and benefits of ICD implant. Alternatively, an electrophysiologist may not have expertise with other specific clinical syndromes and may not have any more data upon which to base an option. The decision may need to be shared by all treating physicians and incorporate the wishes and decisions of the patient and his or her family.

Projected patient longevity, patient functionality, the relative risk of a cardiac arrest, the risk of recurrent syncope, and the relationship of the risk of cardiac arrest to syncope must all be considered. The stakes are high for the patient as the ICD implant carries risks: it can influence employment, participation in activities (including competitive sports), and alter quality of life. However, a single episode of untreated, sustained, ventricular tachycardia may be deadly.

Which syncope patient may benefit from an ICD?

The first step in the patient with syncope is careful assessment: what is causing the symptoms? The evaluation of the patient with syncope is well described in other chapters. Based on a carefully scrutinized history and well-performed physical examination (including a carotid sinus massage in selected patients), it is possible to identify the cause for syncope in many patients. It is also possible in some patients to identify risks for life-threatening arrhythmias and conditions that may benefit from an ICD.

If there is evidence for congestive heart failure based on history or found on physical examination, or if there is evidence for an impaired left ventricular ejection fraction, the patient may be at high risk for cardiac arrest and should be considered for an ICD implant. If the patient has a strong family history of sudden death at an early age (even if the patient is young), or if the patient has evidence for a long QT interval [38], or the Brugada syndrome, he or she may derive benefit from an ICD implant. If the patient has hypertrophic cardiomyopathy [39], infiltrative cardiomyopathy (such as hemachromatosis or sarcoidosis [40]), valvular cardiomyopathy, or evidence for right ventricular dilation (resulting from arrhythmogenic right ventricular dysplasia), the patient may be at risk. Unfortunately, many situations are not straightforward.

Some conditions can be identified, if not already diagnosed, by performing an ECG and an echocardiogram. An ECG is routine for every syncope patient. If the syncope patient shows evidence for a myocardial infarction, a bundle branch block, a distinctly abnormal ECG, or a strong family history of sudden death the level of concern for arrhythmic death should rise.

An echocardiogram should be obtained if there are data suspicious for a cardiac cause of syncope, if there is an abnormal ECG, if there is evidence for cardiovascular abnormalities on the physical examination, or if the patient has risk factors for sudden death. Other testing, such as external and internal (implanted) loop monitoring and use of electrophysiology testing should be based on specific clinical features derived from the history (see Chapters 6 and 19). In some situations, such monitoring is superseded by an ICD implant if the risk of death is too high.

Non-invasive sudden death predictors, including signal-averaged ECG, T-wave alternans, QT dispersion, heart rate variability, and spectral turbulence, have little independent prognostic value alone in the syncope patient but each test may add supportive evidence that a patient is at risk. These

Table 8.2 Current ACC/AHA recommendations for ICD therapy [34]. Patients with syncope.

Class I

Syncope of undetermined origin with clinically relevant, hemodynamically significant, sustained VT or VF induced at electrophysiological study when drug therapy is ineffective, not tolerated, or not preferred (*Level of evidence: B*)

Comment: It is not clear that induction of VF in a syncope patient has clinical relevance in most circumstances. Drug therapy is not as effective as an ICD in patients with poorly tolerated, inducible, sustained VT. An ICD should be considered

Class IIb

Severe symptoms (e.g., syncope) attributable to ventricular tachyarrhythmias in patients awaiting cardiac transplantation (*Level of evidence: C*)

Comment: Depends on how long it will be until transplantation and where the patient will wait for the transplant

Familial or inherited conditions with a high risk for life-threatening ventricular tachyarrhythmias such as long QT syndrome or hypertrophic cardiomyopathy (*Level of evidence: B*)

Comment: These conditions usually come to light with symptoms such as syncope. An ICD is reasonable for these individuals but the weight of the evidence does not place these patients in a Class I category for an ICD

Recurrent syncope of undetermined origin in the presence of ventricular dysfunction and inducible ventricular arrhythmias at electrophysiologic study when other causes of syncope have been excluded (*Level of evidence: C*)

Comment: This seems very similar to the Class I indication except perhaps even a higher risk group. I would favor an ICD in these patients

Syncope of unexplained origin or family history of unexplained sudden cardiac death in association with typical or atypical right bundle branch block and ST-segment elevations (Brugada syndrome) (*Level of evidence: C*)

Comment: A rare cause of syncope

Syncope in patients with advanced structural heart disease in whom thorough invasive and non-invasive investigations have failed to define a cause (*Level of evidence: C*)

Comment: This includes patients with dilated cardiomyopathy who have a negative electrophysiology test

Class III

Syncope of undetermined cause in a patient without inducible ventricular tachyarrhythmias and without structural heart disease (*Level of evidence: C*)

Comment: This is very reasonable but an electrophysiology study may not even need to be performed in these patients

DEFINITIONS

Level of recommendation

The final recommendations for indications for device therapy are expressed in the standard ACC/AHA format as follows:

Class I Conditions for which there is evidence and/or general agreement that a given procedure or treatment is beneficial, useful, and effective

Class II Conditions for which there is conflicting evidence and/or a divergence of opinion about the usefulness/efficacy of a procedure or treatment

Class IIa Weight of evidence/opinion is in favor of usefulness/efficacy

Class IIb Usefulness/efficacy is less well established by evidence/opinion

Class III Conditions for which there is evidence and/or general agreement that a procedure/treatment is not useful/effective and in some cases may be harmful

Strength of evidence

A Data derived from multiple, randomized, clinical trials involving a large number of individuals

B Data derived from a limited number of trials involving a comparatively small number of patients or from well-designed data analyses of non-randomized studies or observational data registries

C Consensus opinion of experts

ICD, implanted cardioverter defibrillator; VF, ventricular fibrillation; VT, ventricular tachycardia.

Table 8.3 ACC/AHA guidelines changes: 1998–2002 [34]. ICDs in patients with syncope.

1998 Recommendations	2002 Recommendations
Class IIb	*Class IIb*
Severe symptoms attributable to sustained ventricular tachyarrhythmias while awaiting cardiac transplantation (*Level of evidence:* C)	Severe symptoms (e.g., syncope) attributable to ventricular tachyarrhythmias in patients awaiting cardiac transplantation (*Level of evidence:* C)
	Syncope of unexplained etiology or family history of unexplained sudden cardiac death in association with typical or atypical right bundle branch block and ST-segment elevations (Brugada syndrome) (*Level of evidence:* C)
	Syncope in patients with advanced structural heart disease in which thorough invasive and non-invasive investigation has failed to define a cause (*Level of evidence:* C)
Class III	*Class III*
Syncope of undetermined cause in a patient without inducible ventricular tachyarrhythmias (*Level of evidence:* C)	Syncope of undetermined cause in a patient without inducible ventricular tachyarrhythmias and without structural heart disease (*Level of evidence:* C)

Table 8.4 When an ICD should be considered in a patient with syncope.

1 The identifiable risk of sudden arrhythmic death is sufficiently high, no other treatment is proven effective, the risk of death from other causes is low, and the patient is aware of restrictions from an ICD

2 Unexplained syncope is present or syncope results from a non-arrhythmic cause and the patient has a separate approved indication for an ICD, or in a patient with structural heart disease and inducible monomorphic ventricular tachycardia at electrophysiology testing

3 Patients with structural heart disease and documented symptomatic ventricular tachycardia

non-invasive approaches fall in and out of favor and none has stood the test of time but T-wave alternans has shown promise regarding its predictive accuracy in determining risk of sudden cardiac death in patients with left ventricular dysfunction with or without coronary artery disease.

Electrophysiologic testing

The electrophysiology test has a role as a risk stratifier (Table 8.1) but not all patients at high risk will benefit [18]. The electrophysiology test has remained a standard modality to identify patients at risk for cardiac arrest. Those who have a positive electrophysiology study and syncope have poorer outcomes with an ICD [41] and a high likelihood of appropriate ICD discharge if the device is implanted [42]. The electrophysiology study remains a well-accepted risk stratifier, but recent data indicate that electrophysiologic testing can be non-specific and insensitive. Results depend on the patient population being studied.

Electrophysiological testing may now be used less often for patients with syncope because they may be candidates for an ICD even if the cause for their syncope is not known. These high-risk patients can be identified simply by knowing the LVEF and New York Heart Association Functional Class. The information gleaned from an electrophysiology test is often valuable and the test should be considered even if an ICD implant is planned in patients with ischemic or non-ischemic cardiomyopathy (the largest number of patients with malignant arrhythmias as cause for syncope).

Patients who have relatively normal left ventricular function who are at risk for sudden cardiac death include those with various, relatively unusual, but important clinical conditions including arrhythmogenic right ventricular dysplasia, hypertrophic cardiomyopathy, Brugada syndrome, catecholaminergic ventricular tachycardia, sarcoidosis (and other infiltrative conditions), and other conditions (e.g., Kearns–Sayre syndrome [43,44]).

The value of the electrophysiology test in these conditions has been questioned but some useful information can be obtained.

An electrophysiology test can be of use for patients with idiopathic ventricular tachycardia who have syncope caused by this [45,46]. For such patients, the electrophysiology test can be used to ablate and cure the ventricular tachycardia and thus prevent syncope. Such a patient would not need an ICD.

Ablation can also be used to prevent recurrent ventricular tachycardias in patients with structural heart disease who already have an ICD but are continuing to have recurrent ICD activations (shocks or antitachycardia pacing). Ablation can reduce the risk of ICD shocks and syncope in patients with structural heart disease and monomorphic ventricular tachycardia. These patients still require an ICD. In such patients, the use of a random or routine electrophysiology test would have little utility and even less if the patient had definite evidence for a ventricular tachycardia identified by some means.

It is important to realize that even if an arrhythmia is present and documented but it appears to be a wide QRS complex tachycardia, it may still be worthwhile to perform an electrophysiology test as the arrhythmia may be a supraventricular tachycardia with aberration. An ICD may be inappropriate for such a patient; it may not treat the arrhythmia properly. An ablation of the supraventricular tachycardia may correct the entire problem.

The predictive accuracy of an electrophysiology test is greatest in patients with coronary artery disease and impaired left ventricular function. That said, the test may be positive in other conditions (such as dilated cardiomyopathy or in patients with mildly impaired left ventricular function) as it still predicts the need for an ICD. We advocate the use of electrophysiologic testing in any patient with syncope who has underlying structural heart disease and therefore may be at risk for a cardiac arrest as long as the cause for syncope is not otherwise known by the history and physical examination.

According to ACC/AHA/NASPE guidelines [34], an ICD is indicated for patients with syncope who have an electrophysiology study that is positive for ventricular tachyarrhythmia, when drug therapy is ineffective, not tolerated, or not preferred (Table 8.2). An ICD should not be implanted in a patient with syncope, ventricular tachycardia, and no structural heart disease (idiopathic ventricular tachycardia is not an indication for an ICD). Based on the 2002 guidelines, an ICD is not indicated in patients with syncope of undetermined origin when there is no inducible tachyarrhythmia and no structural heart disease. ACC/AHA/NASPE guidelines now address syncope in association with the Brugada syndrome, syncope in patients with advanced structural heart disease for whom thorough invasive and non-invasive testing has failed to define a cause, and syncope that is attributable to ventricular tachyarrhythmias in patients awaiting cardiac transplantation.

Syncope of undetermined origin

Even after complete evaluation with appropriate diagnostic testing, including electrophysiology study, it may not be possible to determine the cause for syncope. After appropriate testing is complete, a substantial number of patients with syncope will not have a diagnosis secured and the cause for syncope remains undefined.

Large, long-term, follow-up epidemiologic studies suggest that when appropriate diagnostic approaches are taken in patients with syncope, the chance for sudden cardiac death is relatively low. Nevertheless, there are specific populations, including patients who have a strong family history for sudden cardiac death, who should be considered for an ICD, including patients with dilated non-ischemic cardiomyopathy. There may be a need to consider an ICD as these patients may be at risk for sudden cardiac death.

What to do before the ICD implant

One concern with data that support the prophylactic use of ICDs is that there is a tendency to become lax regarding complete evaluation of the patient. Patients at risk for sudden cardiac death who may require an ICD but who also pass out do not necessarily pass out as a result of a malignant ventricular arrhythmia or even asystole, even if there is evidence for risk. All patients require complete and thoughtful evaluation. They should be given an explanation of the benefits of the therapy given.

Consider a patient with critical aortic stenosis and left ventricular dysfunction. An ICD would not necessarily be full or correct therapy for this patient. It is also possible that the patient may have severe coronary artery disease, left ventricular dysfunction, and neurocardiogenic syncope as the cause for the problem. An ICD will not help this patient, although he or she may benefit from reduction in risk of sudden cardiac death.

The goal of therapy in the patient with syncope who is at risk for sudden cardiac death becomes twofold:
1 to reduce the risk of sudden cardiac death and total death using an ICD; and
2 to reduce symptoms, which may include congestive heart failure and syncope.
Present ICD therapies cannot eliminate episodes of recurrent ventricular tachycardia but they can abort the episodes to prevent cardiac arrest. Nevertheless, it is still possible for a patient to pass out. It is important to recognize this possibility and to treat the underlying conditions that may be responsible. Tilt table testing, electrophysiology testing, and other appropriate evaluation may provide evidence for another cause for syncope. It also may provide another cause for elevation in risk such as a valvular problem in need of repair.

Specific subgroups

Dilated cardiomyopathy
Patients with dilated cardiomyopathy may not benefit as much from ICDs as those patients who have ischemic cardiomyopathy [34]; those who have dilated cardiomyopathy and syncope tend to have a very poor prognosis [28,47]. Small, retrospective, non-randomized, uncontrolled studies have shown that ICD implantation in patients with dilated cardiomyopathy and syncope may be appropriate and, recently, a large multicenter trial has shown the benefit of an ICD in patients with dilated cardiomyopathy, impaired ventricular function and ventricular ectopy regardless of if syncope is present [5]. Patients with dilated cardiomyopathy and syncope are at higher risk of sudden cardiac death than patients with dilated cardiomyopathy and no syncope. Electrophysiology testing may be a poor predictor of future events. Now, with evidence that patients with dilated cardiomyopathy may benefit from an ICD regardless of the syncope history, the decision to implant an ICD may become easier, even without carefully controlled clinical trials. The more difficult group

includes those patients with syncope who are otherwise asymptomatic (i.e., Functional Class I with respect to heart failure).

There is controversy about whether a patient with dilated cardiomyopathy who has syncope but whose electrophysiology study results are negative requires an ICD. A small study compared 14 patients who had syncope, dilated cardiomyopathy, and negative electrophysiology study results with 19 patients who survived cardiac arrest. Appropriate shocks were similar in both groups [48]. Retrospective evaluation suggests that high-risk cardiomyopathy patients with syncope who had an ICD implanted survived longer than those who did not.

Patients with dilated cardiomyopathy, a negative electrophysiology test, and syncope that cannot be explained by any other mechanism should be considered for an ICD implant [49]. This recommendation is now part of the ACC/AHA/NASPE guidelines [34] (Table 8.2).

Arrhythmogenic right ventricular dysplasia (cardiomyopathy)
No single test can diagnose this condition with certainty and there are gradations of its severity. It may be caused by "apoptosis" and thus be progressive. Arrhythmogenic right ventricular dysplasia is the most common cause of death in athletes in the Veneto region of Italy and it is also a cause of death in athletes in the USA and other countries [50]. The diagnosis is complex but requires echocardiographic evidence, magnetic resonance imaging (MRI) evidence, or angiographic evidence of right ventricular dilation and dysfunction. It is not clear that any drug or ablative therapy will prevent the risk of death in a patient with this condition who has syncope.

If diagnosed with certainty, if syncope is not otherwise explained, or even if another cause is suspected but not proven, an ICD should be implanted, because the risk of arrhythmic death is high [51]. Athletic restriction is mandated. Fibrofatty deposits infiltrating the right ventricle may make ICD implantation more difficult and risky. Ventricular perforation and decreased sensing capabilities are possible.

Congenital long QT interval syndrome
This syndrome represents a complex mix of several congenital abnormalities in cardiac sodium or

potassium ion channels. Patients with this condition can have a cardiac arrest from ventricular fibrillation or develop syncope from torsade de pointes. Syncope, "seizures," and cardiac arrest are common clinical presentations. Congenital long QT interval syndrome may be associated with syncope brought about by other causes including neurocardiogenic syncope.

The diagnosis is generally made by ECG, but some patients with an atypical form of the congenital syndrome have reversible long QT interval abnormalities caused by medications or electrolyte disturbances. The condition is sometimes obvious on the ECG and there is a strong family history of sudden death. Unfortunately, some patients have an equivocal ECG and a confusing family history. This makes caring for these patients difficult, especially for the younger patient who may not understand the risks and benefits of an ICD.

It is a challenge to decide which patients with the syndrome will benefit from an ICD. Significant lifelong risks, expense, discomfort, shocks, disability, and restrictions may ensue from the implantation. If unexplained syncope is present and there is evidence for a long QT interval syndrome on the ECG (> 0.450 and definitely if the QT_C exceeds 0.500), despite beta-blockade or other medical treatments and if there is a family history of early sudden death, an ICD should be strongly considered.

Beta-blockade is the first-line approach but some patients may not improve with beta-blocker therapy. Class I antiarrhythmic drugs may benefit those with the long QT III syndrome and beta-blocker may be harmful in this group. Gene-specific therapies are not yet available.

Because of their efficacy, ICDs are being used more frequently. No study has yet shown substantial benefit of an ICD over other therapies. There are no randomized trials to indicate that an ICD is required. There are only a few data indicating that those patients who have an ICD implanted may have a better prognosis than those who do not. This population is usually young and usually has no other cause for death. Unfortunately, the natural history of these conditions is unknown. It is assumed that an ICD will alter the course of the condition and have life-saving benefit but it is not clear that the ICD will be a life-saving therapy for this problem and other congenital syndromes. While the risks of sudden death may be low, they are greater than for the population at large for that age group.

Another difficult population is those who demonstrate lengthening in the QT interval with drug therapy. It is likely that these patients have defects in the potassium channel and may be at risk. If they are, the risk appears to be lower and does not mandate consideration of an ICD. There are many patients who have a slightly prolonged QT interval but may have other causes for syncope. Patients with the congenital long QT interval syndrome also have a tendency to have a positive tilt table test. The reason for this relationship is unclear.

Hypertrophic cardiomyopathy

Several mechanisms can explain syncope in patients with hypertrophic cardiomyopathy, including malignant ventricular arrhythmias, supraventricular arrhythmias, left ventricular outflow tract obstruction, diastolic dysfunction, and neurocardiogenic responses. Patients with unexplained syncope, a family history of sudden death, frequent ventricular ectopy (especially non-sustained ventricular tachycardia) or marked septal thickness > 30 mm should have an ICD implanted. Patients with hypertrophic cardiomyopathy who have an ICD implanted for either primary or secondary prevention have a high rate of appropriate ICD discharges [52]. It remains unclear which patients benefit from having an ICD. Two issues must be considered: how much risk is acceptable, and is the syncope caused by an arrhythmia? The latter issue may be difficult, if not impossible, to determine.

Brugada syndrome

The Brugada syndrome is a recently recognized syndrome consisting of right bundle branch block with ST elevation in the right precordial leads (V_1–V_3) with a normal QT interval that occurs in the absence of structural heart disease [53]. Brugada syndrome can induce sudden death by causing polymorphic ventricular tachycardia. Because there is no known treatment to reduce the risk, an ICD should be implanted when this syndrome is diagnosed, especially if it is accompanied by unexplained syncope.

The ECG findings that characterize the Brugada syndrome were initially thought to be highly predictive of arrhythmic death; however, recent information suggests that the phenotype may be more common than previously recognized and associated with a much lower mortality risk. There are various manifestations of the problem [54]. ST elevation may only become apparent if the patient is given a Class I antiarrhythmic drug challenge (not quinidine). There appears to be a gradation in risk that is not completely understood but, if there is clear-cut evidence of Brugada syndrome on the baseline ECG and the patient has had syncope, an ICD should be considered.

Other ICD indications

An ICD should be considered for patients with unexplained syncope who have valvular heart disease associated with impaired ventricular function, but not mitral valve prolapse or critical aortic stenosis, and not when an obstructive lesion caused the collapse; congenital heart disease of various types (but there are risks) [55]; idiopathic bidirectional ventricular tachycardia; exertional (catecholaminergic) polymorphic ventricular tachycardia, despite the best medical therapy. The reason to implant an ICD is to prevent death but much is unknown about the prognosis of these patients. To better define the arrhythmia issues, and despite the lack of sensitivity of the test, we recommend that an electrophysiology test be performed, in some cases with catecholamine stimulation to improve understanding of the mechanism of the problem. Empiric use of an ICD in a patient with congenital heart disease and syncope, for example, is not encouraged.

Patients needing pacemakers

Before pacemaker implantation for a symptomatic bradyarrhythmia – a bradyarrhythmia that caused syncope – it is worth considering performing a test that evaluates LVEF. If there is left ventricular dysfunction, the patient may be at risk for a cardiac arrest and death, even if syncope was caused by a bradyarrhythmia. In such a case, instead of a pacemaker the patient may benefit from an ICD.

Recurrent syncope with an ICD

Despite the best intent to treat a patient with syncope at risk for sudden cardiac death, syncope may recur. This is one reason to restrict from driving those patients who have syncope and who receive an ICD. There may be several reasons for syncope recurrence:

1 Syncope was caused by another problem and was not a result of an arrhythmia.
2 The device was improperly set so that the arrhythmia was not properly detected.
3 The arrhythmia was properly detected and treated but the patient passed out anyway.
4 The arrhythmia was properly detected but it was non-sustained and caused syncope anyway.
5 There was malfunction of the device.

If a patient who has an ICD passed out, the device must be interrogated to attempt to see if an arrhythmia was detected. If not, an arrhythmia still could have been present.

Disadvantages of ICDs

There are several important potential disadvantages to an ICD that must be considered carefully before an implant is undertaken in any patient for syncope:

1 The ICD requires a lifelong commitment to therapy.
2 This therapy may cause painful ICD shocks that do not necessarily prevent syncope or death and may impair quality of life.
3 The patient with syncope who requires an ICD may have long-standing restrictions with respect to work and driving. These restrictions may extend indefinitely and can have a devastating impact on quality of life.
4 Not all therapies delivered by the ICD are required. Inappropriate activations may have deleterious effects psychologically and may initiate rhythm disturbances (i.e., be proarrhythmic).
5 The ICD will not prevent all causes of death, even cardiac death.
6 There is a substantial cost associated with the ICD implant.
7 The ICD may not provide any benefit for the patient, especially if the cause for syncope is unrelated to an arrhythmia as suspected. This could be extremely devastating to any patient but particularly a younger individual.
8 There can be complications with the implant (pneumothorax, infection, bleeding) and in the long term (lead fracture, sensing and pacing problems).
9 The implant may adversely affect quality of life.

By no means is an ICD a panacea. Those who can benefit, though, represent a heterogeneous group. Well-controlled data that support the need for an

ICD in many syncope patients are difficult to find. Caring for the high-risk syncope patient is a growing challenge.

Cost effectiveness

Despite enthusiasm for ICD therapy, with limited health care resources available, the cost of ICD implantation is a major concern. The costs include, but are not limited to, the device, lead, surgery and initial hospitalization, rehospitalizations(s), and follow-up. The total costs of ICD implantations could have a major financial impact on Medicare, managed care institutions, and health insurance companies. Although the ICD is a very effective therapy, is the ICD cost-effective?

Antiarrhythmic drugs have not been shown to be cost effective. In the ESVEM trial [56], the cost effectiveness of antiarrhythmic drugs used was over $162,000 per life year saved. The only worse alternative would be to deny any therapy and allow an unnecessary death. While this approach may save resources, it is clearly unacceptable.

There can be a dramatic reduction in hospital stays and costs after implants, with a 4.6-fold reduction in cost after implant and a 10-fold difference in hospital stay [57]. Valenti *et al.* [57] assessed hospitalization costs and stays before and after ICD implantation. Hospitalizations after ICD implant decreased from 3.28 ± 2.38 to 0.88 ± 1.23 hospitalizations per patient per year ($P < 0.05$). Cardiac hospitalizations decreased by 90%. Hospital days also decreased. For this reason, the total costs of an ICD may become less than medical therapy over time (at < 1.5 years).

In the AVID trial [2], the cost per life year saved was more than $114,917 by some estimates (see [58]). The reason for this extraordinarily high cost is not completely understood but, in part, may be because of the short-term follow-up and the short 2.9-month survival advantage for the ICD group despite a 37% reduction in mortality. The cost for the index hospitalization was $66,629 for the ICD group and $34,059 for the antiarrhythmic drug therapy group. Recurrent hospitalization charges were $9104 for the ICD group and $11,594 for the antiarrhythmic drug therapy group. Assuming the use of today's practices, the cost effectiveness would be $28,148 per life year saved. Also assuming upfront costs of $45,000 (similar to most up-front costs for ICD implant in most hospitals) rather than $66,629, the cost effectiveness results would be

$5948 per life year saved. The cost effectiveness ratio for AVID has also been calculated to be $66,677 per year of life saved versus antiarrhythmic therapy (95% CI, $30,761 to $154,768) and this number remains stable at 6 and 20 years [59].

The pressure to reduce costs has been particularly intense for high-technology interventions such as ICDs. Many US centers have now begun to use lower cost practices for ICD implantation. These include elimination of a preimplant electrophysiology study, use of local anesthesia and/or conscious sedation, implantation of a single chamber device, a shift in procedure site from the operating room to the electrophysiology laboratory or a procedure room, and reduced length of stay postimplant. Market pressures in the USA are forcing physicians and hospitals to continually update their practice patterns to provide higher quality, lower cost care.

There are clearly major differences in the calculations for the cost per life year saved for ICD therapy, leading to bewildering results. The accuracy of the data remains in question with respect to recent approaches to ICD implantation. Differences in the costs between analyses may be related to the type of patients enrolled in the trials, but other factors must be considered including lack of accuracy of the cost analysis data, differences in mortality of the patients in the trials, difference in the benefit of the ICD, techniques to implant ICDs, longevity of ICD implant, and capabilities of the ICD to offset further problems, including readmission and need for follow-up.

It appears that the ICD can now be more cost effective by using modern, simpler implantation techniques, shorter hospitalizations, and improved, longer lasting devices requiring less follow-up, even in the highest risk patients who stand to derive a mortality benefit of 20–40%. Nevertheless, recent cost effective analyses suggest that the cost per life year saved is still expensive [58,60].

It is not clear that any other therapies are less expensive or nearly as effective. With further streamlining of the implant approach and long-term follow-up, the costs should continue to come down even further. Alternatively, the use of biventricular ICDs may drive the costs up again. Much of medical practice is not dictated by reimbursement rather than what is necessarily best for the patients. It is to be hoped that the two will come into better alignment over time.

Practical concerns in syncope patients

All therapies must be evaluated based on their effects on increasing longevity, but other variables must also be considered: risk, quality of life, and cost. Many therapies tie a patient even more closely to the medical profession and take away some degree of autonomy. The goal to prevent syncope and cardiac death is attainable but, more importantly, the ultimate goal to extend meaningful life is quite complex.

Unfortunately, many patients do not fit exactly into the categories defined by the results of the clinical trials. Often extrapolations of data to specific patients can be lacking about the long-term beneficial results. Recently, enthusiasm of ICD use has spread to patients, often with complex medical problems, for which the ICD may not extend their lives and may simply impair the quality of the remainder of their lives. Patients who have multisystem disease (renal failure, ongoing ischemia, or steroid use) may have problems that complicate the use of the ICD and increase the risk of device implantation.

With the recent wave of enthusiasm for ICD implants, temperance and prudent judgment must be employed. It is conceivable that an elderly man who comes into the ER having tripped on a rug at home (not passing out) may find a physician who wants to top off the visit with an ICD implant. Ironically, depending on the status of the patient, the presence of congestive heart failure, and LVEF, this still might be the right plan. The ICD, however, may not prevent another slip on the rug.

For many patients, an ICD is a godsend. The same is not always true for a young, healthy patient with a condition such as the long QT interval syndrome. In such a patient, the ICD can have devastating consequences. Just the presence of the device can have a major psychological impact, and this, coupled with restrictions (e.g., from athletic activities), can destroy a life in ways many physicians do not understand.

Risks of infection and inappropriate ICD discharges may outweigh the benefit of the ICD in some patients.

The patient with an ICD who still has syncope

A patient who has syncope before an ICD implant may continue to have syncope after the implant or have ICD activations of various sorts. Most ICDs now can record episodes of tachyarrhythmias. They will be stored in the memory of the device for future interrogation and analysis.

For those patients with recurrent syncope after an ICD implant, several possibilities exist:

1 The patient has episodes of ventricular tachycardia but is getting curative ICD activation after the tachycardia causes syncope. This is both good and bad. Patients do not like to feel ICD shocks but they do not like to pass out either.

2 The patient is passing out from a cause other than a ventricular arrhythmia (or a bradycardia). Further work-up may be in order.

3 The ICD or lead system is malfunctioning. This could be discovered on ICD interrogation or by a chest X-ray.

4 The patient is having another tachyarrhythmia not treated by the ICD, such as atrial fibrillation.

5 The patient is having a non-sustained ventricular tachycardia. Therapy is not delivered or it is delivered in sinus rhythm.

6 The patient is having ventricular tachycardia that is underdetected in a properly programmed ICD or is having a ventricular tachycardia below the rate cut-off set for the ICD.

Any one of these possibilities, or others, may exist, but the patient who continues to pass out with an ICD device or who receives frequent activations from their device should be seen by an electrophysiologist. The device should be interrogated so that an understanding may be reached about why the patient passed out to try to correlate the episodes with device activations or with a tachyarrhythmia. Therapies may include institution of an antiarrhythmic drug, catheter ablation, or reprogramming of the ICD. Non-invasive programmed simulation (NIPS) may need to be performed to program the ICD properly.

Case 1

A 59-year-old physician had syncope. He had a prior anterior myocardial infarction (3 years ago) and transient heart failure. The physical examination was unremarkable. An ECG showed a left bundle branch block. Cardiac enzymes were normal. Cardiac catheterization showed LVEF of 0.30 and a 75% mid-left anterior descending lesion. What do you do?

The loss of consciousness is not explained. It could be ventricular tachycardia. It could be caused by a bradycardia or heart block. Electrophysiology study is indicated and was performed. It showed an HV interval of 90 ms (abnormal) and inducible sustained monomorphic ventricular tachycardia (rate 210 b min^{-1}), with associated hemodynamic collapse.

How do you now approach this patient?

1 Angioplasty of the left anterior descending.
2 Electrophysiology-guided drug therapy.
3 Ablate the ventricular tachycardia.
4 Implant an ICD.

As there can be many different causes for syncope, it is important to obtain a complete history and physical examination, and monitor the patient closely in hospital. For this patient, no other obvious cause for the syncope could be found on further evaluation. Based on ACC/AHA guidelines, an ICD is indicated. Bradycardias and tachycardias can be treated with an ICD.

Case 2

A 78-year-old man has a dilated cardiomyopathy, an ejection fraction of 0.32, a left bundle branch block and Functional Class II congestive heart failure. He has recurrent syncope and undergoes an ICD implant. Syncope continues. An electrophysiology study after the implant and to evaluate the syncope showed he had poorly tolerated supraventricular tachycardia below the programmed tachycardia detection interval of the ICD. This was the cause of syncope. After ablation of the supraventricular tachycardia, syncope stopped.

The ICD may have been appropriate based on the clinical characteristics of the patient but, prior to ICD implant, an electrophysiology test is always suggested. Proper programming of the ICD may influence the chance of recurrent syncope if the detection window for ventricular tachycardia is set too high. With modern ICDs, it is possible to program several "zones": ventricular tachycardia (VT) zones, and a ventricular fibrillation (VF) zone. If the cause for the syncope is not clear in a patient with cardiomyopathy and if an electrophysiology study is non-diagnostic, it is best to set a slower VT zone to prevent this possibility. At the same time, an effort must be made to protect the patient against inappropriate shocks by setting the rate of the zone too low and having the ICD trigger for sinus tachycardia.

Conclusions

Syncope is a common problem that may indicate a life-threatening arrhythmic problem. Recent data indicate that ICDs can reduce the risk of sudden and total death in high-risk populations with cardiac disease, whether it is structural or electrical. The ICD will have a more important role in patients with syncope. Evaluation and treatment of these patients prior to ICD implant is crucial. ICDs may be indicated for the underlying disease even though they may not have a role in prevention of syncope, but careful discussion must take place between the patient and the physician regarding ICD implant, its risks and benefits.

Acknowledgment

The author thanks Pamela Nerheim for her help with this chapter.

References

1 Olshansky B. Is syncope the same thing as sudden death except that you wake up? *J Cardiovasc Electrophysiol* 1997;**8**:1098–101.

2 A comparison of antiarrhythmic-drug therapy with implantable defibrillators in patients resuscitated from near-fatal ventricular arrhythmias. The Antiarrhythmics versus Implantable Defibrillators (AVID) Investigators. *N Engl J Med* 1997;**337**:1576–83.

3 Moss AJ, Zareba W, Hall WJ, *et al.* Prophylactic implantation of a defibrillator in patients with myocardial infarction and reduced ejection fraction. *N Engl J Med* 2002;**346**:877–83.

4 Bristow MR, Saxon LA, Boehmer J, *et al.* Cardiac-resynchronization therapy with or without an implantable defibrillator in advanced chronic heart failure. *N Engl J Med* 2004;**350**:2140–50.

5 Kadish A, Dyer A, Daubert JP, *et al.* Prophylactic defibrillator implantation in patients with non-ischemic dilated cardiomyopathy. *N Engl J Med* 2004;**350**:2151–8.

6 Grimm W, Herzum I, Muller HH, Christ M. Value of heart rate variability to predict ventricular arrhythmias in recipients of prophylactic defibrillators with idiopathic dilated cardiomyopathy. *Pacing Clin Electrophysiol* 2003;**26**:411–5.

7 Bauer A, Schmidt G. Heart rate turbulence. *J Electrocardiol* 2003;**36** (Suppl.):89–93.

8 Hohnloser SH, Ikeda T, Bloomfield DM, Dabbous OH, Cohen RJ. T-wave alternans negative coronary patients

with low ejection and benefit from defibrillator implantation. *Lancet* 2003;**362**:125–6.

9 Cohen RJ. Enhancing specificity without sacrificing sensitivity: potential benefits of using microvolt T-wave alternans testing to risk stratify the MADIT-II population. *Card Electrophysiol Rev* 2003;**7**:438–42.

10 Priori SG, Napolitano C, Diehl L, Schwartz PJ. Dispersion of the QT interval: a marker of therapeutic efficacy in the idiopathic long QT syndrome. *Circulation* 1994;**89**:1681–9.

11 Vrtovec B, Delgado R, Zewail A, Thomas CD, Richartz BM, Radovancevic B. Prolonged QT$_c$ interval and high B-type natriuretic peptide levels together predict mortality in patients with advanced heart failure. *Circulation* 2003;**107**:1764–9.

12 Harrison A, Morrison LK, Krishnaswamy P, *et al.* B-type natriuretic peptide predicts future cardiac events in patients presenting to the emergency department with dyspnea. *Ann Emerg Med* 2002;**39**:131–8.

13 Berbari EJ, Lazzara R. The significance of electrocardiographic late potentials: predictors of ventricular tachycardia. *Annu Rev Med* 1992;**43**:157–69.

14 Kuchar DL, Thorburn CW, Sammel NL. The role of signal-averaged electrocardiography in the investigation of unselected patients with syncope. *Aust N Z J Med* 1985;**15**:697–703.

15 Kapoor WN, Hammill SC, Gersh BJ. Diagnosis and natural history of syncope and the role of invasive electrophysiologic testing. *Am J Cardiol* 1989;**63**:730–4.

16 Klein GJ, Gersh BJ, Yee R. Electrophysiological testing: the final court of appeal for diagnosis of syncope? *Circulation* 1995;**92**:1332–5.

17 Linzer M, Prystowsky EN, Divine GW, *et al.* Predicting the outcomes of electrophysiologic studies of patients with unexplained syncope: preliminary validation of a derived model. *J Gen Intern Med* 1991;**6**:113–20.

18 Olshansky B, Mazuz M, Martins JB. Significance of inducible tachycardia in patients with syncope of unknown origin: a long-term follow-up. *J Am Coll Cardiol* 1985;**5**:216–23.

19 Rahimtoola SH, Zipes DP, Akhtar M, *et al.* Consensus statement of the conference on the state of the art of electrophysiologic testing in the diagnosis and treatment of patients with cardiac arrhythmias. *Circulation* 1987;**75**:III3–11.

20 Teichman SL, Felder SD, Matos JA, Kim SG, Waspe LE, Fisher JD. The value of electrophysiologic studies in syncope of undetermined origin: report of 150 cases. *Am Heart J* 1985;**110**:469–79.

21 Linzer M, Yang EH, Estes NA III, Wang P, Vorperian VR, Kapoor WN. Diagnosing syncope. Part 2. Unexplained syncope. Clinical efficacy assessment project of the American College of Physicians. *Ann Intern Med* 1997;**127**:76–86.

22 Zipes DP, DiMarco JP, Gillette PC, *et al.* Guidelines for clinical intracardiac electrophysiological and catheter ablation procedures. A report of the American College of Cardiology/American Heart Association Task Force on Practice Guidelines (Committee on Clinical Intracardiac Electrophysiologic and Catheter Ablation Procedures), developed in collaboration with the North American Society of Pacing and Electrophysiology. *J Am Coll Cardiol* 1995;**26**:555–73.

23 Savage DD, Corwin L, McGee DL, Kannel WB, Wolf PA. Epidemiologic features of isolated syncope: the Framingham Study. *Stroke* 1985;**16**:626–9.

24 Silverstein MD, Singer DE, Mulley AG, Thibault GE, Barnett GO. Patients with syncope admitted to medical intensive care units. *JAMA* 1982;**248**:1185–9.

25 Kapoor WN, Hanusa BH. Is syncope a risk factor for poor outcomes? Comparison of patients with and without syncope. *Am J Med* 1996;**100**:646–55.

26 Olshansky B, Hahn EA, Hartz VL, Prater SP, Mason JW. Clinical significance of syncope in the electrophysiologic study versus electrocardiographic monitoring (ESVEM) trial. The ESVEM Investigators. *Am Heart J* 1999;**137**:878–86.

27 Steinberg JS, Beckman K, Greene HL, *et al.* Follow-up of patients with unexplained syncope and inducible ventricular tachyarrhythmias: analysis of the AVID registry and an AVID substudy. Antiarrhythmics versus implantable defibrillators. *J Cardiovasc Electrophysiol* 2001;**12**:996–1001.

28 Middlekauff HR, Stevenson WG, Stevenson LW, Saxon LA. Syncope in advanced heart failure: high risk of sudden death regardless of origin of syncope. *J Am Coll Cardiol* 1993;**21**:110–6.

29 Schwartz PJ, Camm AJ, Frangin G, Janse MJ, Julian DG, Simon P. Does amiodarone reduce sudden death and cardiac mortality after myocardial infarction? The European Myocardial Infarct Amiodarone Trial (EMIAT). *Eur Heart J* 1994;**15**:620–4.

30 Naccarelli GV, Wolbrette DL, Dell'Orfano JT, Patel HM, Luck JC. Amiodarone: what have we learned from clinical trials? *Clin Cardiol* 2000;**23**:73–82.

31 Bardy G, *et al.* SCD-HeFT. *N Engl J Med* 2005, in press.

32 The ESVEM trial. Electrophysiologic study versus electrocardiographic monitoring for selection of antiarrhythmic therapy of ventricular tachyarrhythmias. The ESVEM Investigators. *Circulation* 1989;**79**:1354–60.

33 Militianu A, Salacata A, Seibert K, *et al.* Implantable cardioverter defibrillator utilization among device recipients presenting exclusively with syncope or near-syncope. *J Cardiovasc Electrophysiol* 1997;**8**:1087–97.

34 Gregoratos G, Abrams J, Epstein AE, *et al.* ACC/AHA/NASPE 2002 guideline update for implantation of cardiac pacemakers and antiarrhythmia devices: summary

article: a report of the American College of Cardiology/ American Heart Association Task Force on Practice Guidelines (ACC/AHA/NASPE Committee to Update the 1998 Pacemaker Guidelines). *J Am Coll Cardiol* 2002; **40**:1703–19.

35 Bigger JT Jr. Prophylactic use of implanted cardiac defibrillators in patients at high risk for ventricular arrhythmias after coronary-artery bypass graft surgery. Coronary Artery Bypass Graft (CABG) PATCH Trial Investigators. *N Engl J Med* 1997;**337**:1569–75.

36 Hohnloser SH, Kuck KH, Dorian P, *et al.* Prophylactic use of an implantable cardioverter-defibrillator after acute myocardial infarction. *N Engl J Med* 2004;**351**:2481–8.

37 Gronefeld G, Connolly SJ, Hohnloser SH. The defibrillator in acute myocardial infarction trial (DINAMIT): rationale, design and specific aims. *Card Electrophysiol Rev* 2003;**7**:447–51.

38 Moss AJ. Long QT syndrome. *JAMA* 2003;**289**:2041–4.

39 Maron BJ, Cecchi F, McKenna WJ. Risk factors and stratification for sudden cardiac death in patients with hypertrophic cardiomyopathy. *Br Heart J* 1994;**72**:S13–8.

40 Paz HL, McCormick DJ, Kutalek SP, Patchefsky A. The automated implantable cardiac defibrillator: prophylaxis in cardiac sarcoidosis. *Chest* 1994;**106**:1603–7.

41 Bachinsky WB, Linzer M, Weld L, Estes NA III. Usefulness of clinical characteristics in predicting the outcome of electrophysiologic studies in unexplained syncope. *Am J Cardiol* 1992;**69**:1044–9.

42 Link MS, Costeas XF, Griffith JL, Colburn CD, Estes NA III, Wang PJ. High incidence of appropriate implantable cardioverter-defibrillator therapy in patients with syncope of unknown etiology and inducible ventricular arrhythmias. *J Am Coll Cardiol* 1997;**29**:370–5.

43 Oginosawa Y, Abe H, Nagatomo T, Mizuki T, Nakashima Y. Sustained polymorphic ventricular tachycardia unassociated with QT prolongation or bradycardia in the Kearns–Sayre syndrome. *Pacing Clin Electrophysiol* 2003; **26**:1911–2.

44 Rashid A, Kim MH. Kearns–Sayre syndrome: association with long QT syndrome? *J Cardiovasc Electrophysiol* 2002;**13**:184–5.

45 Morady F, Kadish AH, DiCarlo L, *et al.* Long-term results of catheter ablation of idiopathic right ventricular tachycardia. *Circulation* 1990;**82**:2093–9.

46 Wellens HJ, Smeets JL. Idiopathic left ventricular tachycardia: cure by radiofrequency ablation. *Circulation* 1993;**88**:2978–9.

47 Middlekauff HR, Stevenson WG, Saxon LA. Prognosis after syncope: impact of left ventricular function. *Am Heart J* 1993;**125**:121–7.

48 Knight BP, Goyal R, Pelosi F, *et al.* Outcome of patients with non-ischemic dilated cardiomyopathy and unex- plained syncope treated with an implantable defibrillator. *J Am Coll Cardiol* 1999;**33**:1964–70.

49 Cappato R, Negroni S, Bentivegna S, *et al.* Role of implantable cardioverter defibrillators in dilated cardiomyopathy. *J Cardiovasc Electrophysiol* 2002;**13**:S106–9.

50 Bauce B, Nava A, Rampazzo A, *et al.* Familial effort polymorphic ventricular arrhythmias in arrhythmogenic right ventricular cardiomyopathy map to chromosome 1q42–43. *Am J Cardiol* 2000;**85**:573–9.

51 Corrado D, Leoni L, Link MS, *et al.* Implantable cardioverter-defibrillator therapy for prevention of sudden death in patients with arrhythmogenic right ventricular cardiomyopathy/dysplasia. *Circulation* 2003; **108**:3084–91.

52 Maron BJ, Shen WK, Link MS, *et al.* Efficacy of implantable cardioverter-defibrillators for the prevention of sudden death in patients with hypertrophic cardiomyopathy. *N Engl J Med* 2000;**342**:365–73.

53 Brugada J, Brugada R, Brugada P. Determinants of sudden cardiac death in individuals with the electrocardiographic pattern of Brugada syndrome and no previous cardiac arrest. *Circulation* 2003;**108**:3092–6.

54 Priori SG, Napolitano C, Gasparini M, *et al.* Natural history of Brugada syndrome: insights for risk stratification and management. *Circulation* 2002;**105**:1342–7.

55 Alexander ME, Cecchin F, Walsh EP, Triedman JK, Bevilacqua LM, Berul CI. Implications of implantable cardioverter defibrillator therapy in congenital heart disease and pediatrics. *J Cardiovasc Electrophysiol* 2004;**15**: 72–6.

56 Hlatky MA, Boothroyd DB, Johnstone IM, *et al.* Long-term cost-effectiveness of alternative management strategies for patients with life-threatening ventricular arrhythmias. Electrophysiologic Study Versus Electrocardiographic Monitoring (ESVEM) investigators. *J Clin Epidemiol* 1997;**50**:185–93.

57 Valenti R, Schlapfer J, Fromer M, Fischer A, Kappenberger L. Impact of the implantable cardioverter-defibrillator on rehospitalizations. *Eur Heart J* 1996;**17**:1565–71.

58 Hlatky MA, Sanders GD, Owens DK. Cost-effectiveness of the implantable cardioverter defibrillator. *Card Electrophysiol Rev* 2003;**7**:479–82.

59 Larsen G, Hallstrom A, McAnulty J, *et al.* Cost-effectiveness of the implantable cardioverter-defibrillator versus antiarrhythmic drugs in survivors of serious ventricular tachyarrhythmias: results of the Antiarrhythmics Versus Implantable Defibrillators (AVID) economic analysis substudy. *Circulation* 2002;**105**:2049–57.

60 Chen L, Hay JW. Cost-effectiveness of primary implanted cardioverter defibrillator for sudden death prevention in congestive heart failure. *Cardiovasc Drugs Ther* 2004; **18**:161–70.

CHAPTER 9

Neurologic causes of syncope

Phillip A. Low, MD

Introduction

An abrupt loss of consciousness with loss of postural tone followed by complete recovery is more common in subjects without than in those with neurologic disease. However, a significant proportion of patients who carry the diagnosis of vasovagal or neurocardiogenic syncope have some underlying dysautonomia. Occasionally, more severe peripheral or central neurologic denervation can be responsible for syncope. Rarely, a humoral vasodilator, usually secreted by a tumor, can cause transient blood pressure (BP) alterations and precipitate syncope. The focus of this chapter is on the causes, pathophysiology, and management of neurologic causes of syncope.

Neurologic causes of syncope

Orthostatic hypotension

Neurologic causes of syncope are shown in Table 9.1. Syncope is common in patients with neurogenic orthostatic hypotension (OH) [1]. Neurogenic OH needs to be distinguished from the fall in BP during presyncope. Indeed, the term OH should *not* be used for the fall in BP during presyncope. In symptomatic OH, there is usually premonitory symptoms of cerebral hypoperfusion such as lightheadedness, blurring or tunneling of vision, mental fogging or haziness, and diffuse weakness or heaviness of the legs. Elderly subjects may have subtle orthostatic cognitive symptoms, which they (and the physician) may fail to ascribe to OH, so that syncope occurs [2] (Fig. 9.1). Typically, once they learn to recognize the premonitory symptoms, they can usually avoid syncope.

OH is a consistent feature in established multisystem atrophy (MSA), a condition characterized by OH, male erectile dysfunction, neurogenic bladder, and parkinsonism or spinocerebellar ataxia [3]. OH is not typically present in Parkinson's disease (PD) although it can occur following orthostatic stress (such as raised ambient temperature, a meal, or exercise) or medications such as levodopa or cardidopa ingestion, which has a central hypotensive action [4]. These patients differ from those with MSA in several essential respects. First, they have a rest tremor, which is usually absent in MSA. Second, in contrast to MSA, they are levodopa responsive and have levodopa-induced dyskinesia. Their autonomic failure tends to be less generalized than MSA. It is important to make this distinction because patients with Parkinson's disease and autonomic failure (PD-AF) have a prognosis that is closer to PD than MSA [5]. These patients generally have florid orthostatic hypotension but with a more restricted distribution of autonomic failure. For instance, cardiovagal function is often at least partially preserved and sweat loss is generally less extensive than in patients with MSA. Patients with diffuse Lewy body disease have characteristic symptoms of dementia, psychiatric symptoms, and vivid dreams. Some patients have OH [6,7]. The condition can be hard to differentiate from MSA, and both conditions can be lumped together as a synucleinopathy.

Wernicke–Korsakoff syndrome typically occurs in alcoholics and is brought about by vitamin B_1 deficiency [8]. Patients have a combination of cranial nerve lesions, nystagmus, ataxia, and neuropathy. The OH is caused by a lesion of the medulla. A thalamic lesion is consistently present. Recognition

Table 9.1 Neurologic causes of syncope.

Syncope resulting from orthostatic hypotension

Brain disease
Multisystem atrophy (MSA)
Parkinson's disease with autonomic failure
Diffuse Lewy body disease (some cases)
Wernicke–Korsakoff syndrome

Spinal cord disease
Traumatic tetraplegia (above T5)
Spinal cord tumors

Autonomic neuropathies
The autoimmune autonomic neuropathies (acute,
    subacute, chronic)
Paraneoplastic autonomic neuropathy
Guillain–Barré syndrome
Porphyria
Amyloid
Diabetic autonomic neuropathy
Familial dysautonomia (Riley–Day syndrome)

Loss of vasoconstrictor tone
Dopamine-β-hydroxylase deficiency

Syncope with underlying limited autonomic neuropathy

Syncope with underlying hyperadrenergic state

Intracranial causes of syncope
Mechanical obstruction (e.g., third ventricle cyst);
Arnold–Chiari malformation
Brainstem ischemia

Syncope associated with episodic vasodilation
Mastocytosis
Pheochromocytoma
Carcinoid syndrome
Hyperbradykininsm
Hyperepinephrinemia
Vasoactive intestinal polypeptide secreting tumor

Reflex syncope
Carotid sinus syncope
Micturition syncope
Cough syncope
Swallow syncope

---

of the syndrome is critically important, because intravenous infusion of glucose–saline without vitamin B_1 will aggravate or precipitate the neurologic lesion.

Complete spinal cord lesions above T5 regularly result in OH. The splanchnic-mesenteric bed, supplied by the splanchnic outflow, is denervated by lesions above T5. Lesions below T5 are not associated with OH, highlighting the great importance of the splanchnic-mesenteric bed in the maintenance of postural normotension [9]. This baroreflex-responsive venous-capacitance bed contains 20% of total blood volume and increases 200–300% following a meal [10].

Motor, sensory, and autonomic fibers are involved to varying degrees in the peripheral neuropathies [11]. When autonomic nerve fibers are disproportionately affected, the term autonomic neuropathy is used. The most common cause of autonomic neuropathy in developed countries is diabetic neuropathy [9,12]. Autonomic impairment occurs *pari passu* with somatic sensory nerve fibers and, to a lesser degree, somatic motor fibers [9,13]. The other causes of autonomic neuropathy are autoimmune (acquired autoimmune, paraneoplastic, Guillain–Barré syndrome), amyloidosis, porphyria, and familial dysautonomia. The great importance of recognizing these neuropathies is that specific tests are available for the majority of them.

Subacute autoimmune autonomic neuropathy is characterized by the subacute onset of widespread autonomic failure (hence the original term pandysautonomia). There is a postviral onset in over half of cases [14]. With the availability of autonomic function tests, milder cases are increasingly recognized [15]. The most common clinical autonomic deficits are the triad of OH, gastrointestinal motor deficits, and thermoregulatory failure [14]. The neuropathy is associated with a high titer of ganglionic antibody in half of cases [16]. The titers of this antibody parallel the severity of autonomic failure, suggesting that the antibody might be pathogenetically involved. Recently, we have demonstrated that some cases with the phenotype of pure autonomic failure may be caused by autoimmune autonomic neuropathy [17]. Hence, autoimmune autonomic neuropathy can present phenotypically as acute (acute pandysautonomia), subacute, or chronic (pure autonomic failure) autonomic neuropathies.

There is a panel of paraneoplastic autoantibodies that are closely linked to certain cancers. The most

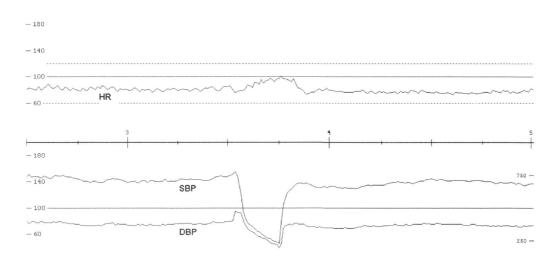

Fig. 9.1 Woman, 74 years of age, with orthostatic hypotension. On head upright tilt (HUT) there was the rapid development and progression of blood pressure decrement and syncope.

common autonomic syndrome is a subacute autonomic neuropathy. The most common cancer is small cell lung carcinoma (SCLC) (which can be occult). Other common cancers are breast and ovary. Often, the only clue to the presence of a neoplasm is high titers of these paraneoplastic antibodies. These include ANNA-1–3, PCA-1–2, CRMP-5, and calcium-channel antibodies [11,18].

Guillain–Barré syndrome is characterized by rapid, ascending (from lower limbs to upper limbs, respiration and facial) motor paralysis, often postviral, with increased cerebrospinal fluid protein and areflexia [19]. Cranial nerve and respiratory paralysis are common. OH and dysautonomia, including "autonomic storms," characterized by tachycardia, hypertension, and a hyperadrenergic state are not uncommon in Guillain–Barré syndrome. BP can be quite erratic, rendering pharmacologic management difficult [20].

Partial autonomic failure

The majority of patients who have vasovagal syncope have no evidence of autonomic impairment. However, there is a subset of patients who have laboratory evidence of a length-dependent autonomic neuropathy [3]. These patients do not have OH but have a slow gradual fall in BP for 1–3 min preceding syncope [21]. Beat-to-beat BP recordings of the Valsalva maneuver show a loss of baroreflex-

mediated vasoconstrictor response (late phase II; Fig. 9.2). The same patient (Fig. 9.1) developed syncope during head upright tilt (HUT). In the thermoregulatory sweat test or the quantitative sudomotor axon reflex test (QSART), there is distal anhidrosis. Some of these patients are known to have a peripheral neuropathy, demonstrable on nerve conduction studies. Some patients do not have a large fiber neuropathy and are referred to as having distal, small fiber neuropathy. Some elderly subjects with syncope fall into this category. The mechanism of syncope in these patients is presumed to occur as follows. Partial autonomic failure results in a moderate fall in BP. This fall in blood and pulse pressure triggers baroreflexes (which are still partially intact) with a resulting superimposed vasovagal component (augmentation of reflex syncope), recognizable by the abrupt bradycardia associated with syncope (Table 9.2; Fig. 9.2).

Syncope with underlying hyperadrenergic state

Certain autonomic neuropathies go through a phase of a hyperadrenergic state with an increased risk of syncope. These include diabetic neuropathy and the postural tachycardia syndrome (POTS) [22]. The hyperadrenergic state is characterized by an excessive orthostatic increase in heart rate and plasma norepinephrine (≥ 600 pg/mL) [23]. The diabetic

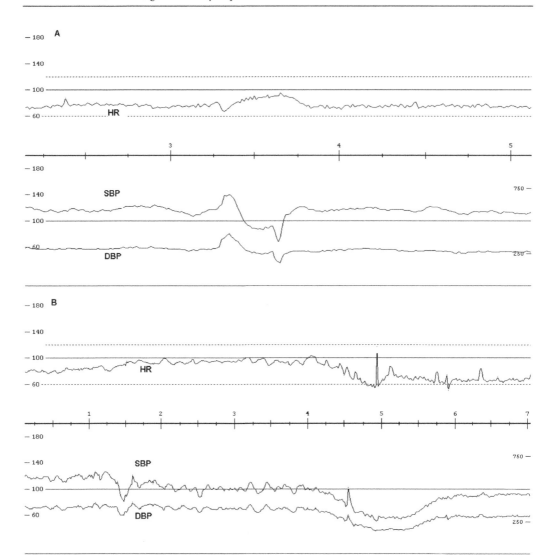

Fig. 9.2 Man, 57 years of age, with mild autonomic impairment. Reflex vasoconstriction is absent in the Valsalva maneuver (A). To head upright tilt (HUT) (B) there is a gradual fall in blood pressure and development of neurocardiogenic syncope.

Table 9.2 Neurologic mechanisms of syncope.

1 Reflex syncope
2 Dysautonomia with hyperadrenergic state →
augmentation of reflex syncope
3 Autonomic failure with sympathetic dysfunction →
augmentation of reflex syncope
4 Neurogenic orthostatic hypotension → progressive
cerebral hypoperfusion
5 Central mechanisms of brainstem oligemia

state is termed hyperadrenergic diabetic neuropathy and when OH is present, hyperadrenergic OH [24]. Dysautonomia is an integral component of diabetic neuropathy and is associated with increased mortality, especially when associated with vascular complications. Recent studies on cardiac sympathetic innervation have provided a theoretical basis for arrhythmias. Single-photon emission computed tomography (SPECT) and positron emission tomography (PET) using ^{123}I-metaiodobenzylguanidine (^{123}I-MIBG) and ^{11}C-hydroxyephedrine

(^{11}C-HED) have shown that cardiac sympathetic dysfunction is commonly present in both type 1 and type 2 diabetes [25]. The pattern of sympathetic disturbances is heterogeneous, with denervation affecting mainly the posterior myocardial region, with some focal hyperinnervation of the proximal segment [26].

A similar state occurs in POTS [27–29]. Of interest is that both conditions can be associated with a contracted plasma volume [24,28,30].

Intracranial causes of syncope

There are a number of intracranial causes of syncope [31]. One such example is a colloid cyst of the third ventricle. In certain positions, the cyst occludes cerebrospinal fluid pathways and results in syncope. Syncope can be triggered by stimulation of any of the limbic structures and can occur with emotive stress, pain, seizures as in certain cases of partial complex seizures, with mass lesions as in colloid cyst of the third ventricle, and in Arnold–Chiari malformations [32]. Brainstem ischemia can cause syncope. The most common is vertebrobasilar transient ischemic attack. The clinical features of diplopia, vertigo, ataxia, cranial nerve and corticospinal tract involvement allow easy diagnosis. However, the rare case can occur with much less florid neurologic manifestations.

Reflex syncope

There are a number of causes of reflex syncope, all characterized by abrupt onset and rapid recovery. They differ in the stimulus and receptor. These syndromes are covered in greater detail elsewhere in this book (Chapter 2). These are types of neurocardiogenic syncopes with identifiable triggers. These include carotid sinus pressure in carotid sinus supersensitivity and vagal stimulation in patients with vagal supersensitivity. Other triggers include the stimulation of areas supplied by the trigeminal and glossopharyngeal nerves [33,34]. Some patients develop syncope with coitus, micturition, vigorous coughing, or even swallowing [33,34]. Figure 9.3 shows the BP and heart rate changes in response to swallowing water.

Micturition syncope typically occurs in young, muscular males, occurring at the end of micturition or shortly thereafter. The onset is abrupt and recovery is rapid. Several mechanisms are probably operative. Typically, the patient arises from sleep in a warm bed, warm and vasodilated. Nocturnal BP is reduced. A full bladder is uncomfortable inducing vasoconstriction. Bladder emptying removes this stimulus and results in vasodilation. Vasodilation can be augmented by alcohol or sleep in a warm bed. The supine posture results in a diuresis, reducing blood volume. Micturition itself results in vagal

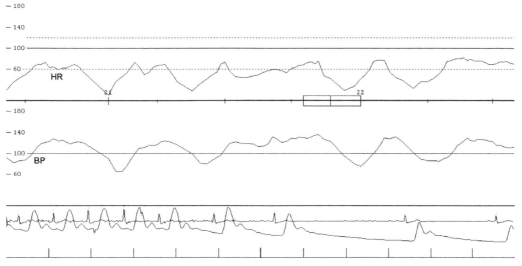

Fig. 9.3 Man, 51 years of age, with swallow-induced syncope. In the recording, each epoch of bradycardia is associated with hypotension, and was induced by repeated swallowing. The box selects the epoch for which electrocardiogram and beat-to-beat blood pressure recordings are shown below.

stimulation and the performance of a Valsalva maneuver resulting in reduced preload. Micturition syncope can less commonly occur in women [35], the majority of whom have orthostatic hypotension.

Rare causes of syncope

There are certain rare causes of syncope. These include dopamine-β-hydroxylase deficiency as a rare cause of orthostatic hypotension and rare tumors that secrete epinephrine, norepinephrine, serotonin, vasoactive intestinal polypeptide, bradykinin, histamine, and prostaglandins. Dopamine-β-hydroxylase deficiency is characterized by OH (resulting from the inability to synthesize norepinephrine from dopamine) and bilateral ptosis [36,37]. Retrograde ejaculation occurs, because ejaculation is a sympathetic function. The clue to one of these rare tumors is the presence of flushing or BP fluctuations. In pheochromocytoma, hypertension is usual but OH can occur and norepinephrine and its metabolites are increased. Hyperepinephrinemia can cause tremulousness, flushing, and variable BP [38]. Carcinoid syndrome is suggested by flushing, diarrhea, and hypotension, and syncope can occur. Histamine and prostaglandin D_2 levels are increased. A vasoactive, intestinal, polypeptide-secreting tumor causes flushing, diarrhea, and fluctuating BP [39]. Hyperbradykininism causes facial erythema, tachycardia, and acral discoloration associated with high bradykinin levels [40].

Pathophysiology of syncope in neurologic disease

Mechanisms of syncope in neurologic disease differ in different conditions (Table 9.2). For the patient with severe generalized autonomic failure and absent baroreflex and other reflexes that maintain BP, syncope is common at the onset of development of neurogenic OH. The mechanism of syncope is one of progressive cerebral hypoperfusion. On HUT, there is the immediate development of OH, with progressive further decline in BP with continuation of HUT (Fig. 9.1). Heart rate is fixed. During the Valsalva maneuver, there is a pronounced vasodepressor response during the maneuver (increased early phase II), absence of a vasoconstrictor response, and with cessation of the maneuver, an absence of a BP overshoot. As OH becomes chronic, syncope becomes much less common for several reasons. Patients with chronic orthostatic hypotension may be remarkably tolerant of very low orthostatic blood pressures, developing no symptoms, especially when the condition becomes more chronic. This improvement in orthostatic tolerance appears to be related to an expansion of the autoregulated range of lower blood pressures [41,42]. Within this range, cerebral blood flow remains constant in the face of changing systemic blood pressure by a change in cerebral arteriolar tone. Thomas and Bannister [42] demonstrated that cerebral blood flow was maintained in response to head-up tilt down to a systolic pressure of 60 mmHg. Recent studies have combined transcranial Doppler (TCD) with cerebral blood flow recordings. Flow velocity, measured by TCD, becomes reduced when cerebral arteriolar tone increases. It was demonstrated that blood flow was maintained by a change in cerebral arteriolar tone [41]. Patients also learn to recognize the subtle symptoms of orthostatic intolerance and take the necessary maneuvers to prevent syncope. Especially in the elderly, lightheadedness or blurred vision may be delayed. Instead, mental blunting or confusion may be the sole manifestation of hypoperfusion.

Although investigators have emphasized autonomic failure, many of the problems in neurogenic OH relate to residual autonomic and especially sympathetic tone [43]. It is this residual tone, coupled with the loss of regulatory reflexes, that is responsible for the supine hypertension. Patients with limited autonomic neuropathy will often have a pattern on HUT of a gradual fall in BP associated with normal or excessive heart rate increment. Several minutes into the study, they develop neurocardiogenic syncope with an abrupt fall in BP and heart rate [21]. The pathophysiology of syncope is as follows: limited autonomic failure → impaired total systemic vascular resistance → gradual fall in BP → ↑ sympathetic tone → reflex syncope (Table 9.2). The diagnosis of limited autonomic failure leads to appropriate treatment aimed at enhancing vasomotor tone or enhancing vascular reflexes.

A third mechanism of neurogenic syncope is syncope associated with hyperadrenergic states. Cryer *et al.* [24] described what they termed an unusual subset of diabetic autonomic neuropathy, which they called hyperadrenergic orthostatic hypotension. These patients and those with POTS [28] have high resting heart rate, orthostatic tachycardia, an excessive norepinephrine response, and propensity to syncope. The likely mechanism of syncope is: partial autonomic failure → impaired total systemic vascular resistance → OH + hyperresponsive sympathetic nervous system → ↑↑ sympathetic tone → reflex syncope (Table 9.2). OH is not mandatory. For patients with neuropathic POTS the steps are: limited autonomic failure → impaired total systemic vascular tone + hyperresponsive sympathetic nervous system → ↑↑ sympathetic tone → reflex syncope. The treatment of hyperadrenergic syncope can be difficult. There are also concerns that, in the diabetic patient, the combination of having islands of hyperinnervated myocardium [26,44] and high catecholamine levels can be responsible for fatal arrhythmias [25]. Volume contraction is typical of hyperadrenergic states so that volume expansion is mandatory [28]. Some patients with β-receptor supersensitivity respond to beta-blockers, but the hyperadrenergic state may be central in origin and may require a centrally acting α_2-agonist such as clonidine.

Finally, all the reflex syncopes are triggered by activating a presumably supersensitive receptor resulting in activating different afferent pathways, central integration with the same final common efferent pathways.

Approach to evaluation and management of neurogenic syncope

Step 1: Is it syncope?

The approach to the management of syncope should proceed in a number of graduated steps. Step 1 is to determine if syncope is present. The main differential diagnosis is cardiac arrhythmia, seizure disorder, hypoglycemia, pseudosyncope, and transient ischemic attack. Cardiac arrhythmia or other cardiac disease is evaluated by the history of heart disease, irregularities of heart rate, precipitation by certain activities, especially exertion, and studied with electrocardiogram (ECG), Holter monitor, and, if warranted, by cardiac electrophysiologic studies. The similarities are usually only superficial.

A seizure disorder is recognized by the prodrome,

motor or other neurologic manifestations, and by the postictal manifestations. The aura is typical of a temporal lobe focus and is distinctly neurologic instead of symptoms of hypoperfusion. Examples are an unusual odor or perception. The motor accompaniments of clonic–tonic jerks are caused by secondary generalization (from a focal seizure to grand mal seizure). The focal manifestations are typically much more subtle, such as twitching of the eyelids or of the corner of the mouth. Bladder or bowel incontinence suggests a seizure disorder rather than syncope. The recovery period tends to be brief and complete with syncope and protracted in seizures. The presence of a few clonic jerks after loss of consciousness is not uncommon in syncope and should not be confused with seizures.

Hypoglycemia coma is usually not difficult to differentiate from syncope. The patient is usually drowsy before the loss of consciousness, there is clear evidence of sympathetic overreaction, and blood glucose is diagnostic. When it occurs in a diabetic subject, diagnosis is usually straightforward. More challenging is hypoglycemia that occurs in an islet-secreting tumor.

Pseudosyncope can be difficult to differentiate from true syncope. Suspicious clinical circumstances include a high frequency of episodes, unassociated with injuries, secondary gain, and the lack of cardiovascular alterations. A tilt study should be carried out. Pseudosyncope is unassociated with BP or heart rate alterations. The definitive test would require the concomitant recording of an electroencephalogram (EEG) and TCD. If the loss of consciousness is unassociated with cardiovascular, TCD, or EEG alterations of syncope, then a diagnosis of pseudosyncope can be made with confidence. A transient ischemic attack is differentiable by the presence of focal deficits. Vertebrobasilar transient ischemic attacks may more closely mimic syncope for the non-neurologist.

Step 2: What is the mechanism of syncope?

The history and examination should be focused on determining if the patient has an underlying neurologic basis for syncope. The clinical evaluation needs to be supplemented by laboratory evaluation (Table 9.3). Routine evaluation consists of detailed neurologic and autonomic history, examination,

Table 9.3 Laboratory evaluation for neurologic causes of syncope.

Test	Rationale
Routine studies	
Chest X-ray	Carcinoma of lung
ECG	Cardiac arrhythmia and heart disease
Routine tests including glucose, creatinine, and screen for connective tissue disease	
Autonomic reflex screen	Diagnose autonomic failure and POTS
Plasma catecholamines	Supine and orthostatic norepinephrine
24-h urinary sodium	Plasma volume status
If OH present or autonomic neuropathy suspected	
Paraneoplastic panel	Cancer responsible for autonomic failure
Imaging studies (CT chest, abdomen and pelvis; mammography)	
Ganglionic antibody	Autonomic neuropathy
Fat aspirate for amyloid	Amyloid neuropathy
EMG/conduction studies	Peripheral neuropathy
EPG/IEPG	Paraproteinemia
MRI of brain/cervical spine	MSA and related conditions
Thermoregulatory sweat test	Pattern of autonomic sudomotor deficit

CT, computed tomography; ECG, electrocardiogram; EMG, electromyogram; MRI, magnetic resonance imaging; MSA, multisystem atrophy; OH, orthostatic hypotension; POTS, postural tachycardia syndrome.

Table 9.4 The autonomic reflex screen.

Test	Autonomic system evaluated
1 QSART distribution	Postganglionic sympathetic sudomotor status
2 HR response to deep breathing	Cardiovagal function
3 Valsalva ratio	Cardiovagal function
4 B/B BP responses to VM	Adrenergic function
5 B/B BP responses to HUT	Adrenergic function

B/B BP, beat-to-beat blood pressure; HUT, head upright tilt; QSART, quantitative sudomotor axon reflex test; VM, Valsalva maneuver.

ECG, and chest X-ray. An autonomic reflex screen (Table 9.4) is carried out for two reasons:
1 to evaluate adrenergic, cardiovagal, and sudomotor function to determine if autonomic failure including OH is present; and
2 to detect the presence of orthostatic intolerance. The duration of HUT is 5–10 min, adequate for demonstrating the presence of OH and orthostatic intolerance but not for the diagnosis of syncope.

If OH is detected or an autonomic neuropathy is suspected, additional tests are undertaken (Table 9.3). The neurodegenerative causes of orthostatic hypotension (such as MSA and related conditions) are highly characteristic clinically and on laboratory testing. The patient has parkinsonism and/or ataxia and has the triad of neurogenic bladder, generalized autonomic failure (including OH), and widespread anhidrosis on the thermoregulatory sweat test. Parkinson's disease with autonomic failure has classic PD symptoms including rest tremor, levodopa responsiveness, and levodopa-induced dyskinesia. The patient has OH (which

Table 9.5 Paraneoplastic antibodies, associated cancers, and neurologic syndromes.

Antibody	Common cancers	Clinical syndrome
ANNA-1 (Hu)	SCLC	Autonomic neuropathy; sensory neuronopathy; gastrointestinal dysmotility
ANNA-2	SCLC; breast	Sensory neuronopathy; autonomic neuropathy
ANNA-3	SCLC	Subacute, multifocal sensory or sensorimotor neuropathy; cerebellar ataxia, myelopathy, brainstem and limbic encephalopathy
PCA-1; Purkinje (Yo)	Ovarian; breast	Neuropathy; subacute cerebellar degeneration; motor neuron disease
PCA-2	SCLC	Limbic encephalitis; cerebellar ataxia; LEMS; autonomic neuropathy; neuropathy
Ganglionic (A$_3$)	SCLC	Autonomic neuropathy (idiopathic; paraneoplastic)
Acetylcholine receptor (A$_1$)	Thymoma	Myasthenia gravis; subacute autonomic neuropathy
Voltage gated Ca^{2+}	SCLC	Myasthenic syndrome; subacute autonomic neuropathy
CRMP-5	SCLC	Autonomic neuropathy; sensorimotor neuropathy; cerebellar ataxia, LEMS, subacute dementia; inflammatory CSF

CRMP-5, collapsin response mediator protein-5; CSF, cerebrospinal fluid; LEMS, Lambert–Eaton myasthenic syndrome; SCLC, small cell carcinoma of the lung.

can be profound) but has usually less impaired cardiovagal and sudomotor impairment (i.e., less generalized autonomic failure) [5]. These patients have reduced cardiac adrenergic innervation in contrast to those with MSA (who are normal). Neuropathologically, PD-AF patients have less brainstem neuropathology that is closer to PD than MSA [45].

The autonomic neuropathies can be highly characteristic clinically, as are the reflex syncopes. Laboratory evaluation of etiology is extremely helpful in the group. Patients who have a paraneoplastic basis of subacute autonomic neuropathy will have the diagnosis made in almost all cases if an adequate paraneoplastic panel (Table 9.5) and imaging studies of the chest, breast, abdomen, and pelvis are made. Autoimmune autonomic neuropathy is diagnosed on the basis of the characteristic clinical picture (subacute postviral onset and triad of OH, gastrointestinal dysmotility, and anhidrosis) and confirmed in 50% of cases by positive ganglionic antibody [16]. Amyloid neuropathy is associated with monoclonal gammopathy and demonstration of amyloid deposits in subcutaneous fat (80% yield) or nerve biopsy (> 90% yield) [15]. Familial dysautonomia is not likely to present in adult life. Genetic testing is now available [46].

Many patients will have evidence of denervation on autonomic testing without florid autonomic neuropathy. These patients have at least partially intact baroreflexes that can be dysfunctional. The failure of vasomotor tone and intact/dysfunctional reflexes appear to predispose them to syncope. As subjects age, there is a progressive impairment of vasomotor tone seen in BP control in response to HUT and to the Valsalva maneuver [47]. These patients often respond exquisitely well to small doses of vasoconstrictors.

The patient with hyperadrenergic state is recognized clinically and on laboratory testing. Some patients have a resting tachycardia. Occasionally, patients have autonomic storms characterized by tachycardia, tremulousness, sweating, and nausea that are distinct from panic attacks. They may have a resting tachycardia. On autonomic testing there are changes in catecholamines, the Valsalva maneuver, and HUT. There is an exaggerated orthostatic norepinephrine response (to > 600 pg/mL). On the Valsalva maneuver, the BP phase IV (overshoot) response is exaggerated (often to > 200 mmHg systolic BP). On HUT there is often an excessive heart rate increment (to > 120 b min^{-1}). The most common diseases that cause the hyperadrenergic state are POTS and diabetic autonomic neuropathy.

I routinely measure supine and standing catecholamine levels. The rare case of dopamine-β-hydroxylase deficiency would presumably be diagnosed by the low dopamine-β-hydroxylase to norepinephrine level. I do not routinely measure serum vasodilators. In the patient with flushing and fluctuating BP, additional tests could then be carried out (24-h urinary metanephrine, 5-HIAA, histamine, prostaglandin D_2, serum vasoactive intestinal polypeptide [VIP], bradykinin).

Step 3 is pathophysiologically based treatment. A detailed description of this is beyond the scope of this chapter and only a brief description is provided. More detailed coverage is available [15,48,49].

Patients with POTS can have vasodepressor syncope but have preceding tachycardia. The different types of POTS require different management strategies [50,51]. All patients, especially the hypovolemic patient, requires volume expansion and increased salt intake. The neuropathic POTS subject responds to low-dose midodrine [52]. Beta-receptor supersensitivity responds to low-dose beta-blockers. Resistance training followed by endurance training can be beneficial.

The reflex syncopes are types of neurocardiogenic syncopes with identifiable triggers. These include carotid sinus pressure in carotid sinus supersensitivity and vagal stimulation in patients with vagal supersensitivity. Other triggers include the stimulation of areas supplied by the trigeminal and glossopharyngeal nerves. Some patients develop syncope with coitus, micturition, or vigorous coughing. Another form of reflex syncope is caused by CNS structural lesions such as an Arnold–Chiari malformation or third ventricle cyst.

In summary, it is important to improve understanding of the pathophysiology of syncope, seeking out neurologic causes that require a different approach to treatment. The patient with OH, limited autonomic failure, hyperadrenergic state, paraneoplastic, or intracerebral cause clearly needs specific management.

References

1 Low PA. Neurogenic orthostatic hypotension. In: Johnson JT, Griffin JW, eds. *Current Therapy in Neurologic Disease*, 4th edn. St. Louis: Mosby Year Book, 1993: 21–6.

2 Low PA, Opfer-Gehrking TL, McPhee BR, *et al.* Prospective evaluation of clinical characteristics of orthostatic hypotension. *Mayo Clin Proc* 1995;**70**;617–22.

3 Low PA, Bannister R. Multiple system atrophy and pure autonomic failure. In: Low PA, ed. *Clinical Autonomic Disorders: Evaluation and Management*, 2nd edn. Philadelphia: Lippincott-Raven, 1997: 555–75.

4 Low PA, Allsop JL, Halmagyi GM. Huntington's chorea: the rigid form (Westphal variant) treated with levodopa. *Med J Aust* 1974;**1**:393–4.

5 Sandroni P, Ahlskog JE, Fealey RD, Low PA. Autonomic involvement in extrapyramidal and cerebellar disorders. *Clin Auton Res* 1991;**1**:147–55.

6 Pakiam AS, Bergeron C, Lang AE. Diffuse Lewy body disease presenting as multiple system atrophy. *Can J Neurol Sci* 1999;**26**:127–31.

7 Thaisetthawatkul P, Boeve BF, Benarroch EE, *et al.* Autonomic dysfunction in dementia with Lewy bodies. *Neurology* (in press).

8 Low PA, Walsh JC, Huang CY, McLeod JG. The sympathetic nervous system in alcoholic neuropathy: a clinical and pathological study. *Brain* 1975;**98**:357–64.

9 Low PA, Walsh JC, Huang CY, McLeod JG. The sympathetic nervous system in diabetic neuropathy: a clinical and pathological study. *Brain* 1975;**98**:341–56.

10 Fujimura J, Camilleri M, Low PA, Novak V, Novak P, Opfer-Gehrking TL. Effect of perturbations and a meal on superior mesenteric artery flow in patients with orthostatic hypotension. *J Auton Nerv Syst* 1997;**67**:15–23.

11 Low PA, Vernino S, Suarez GA. Autonomic dysfunction in peripheral nerve disease. *Muscle Nerve* 2003;**27**:646–61.

12 Low PA. Diabetic autonomic neuropathy. *Semin Neurol* 1996;**16**:143–51.

13 Dyck PJ, Karnes JL, O'Brien PC, Litchy WJ, Low PA, Melton LJ III. The Rochester Diabetic Neuropathy Study: reassessment of tests and criteria for diagnosis and staged severity. *Neurology* 1992;**42**:1164–70.

14 Suarez GA, Fealey RD, Camilleri M, Low PA. Idiopathic autonomic neuropathy: clinical, neurophysiologic, and follow-up studies on 27 patients. *Neurology* 1994;**44**:1675–82.

15 Low PA, McLeod JG. Autonomic neuropathies. In: Low PA, ed. *Clinical Autonomic Disorders: Evaluation and Management*, 2nd edn. Philadelphia: Lippincott-Raven, 1997: 463–86.

16 Vernino S, Low PA, Fealey RD, Stewart JD, Farrugia G, Lennon VA. Autoantibodies to ganglionic acetylcholine receptors in autoimmune autonomic neuropathies. *N Engl J Med* 2000;**343**:847–55.

17 Klein CM, Vernino S, Lennon VA, *et al.* The spectrum of autoimmune autonomic neuropathies. *Ann Neurol* 2003;**53**:752–8.

18 Lee HR, Lennon VA, Camilleri M, Prather CM. Paraneoplastic gastrointestinal motor dysfunction: clinical and laboratory characteristics. *Am J Gastroenterol* 2001;**96**:373–9.

19 Asbury AK, Arnason BG, Karp HR, McFarlin DE. Criteria

for diagnosis of Guillain–Barré syndrome. *Ann Neurol* 1978;**3**:565–6.

20 Ropper AH, Wijdicks EFM. Blood pressure fluctuations in the dysautonomia of Guillain–Barré syndrome. *Arch Neurol* 1990;**27**:337.

21 Sandroni P, Opfer-Gehrking TL, Benarroch EE, Shen WK, Low PA. Certain cardiovascular indices predict syncope in the postural tachycardia syndrome. *Clin Auton Res* 1996;**6**:225–31.

22 Schondorf R, Low PA. Idiopathic postural tachycardia syndrome. In: Low PA, ed. *Clinical Autonomic Disorders: Evaluation and Management*. Boston: Little, Brown and Co, 1993: 641–52.

23 Jacob G, Ertl AC, Shannon JR, Robertson RM, Robertson D. Idiopathic orthostatic tachycardia: the role of dynamic orthostatic hypovolemia and norepinephrine. *Circulation* 1996;**94** (Suppl. I):627.

24 Cryer PE, Silverberg AB, Santiago JV, Shah SD. Plasma catecholamines in diabetes: the syndromes of hypoadrenergic and hyperadrenergic postural hypotension. *Am J Med* 1978;**64**:407–16.

25 Schnell O. Cardiac sympathetic innervation and blood flow regulation of the diabetic heart. *Diabetes Metab Res Rev* 2001;**17**:243–5.

26 Stevens MJ. New imaging techniques for cardiovascular autonomic neuropathy: a window on the heart. *Diabetes Technol Ther* 2001;**3**:9–22.

27 Robertson D. The epidemic of orthostatic tachycardia and orthostatic intolerance. *Am J Med Sci* 1999;**317**:75–7.

28 Rosen SG, Cryer PE. Postural tachycardia syndrome: reversal of sympathetic hyperresponsiveness and clinical improvement during sodium loading. *Am J Med* 1982;**72**:847–50.

29 Streeten DH. Pathogenesis of hyperadrenergic orthostatic hypotension: evidence of disordered venous innervation exclusively in the lower limbs. *J Clin Invest* 1990;**86**:1582–8.

30 Jacob G, Biaggioni I, Mosqueda-Garcia R, Robertson RM, Robertson D. Relation of blood volume and blood pressure in orthostatic intolerance. *Am J Med Sci* 1998;**315**:95–100.

31 Low PA, Benarroch EE, Suarez GA, Dotson RM. Clinical autonomic disorders. In: Joynt RJ, Griggs RC, eds. *Clinical Neurology*. Philadelphia: Lippincott-Raven, 1997: 1–91.

32 Benarroch EE, Chang SF. Central autonomic disorders. *J Clin Neurophysiol* 1993;**10**:39–50.

33 Strasberg B, Sagie A, Erdman S, Kusniec J, Sclarovsky S, Agmon J. Carotid sinus hypersensitivity and the carotid sinus syndrome. *Prog Cardiovasc Dis* 1989;**31**:379–91.

34 Weiss S, Baker JP. The carotid sinus reflex in health and disease: its role in the causation of fainting and convulsions. *Medicine* 1933;**12**:297–354.

35 Kapoor WN, Peterson JR, Karpf M. Micturition syncope: a reappraisal. *JAMA* 1985;**253**:796–8.

36 Biaggioni I, Goldstein DS, Atkinson T, Robertson D. Dopamine-β-hydroxylase deficiency in humans. *Neurology* 1990;**40**:370–3.

37 Mathias CJ, Bannister RB, Cortelli P, *et al.* Clinical autonomic and therapeutic observations in two siblings with postural hypotension and sympathetic failure due to an inability to synthesize noradrenaline from dopamine because of a deficiency of dopamine-β-hydroxylase. *Q J Med* 1990;**75**:617–33.

38 Streeten DH, Anderson GH Jr, Lebowitz M, Speller PJ. Primary hyperepinephrinemia in patients without pheochromocytoma. *Arch Intern Med* 1990;**150**:1528–33.

39 Verner JV, Morrison AB. Islet cell tumor and a syndrome of refractory watery diarrhea and hypokalemia. *Am J Med* 1958;**2**:374–80.

40 Streeten DH, Kerr CB, Kerr LP, Prior JC, Dalakos TG. Hyperbradykininism: a new orthostatic syndrome. *Lancet* 1972;**2**:1048–53.

41 Brooks DJ, Redmond S, Mathias CJ, Bannister R, Symon L. The effect of orthostatic hypotension on cerebral blood flow and middle cerebral artery velocity in autonomic failure, with observations on the action of ephedrine. *J Neurol Neurosurg Psychiatry* 1989;**52**:962–6.

42 Thomas DJ, Bannister R. Preservation of autoregulation of cerebral blood flow in autonomic failure. *J Neurol Sci* 1980;**44**:205–12.

43 Shannon JR, Jordan J, Diedrich A, *et al.* Sympathetically mediated hypertension in autonomic failure. *Circulation* 2000;**101**:2710–5.

44 Stevens MJ, Dayanikli F, Raffel DM, *et al.* Scintigraphic assessment of regionalized defects in myocardial sympathetic innervation and blood flow regulation in diabetic patients with autonomic neuropathy. *J Am Coll Cardiol* 1998;**31**:1575–84.

45 Benarroch EE, Schmeichel AM, Parisi JE. Involvement of the ventrolateral medulla in parkinsonism with autonomic failure. *Neurology* 2000;**54**:963–8.

46 Slaugenhaupt SA, Blumenfeld A, Gill SP, *et al.* Tissue-specific expression of a splicing mutation in the *IKBKAP* gene causes familial dysautonomia. *Am J Hum Genet* 2001;**68**:598–605.

47 Denq JC, O'Brien PC, Low PA. Normative data on phases of the Valsalva maneuver. *J Clin Neurophysiol* 1998;**15**: 535–40.

48 Fealey RD, Robertson D. Management of orthostatic hypotension. In: Low PA, ed. *Clinical Autonomic Disorders: Evaluation and Management*, 2nd edn. Philadelphia: Lippincott-Raven, 1997: 763–75.

49 Low PA. Neurogenic orthostatic hypotension. In: Johnson R, ed. *Current Therapy in Neurologic Disease*, 4th edn. Philadelphia: Mosby Year Book, 1994.

50 Low PA, Opfer-Gehrking TL, Textor SC, *et al.* Postural tachycardia syndrome (POTS). *Neurology* 1995;**45**:S19–S25.

51 Low PA, Schondorf R, Novak V, Sandroni P, Opfer-Gehrking TL, Novak P. Postural tachycardia syndrome. In: Low PA, ed. *Clinical Autonomic Disorders: Evaluation and Management*, 2nd edn. Philadelphia: Lippincott-Raven, 1997: 681–97.

52 Ward C, Kenny RA. Observations on midodrine in a case of vasodepressor neurogenic syncope. *Clin Auton Res* 1995;**5**:257–60.

CHAPTER 10

Structural and obstructive causes of cardiovascular syncope

Blair P. Grubb, MD, *& Yousuf Kanjwal,* MD

Introduction

Conditions that impair cardiac output can cause syncope. Specific conditions that impair left ventricular outflow include: aortic stenosis, hypertrophic cardiomyopathy, obstruction of prosthetic heart valves, and cardiac tumors. Alternatively, blood flow may be impaired by other means. These include pulmonary hypertension and embolism, cardiac tamponade, and aortic dissection.

Obstructive causes for syncope

(Table 10.1)

Aortic valve stenosis (AS) results in an inability of the valve to open fully, thus impeding left ventricular emptying and reducing cardiac output. The obstruction may be at the level of the valve, below the valve (subvalvular), or, rarely, above the valve (supravalvular) [1]. The most frequent causes of AS are congenital malformation, rheumatic fever, or valve calcification (senile or degenerative AS) [2]. Congenital AS is discussed in Chapter 16.

Table 10.1 Obstructive causes of syncope.

Aortic stenosis
Hypertrophic cardiomyopathy
Obstruction of prosthetic heart valves
Cardiac tumors
Pulmonary hypertension
Pulmonary embolism
Cardiac tamponade
Aortic dissection

Rheumatic AS occurs because of adhesions and fusion of the cusps and commissures, with subsequent retraction and stiffening of the cusps. Rheumatic AS is uncommon in the developed world and congenital bicuspid aortic valve, seen in approximately 2% of births, has become a much more common cause of AS [3]. The altered blood flow pattern across the malformed valve produces a progressive trauma to the valve cusps leading to fibrosis and calcification. Approximately 30% of patients with bicuspid valves will develop AS before age 70 years [2].

Senile or degenerative changes to the valve are an increasingly frequent cause of AS. Approximately 40% of those over age 60 years have mild aortic valve calcification on echocardiography [4]. By age 85 years the proportion is 75%. Critical AS becomes increasingly frequent with age, affecting 2% of people over the age of 75 years and 6% of those older than 85 years. Senile, degenerative AS was thought to be caused by repeated minor trauma to the valve, leading to calcium deposition and fibrosis but recent observations suggest that it may be the result of an immune reaction to antigens present in the valve [5].

Aortic stenosis may be relatively asymptomatic even in severe cases. Syncope may be the presenting symptom in up to one-quarter of patients [6]. While most commonly seen following exertion, syncope may also be seen after rapid changes in position (such as standing) or following exposure to intense heat (such as a hot bath or sauna). Often this is brought about by systemic vasodilation that occurs in the presence of a fixed or inadequate cardiac output. Stimulation of left ventricular mechanoreceptors by elevated intracavitary pressure may result in reflex vasodilation (similar to that felt to occur in neurocardiogenic syncope) leading to hypotension, bradycardia, and cerebral hypoperfusion [7]. Syncope may occur at rest because of a ventricular tachyarrhythmia resulting from AS [8]. Other causes of syncope in AS are atrial fibrillation and transient atrioventricular block. During atrial fibrillation, the hypertrophied left ventricle loses its much needed "booster pump" that is especially important as AS causes diastolic dysfunction that results in reduction in diastolic filling.

The diagnosis of AS is made through auscultation of a systolic murmur that usually peaks in mid-systole and is heard best in the second intercostal space. An absent A2, a late peaking murmur, absence of a previous murmur, a thrill, a prolonged and late carotid impulse ("pulsus tardis et parvis") portends a poor prognosis [9]. After physical examination, electrocardiogram and chest X-ray, echocardiography with Doppler ultrasound is the most useful diagnostic tool [10]. It can demonstrate a grossly thickened, poorly mobile valve with a large valve pressure gradient and a small valve area.

Confusion sometimes occurs regarding the gradient measurements by continuous wave Doppler. The measurement is not the same as pressure gradient measurements assessed during cardiac catheterization. The peak measured by Doppler is the peak instantaneous gradient. This is usually higher than the peak-to-peak gradient measured during catheterization. Cardiac catheterization is often the employed "gold standard" for gradient determination, aortic valve area, and the possible presence and severity of coronary atherosclerosis. Severe AS is present when the peak-to-peak catheter gradient exceeds 50 mmHg or the Doppler instantaneous gradient exceeds 70–80 mmHg. The prognosis of patients with severe AS is poor, with a 50% mortality at 5 years and a 90% mortality at 10 years. Syncope adds to the poor prognosis. The mean survival after syncope in patients with AS is approximately 2 years. Most AS patients with syncope die within 3 years [11,12]. The most effective therapy for AS is valve replacement. Syncope, if it occurs after valve replacement in patients with AS, is caused by AV block or ventricular tachyarrhythmias.

Patients with critical mitral stenosis have a propensity toward left atrial thrombus formation (Fig. 10.1). While these thrombi are often flat against the atrial wall, they may on occasion be mobile and behave much like a "ball-valve" thrombus [13]. Occlusion of the already stenotic mitral valve may result in syncope or, more rarely, in sudden death (Fig. 10.2).

Hypertrophic cardiomyopathy (HCM), an important cause for syncope, is a heterogeneous, inherited group of disorders manifest as a pathologic thickening of the left ventricular wall in the presence of a non-dilated cavity [14]. It occurs independent of any systemic or cardiac disease that could be responsible for producing the degree of hypertrophy present. HCM is an autosomal dominant genetic disorder with a high degree of penetrance [15]. Several forms exist. Mutations of the cardiac β-myosin heavy-chain (β-*MHC*) gene cause HCM. Up to 50% of cases of HCM may be caused by spontaneous mutations. Between 1 in 500 and 1 in 1000 people in the general population have this condition.

While the classic form of HCM is associated with asymmetric hypertrophy of the interventricular septum and obstruction (Fig. 10.2), other patterns occur (indeed, outflow tract obstruction is present in only 25%). These include isolated areas of hypertrophy involving apex or posterior left ventricle, right ventricular involvement, and concentric left ventricular hypertrophy [16]. The normal parallel arrangement of myocytes is altered with fibrosis and gross muscle bundle disorganization at oblique and perpendicular angles to each other. The process disturbs systolic and diastolic function. There is early and complete left ventricular emptying with cavity obliteration at the end of systole. Obstruction to left ventricular outflow is possible and can be intermittent depending on contractility, ventricular volume, hydration status, and catecholamine level. Mitral regurgitation can also occur [17]. The abnormal cellular arrangement may result in ventricular tachycardia, while atrial fibrillation may cause a loss of the atrial contribution to already compromised ventricular filling.

Patients with HCM may die suddenly and HCM is one of the most common causes of sudden death among athletes (even though the overall risk is small) [18]. The annual mortality for adult HCM

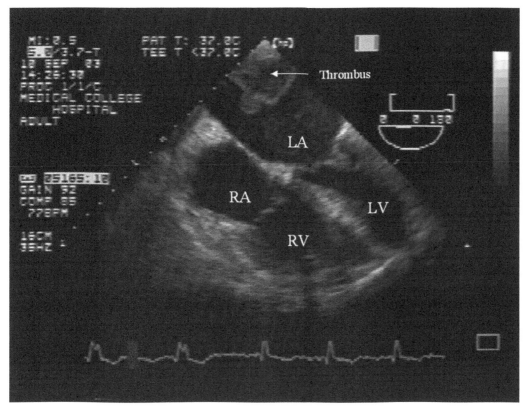

Fig. 10.1 Echocardiogram of a left atrial thrombus. LA, left atrium; LV, left ventricle; RA, right atrium; RV, right ventricle.

patients is 1–2.5%, while for children and adolescents it may be as high as 6%. Thirty-six percent of young athletes who die suddenly have definite or probable HCM [18].

Proposed risk factors for sudden cardiac death (SCD) in HCM are youth, a family history of SCD, extreme thickness of the left ventricle (septal thickness > 30 mm), and ventricular tachycardia [19]. Exercise-induced hypotension may be a risk factor for a poor prognosis. Syncope is reported to occur in 15–20% of HCM patients with or without exertion. In some patients, outflow tract obstruction limits blood flow, while in others, abnormal mechanoreceptor activation may cause systemic vasodilation. Syncope can result in either case.

Treatment includes: negative inotropic drugs such as beta-blockers, calcium-channel blockers, and disopyramide. Amiodarone has been used to prevent atrial fibrillation and ventricular tachycardia (but is not shown to be very effective). Dual-chamber pacing has been reported to decrease the

obstructive gradient in some patients but its use remains controversial [14]. Increasingly, implantable cardioverter defibrillators (ICDs) are being used to decrease the patient's risk of arrhythmic death [19] (see Chapter 8). Surgical therapy involving septal myomectomy has been used to relieve severe symptoms resulting from outflow tract obstruction.

Patients with syncope and HCM require careful evaluation that includes: echocardiogram, Holter and other risk assessments (e.g., stress test, electrophysiologic study).

Mobile tumors in the left atrium may occlude the mitral valve intermittently and obstruct forward blood flow to impede cardiac output [20]. Syncope often occurs when the patient changes position. This can alter the degree of obstruction present. Myxomas, the most common primary cardiac tumors, account for approximately one-quarter of cardiac tumors (Fig. 10.3). While myxomas can occur in any cardiac chambers, 75% occur in the

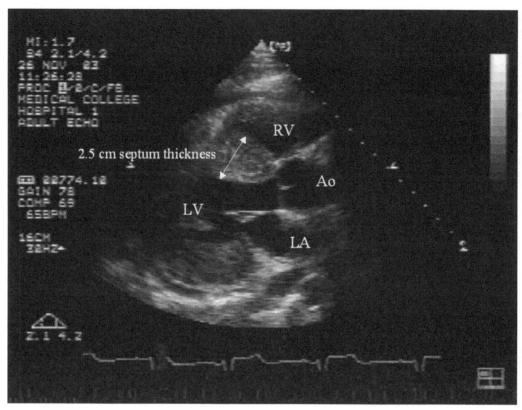

Fig. 10.2 Echocardiogram of hyspertrophic cardiomyopathy. Ao, aorta; LA, left atrium; LV, left ventricle; RV, right ventricle.

left atrium; 5% are bi-atrial [21]. They can present as a systemic autoimmune disease. On occasion, malignancies from other sites may spread to the heart and behave similar to a myxoma; the most common origins are breast and lung cancer, lymphoma and melanoma, but they can also arise from the liver, larynx, and by direct extension from the pericardium and adjacent structures. Other tumors that can cause obstruction and syncope include: lipomas, angiosarcomas, leiomyosarcomas, rhabdomyomas, and malignant hemangiosarcomas [22]. Cardiac fibromas can mimic HCM. Increased plasma concentration of atrial natiuretic factor with changes in serum sodium, hypotension, and syncope has been seen with squamous cell carcinoma invasion of the right and left atria.

Obstruction of a mechanical prosthetic heart valve, especially in the aortic and mitral valve position, may precipitate syncope [23]. Usually, the obstruction is caused by a thrombus or fibrous pannus (Fig. 10.4). These appear to occur more frequently in tilting disk style valves. In addition to syncope, patients with prosthetic valve obstructions may present with unexplained heart failure, angina, hypotension, peripheral embolism, or cardiogenic shock. A high level of suspicion, a careful physical examination, and an echocardiogram are keys to the diagnosis.

As many as 13% of patients with pulmonary embolism present with syncope [24]. Syncope may be the first symptom of pulmonary embolism resulting from a sudden reduction in cardiac output [25]. When consciousness resumes, the patient can display peripheral and central cyanosis, right heart failure, and hypotension [26]. There are several potential reasons why this can occur. Cardiac output can be reduced because of obstruction of the pulmonary arteries. Syncope may result from a reflex (vagal) response to mechanoreceptor activation from a sudden, right ventricular volume overload. Typical risk factors and typical signs of pulmonary embolism may or may not be present

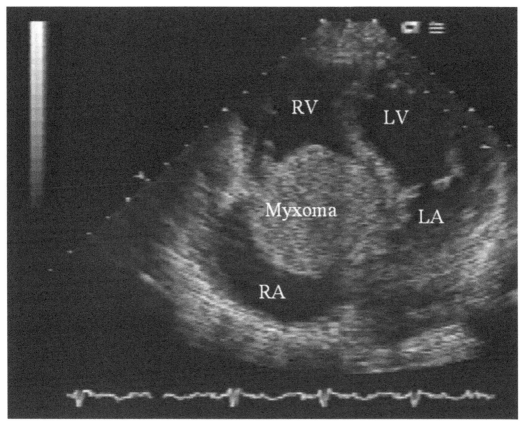

Fig. 10.3 Echocardiogram of a large atrial myxoma. LA, left atrium; LV, left ventricle; RA, right atrium; RV, right ventricle.

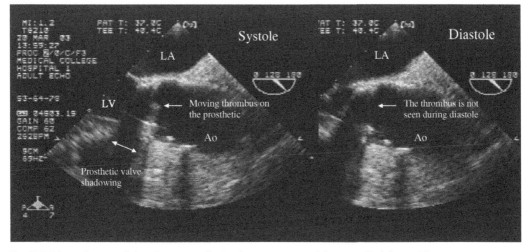

Fig. 10.4 Echocardiogram of thrombus on prosthetic valve. Ao, aorta; LA, left atrium; LV, left ventricle.

when a patient with extensive pulmonary emboli presents in an emergency situation with syncope [26]. A high level of suspicion and a proper diagnostic approach is critical to institute life-saving therapy. Right heart failure, a hallmark of extensive pulmonary embolism causing syncope, can be manifest by high brain natiuretic peptide (BNP) levels, even though BNP levels do not predict prognosis in this condition [27].

Patients with cardiac papillary fibroelastoma can present with acute pulmonary embolism similar to other right-sided tumors. Indwelling right-sided catheters can lead to extensive pulmonary emboli.

The magnitude of pulmonary artery obstruction required to produce syncope is great and should prompt rapid institution of definitive therapy with anticoagulation, thrombolytic therapy, and surgical or percutaneous embolectomy. The mortality is high with any therapeutic approach [28].

Pulmonary hypertension is most commonly caused by chronic cardiac or pulmonary disease. Idiopathic or "primary" pulmonary hypertension and *in situ* pulmonary thromboembolic disease may occur in the absence of any other cause [29]. In either the primary or secondary forms of the disorder, there is a high pulmonary vascular resistance so that cardiac output becomes compromised.

Presyncope or syncope may occur because of the inability of the right ventricle to move sufficient blood through the obstructed pulmonary vasculature to meet the body's needs [30]. Commonly, the reflex response to right ventricular pressure overload is asystole and marked peripheral vasodilation that causes hemodynamic collapse by a neurocardiogenic mechanism. Asystole can be preceded by marked sinus tachycardia. The approach to therapy is not to slow the rate but to improve pulmonary hemodynamics.

Syncope may occur in as many as 55% of patients with pulmonary hypertension and is more common in patients with the primary form [30]. Chronic right ventricular pressure overload may result in either right ventricular hypertrophy and/or right atrial enlargement. These conditions can predispose the patient to supraventricular and/or ventricular arrhythmias, another cause for syncope and sudden death in this population.

Acute or chronic cardiac tamponade may trigger syncope. The common presentation is hypotension and bradycardia rather than tachycardia [31].

Almost any disease that affects the pericardium may produce a pericardial effusion [32]. Similarly, tamponade may occur resulting from any pericardial effusion (Fig. 10.5). Acute cardiac tamponade may develop so suddenly that there are few if any prodromic signs. It is most often the result either of trauma (either penetrating or blunt), or of rupture of the heart or aorta because of an aneurysm, myocardial infarction, or aortic dissection.

Acute tamponade may arise as a complication of a procedure such as electrophysiology testing, radiofrequency catheter ablation, pacemaker or implantable defibrillator placement, cardiac catheterization, angioplasty, or central line placement [31]. Syncope occurs very quickly in these patients, usually occurring at (or very soon after) the moment of perforation or rupture.

Subacute cardiac tamponade may occur as a result of a vast number of conditions. The most common causes are idiopathic, viral, malignancy, and renal insufficiency [32]. Syncope may occur as a consequence of decreased cardiac filling with subsequent hypotension or a neurocardiogenic reflex with precipitous hypotension and bradycardia. This may be compounded by other issues such as dehydration, blood loss, or any condition causing vasodilation (excess heat or drugs) or an arrhythmia (perhaps even initiated by the process causing the effusion).

The diagnosis is often suspected from the clinical setting and physical signs such as a marked elevation of the jugular venous pressure, pulsus paradoxus, systemic hypotension, muffled cardiac sounds, and cold diaphoretic extremities. Whenever cardiac tamponade is suspected, two-dimensional echocardiography should be performed as soon as possible, which will usually confirm the diagnosis. Right heart catheterization should be performed if the diagnosis is in question, with careful comparison of right atrial and pulmonary wedge pressures. In patients with significant hemodynamic compromise, drainage of pericardial fluid, by either pericardiocentesis or open surgical drainage, should be performed.

While most commonly seen in men aged 50–70 years, aortic dissection has also been reported in the elderly and in children [33]. The condition usually presents with sudden severe pain that is variously described as cutting, tearing, or ripping. There are two aspects of the pain that help distinguish it from

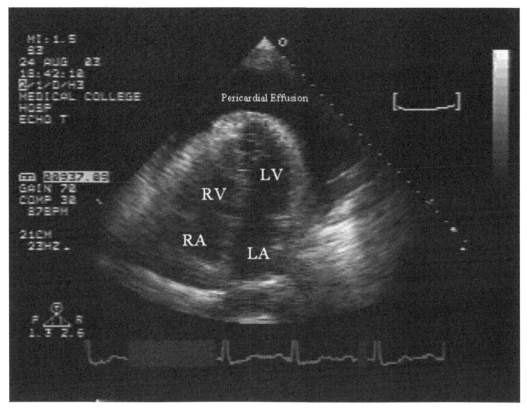

Fig. 10.5 Pericardial effusion and tamponade. LA, left atrium; LV, left ventricle; RA, right atrium; RV, right ventricle.

other conditions. Rather than increasing over time, the pain is most intense at the beginning. In addition, the pain is often located either sequentially or simultaneously over the anterior chest, the intrascapular area, and the epigastrium or lumbar areas [34].

Syncope is the most common neurologic event to accompany dissection and carries with it a poor prognosis [33]. It may result as a consequence of the severe pain or because of a mechanical disturbance resulting from dissection back into the pericardium with subsequent tamponade or flow through the cerebral vessels.

Aortic dissection is suggested in patients who present following collapse associated with severe chest and back pain. While the patient appears to be in shock, the blood pressure may be normal or elevated (although approximately 20% present with hypotension). Other signs of aortic dissection include aortic regurgitation, pulse deficits, and local neurologic disturbances. Control of blood pressure should be rapidly obtained with sodium nitroprusside or a beta-blocker such as labetalol [35]. A chest X-ray will show an abnormal aortic shadow in 80–90% of cases. Confirmation of the diagnosis is made either by transesophageal echocardiography or computed tomography following contrast administration. Magnetic resonance imaging may also be helpful, but often takes longer to perform. For those patients with dissections of the ascending aorta, surgery is recommended, whereas those with descending dissections are usually treated medically.

Conclusions

Structural or obstructive causes should be considered in patients presenting with syncope. Often, these conditions can be uncovered through the use of two-dimensional echocardiography and Doppler ultrasonography (and on occasion transesophageal echocardiography).

References

1 Roberts WC. Valvular, subvalvular and supravalvular aortic stenosis. *Cardiovasc Clin* 1973;**5**:97–101.

2 Braunwald E, Goldblatt A, Aygen NM, Rockoff SD, Morrow AG. Congenital aortic stenosis. I. Clinical and hemodynamic findings in 100 patients. *Circulation* 1963;**27**:426–62.

3 Passik CS, Ackerman DM, Pluth JR, Edwards WD. Temporal changes in the causes of aortic stenosis: a surgical pathologic study of 646 cases. *Mayo Clin Proc* 1987;**62**:119–23.

4 Lindross K, Kupari M, Heikkila J, Tilvis R. Prevalence of aortic valve abnormalities in the elderly: an echocardiographic study of a random population. *J Am Coll Cardiol* 1993;**21**:1220–5.

5 Olsson N, Dalsgarro CJ, Haegerstrand A, *et al.* Accumulation of T lymphocytes and expression of interleukin-2 receptors in non-rheumatic stenotic aortic valves. *J Am Coll Cardiol* 1994;**23**:1162–70.

6 Schwartz LS, Goldfisher J, Sprague GL, Schartz SP. Syncope and sudden death in aortic stenosis. *Am J Cardiol* 1969;**23**:647–58.

7 Grech ED, Ramsdale DR. Exertional syncope in aortic stenosis: evidence to support inappropriate left ventricular baroreceptor response. *Am Heart J* 1991;**121**:603–6.

8 Kulbertus HE. Ventricular arrhythmias, syncope and sudden death in aortic stenosis. *Eur Heart J* 1988;**9**(Suppl. E):51–2.

9 Selzer A. Changing aspects in the natural history of valvular aortic stenosis. *N Engl J Med* 1987;**31**:91–8.

10 Rahimtoala SH. Valvular heart disease: a perspective. *J Am Coll Cardiol* 1983;**1**:199–215.

11 Hoagland PM, Cook EF, Wynne J, Goldman L. Value of non-invasive testing in adults with suspected aortic stenosis. *Am J Med* 1986;**80**:1041–58.

12 Roger VL, Tajik AJ, Reader GS, *et al.* Effect of Doppler echocardiography on utilization of hemodynamic cardiac catheterization in the perioperative evaluation of aortic stenosis. *Mayo Clinic Proc* 1996;**71**:141–9.

13 Fraser AG, Angelini GD, Ikram S, Butchart EG. Left atrial ball thrombus: echocardiographic features and clinical implications. *Eur Heart J* 1988;**9**:672–7.

14 Nishimura RA, Holmes DR Jr. Hypertrophic cardiomyopathy. *N Engl J Med* 2004;**350**(13):1320–7.

15 Maron BJ. Hypertrophic cardiomyopathy. *JAMA* 2002; **287**:1308–20.

16 Wigle ED, Sasson Z, Henderson MA, *et al.* Hypertrophic cardiomyopathy: the importance of the site and the extent of the hypertrophy – a review. *Prog Cardiovasc Dis* 1985;**28**:1–83.

17 Braunwald E, Seidman CE, Sigwart V. Contemporary evaluation and management of hypertrophic cardiomyopathy. *Circulation* 2002;**106**:1312–6.

18 Maron BJ. Sudden death in young athletes. *N Engl J Med* 2003;**349**:1064–75.

19 Maron BJ, Shen WK, Link MS, *et al.* Efficacy of implantable cardioverter-defibrillators for the prevention of sudden death in patients with hypertrophic cardiomyopathy. *N Engl J Med* 2000;**342**:365–73.

20 Salcedo EE, Cohen GI, White RD, David MB. Cardiac tumors: diagnosis and management. *Curr Probl Cardiol* 1992;**17**:73–137.

21 Fine G. Primary tumors of the pericardium and heart. *Cardiovasc Clin* 1973;**5**:207–8.

22 Burke AP, Cowan D, Virmani R. Primary sarcomas of the heart. *Cancer* 1991;**67**:2066–70.

23 Hausmann D, Mugge A, Daniel NG. Valve thrombosis: diagnosis and management. In: Butchart EG, Bodnar G, eds. *Current Issues in Heart Valve Disease: Thrombosis, Embolism, and Bleeding*. London, UK: ICR, 1992: 387–401.

24 Thames M, Alpert J, Dalen J. Syncope in patients with pulmonary embolism. *JAMA* 1997;**238**:2509–11.

25 Wilk J, Nardone A, Jennings C, *et al.* Unexplained syncope: when to expect pulmonary embolism. *Geriatrics* 1995;**50**(10):46–50.

26 Ryo JH, Olson EJ, Pellikka PA. Clinical recognition of pulmonary embolism: problem of unrecognized and asymptomatic cases. *Mayo Clin Proc* 1998;**73**:873–9.

27 Riberio A, Lindmarker P, Johnsson H, *et al.* Pulmonary embolism: one year follow up with echocardiography Doppler and five year survival analysis. *Circulation* 1999; **99**:1325–30.

28 Peterson KL. Acute pulmonary thromboembolism: has its evaluation been redefined? *Circulation* 1999;**99**:1280–3.

29 Fedullo PF, Auger WR, Kerr KM, Rubin LT. Chronic thromboembolic pulmonary hypertension. *N Engl J Med* 2001;**345**:1465–72.

30 Fishman AP. Pulmonary hypertension and cor pulmonale. In: Fishman AP, ed. *Pulmonary Diseases and Disorders*, 2nd edn. New York, NY: McGraw Hill, 1988: 999–1048.

31 Reddy PS, Curtis EI, O'Toole SD, Shaver JA. Cardiac tamponade: hemodynamic observations in man. *Circulation* 1978;**58**:265–72.

32 Shabetai R. *The Pericardium*. New York, NY: Grune & Stratton, 1981:206–8.

33 Crawford ES. The diagnosis and management of aortic dissection. *JAMA* 1990;**264**:2537–41.

34 Roberts WC. Aortic dissection: anatomy, consequences and causes. *Am Heart J* 1981;**101**:195–214.

35 Glower DD, Fann JI, Speier RH, *et al.* Comparison of medical and surgical therapy of uncomplicated descending aortic dissection. *Circulation* 1990;**82**(Suppl. 4):39–46.

CHAPTER 11

Inherited arrhythmic and related causes of syncope

Blair P. Grubb, MD, *& Brian Olshansky,* MD

Introduction

Syncope can result from ventricular arrhythmias that occur as a consequence of ultrastructural changes in the ion channels of cardiac myocytes which disturb normal repolarization or from larger disturbances in cardiac architecture. Examples of the former include the congenital long QT syndrome (LQTS), short QT syndrome, and Brugada syndrome; the latter is represented by arrhythmogenic right ventricular cardiomyopathy.

Long QT syndromes

The long QT syndrome(s) may be primary (or congenital) or secondary to other causes (commonly, drugs that prolong cardiac repolarization) [1]. Drug-induced LQTS occurs much more frequently than its congenital counterpart, and the list of pharmacologic agents capable of lengthening cardiac repolarization continues to increase [2]. There is a steadily growing risk of unintended iatrogenic LQTS; namely, prolongation of cardiac repolarization to such a point that polymorphic ventricular tachycardia occurs. Polymorphic ventricular tachycardias tend to be more unstable than monomorphic tachycardias, have much faster rates, and are generally of shorter duration than monomorphic ventricular tachycardias (or degenerate to ventricular fibrillation) [3]. They lower cardiac output to a greater extent, resulting in near-syncope and syncope. The type of polymorphic ventricular tachycardia most commonly associated with LQTS is characterized by peaks and troughs in the QRS complex that appear to twist around the baseline (torsade de pointes) [4]. Physicians need to pay greater attention to the possibility of drug-induced LQTS, especially when multiple drugs are used together. Therapy is aimed at initially stabilizing the patient, then identifying and stopping the responsible medication.

The primary or congenital LQTSs are a group of disorders, generally familial and present from childhood, characterized by prolonged cardiac repolarization time. This is reflected by a long QT interval and/or prominent U waves on a 12-lead electrocardiogram (ECG) (Fig. 11.1) [5]. The two principal clinical presentations have been described. The first was reported in 1957 in a family with several children who suffered from congenital nerve deafness and who were noted to have QT prolongation. These individuals had a high incidence of syncope and sudden death, with an inheritance pattern suggestive of an autosomal recessive trait (the Jervell–Lange-Nielsen syndrome) [6]. Several years later a similar, more frequent condition not associated with deafness and an autosomal dominant inheritance was reported (the Romano–Ward syndrome) [7,8].

Recent investigations into the molecular genetics of the disorder have revealed that they occur because of inherited defects in membrane ion channel molecular structure and function [1]. At least six different gene mutations have been identified and appear to be associated with distant patterns of clinical, genotypic, and phenotypic presentation. While the hallmark of the condition is a prolonged QT, there are some individuals in whom the base-

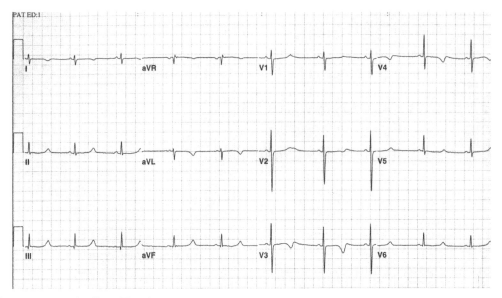

Fig. 11.1 An example of long QT syndrome.

line QT interval may be within normal limits. Individuals may present with syncope, sudden death, or the incidental finding of QT prolongation on ECG. Syncope often starts to occur when the patient is young, frequently between 5 and 15 years of age [9]. Although in the majority of LQTS patients syncope (or sudden death) tends to be initiated by exercise (LQT1) or acute arousal type emotions (LQT2), a small subgroup may experience events associated with bradycardia during sleep or at rest (LQT3) [10] (Table 11.1). Diagnostic criteria have been published to aid in determining the diagnosis of LQTS, with a scoring system that places patients into high, intermediate, or low risk of having LQTS (Table 11.2). Several factors appear to select out individuals at increased risk of sudden death: a prior episode of aborted sudden death, a family history of sudden death, syncope beginning at a young age, a very prolonged QT interval (> 600 ms), and if the individual suffers from the recessive form of LQTS associated with congenital deafness (Jervell–Lange-Nielsen syndrome).

For the most part, individuals suffering from LQTS should avoid competitive sports and even very vigorous exercise [11]. Extreme care should be taken to avoid exposure to drugs known to prolong

Table 11.1 Clinical triggers in long QT syndrome.

Type	Triggers
LQT1	Stress, exercise
LQT2	Noise
LQT3	Sleep, rest
LQT6	Drugs, exercise

LQT, long QT syndrome.

QT interval. First-line therapy for most patients is a beta-blocking drug (except in the LQT3 or bradycardic form, where pacemaker or implanted cardioverter defibrillator [ICD] placement is warranted). ICD placement should be considered in patients with multiple risk factors for sudden death or those who have syncope despite beta-blockade [1].

The expanding information on the nature of the genetically produced ion channel disorders that cause LQTS may lead to novel and more specific therapies in the near future.

Long QT syndrome may also be caused in otherwise normal individuals by exposure to drugs that

Table 11.2 Diagnostic criteria for long QT syndrome (LQTS) [1,11].

Electrocardiographic criteria	Points
Corrected QT interval*	
> 0.48 s	3
0.46–0.47 s	2
0.45 s (in men)	1
Torsade de pointes†	2
T-wave alternans	1
Notched T-wave 3 leads	1
Low heart rate for age	0.5
Clinical history	
Syncope	
during stress	2
without stress	1
Congenital deafness	0.5
Family history‡	
LQTS in family members	1
Unexplained sudden death (under 30 years of age) among immediate family members	0.5

* The corrected QT interval (QT$_c$) is $QT_c = {}^{QT}/_{\sqrt{RR}}$
Torsade de pointes and syncope are mutually exclusive.
† A resting heart rate before the second percentile for age.
‡ The same family member should not be counted in both groups.

prolong repolarization (acquired LQTS). The most common agents responsible are the antiarrhythmic drugs (quinidine being the classic example but also other type IA and type III antiarrhythmics) that cause prolongation of the QT interval prior to the onset of the arrhythmia [2]. Other risk factors include bradycardia, hypomagnesemia, and hypokalemia. QT prolongation by the class IA agents appears to be an idiosyncratic reaction that occurs among a small predisposed subgroup of individuals (although no specific inheritance pattern has been seen) [4]. Commonly, the type III agents, such as sotalol, cause a dose-dependent prolongation in the QT interval. There are a number of other drugs that may prolong QT duration, including phenothiazines, pentamidine, cocaine, certain antibiotics, cocaine, and terfenadine, to name but a few

[12]. Other causes of acquired LQTS include liquid protein diets, myocardial ischemia, and acute central nervous system injury [2,5].

Recently, it has been found that there is also a "short QT syndrome" which may also lead to arrhythmias, syncope, and sudden death [13]. An autosomal dominant inheritance pattern has been seen, and a gene defect resulting in hyperactivity of potassium ion channels has also been identified [14]. It has been postulated that lone atrial fibrillation may possibly be related to short QT syndrome [15].

The Brugada syndrome

It has been known for many years that men from specific oriental populations are at risk for sudden cardiac death during sleep. This was called Pokkuri or Bangangut [15]. In 1992, Brugada and Brugada [16] described eight patients who had recurrent episodes of aborted sudden death who did not have any demonstrable structural heart disease. Their ECGs all showed ST segment elevation in the precordial leads V$_1$–V$_3$ with a QRS morphology resembling a right bundle branch block (and resembling J point elevation).

The syndrome appears to be genetic with an autosomal dominant transmission [15]. Patients with Brugada syndrome may develop episodes of polymorphic ventricular tachycardia (not dissimilar to LQTS) that may end spontaneously and thus cause syncope, or may degenerate into ventricular fibrillation and lead to sudden death [17]. The disorder appears to occur as a result of an early inactivation of the myocardial sodium channel causing early epicardial repolarization (resulting in the ST segment elevation seen on ECG). This produces a "dispersion of refractoriness" necessary for the polymorphic VT to occur. Sodium channel blocking drugs enhance this tendency, as does an increase in vagal stimulation. Conversely, exercise decreases it.

Interestingly, the ECG may change over time from fully normal to one with typical Brugada characteristics. In patients who are thought to have Brugada syndrome with a normal ECG, the intravenous infusion of a sodium channel blocking

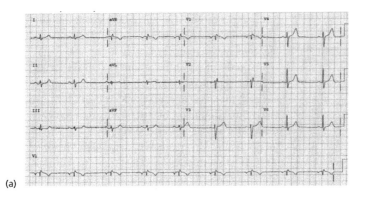

(a)

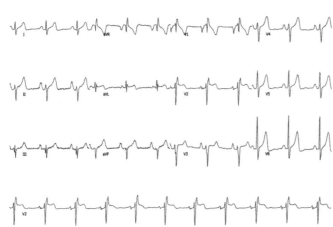

(b)

Fig. 11.2 An electrocardiogram of Brugada syndrome. (a) Before procainamide. (b) After procainamide. The classic pattern is not apparent until after procainamide infusion.

agent (a type I antiarrhythmic such as procainamide) will provide the typical ECG changes and help to establish the diagnosis (Fig. 11.2a,b) [15].

While the prognosis of asymptomatic patients with the Brugada syndrome is unclear, those who have syncope or a family history of sudden death (or have themselves already suffered an aborted sudden death episode) have a high mortality. A recent study reported that the strongest predictor of outcome in patients with an ECG diagnostic of Brugada syndrome was inducibility of arrhythmias by programmed stimulation performed during electrophysiologic study [17]. Because no antiarrhythmic agent has been shown to be effective,

high-risk patients with Brugada syndrome should undergo ICD placement [15,17].

Arrhythmogenic right ventricular cardiomyopathy

In 1996, the World Health Organization introduced the term "arrhythmogenic right ventricular cardiomyopathy" (ARVC) to describe a group of disorders that produce ventricular tachycardia and share similar histopathologic patterns, but have different clinical presentations and outcomes [18]. The most common and well known of these is "arrhythmogenic right ventricular dysplasia"

(ARVD), a condition that results from either a segmental or diffuse lack of myocardium in the free wall of the right ventricle, which is replaced by fibrous and/or fatty tissue [19]. Two different pathologic forms have been identified [20]. The first (or classic) form demonstrates myocardial thinning and myocyte atrophy with replacement by a mixture of fat and fibrous tissue [21]. It most commonly involves the right ventricular outflow tract infundibulum as well as the lateral apical region (sometimes called the "triangle of dysplasia") [22]. Lymphocytic infiltrates and aneurismal dilation is common. The second type (pure adipose form) is characterized by a significant (near total) replacement of the right ventricle by fatty tissue, especially in the infundibulum and apex [23]. As opposed to the classic form, there is an absence of inflammatory infiltrates, fibrosis, or myocyte atrophy in the affected myocardium. In either case, the resultant myocardial disruption results in disturbed conduction and repolarization that gives rise to ventricular arrhythmias [20].

ARVD is much more common in males and generally presents in adolescents or young adults (mean age 33 ± 14 years). The prevalence is not exactly known, but current estimates place it at 6 in 10,000 [20]. In some localities (such as northern Italy) the prevalence may be as high as 4.4 in 1000, and may account for 20% of the sudden deaths in young adults and 25% of sudden cardiac deaths among athletes [24–26].

The most common presenting symptoms are palpitations, syncope, and sudden death [20]. The most common arrhythmia is ventricular tachycardia of right ventricular origin with a left bundle branch pattern. Diagnosis is based on a series of major and minor criteria based on histologic, structural, arrhythmic, electrocardiographic, and genetic factors. Of the potential diagnostic modalities, magnetic resonance imaging with T_1-weighted spin echo sequences are the most useful [27].

Other forms of ARVC have also been described. Naxos disease has been described on the Greek island of Naxos [28]. Patients also demonstrate palmoplantar keratomas and "woolly" (curly) hair, as well as ARVD. Venetian cardiomyopathy (also known as right ventricular cardiomyopathy) clearly resembles ARVD, but with a higher degree of familial penetrance. Uhl's anomaly demonstrates a characteristic dilated and nearly transparent, right ventricular free wall, caused by apposition of the right ventricular endocardium with the epicardium without intervening myocardium [29]. Death usually occurs resulting from congestive heart failure or cardiac arrhythmias [30–32].

The treatment of ARVD is still evolving, and is principally directed at preventing or terminating ventricular arrhythmias [20,33]. Antiarrhythmic drug therapy (in particular, sotalol) has been advocated, but there are few data on its effectiveness [34]. Radiofrequency catheter ablation has also been proposed; however, its use is inherently limited by the vast amount of the heart that has the potential to be arrhythmogenic [35]. Those patients with ARVD and syncope who have been shown to have ventricular tachycardia (either by monitoring or induced by programmed stimulation during electrophysiologic study) should undergo ICD implantation [36]. The long-term prognosis of ARVD patients who receive ICDs is unclear; however, long-term follow-up studies are currently underway.

Conclusions

The inherited arrhythmic causes of syncope (LQTS, Brugada syndrome, right ventricular dysplasia) constitute a diverse group of potentially lethal disorders where syncope may be the only warning a patient may have prior to sudden death. Proper recognition and diagnosis of these causes of syncope is critical in preventing potentially tragic outcomes. Ongoing research into the genetics of these disorders may someday provide a reliable testing modality for early identification and treatment.

References

1 Moss AJ. Long QT syndrome. *JAMA* 2003;**289**:2041–127.
2 Khan IA. Clinical and therapeutic aspects of congenital and acquired long QT syndrome. *Am J Med* 2002;**112**:58–66.
3 Fontaine G, Frank G, Grosgogeat Y. Torsades de pointes:

definition and management. *Mod Concepts Cardiovasc Dis* 1982;**51**:103–8.

4 Keren A, Tzivoni D, Gavish D, *et al.* Etiology, warning signs and therapy of torsade de pointes. *Circulation* 1981;**64**:1167–71.

5 Bhandri AK, Scheinmann M. The long QT syndrome. *Mod Concepts Cardiovasc Dis* 1985;**54**:45–50.

6 Terrell A, Lange-Nielsen F. Congenital deaf mutism, functional heart disease with prolongation of the QT interval and sudden death. *Am Heart J* 1957;**54**:59–78.

7 Ward OC. A new familial cardiac syndrome in children. *J Irish Med Assoc* 1964;**54**:103–6.

8 Romano C. Congenital cardiac arrhythmia. *Lancet* 1965;**1**:658–9.

9 Moss AJ, Schwartz PJ, Crampton RS, *et al.* The long QT syndrome: prospective longitudinal study of 328 families. *Circulation* 1991;**84**:1136–44.

10 Schwartz PJ, Priori SG, Spazzolini C, *et al.* Genotype–phenotype correlation in the long QT syndrome: gene specific triggers for life-threatening arrhythmias. *Circulation* 2001;**103**:89–95.

11 Schwartz PJ. Stress and sudden death: the case of the long QT syndrome. *Circulation* 1991;**83**(Suppl. 2):71–80.

12 Stratman HG, Kennedy HL. Torsades de pointes associated with drugs and toxins: recognition and management. *Am Heart J* 1987;**113**:1470–82.

13 Gussak I, Brugada P, Brugada J, *et al.* Idiopathic short QT interval: a new clinical syndrome? *Cardiology* 2000; **94**:99–102.

14 Gaita F, Giustetto C, Bianchi F, *et al.* Short QT syndrome: a familial cause of sudden death. *Circulation* 2003; **108**:965–70.

15 Antzelevitch C. The Brugada syndrome. *J Cardiovasc Electrophysiol* 1998;**9**:513–6.

16 Brugada P, Brugada J. Right bundle branch block, persistent ST segment elevation and sudden death: a distinct clinical and electrocardiographic syndrome: a multicenter report. *J Am Coll Cardiol* 1992;**20**:1391–6.

17 Brugada J, Brugada R, Brugada P. Right bundle branch block and ST segment elevation in leads V_1 through V_3: a marker for sudden death in patients without demonstrable structural heart disease. *Circulation* 2000;**101**:510–5.

18 Richardson PJ, McKenna WJ, Bristow M, *et al.* Report of the 1995 World Health Organization/International Society and Federation of Cardiology Task Force on the definition and classification of cardiomyopathies. *Circulation* 1996;**93**:841–2.

19 Conado D, Basso C, Thiene G, *et al.* Spectrum of clinicopathologic manifestations of arrhythmogenic right ventricular dysplasia: a multicenter study. *J Am Coll Cardiol* 1997;**30**:1512–20.

20 Fontaine G, Fontraliran F, Frank R. Arrhythmogenic right ventricular cardiomyopathies: clinical forms and main differential diagnosis. *Circulation* 1982;**65**: 1532–5.

21 Ibsen HHW, Baandrup U, Simonsen EE. Familial right ventricular dilated cardiomyopathy. *Br Heart J* 1985; **54**:156–9.

22 Fontaine G, Fontaliran F, Rosas Andrade F, *et al.* The arrhythmogenic right ventricle: dysplasia versus cardiomyopathy. *Heart Vessels* 1995;**10**:227–35.

23 Fontaine G, Fontaliran F, Hebert JL, *et al.* Arrhythmogenic right ventricular dysplasia. *Annu Rev Med* 1999;**50**:17–35.

24 Maron BJ, Shirani J, Poliac LC, Mathenge R, Roberts WC, Mueller FO. Sudden death in young competitive athletes: clinical, demographic, and pathological profiles. *JAMA* 1996;**276**:199–204.

25 Thiene G, Nava A, Corrado D, Rossi L, Pennelli N. Right ventricular cardiomyopathy and sudden death in young people. *N Engl J Med* 1988;**318**:129–33.

26 Corrado D, Thiene G, Nava A, Rossi L, Pennelli N. Sudden death in young competitive athletes: clinicopathologic correlations in 22 cases. *Am J Med* 1990; **89**:588–96.

27 Kayser HWM, van der Wall EE, Sivananthan MU, Plein S, Bloomer TN, de Roos A. Diagnosis of arrhythmogenic right ventricular dysplasia: a review. *RadioGraphics* 2002; **22**(3):639–48.

28 Cooner AS, Protonotarios N, Tsatsopoulou A, *et al.* Gene for arrhythmogenic right ventricular cardiomyopathy with diffuse non-epidermolytic palmoplantar keratoma and woolly hair (Naxos disease) maps to 17q21. *Circulation* 1998;**97**:2049–58.

29 Uhl H. A previously undescribed congenital malformation of the heart: almost total absence of the myocardium of the right ventricle. *Bull Johns Hopkins Hosp* 1952;**91**:197–209.

30 Gerlis LM, Schmidt-Ott SC, Ho SY, Anderson RH. Dysplastic conditions of the right ventricular myocardium: Uhl's anomaly versus arrhythmogenic right ventricular dysplasia. *Br Heart J* 1993;**69**:142–50.

31 Marcus FI, Fontaine GH, Frank R, Gallagher JJ, Reiter MJ. Long-term follow-up in patients with arrhythmogenic right ventricular disease. *Eur Heart J* 1989;**10** (Suppl. D):68–73.

32 Blomstrom-Lundqvist C, Sabel KG, Olsson SB. A long-term follow-up of 15 patients with arrhythmogenic right ventricular dysplasia. *Br Heart J* 1987;**58**:477–88.

33 Leclercq JF, Coumel PH. Characteristics, prognosis and treatment of the ventricular arrhythmias of right ventricular dysplasia. *Eur Heart J* 1989;**10**(Suppl. D): 61–7.

34 Haverkamp W, Martinez-Rubio A, Hief C, *et al*. Efficacy and safety of D,L-Sotalol in patients with ventricular tachycardia and in survivors of cardiac arrest. *J Am Coll Cardiol* 1997;**30**:487–95.

35 Fontaine G, Frank R, Tonet J, Grosgogeat Y. Identification of a zone of slow conduction appropriate for VT ablation: theoretical and practical considerations. *PACE* 1989;**12**(II):262–7.

36 Link MS, Wang PJ, Haugh CJ, *et al*. Arrhythmogenic right ventricular dysplasia: clinical results with implantable cardioverter defibrillators. *J Interv Card Electrophysiol* 1997;**1**:41–8.

CHAPTER 12

Psychiatric disorders in patients with syncope

Angele McGrady, PhD, MEd, LPCC, *& Ronald McGinnis,* MD

Introduction

Psychological symptoms and psychiatric disorders are common in the general population and have been associated with patients' presentation of dizziness, lightheadedness, and syncope. Psychopathology may be the main factor contributing to the syncope, a co-occurring disorder or symptoms that develop in response to a primary debilitating medical condition causing the syncope. Some psychiatric disorders that are described in the American Psychiatric Association's Diagnostic and Statistical Manual of Mental Disorders include dizziness and syncope as symptoms [1]. These include: anxiety disorders; generalized anxiety and panic disorder as well as the somatoform disorders; and somatization, conversion, and hypochondriasis. Substance abuse disorders related to use or withdrawal can cause or exacerbate syncope, and mood disorders such as major depressive disorder have also been associated with syncope. As is the case with many psychiatric disorders, the degree of comorbidity is high, with anxiety, substance abuse, and mood disorders often contributing symptoms in individual patients. Based on this comorbidity between syncope and psychiatric disorders, a combined approach to the management of syncope is recommended [2].

Theoretical framework

Psychological stress has been implicated in the etiology of syncope. Early studies proposed that syncope is preceded by stressful situations, such as anticipation or threat of bodily or psychological harm. The person might fear humiliation or embarrassment, yet denies their fear and escapes by fainting [3]. Some individuals have a propensity for lability in autonomic responses, perhaps genetically programmed. Acute increases in sympathetic neural activity are followed by parasympathetic dominance, leading to sudden decreases in blood pressure (BP) and syncope. Stress may be related to autonomic responses via the vagal system to elicit syncope and even death [4].

Early theories of the diphasic reaction as a basis for syncope were expanded to describe the initial significant increase in heart rate and BP as the person reacts to a psychological stressor, followed by vagal dominance, rapidly decreasing heart rate and BP [5]. The sympathetic "fight–flight" reaction is followed quickly by the parasympathetic conservation–withdrawal response. Differences in responses to laboratory stress in subjects with high or low heart rate reactivity were investigated [6]. Those who react to laboratory stress with high sympathetic cardiac reactivity also had high plasma cortisol in comparison to low reactors; this pattern of reactivity may be related to depression of the immune system and higher risk for illness in patients with autonomic dysfunction. A group of 52 patients were monitored during tilt in an effort to describe parallel physiological changes in tilt-positive and tilt-negative subjects. In addition to the expected lower BP and heart rate in the tilt-positive group compared with the tilt-negative group, skin conductance level decreased only in the tilt-positive response group compared with the tilt-negative response group, suggesting withdrawal of sympathetic activity in the former [7].

Psychiatric disorders in patients with syncope

The Diagnostic Interview Schedule (DIS) was used to evaluate more than 400 patients with syncope. Twenty-five percent of patients with unexplained syncope had one or more psychiatric illness, in comparison with only 7.3% of patients with cardiac syncope. Major depressive disorder, generalized anxiety disorder, and alcohol dependence were the most common conditions [8]. Another study compared 40 patients who had unexplained syncope with age- and sex-matched controls referred for arrhythmia. Patients with syncope more frequently had anxiety disorders than the controls and tended to use avoidance or withdrawal types of coping with stressful life events. The presence of a psychiatric disorder was associated with a higher risk of recurrence of syncope [9]. In addition to diagnosed or subsyndromal psychiatric conditions, patients with autonomic dysfunctions are troubled by other symptoms such as fatigue, dizziness, and headache. Patients worry about worsening of symptoms, personal injury, and long-term disability; they may feel hopeless when a diagnosis is elusive and these concerns may well intensify anxiety and increase risk for depression [10].

Anxiety disorders

Generalized anxiety disorder is characterized by at least 6 months of excessive anxiety and worry, manifested by autonomic physiological sensations that impair normal functioning. Worry may become all-consuming, decreasing concentration and producing distorted thinking. Persons with panic disorder experience recurrent unexpected panic attacks, which may be debilitating and compromise quality of life [1]. Anxiety is a common symptom of patients with autonomic dysfunction. In a series of 35 tilt-positive adolescents, 25% had anxiety as a symptom of postural orthostatic tachycardia syndrome, although not as the cause of their symptoms [11]. Tilt-positive subjects, particularly women, had higher anxiety scores (Beck Anxiety Inventory) than did tilt-negative subjects [12]. Reduced, vagally mediated, heart rate variability (HRV) was observed in subjects with generalized anxiety disorder. Interestingly, lower HRV was associated with consciously induced worry in subjects with an anxiety disorder as well as non-anxious controls, while relaxation increased variability in all subjects [13].

Blood phobics who manifested extreme fear at the sight of blood exhibited the diphasic physiological reaction to disturbing pictures of bloody injury. The controls exhibited signs of stress (increased heart rate and BP), but there was a slow and gradual decline back to the prestress levels after the video. During a standard exercise stress test, all subjects showed the expected increases in heart rate and BP and slow decreases after cessation of exercise. So, in individuals with a phobic response to blood, the diphasic reaction is evident only in this specific situation, not as a general response to stress nor is it automatic after significant increases in BP and heart rate [5]. Patients with panic disorders showed the highest heart rates and lowest HRV in response to stress, whereas phobics who fainted at the sight of blood evidenced higher HRV than those who panic, but still lower than non-anxious controls [14].

Substance abuse disorders

Alcohol dependence and abuse in addition to other substances are among the most prevalent mental disorders in the population and are projected to increase in the future. Not only are these disorders common, but they are frequently found concurrently with anxiety and mood disorders. Relationships of substance abuse in patients with syncope include co-occurrence, self-medication, direct physiologic effects of the substance, and withdrawal phenomena. Acute intoxication with alcohol, sedatives, opiates, or anxiolytics have been associated with unsteady gait, incoordination, and falls. Stimulants such as cocaine and amphetamines acutely increase anxiety, heart irregularities, and may lead to blood pressure fluctuations. Withdrawal effects of alcohol and anxiolytics can lead to autonomic hyperactivity, anxiety, and even seizures resulting in loss of consciousness.

Chronic effects of alcohol lead to many medical conditions that may have deleterious effects in patients with syncope. Poor nutrition, anemia, loss of intravascular volume secondary to vomiting and diarrhea, blood loss, liver disease, and central nervous system effects leading to cognitive impairment and degenerative changes in the cerebellum may all increase symptoms of syncope.

Patients dealing with ongoing medical problems and secondary anxiety often resort to sedatives and alcohol as a means to self-medicate. Although initially effective in reducing secondary symptoms of anxiety, chronic use of these substances leads to tolerance, dependence, and disability. Denial of underlying anxiety symptoms as well as the misuse of substances leads to a vicious cycle of substance abuse and secrecy.

Mood disorders

The mood disorders consist of major depressive disorder, dysthymia, and bipolar disorder. Major depressive disorder is one of the most common psychiatric disorders, with a lifetime prevalence of approximately 17%. It is characterized by symptoms of fatigue, sleep disturbance, lack of interest and pleasure, depressed mood, poor concentration, feelings of worthlessness, and thoughts of death or suicide. Major depression has been associated with many medical illnesses and has been found in a significant number of patients with syncope [8]. It is unclear whether major depression predisposes to syncope or rather coexists as it does with other psychiatric and medical illnesses. There is some indication that central neurohumoral abnormalities, found in major depression, may cause autonomic dysregulation and result in syncope or presyncope [15].

There has also been some indication that there is a relationship between BP and mood. Patients referred for tilt table testing were examined with the Beck Depression Inventory. The tilt-positive group was younger and had significantly higher mean depression scores compared with the tilt-negative group [7].

Low BP has been associated with higher depression scores in older men [16] as well as predicting the development of depressive symptomatology at follow-up in a 2-year longitudinal study [17]. Low BP may be associated with fatigue, a prominent symptom of depression. Mood symptoms of fatigue, anorexia, weight loss, lack of motivation, and pessimism significantly increase patients' disability and often reduce compliance with treatment.

Major depression has been shown to greatly increase morbidity and mortality in many medical illnesses such as coronary artery disease, disabilities, stroke, and AIDS. Untreated major depression complicates diagnosis, treatment, and outcomes in patients with syncope, while treatment of depression in these patients has been associated with improvement in mood and syncopal symptoms. Thus, it becomes very important to screen for depression and treat appropriately to ensure better patient outcomes.

Somatoform disorders

This category of disorders includes three conditions linked to syncope: somatization disorder, conversion, and hypochondriasis. Cardiovascular symptoms presented by patients with somatoform disorders cannot be explained by physical findings because psychological distress is expressed through physical symptoms [18]. The ICD 10 system of classification includes somatoform autonomic dysfunction (symptoms attributed to dysregulation of the autonomic nervous system). Fainting during tilt occurs without evidence of severe bradycardia, hypotension, or other diagnostic hemodynamic indicators. Outside of the clinic, fainting episodes occur at times of stress and commonly in the presence of others [19].

Putative causes of subjects' overreaction or amplification of symptoms are varied and complex. The multiplicity of symptoms in autonomic dysfunction (i.e., dizziness, headache, nausea, anxiety, and depression in addition to syncope) cause some patients to conclude that a serious, life-threatening illness must be present. The subjects may have a more reactive physiology that increases the likelihood of numerous symptoms [20]. High hypnotic ability focuses subjects on physical symptoms and tends to increase the frequency of catastrophizing attributions [21]. In addition, reporting only somatic symptoms directs the physician's attention away from psychological distress and appropriate questioning about distress, depressive, or anxious thoughts [22]. In its extreme form, the chronic somatizer will refuse to believe that emotion influences physiological distress. Perhaps these individuals have had more experience with illness in childhood or adolescence and fear any sign of emergent disease [23]. The frightening experience of sudden loss of consciousness lowers the threshold for anxiety about further episodes. In time, abnormal illness behavior predominates so that, despite reassurance, the patient continues to believe that there is something seriously amiss in the physiological domain. This conceptualization of symptoms leads the person to assume the sick role, becoming dependent on others [24].

Children may use syncope as a way of coping (through withdrawal) or adapting to emotionally distressing life events. Feelings about stressful situations are avoided and internalized, then manifested as somatic symptoms [25]. Under certain circumstances, neither medical illness nor psychopathology can explain syncope. For example, an episode of "epidemic" fainting in school-aged girls was carefully studied. Neither medical nor psychological factors were pivotal in explaining the outbreak. Instead, social factors were identified as the prime agents responsible for spreading the syncopal attacks [26].

Evaluation of the patient

As in many chronic medical conditions, the need for a thorough medical history is essential. Understanding the medical–psychiatric interactions in syncope, the evaluator's history should include not only psychiatric symptoms but also diagnosed illnesses, family history, personal past history, and evaluation of substances of abuse. This becomes not only important during initial evaluation of the patient, but also during ongoing care. Given that the treatment of mental disorders is often separate from therapy of medical illness by separate providers and third party reimbursement, ongoing care should include regular updates of psychiatric diagnosis and treatment.

Many patients consider psychiatric diagnoses as having a great stigma attached to them. They also fear that if a clinician sees them as having a mental disorder, he or she will think that all their problems are not real and "in their head." Most patients can benefit initially from a discussion of the biologic and psychologic factors that may be related to their symptoms. In the context of a medical–psychiatric interaction model, patients are more likely to feel comfortable discussing the psychological nature of their syncopal symptoms.

A past history of treatment for depression, anxiety, or substance abuse often gives clues to successful treatments and the degree of chronicity of the disorder. Psychiatric hospitalizations and a history

of suicide attempts should also be noted. Such a history places the patient at higher risk for future disability secondary to psychiatric illness.

Many of the psychiatric disorders including anxiety, depression, and substance abuse have familial tendencies and genetic predispositions. It is not uncommon to see three generations suffering from the same disorder. Family history not only gives information for diagnosing current conditions, but also may give an indication about successful treatments and co-occurring conditions. Unless the examiner specifically asks about depression, anxiety, or substance abuse in the family, patients will rarely offer this information on their own. Stigma and the perpetuation of family secrets tend to keep many family patterns hidden if not directly elicited.

A patient's personal history is also important in the development of several psychiatric disorders. A history of experiencing traumatic abuse has been associated with the later development of mood, anxiety, and somatization disorders. Past abuse may be emotional, physical, or sexual. An abuse history as part of a routine evaluation not only reveals relevant information, but it also affords the patient an opportunity to disclose past trauma and open the door for treatment.

Eliciting history and current use of substances of abuse remains a challenging but critical part of the evaluation of every patient with syncope. Substance abuse is often classified as an illness of shame and secrecy. Denial and minimization of use adds to the difficulty in obtaining reliable information. The evaluator's own discomfort in asking about substance abuse and not having a reliable routine of evaluation further limit obtaining useful data. Patients should be assessed for alcohol and other substances of abuse, including amount, frequency, and last use. Information regarding past and present use of abusable prescription medications and intravenous use of drugs allows the clinician to identify and treat a major confounding illness in both the treatment of psychiatric and medical disorders. Patients who fail to respond to treatment of psychiatric disorders including anxiety and depression may often have a reoccurring substance abuse disorder.

Practitioners treating patients with autonomic dysfunction are well advised to screen, assess, and diagnostically evaluate them for emotional conditions. Well-validated, self-report inventories are available for the assessment of anxiety, depression, general distress, and quality of life; these inventories can be purchased from the Psychological Corporation and easily used by practitioners.

The PRIME-MD (primary care evaluation tool for mental disorders) [27] contains screening questions for anxiety, mood, somatoform disorders, and substance abuse as well as other conditions. If patient answers positively to the screening questions, the clinician follows up with more detailed queries and evaluation tools.

The Beck Depression Inventory (updated as BDI-II) is a 21-item, self-report, valid and reliable diagnostic test for assessment of depression [28]. Caution is necessary if the practitioner wishes to use a shorter inventory such as the short-form, 13-item BDI [29]. The short Beck contains a relatively high number of somatic items, yielding more false-positive scores [30]. Patients with unexplained physical symptoms (e.g., patients with autonomic dysfunction) would score highly, even if they did not endorse many mood symptoms. The Hamilton Depression Inventory consists of 38 questions requiring approximately 10 min; however, the scoring is more time intensive than the BDI-II [31]. We recommend the use of the BDI-II for adults; for adolescents, the Reynolds Depression Inventory is a good choice [32]. The Zung Self-Rating Depression Scale contains nearly equal numbers of somatic and affective items related to depression; the two subscales can be scored separately [33]. A group of 17 subjects without a DSM-IV Axis I diagnosis had their BP measured after a standard meal. The postprandial drop in systolic BP correlated only with the score on the somatic items of the Zung. In response to orthostatic stress, however, the systolic BP drop was correlated only with the score on the affective items of the Zung scale [34].

The Beck Anxiety Inventory, comprising 21 items, covering physiological symptoms associated with anxiety such as numbness, tingling, dizziness, and sweating, and items related to psychological symptoms of anxiety such as fear of the worst, fear of losing control, or going crazy [35]. A scale that is specific to phobic symptoms elicited by blood and injections is the BISS (blood injection symptom scale). Symptoms were divided into three subscales: faintness, anxiety, and tension. This scale may be useful in assessing severity of symptoms and following improvement as a result of treatment [36].

In children and adolescents with syncope, some assessment, even if informal, of parents' psychological health should be attempted. For girls, father's shortness of breath and distress was related both to frequency of syncope and number of visits to the emergency room. For boys, mother's psychological distress, particularly depressive symptoms and anxiety-mediated shortness of breath, was correlated to their son's syncope [37].

Treatment of psychiatric disorders in patients with syncope

Education and support groups are an integral part of comprehensive treatment of patients with syncope. Reading materials such as those available from the National Dysautonomia Research Foundation are recommended. This organization provides a newsletter, a website, www.ndrf.org, and a referral network for support groups and sponsors a yearly meeting. For practitioners and researchers, the American Autonomic Society is a scientific research organization that offers a scientific journal and an annual meeting.

Behavioral interventions

Behavioral interventions in management of syncope include behavior therapy, psychophysiological therapies such as biofeedback, changes in posture, and dietary recommendations. Simple suggestions should precede more elaborate, time-consuming, and expensive interventions. A 250-mg dose of caffeine prior to the donation of blood blunts the vasovagal reaction (dizziness, lightheadedness, and fainting), by way of the pressor and, perhaps, other effects of caffeine, which remains in the body long enough to prevent parasympathetic dominance and fainting [38].

Daily tilt sessions were provided for 42 patients with history of vasodepressor or cardioinhibitory syncope. Sessions began while patients were in the hospital and were followed by 30 min/day home practice of upright standing against a wall. Two-thirds of the patients were free of syncope after treatment [39]. Leg crossing and muscle tensing for 30 s at the beginning of a tilt table-induced impending faint was tested in 21 subjects with syncope.

Twenty of the 21 subjects dramatically increased their BP while tensing and did not faint. At 10 months' follow-up, 13 of 20 subjects were applying the maneuver daily and could postpone or prevent syncope [40]. Increases in cerebral blood flow during muscle tension in subjects who faint in response to blood injury have also been documented [41]. The detailed treatment plan for muscle tensing is provided in several case studies, two of which combined systematic desensitization with muscle tensing. Treatment and continued practice successfully eliminated panic and fainting during medical procedures [42].

Cognitive–behavioral techniques may also be added to muscle tensing and desensitization [43]. For subjects agreeable to hypnotherapy, multidimensional therapy including hypnosis can assist subjects to decrease high levels of fear and anxiety of injections [44]. Social skills training was added to cognitive–behavioral therapy and response prevention in a case of a woman who feared death from injections. Extensive homework assignments comprised relaxation exercises, exposure and monitoring level of distress using the Subjective Units of Distress Scale (SUDS). The subject successfully received multiple injections after treatment [45].

Biofeedback is a behavioral therapy that consists of providing information to a subject about a specific physiological response such as muscle tension, hand temperature, or heart rate. Biofeedback is commonly combined with relaxation therapy in an 8–12 session protocol; home practice relaxation is an integral part of the treatment [46]. Biofeedback assisted relaxation has been successfully used either as sole treatment or as a component of therapy for such stress-related disorders as migraine headaches and essential hypertension [46]. Biofeedback gives the subject a sense of control over their physiology, while relaxation decreases sympathetic activity and increases heart rate variability [13].

Biofeedback was provided to a series of 10 patients with syncope or near-syncope and headache. Six of 10 patients sustained a significant decrease in symptoms at the end of 10 sessions of electromyography, thermal biofeedback, and progressive and autogenic relaxation. The patients with true syncope (six of the seven) decreased their syncopal episodes by at least 50% [47]. In a subsequent controlled study, findings confirmed those of the case

series. In the treated group, significant decreases were observed in the headache index and in loss of consciousness in those who experienced true syncope with no benefit to the wait list control group. After training in biofeedback and relaxation, patients were given symptom-specific recommendations. Protocol modifications are necessary in biofeedback therapy of syncope, because during the sympathetic arousal phase, BP and heart rates are elevated in contrast to the significant declines that follow. Thus, subjects are instructed to use passive relaxation during the sympathetically mediated stress response or at the first sign of a headache, to use progressive relaxation if dizzy or lightheaded, and to use muscle tensing when loss of consciousness was the primary concern. Successful patients were able to recognize the sensations of headache prodrome or presyncope, to have command of multiple techniques, and to implement them as needed [48].

Another modification of standard biofeedback assisted relaxation therapy was successfully applied to aviators challenged by severe motion sickness and post-flight hypotension [49,50]. Autogenic Feedback Training utilizes more than one feedback signal at a time in an effort to "condition multiple responses simultaneously." A tilt table was used as the training stimulus. Pilot-astronauts learned to anticipate symptoms and to prevent the activation of the sympathetic nervous system that occurs at the beginning of motion sickness. Inducing the relaxation response at will also reduced the lability of the autonomic nervous system so that if physiological responses to motion occurred, they could be controlled before efficiency became compromised [50].

Cognitive–behavioral therapy (CBT) is a mode of psychotherapy that views thoughts as the major determinants of emotion and behavior. Errors in thinking, catastrophizing, and overgeneralization are countered by rational thinking [51]. To our knowledge there are no reports of trials of CBT in autonomic dysfunction, but the therapy is widely used for psychiatric disorders. In a review of CBT for somatization disorder, outcome measures were physical symptoms, psychological distress, and functionality. Physical symptoms were the most responsive to CBT, followed by improvements in function and reduction of psychological symptoms

[52]. Thus, CBT is appropriate for the anxiety, mood, and somatoform disorders that accompany autonomic dysfunction.

Medical treatment

The therapeutic use of medications in the treatment of psychiatric disorders has become more and more common over the last several decades. Many different types of medications are used for the treatment of anxiety, mood, and psychiatric disorders. It is also common for the same type of medication to have multiple uses. For example, antidepressants are useful as antianxiety agents while antipsychotics have antimanic effects. The medications have therapeutic as well as side-effects and toxicity, which can complicate their use in patients with syncope. In addition, some medications that are commonly used for psychiatric disorders have demonstrated effectiveness in the treatment of some types of syncopal disorders [53]. Some general guidelines for the use of pharmacologic agents are provided herein, but we recommend that the reader refer to other texts for a more complete understanding of the complexities of dosing and combining medications.

Antidepressants

The major types of antidepressants include selective serotonin reuptake inhibitors (SSRIs), monoamine oxidase inhibitors (MAOIs), tricyclic and tetracyclics (TCAs) and trazodone, nafazadone, amfebutamone, mirtazapine, and venlafaxine. All of the medications are effective antidepressants and many have antianxiety effects so are useful in treatment of the anxiety disorders. SSRIs, which include fluoxetine, paroxetine, sertraline, fluvoxamine, citalopram, and excitalopram, have specific receptor activity and have a favorable safety and side-effect profile. SSRIs are not associated with α-adrenergic antagonism and rarely have been associated with orthostatic hypotension [54]. In addition, SSRIs have been found to be useful in the treatment of patients with neurally mediated cardiovascular disorders and may prove advantageous in the medical treatment of depression in patients who experience syncope [53,55].

Monoamine oxidase inhibitors are effective in the treatment of depression and panic disorder. The irreversible MAOIs (phenelzine, isocarboxazid, and tranylcypromine) have more severe and frequent side-effects than other antidepressants. Orthostatic hypotension is very common with the MAOIs; the subsequent dizziness and syncope make these agents difficult to use in syncopal patients. Dietary interactions leading to hypertensive reactions and multiple potential drug interactions also limit the use of these medications.

Tricyclic and tetracyclic medications include imipramine, desipramine, amitriptyline, nortriptyline, clomipramine, trimipramine, doxepin, protriptyline, amoxapine, and maprotiline. These medications differ in their effects on the reuptake of serotonin, norepinephrine as well as cholinergic, α-adrenergic, and histaminergic receptor blockade. TCAs are effective in the treatment of depression and panic disorders that is attributed to their effect on serotonin and norepinephrine. Side-effects and toxicity are related to their effects on cholinergic (dry mouth, constipation), histaminergic (sedation, weight gain), and α-adrenergic (postural hypotension, dizziness) receptors. This later side-effect makes these medications a challenge to use in patients with syncope. Desipramine, nortriptyline, protriptyline, and maprotiline have the least amount of α_1-receptor activity, although they all remain active at this receptor and may cause orthostatic hypotension. Amitriptyline has the strongest affinity for α_1-receptors and may be linked to falls and injury in older individuals [56].

Trazodone is an antidepressant that has both serotonergic agonist and antagonist effects. It is effective in depression and has antianxiety effects as well. Trazodone is significantly sedating and is often used a hypnotic agent. Unfortunately, trazodone has α_1-adrenergic receptor blockade that causes orthostatic hypotension. Trazodone-related syncope in the elderly has been described and limits its use in these patients [57]. Nefazodone, an analogue of trazodone, also acts as a serotonin agonist and antagonist but has less sedation and α_1-adrenergic blockade lending to rare orthostatic hypotension. Recent discovery of life-threatening hepatic failure in patients treated with nefazodone may make it less commonly prescribed [58].

Amfebutamone is a unique antidepressant that has primarily dopaminergic effects and does not affect serotonin, histamine, acetylcholine, or α_1-receptors. It does not trigger orthostatic hypotension and has a favorable cardiovascular profile. It has not been shown to be effective in anxiety disorders but is effective in depression and attention deficit hyperactivity disorder. Seizures and neurologic toxicity has been found in high doses and in patients with eating disorders and should not be used in these patients.

Mirtazapine has a pharmacology profile that is different than other antidepressants. It leads to increased norepinephrine and serotonin release through blockade of presynaptic α_2-autoreceptors and heteroreceptors. It also acts as an antagonist on certain serotonin receptors. It has potent antihistaminic activity that leads to sedation and weight gain. There are no significant increases in cardiovascular side-effects such as blood pressure changes compared with placebo. Unique mode of action and side-effect profile may make mirtazapine an effective adjunctive agent for the treatment of depression in patients with syncope.

Venlafaxine is an effective antidepressant that has selective blockade of reuptake of both serotonin and norepinephrine. It has no effect on cholinergic, histaminergic, or α-adrenergic receptors and thus has a less adverse side-effect profile than the TCAs. Modest increases in blood pressure have been reported with venlafaxine treatment and sustained hypertension at higher doses has also been reported. There is also some indication that venlafaxine may prove useful in patients with refractory orthostatic hypotension, leading to its effective use for depression and anxiety treatment in patients with syncope [59].

Antianxiety agents

SSRIs, TCAs, MAOIs, and other antidepressants can also be used as effective treatments for anxiety disorders. In addition to the antidepressants, the benzodiazepines and buspirone are commonly used medications for anxiety disorders either as a primary or adjunctive treatment. The benzodiazepines have been available since the 1950s and include chlordiazepoxide, diazepam, alprazolam, lorazepam, oxazepam, clorazepate, clonazepam and the hypnotics triazolam, temazepam, flurazepam, and estazolam. All are sedating, anticonvulsant, and have muscle relaxant activity. They exert their effects through action on the benzodiazepine receptor and GABA activity.

Benzodiazepines are effective in the treatment of generalized anxiety disorder and panic disorder. They are generally well tolerated with minimal side-effects. They have been associated with being sedated, slowed down, and having ataxia or slurred speech. These side-effects may complicate the care of a patient with syncope. Abuse potential of these medications does not seem to be a problem in the general population. Patients with a history of substance abuse or alcohol dependence may be more likely to abuse these medications. Rebound anxiety and withdrawal symptoms are common with abrupt discontinuation. Buspirone was the first non-benzodiazepine, non-sedating, antianxiety medication to be developed. It exerts its effects as a partial agonist on postsynaptic serotonin receptors and is effective in the treatment of generalized anxiety disorder but not panic disorders. It is a novel drug that is free of many of the side-effects of the benzodiazepines and does not appear to have any effects on BP. Unlike the benzodiazepines, buspirone does not relieve anxiety immediately and will require several weeks to achieve an effect, much like antidepressant medications.

Anticonvulsants and lithium

The anticonvulsants carbamazepine and valproate have become common treatments for bipolar disorder and the newer anticonvulsants oxcarbazepine and lamotrigine have also been used, largely replacing lithium as first-line treatment. Valproate is generally well tolerated with a low incidence of side-effects. Carbamazepine can have neurological toxicity with ataxia, fatigue, and dizziness, which may complicate treatment in a patient with syncope. Lithium use requires close monitoring because of a narrow therapeutic window and multiple endocrine, renal, and neurologic toxicities. Although it does not primarily lead to hypotension, lithium use in a patient with ongoing syncope would be a challenge with the choice of an anticonvulsant providing less overall risk.

Antipsychotic medications are used for schizophrenia, schizo-affective disorder and as an adjunct for bipolar disorder or in patients with psychotic depressions. Older antipsychotic medications such as chlorpromazine or thioridazine can cause orthostatic hypotension through α_1-adrenergic blockade. Higher potency typical agents such as haloperidol cause little blood pressure dysregulation. In the newer atypical antipsychotics, clozapine has demonstrated significant orthostatic hypotension and tachycardia.

Overall, there are many psychotropic medications available for the treatment of mood, anxiety, and psychotic disorders and there are many more currently in development. When treating patients with underlying syncope, it becomes important to select agents with a beneficial safety profile and minimal effects on BP regulation. Fortunately, there are many choices that can benefit these patients.

Conclusions

Frequent comorbidity exists between autonomic dysfunction and psychiatric conditions, in particular major depression, anxiety, somatoform disorders, and substance abuse. Patients must be evaluated with a thorough history, screening tools, and in-depth diagnostic interviews if needed. Treatment of psychiatric conditions in syncopal patients may comprise of education, support groups, psychopharmacology, behavioral, psychophysiologic, and psychotherapeutic therapies. Knowledge of side-effects of psychiatric medicines common to autonomic dysfunction, particularly dizziness, headache, and nausea is important. Behavioral therapies assist patients in gaining a sense of control over their physiological and emotional responses to life stress and emotional reactions to their illness. Patients must be carefully monitored and managed while acknowledging the distress inherent in their multiple, disruptive symptoms, their fear of disability, and their suboptimal quality of life.

References

1 American Psychiatric Association. *Diagnostic and Statistical Manual of Mental Disorders*, 4th edn. Text revision. Washington, DC: American Psychiatric Association, 2000.

2 Koenig D, Linzer M, Pontinen M, Divine GW. Syncope in young adults: evidence for a combined medical and psychiatric approach. *J Intern Med* 1992;**232**:169–76.

3 Sledge WH. Antecedent psychological factors in the onset of vasovagal syncope. *Psychosom Med* 1978;**40**:568–79.

4 Stevens H. Syncope, seizures and stress. *Stress Med* 1987;**3**:41–9.

5 Dahllöf O, Lars-Göran O. The diphasic reaction in blood phobic situations: individually or stimulus bound? *Scand J Behav Ther* 1998;**7**:7–94.

6 Cacioppo JT. Social neuroscience: atonomic, neuroendocrine, and immune responses to stress. *Psychophysiology* 1994;**1**:13–128.

7 McGrady A, Kern-Buell C, Bush E, Khuder S, Grubb BP. Psychological and physiological factors associated with tilt table testing for neurally mediated syncopal syndromes. *Pacing Clin Electrophysiol* 2001;**24**:296–301.

8 Kapoor WN, Fortunato M, Hanusa BH, Schulberg HC. Psychiatric illnesses in patients with syncope. *Am J Med* 1995;**99**:505–12.

9 Kouakam C, Lacroix D, Klug D, Baux P, Marquie C, Kacet S. Prevalence and prognostic significance of psychiatric disorder in patients evaluated for recurrent unexplained syncope. *Am J Cardiol* 2002;**89**:530–5.

10 Shaffer C, Jackson L, Jarecki S. Characteristics, perceived stressors, and coping strategies of patients who experience neurally mediated syncope. *Heart Lung* 2001;**30**:244–9.

11 Karas B, Grubb BP, Boehm K, Kip K. The postural orthostatic tachycardia syndrome: a potentially treatable cause of chronic fatigue, exercise intolerance and cognitive impairment in adolescents. *PACE* 2000;**23**:344–51.

12 Cohen TJ, Thayapran N, Ibrahim B, Quan C, Quan W, Von Zur Muhlen F. An association between anxiety and neurocardiogenic syncope during head-up tilt table testing. *Pacing Clin Electrophysiol* 2000;**23**:837–41.

13 Thayer JF, Friedman BH, Borkovec TD, Johnsen BH, Molina S. Autonomic characteristics of generalized anxiety and worry. *Biol Psychiatry* 1996;**39**:255–66.

14 Friedman BH, Thayer JF. Anxiety and autonomic flexibility: a cardiovascular approach. *Biol Psychology* 1998;**49**:303–23.

15 Linzer MF, Felder A, Hackel A, *et al.* Psychiatric syncope: a new look at an old disease. *Psychosomatics* 1990;**31**:181–8.

16 Barrett-Connor E, Palinkas LA. Low blood pressure and depression in older men: a population based study. *BMJ* 1994;**308**;446–9.

17 Paterniti S. Low blood pressure and risk of depression in the elderly: a prospective community-based study. *Br J Psychiatry* 2000;**176**:464–7.

18 Kirmayer LJ, Robbins JM, Paris J. Somatoform disorders: personality and the social matrix of somatic distress. *J Abnorm Psychol* 1994;**103**:125–36.

19 Grubb BP, Gerard G, Wolfe DA. Syncope and seizures of psychogenic origin: identification with head upright tilt table testing. *Clin Cardiol* 1992;**15**:839–42.

20 Barsky AJ, Borus JF. Functional somatic syndromes. *Ann Intern Med* 1999;**130**:910–21.

21 Wickramasekera I. Somatization: concepts, data, and predictions from the high risk model of threat perception. *J Nerv Ment Dis* 1995;**183**:15–23.

22 Porter SC, Fein JA, Ginsburg KR. Depression screening in adolescents with somatic complaints presenting to the emergency department. *Ann Emerg Med* 1997;**29**:141–5.

23 Taylor RE, Mann AH. Somatization in primary care. *J Psychosom Res* 1999;**47**:61–6.

24 Lewis P, Lubkin I, Larsen PD. *Illness Roles in Chronic Illness: Impact and Interventions*. Sudbury, MA: Jones & Bartlett, 1998.

25 Byars KC, Brown RT, Campbell RM, Hobbs SA. Psychological adjustment and coping in a population of children with recurrent syncope. *Dev Behav Pediatr* 2000;**21**:189–97.

26 Lee PW, Leung P, Fung AS, Low LC, Tsang MC, Leung WC. An episode of syncope attacks in adolescent schoolgirls: investigations, intervention and outcome. *Br J Med Psychol* 1996;**3**:247–57.

27 Spitzer RL, Williams JBW, Kroenke K, *et al*. Utility of a new procedure for diagnosing mental disorders in primary care: the PRIME-MD 1000 Study. *JAMA* 1994;**272**: 1749–56.

28 Beck AT, Steer RA, Ball R, Ranieri WF. Comparison of Beck Depression Inventories-IA and II in psychiatric outpatients. *J Pers Assess* 1996;**67**:588–97.

29 Beck AT, Beck RW. Screening depressed patients in family practice: a rapid technique. *Postgrad Med* 1972; **52**:81–5.

30 Volk RJ, Pace TM, Parchman ML. Screening for depression in primary care patients: dimensionality of the short form of the Beck Depression Inventory. *Psychol Assess* 1993;**5**:173–81.

31 Kobak KA, Reynolds WM. The Hamilton Depression Inventory. In: Maruish ME, ed. *Handbook of Psychological Assessment in Primary Care Settings*. Mahwah, NJ: Lawrence Erlbaum, 2000: 423–62.

32 Reynolds WM. *Reynolds Adolescent Depression Scale*. Odessa, FL: Psychological Assessment Resources, 1986.

33 Zung WWK. A self-rating depression scale. *Arch Gen Psychiatry* 1965;**12**:63–70.

34 Schwartz S, Feller A, Perimuter L. Postprandial systolic blood pressure and subsyndromal depression. *Exp Aging Res* 2001;**27**:309–18.

35 Beck AT, Epstein N, Brown G, Steer RA. An inventory for measuring clinical anxiety: psychometric properties. *J Consult Clin Psychol* 1988;**56**:893–7.

36 Page AC, Bennett KS, Carter O, Smith J, Woodmore K. The blood-injection symptom scale (BISS): assessing a structure of phobic symptoms elicited by blood and injections. *Behav Res Ther* 1997;**35**:457–64.

37 Morris JAB, Blount RL, Brown RT, Campbell RM. Association of parental psychological and behavioral factors

and children's syncope. *J Consult Clin Psychol* 2001;**69**: 851–7.

38 Sauer LA, France CR. Caffeine attenuates vasovagal reactions in female first-time blood donors. *Health Psychol* 1999;**18**:403–9.

39 Reybrouck T, Heidbuchel H, Gewillig M, Van de Werf F. Tilt training: a new treatment for recurrent neurocardiogenic syncope and severe orthostatic intolerance. *Pacing Clin Electrophysiol* 1998;**21**:193–6.

40 Krediet CT, van Dijk N, Linzer M, van Lieshout JJ, Wieling W. Management of vasovagal syncope: controlling or aborting faints by leg crossing and muscle tensing. *Circulation* 2002;**106**:1684–9.

41 Foulds JW, Patterson K, James-Brooks N. The effects of muscle tension on cerebral circulation in blood phobic and non-phobic subjects. *Behav Res Ther* 1990;**28**:481–6.

42 Anderson KW, Taylor S, McLean PD. Panic disorder associated with blood-injury reactivity: the necessity of establishing functional relationships among maladaptive behaviors. *Behav Ther* 1996;**27**:463–72.

43 Van Dijk N, Velzeboer SCJM, Destrèe-Vonk A, Linzer M, Wieling W. Psychological treatment of malignant vasovagal syncope due to blood phobia. *Pacing Clin Electrophysiol* 2001;**24**:122–4.

44 Medd DY. Fear of injections: the value of hypnosis in facilitating clinical treatment. *Contemp Hypnosis* 2001; **18**:100–6.

45 Panzarella C, Garlipp J. Integration of cognitive techniques into an individualized application of behavioral treatment of blood-injection-injury phobia. *Cogn Behav Pract* 1999;**6**:200–11.

46 Schwartz M, Andrasik F. *Biofeedback: A Practitioner's Guide*, 3rd edn. New York, NY: Guilford, 2003.

47 McGrady AV, Bush EG, Grubb BP. Outcome of biofeedback-assisted relaxation for neurocardiogenic syncope and headache: a clinical replication series. *Appl Psychophysiol Biofeedback* 1997;**22**:63–72.

48 McGrady A, Kern-Buell C, Bush E, Devonshire R, Claggett AL, Grubb BP. Biofeedback-assisted relaxation therapy in neurocardiogenic syncope: a pilot study. *Appl Psychophysiol Biofeedback* 2003;**28**:183–92.

49 Cowings PS. Autogenic feedback training: a presentative method for motion and space sickness. In: Crampton GH, ed. *Motion and Space Sickness*. Boca Raton, FL: CRC Press, 1990: 353–72.

50 Cowings PS, Toscano WB, Miller NE, *et al*. Autogenic feedback training: a potential treatment for orthostatic intolerance in aerospace crews. *J Clin Pharmacol* 1994; **34**:599–608.

51 Beck JS. *Cognitive Therapy: Basics and Beyond*. New York, NY: Guilford, 1996.

52 Kroenke K, Swindle R. Cognitive–behavioral therapy for somatization and symptom syndromes: a critical review

of controlled clinical trials. *Psychother Psychosomat* 2000; **69**:205–15.

53 Kosinski D, Grubb BP, Temesy-Armos P. The use of serotonin reuptake inhibitors in the treatment of neurally mediated cardiovascular disorders. *J Serotonin Res* 1994; **1**:85–90.

54 Schatzberg A, Nemeroff CA, eds. *The American Psychiatric Publishing Textbook of Psychopharmacology*, 3rd edn. Washington, DC: American Psychiatric Publishers, 2004.

55 Grubb BP, Wolfe DA, Samoil D, Temesy-Armos P, Hahn H, Elliot L. Usefulness of fluoxetine hydrochloride for prevention of resistant upright tilt induced syncope. *PACE* 1993;**16**:458–64.

56 Ray WA. Psychotropic drugs and injuries among the elderly: a review. *J Clin Psychopharmacol* 1992;**12**:386–96.

57 Nambudiri DZ, Mirchandani IC, Young RC. Two more cases of trazadone-related syncope in the elderly [Letter]. *J Geriatr Psychiatr Neurol* 1989;**2**:225.

58 *Physician's Desk Reference*. Montvale, NJ: Thomson PDR, 2003.

59 Grubb BP, Kosinski D. Preliminary observations on the use of venlafaxine hydrochloride in refractory orthostatic hypotension. *J Serotonin Res* 1996;**6**:89–94.

Recommended reference texts for office use

Sadock BJ, Sadock VA. *Kaplan & Sadock's Synopsis of Psychiatry*, 9th edn. Philadelphia, PA: Lippincott Williams & Wilkins, 2003.

Schatzberg A, Nemeroff CA, eds. *The American Psychiatric Publishing Textbook of Psychopharmacology*, 3rd edn. Washington, DC: American Psychiatric Publishers, 2004.

CHAPTER 13

Postural tachycardia, orthostatic intolerance, and the chronic fatigue syndrome

Blair P. Grubb, MD, *Hugh Calkins,* MD, *& Peter C. Rowe,* MD

Introduction

The last two decades have given birth to a sudden and near-explosive increase in our knowledge of disorders that affect the autonomic nervous system. At first these investigations focused primarily on neurocardiogenic (or reflex) syncope, largely a result of the development of head-up tilt table testing as a fairly reliable method of provoking episodes of autonomic nervous system decompensation. This not only allowed for a long sought after diagnostic tool, but also provided a stable environment during which a number of measurements and tests could be performed. In the course of these investigations it became evident that a subgroup of patients had a somewhat different form of autonomic disturbance that resulted in persistent postural tachycardia and orthostatic intolerance. More detailed observations of these patients uncovered a consistent set of clinical histories and tilt responses associated with similar complaints of postural tachycardia, exercise intolerance, extreme fatigue, dizziness, lightheadedness, near-syncope, and visual blurring [1]. This disorder has been referred to as the postural orthostatic tachycardia syndrome (POTS) or orthostatic intolerance syndrome. This condition has also been implicated in the pathogenesis of symptoms in the chronic fatigue syndrome (CFS) in a subset of patients. This chapter presents a review of the pathophysiology, diagnosis, and management of this disorder as well as its potential relation to CFS.

Historical perspective

To be able to tolerate the demands of an active lifestyle, almost everyone will face situations that require long periods of standing (sometimes lasting hours), without significant problems. There are a multitude of disorders that have the potential to reduce an individual's ability to stand for prolonged periods. To remain upright without symptoms, an individual must maintain a continuous and adequate flow of oxygen to the brain. Conditions such as dehydration, anemia, the effects of pharmacotherapy (either medicinal or secretional), and heart failure may compromise both the ability to stand as well as the capacity to exercise [2]. However, in the absence of these (and similar) causes, the possibility of a failure of autonomically mediated control of the circulation may be present. The mechanisms by which circulatory control is maintained have already been discussed in detail in Chapters 3 and 4.

By the mid-19th century, physicians had begun to report on patients with a disorder that was characterized by palpitations, exercise intolerance, and extreme fatigue, which would occur suddenly without an obvious cause (such as dehydration, blood loss, or prolonged immobility) [3]. During the American Civil War, cases of orthostatic intolerance and postural tachycardia were clearly described by Da Costa [4] who referred to the condition as *irritable heart syndrome.*

By the time of the First World War there were a

series of reports of ailments employing a variety of labels such as *neuroregulatory asthenia*. Most notable was Thomas Lewis' [5] investigations into a condition that he referred to as the *effort syndrome*. He stated that fatigue was "an almost universal complaint" among these patients along with exercise intolerance with concomitant complaints of palpitations, chest pain, sweating, syncope, and near-syncope. Lewis also reported that these patients displayed an impressive postural tachycardia with heart rates going from 85 b min^{-1} supine to close to 120 b min^{-1} when standing or carrying out minor activity (occurring in the absence of anemia, dehydration, or other known disease process). In some of these patients the blood pressure fell significantly, while in others only a modest decline occurred. Lewis postulated that in these individuals, "the potential reservoir in the veins takes up the blood, the supply to the heart falls away, and the arterial pressure falls rapidly," often with a compensatory tachycardia. The reduction in blood pressure he thought, "may be sufficient to produce cerebral anaemia." The clinical significance of measuring orthostatic changes in heart rate and blood pressure was almost simultaneously reported by Sewall in 1919 [6]. He described several individuals with an increase in heart rate > 28 b min^{-1} without a significant fall in blood pressure, associated with symptoms of orthostatic intolerance.

By the mid-1920s, two papers appeared describing orthostatic tachycardia with only a modest decline in blood pressure that was associated with an orthostatic reduction in cardiac output (by 19–28.6%) and stroke volume (by 47.5–54.9%). In 1934, Nylin [7] confirmed these findings in a group of similar patients, while also reporting a significant orthostatic reduction in the radiologic image size of the heart. Bjure and Laurell [8] referred to this disorder as orthostatic arterial anemia (although none of the patients was anemic on laboratory analysis) and reported that immersion of the legs in cold water (35°C) significantly reduced their postural tachycardia and hypotension and reversed the fall in cardiac output (as well as their fatigue, headache, dizziness, and near-syncope). They later reported that either abdominal or lower limb compression had similar (although a less reliable) effect [9]. They also postulated that the orthostatic tachycardia and hypotension was caused by pooling in the lower extremities and abdomen of these patients.

By the time of the Second World War, MacLean *et al.* [10] described a group of patients who demonstrated a pronounced orthostatic tachycardia (with only a modest fall in blood pressure) who had exercise intolerance, palpitations, and fatigue. They also demonstrated that prevention of blood flow to the legs by applying tourniquets to both thighs could prevent the orthostatic tachycardia from occurring. In a separate paper they also found that a high salt intake along with sleeping with the head of the bed elevated approximately 40 cm would lessen the severity of the symptoms [11]. In both papers, MacLean *et al.* postulated that the mechanism responsible for these findings was a reduction in venous return to the heart because of a lack of appropriate vasoconstriction at the capillary venous level.

In the 1960s, Frolich *et al.* [12] described two patients who had pronounced postural tachycardia (a rise in heart rate of > 40 b min^{-1} on standing without hypotension) associated with postural palpitations, anxiety, dizziness, and near-syncope. Both patients exhibited an exaggerated response to intravenous isoproterenol and had a reduction in symptoms after being placed on beta-blocker therapy. Later, Rosen and Cryer [13] used the term *postural tachycardia syndrome* in reference to a patient who displayed a > 44 b min^{-1} rise in heart rate upon standing (without hypotension) who also complained of postural palpitations, fatigue, and exercise intolerance. Similarly, Fouad *et al.* [14] reported on patients complaining of orthostatic intolerance who displayed a pronounced postural tachycardia with only modest hypotension, labeling the disorder *idiopathic hypovolemia*. Streeten *et al.* [15] then investigated a virtually identical group of patients by giving sodium pertechnetate ^{99}Tc-labeled red cells then performing gamma camera counting over the lower extremities while supine and upright. They displayed marked venous pooling in the lower extremities while upright. Later, Streeten [16] reported on a similar group of patients who also experienced an exaggerated response to isoproterenol infusion.

Shortly thereafter, Hoeldtke *et al.* [17,18] described 13 patients, complaining of exercise intolerance, extreme fatigue, anxiety, and cognitive impairment, who demonstrated a marked postural tachycardia. Schondorf and Low [19] performed an extensive analysis of 16 patients with profound exercise intolerance, severe fatigue, lightheadedness, and bowel hypomotility. Several of these patients had been previously labeled as having panic attacks or chronic anxiety. Yet during head-up tilt table testing these patients demonstrated markedly abnormal cardiovascular responses with heart rates that would dramatically rise to as much as 120–170 b min^{-1}, often within the first 2–5 min of upright tilt. Although some of these patients exhibited a mild reduction in blood pressure, most remained normotensive and some actually became hypertensive [20].

This concept was further amplified in an article by Khurana [21] who reported on a series of eight patients with pronounced orthostatic tachycardia who also had disturbed sudomotor function with diminished function throughout the lower extremities (thought most likely a result of deinnervation). Grubb et al. [1] thereafter reported on a total of 28 patients who had been referred for evaluation of extreme fatigue, exercise intolerance, and cognitive impairment associated with significant postural tachycardia. During head-up tilt table testing, each patient demonstrated a minimum 30 b min^{-1} increase in heart rate during the first 10 min of upright posture. The peak heart rate seen in almost all cases exceeded 120 b min^{-1} within the first 10 min of upright tilt. A modest mean decline of 20 mmHg was observed during tilt; however, in no patient did the systolic pressure fall below 85–90 mmHg. Karas et al. [22] have reported nearly identical findings in a group of adolescent patients, suggesting there is a wide age distribution of patients who are affected by the disorder.

Many investigators have used the term "*postural tachycardia syndrome*" (POTS) to describe the constellation of associated signs and symptoms these patients experience. Most have felt that it represents a mild (yet significant) disturbance in autonomic nervous system function (i.e., a dysautonomia). Over time it became increasingly apparent that the condition was probably composed of a heterogeneous group of disorders with similar clinical characteristics.

Several investigators observed that in some patients there appeared to be a strong familial predisposition toward the development of these disorders. This suspicion was recently given credence in a brilliant study by investigators at Vanderbilt who determined the exact genetic basis for the disorder in one severely affected family [23]. The gene defect results in a poorly functioning norepinephrine reuptake transporter protein that allows for excessive serum norepinephrine levels. Some investigators have felt that there may be multiple different genetic forms of POTS and detailed investigations are currently underway [24]. Rowe et al. [25] proposed a potential link between Ehlers–Danlos III syndrome (joint hypermobility syndrome) and POTS.

At the same time, other investigators have noted that many patients have developed symptoms after a febrile illness (presumed to be viral), suggesting that a possible immune-mediated mechanism might be involved. Confirmation of this basic concept was recently made in a landmark study by investigators at the Mayo Clinic who found that some patients with autonomic neuropathies were found to have high serum levels of autoantibodies to acetylcholine receptors in the peripheral autonomic ganglia [26]. The levels of these antibodies seemed to correlate with the severity of the illness.

Recent studies have suggested that there potentially may be an overlap between POTS and "inappropriate" sinus tachycardia [27]. Support for this concept has recently been provided by Shen et al. [28] who noted that radiofrequency ablation of the sinus node had little effect on symptoms in patients with POTS, and on occasion made people worse. The present authors have noted that some women develop POTS after pregnancy, with the onset of symptoms occurring in the early postpartum period [29]. POTS may also be a paraneoplastic manifestation of adenocarcinomas, with the tumors producing autoantibodies to acetylcholine receptors similar to those seen following viral infections [30].

Future investigations will no doubt uncover further subgroups with similar (while at the same time distinct) pathophysiologies, a situation not unlike that found to exist in the long QT syndromes.

Definitions and prevalence

A great variety of different terms have been employed to describe these disorders and have made reading

Table 13.1 The grading of orthostatic intolerance. (Adapted from [34].)

Grade 0

Normal orthostatic tolerance

Grade I

Orthostatic symptoms are infrequent or occur only under conditions of
  increased orthostatic stress

Subject is able to stand > 15 min on most occasions

Subject typically has unrestricted activities of daily living

Grade II

Orthostatic symptoms are frequent, developing at least once a week

Orthostatic symptoms commonly develop with orthostatic stress

Grade III

Orthostatic symptoms develop on most occasions and are regularly unmasked
  by orthostatic stresses

Subject is able to stand < 1 min on most occasions

Patient is seriously incapacitated, being bed- or wheelchair-bound because of
  orthostatic intolerance

Syncope/presyncope is common if patient attempts to stand

Symptoms may vary with time and state of hydration and circumstances.
Orthostatic stresses include prolonged standing, a meal, exertion, and head
stress.

both the historical and current literature somewhat confusing. While the term orthostatic intolerance has frequently been used in conjunction with POTS, its definition is nevertheless unique [31]. Orthostatic intolerance is currently defined as the provocation of symptoms upon standing that are relieved when becoming supine [32]. These patients will often complain of exercise intolerance, extreme fatigue, lightheadedness, diminished concentration, tremulousness, nausea, headache, near-syncope, and occasionally syncope [33]. Because the degree of autonomic failure these patients exhibit is not severe and the physical findings more subtle, patients are often misdiagnosed as having a form of panic disorder or chronic anxiety [34].

In many of these patients, regular daily activities such as housework, bathing, or even eating may greatly exacerbate symptoms and may thus limit even the most fundamental of normal activities [35]. Interestingly, the severity of symptoms is more prominent in these patients than in those with more pronounced autonomic failure syndromes such as pure autonomic failure [33]. Recent studies have demonstrated that many patients with POTS demonstrate a degree of functional impairment similar to patients with chronic obstructive pul-

monary disease or congestive heart failure [36]. Recently, a grading system for the severity of orthostatic intolerance has been developed (similar to that used in heart failure), which is summarized in Table 13.1 [34].

The impact of this disorder is considerable. Several authors have estimated that there are approximately 500,000–1,000,000 patients with POTS in the USA alone, of whom up to 25% are disabled and unable to work [36,37]. The potential economic burden of this condition is great, not only in direct costs related to health care but also as a result of indirect costs related to work absence and disability. Orthostatic intolerance has been reported to cause approximately 4.8 million days of work absence annually in Germany, nearly 2 million more days than were lost as a result of hypertension (3.2 million days of work absence) over the same time frame [38]. Often, the patients are young and in what would normally have been one of the most productive periods of their lives.

Orthostatic intolerance may also impair work performance and safety. An assessment of 1000 falls during work showed orthostatic intolerance to be a potential causal factor in at least 50 cases [39]. Thus, POTS could pose a substantial safety

Table 13.2 Criteria for postural tachycardia syndrome.

1 Heart rate increase of ≥ 30 b min⁻¹ within 10 min of standing or head up tilt *or*

2 Heart rate ≥ 120 b min⁻¹ within 10 min of standing or upright tilt

3 Consistent symptoms of orthostatic intolerance

4 Absence of a known cause of autonomic neuropathy

5 Serum norepinephrine > 600 pg/mL (hyperadrenergic form)

risk in occupations such as construction workers, scaffolders, roofers, and those working with heavy machinery.

POTS is currently defined as the development of orthostatic intolerance symptoms accompanied by a heart rate increase of at least 30 b min⁻¹ (or a rate that exceeds 120 b min⁻¹) that occurs within the first 10 min of standing or head-up tilt, which occurs in the absence of other chronic debilitating disorders, prolonged bed rest, or medications that impair autonomic reflexes (Table 13.2) [31]. Low *et al.* [34] have stated that in regard to the usual age range of most patients with POTS (15–50 years), an increment of 30 b min⁻1 exceeds the 99th percentile for control subjects from 10 to 13 years.

Most groups have focused on postural tachycardia as an excessive increase in heart rate representing the earliest and most consistent, easily measured finding of orthostatic intolerance. However, it is important to realize that most patients with orthostatic intolerance do not have orthostatic hypotension (a fall of > 20/10 mmHg). Rather, most of these patients will have only a modest decline in blood pressure, no decline at all, or even an increase in blood pressure when they assume an upright posture. Nevertheless, focusing on heart rate has the drawback of overlooking non-orthostatic autonomic symptoms such as paroxysmal disturbances in sweating, blood pressure regulation, thermoregulatory and bowel function. Many patients report that problems such as bowel hypomotility are more troubling than are the hemodynamic and heart rate disturbances.

Classification and clinical features

POTS appears to be a syndrome composed of a heterogeneous group of different disorders associated with similar clinical manifestations. While a variety of different classifications have been proposed, the one presented here seems to be both clinically useful and consistent with current scientific evidence. Any such system of classification is, by its very nature, somewhat arbitrary and open to constant discussion, debate, and revision over time.

At present, the authors classify POTS as being primary or secondary. The primary disorders are idiopathic and not associated with other diseases. The secondary forms are usually seen in association with a particular disease or have been found to arise from a known structural or biochemical abnormality (Fig. 13.1).

The primary forms are divided into two major subtypes. The first and largest subtype is referred to as the *partial dysautonomic* form [37]. These patients appear to have a mild form of peripheral autonomic neuropathy manifested by an inability of the peripheral vasculature to constrict adequately in response to orthostatic stress. They demonstrate an increase in heart rate and contractility while upright that represents a compensatory mechanism

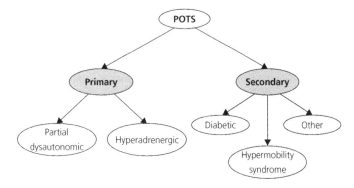

Fig. 13.1 Postural orthostatic tachycardia syndrome (POTS). From Kanjwal *et al*. The postural orthostatic tachycardia syndrome: definitions, diagnosis, and management. *PACE* 2003;**26**:1748, with permission.

which attempts to maintain systemic blood pressure and cerebral perfusion at adequate levels [1]. While in the early stages of this form of POTS, the increase in heart rate and contractility may be fully compensatory, as the disorder progresses greater and greater degrees of peripheral venous pooling occur, and patients become increasingly dependent on their skeletal muscle pumps to maintain adequate venous return. As upright venous pooling increases there is a progressive fall in ventricular preload with more baroreceptor unloading resulting in an increase in sympathetic outflow. Some researchers have used microneurography and heart rate variability analysis to measure sympathetic nerve activity in this form of POTS, finding that they demonstrate an overall increase in adrenergic tone at rest and an enhanced postganglionic sympathetic response to upright posture [32]. However, serum catecholamine levels are usually normal or are only slightly elevated with upright posture. In a remarkable series of studies, Goldstein et al. [40] compared POTS patients with those with neurocardiogenic syncope (NCS), measuring neurochemical indices of cardiac release, reuptake of norepinephrine based on cardiac norepinephrine spillover, cardiac extraction of circulating ^{3}H-norepinephrine, and measurement of left ventricular myocardial innervation density using 6-[^{16}F]-fluorodopamine positron emission scanning. They discovered that POTS and NCS involve substantial, different, tonic abnormalities of cardiac sympathetic function. In NCS they found abnormal, tonically decreased cardiac norepinephrine release, decreased cardiac sympathetic nerve traffic as well as a tonic restraint of sympathetic outflow attenuated increments in sympathetic outflow to skeletal muscles during orthostasis. In contrast, POTS patients demonstrated increased norepinephrine release from intact cardiac sympathetic nerves. Interestingly, they also found that POTS patients had relative tachycardia even during supine rest, in part because of increased norepinephrine delivery to adrenoreceptors on myocardial pacemaker cells. They concluded that in these POTS patients cardiac sympathetic stimulation mainly reflects compensatory activation in response to excessively decreased venous return to the heart. The patients' symptoms would be related to a relative state of volume depletion with additional symptoms from

cardiac sympathetic activation such as palpitations or atypical chest pain.

Stewart [41] has challenged the concept that the blood pooling seen in POTS patients is brought about by an increased venous capacitance. POTS patients were compared with controls using strain gauge plethysmography during supine posture and progressive head-up tilt. He found that venous compliance in POTS was similar to controls and felt that pooling in POTS was caused by blunted arterial vasoconstriction, which produces passive redistribution of blood within peripheral venous capacitance beds. Interestingly, a number of authors have reported that one of the most prominent clinical manifestations of the partial dysautonomic form of POTS is the development of a deep, mottled (almost bluish) discoloration of the lower extremities upon standing (sometimes referred to as acral cyanosis) [34]. Tani et al. [42] have provided compelling evidence that POTS patients have excessive splanchnic-mesenteric blood pooling while supine and at rest (the splanchnic vascular bed normally contains up to 30% of blood volume). They postulated that a limited autonomic neuropathy resulting in peripheral denervation may be the cause of the increased resting flow and reduced mesenteric resistance in these patients. Recent studies using transcranial Doppler ultrasonography have suggested that the development of some symptoms may occur because of an impairment of cerebrovascular autoregulation of blood flow [43,44].

The age at presentation ranges between 14 and 50 years. There is a fairly consistent female to male ratio of 2–5 : 1, suggesting that reproductive hormones may be important etiologically [45]. Indeed, onset of POTS prior to menarche or after menopause is uncommon. A significant number of patients report that their symptoms began suddenly after an acute febrile illness (often presumed to be viral). Other reported precipitating factors have been pregnancy, immunization, sepsis, surgery, and trauma [46]. Often, these patients present complaining of palpitations, lightheadedness, exercise intolerance, extreme fatigue, visual blurring or tunneling, and a sense of weakness (often more pronounced in the legs). A surprising number of patients complain of a significant degree of cognitive impairment. Using a complex battery of functional tests, Duschek *et al.* [47] have demonstrated that there is a significant reduction in cognitive and psychomotor performance that accompanies even moderate degrees of hypotension (mean BP 108/69 mmHg), as compared with normotensive controls. Less frequent complaints of POTS patients are anxiety, bloating, nausea, altered bowel function, chest wall pain, abnormal sweating, a feeling of always being cold, and pain in the extremities [48]. Occasionally, patients will report a resting tachycardia or will awaken from sleep (usually in the early morning hours) complaining of palpitations [49]. A number of patients complain of muscular headaches associated with upright posture which begin in the occipital region of the skull and radiate to the shoulders [1]. A common feature of this form of POTS is the cyclic nature of symptoms. Symptoms often worsen 4–5 days prior to menstruation. Many patients will report some degree of depression, a symptom that several investigators have linked to hypotension and cognitive impairment secondary to reduced cerebral blood flow (which tends to improve with correction of the hypotension and restoration of cerebral blood flow to normal) [50–52]. Some patients may report occasional symptoms at rest associated with changes in blood pressure and heart rate unrelated to arrhythmias. Holter monitoring typically shows a sinus tachycardia; however, sinus bradycardia has also been seen.

It is currently felt that many of the patients with the partial dysautonomic form of POTS may have an immune-mediated pathogenesis. Vernino *et al.* [26] have identified serum autoantibodies to α_3-acetylcholine receptors of the peripheral autonomic ganglia in patients with postviral neuropathic dysautonomia. It is suspected that there are probably other types of autoantibodies present, yet these still await identification. Stewart [53] has proposed a potential link between altered vasoreactivity and antecedent inflammatory disease involving the chronic elaboration of cytokines with potent vasoactive properties (such as interleukin 1 [IL-1], IL-6, and tumor necrosis factor-alpha). Other investigators have suggested a possible link with mitochondrial disorders [54]. Other potential causes may also exist, as some patients with the partial dysautonomic form do not report any antecedent illness and give a long history of symptoms

dating from adolescence [55]. Further studies are attempting to better understand the pathophysiology at work in these patients.

A second (and much less frequent) subtype of POTS has been identified where patients seem to manifest a form of β-adrenergic receptor hypersensitivity, a disorder referred to as hyperadrenergic POTS [46]. While these patients share many characteristics with those with the partial dysautonomic form of POTS, they have several unique features. Patients more commonly report a long, slow onset of symptoms rather than a dramatic, abrupt one.

Hyperadrenergic POTS patients often complain of extreme tremulousness, anxiety when upright, and cold, sweaty extremities [35]. Some patients may experience a significant increase in urinary output after a short time upright. Over half of these patients will have true migraine headaches that include a definite prodrome and unilateral (often frontal) onset with photophobia and nausea. Often, these patients will display orthostatic hypertension during standing or tilt and an exaggerated response to low-dose isoproterenol infusions while supine (an increase of > 30 b min^{-1} after receiving 1 µg min^{-1} isoproterenol) [56]. It is unclear whether this hypersensitivity is primary in nature or a manifestation of deinnervation sensitivity. Many of these patients appear to have experienced excessive sympathetic activation in some neuronal distribution nearly all the time, which is not appropriately modulated by baroreflex activity [57]. As opposed to the partial dysautonomic POTS patients, the serum catecholamine levels of the hyperadrenergic patients are often significantly elevated during upright posture (serum norepinephrine levels are often > 600 ng mL^{-1}) [58].

One study has identified a specific genetic abnormality in a small group of patients with hyperadrenergic POTS [23]. In these individuals, a single point mutation results in a dysfunction of the reuptake transported protein that clears norepinephrine from the intrasynaptic cleft. The resultant inability to adequately control norepinephrine clearance produces a state of excessive sympathetic activation to a variety of sympathetic stimuli that results in a "hyperadrenergic" state [59]. Studies are cuurently underway to determine the exact frequency of this mutation in affected patients. It is certainly quite possible that other abnormalities in neurophysiologic control exist that could produce similar physiological manifestations. It is also likely that other primary forms of POTS will be elaborated over time, as some patients do not fit well into either of the aforementioned groups. The majority of POTS patients appear to have the partial dysautonomic form, while only a fairly small proportion (< 10%) have the hyperadrenergic type.

The term secondary POTS is employed to describe conditions that produce peripheral autonomic deinnervation but with preserved cardiac innervation. The most frequent of these is diabetes mellitus, but it can also be seen in disorders such as sarcoidosis, amyloidosis, alcoholism, chemotherapy (especially with the vinca alkaloids), Sjögren's syndrome, lupus, and heavy metal poisoning [34]. Emerging evidence has revealed that an important cause of secondary POTS is the connective tissue disorder currently referred to as the joint hypermobility syndrome (previously known as type III Ehlers–Danlos syndrome) [60]. This inherited abnormality of connective tissue is characterized by soft, velvety skin with variable hyperextensibility, joint hypermobility, and connective tissue fragility. Vascular abnormalities including easy bruisability, premature varicose veins, and orthostatic acrocyanosis are also commonly observed in this condition, as well as easy fatiguability and diffuse muscle and joint pain. Rowe et al. [25] found a close connection between orthostatic intolerance, CFS, and type III Ehlers–Danlos syndrome (EDS). They proposed that the high rate of orthostatic intolerance in EDS could be attributed to the abnormal connective tissue present in the dependent blood vessels, which permit the veins to distend excessively in response to normal hydrostatic pressures leading to a marked increase in venous pooling with a resultant compensatory tachycardia. They went on to confirm that joint hypermobility was found in 60% of adolescents with CFS compared with just 24% of healthy controls [60]. This concept was confirmed by Gazit et al. [61] who compared responses of patients with the joint hypermobility syndrome (JHS/EDS III) with those of normal control subjects to an extensive battery of autonomic nervous system tests. Orthostatic hypotension, POTS, and/or orthostatic intolerance were found in 78% of patients with joint hypermobility syndrome compared with 10% of control subjects.

They also felt that excessive vessel distensibility allowed excessive blood pooling in dependent areas of the body in these patients. They also noted that the connective tissue in blood vessels, as well as in articular ligaments, contain mainly type I and type III collagen, and that defects in these collagens have been reported in skin biopsies of patients with the joint hypermobility syndrome. A significant number of the patients with refractory POTS seen in the autonomic disorders clinic at the Medical College of Ohio have been found to meet the criteria for the joint hypermobility syndrome, suggesting that this subgroup may constitute a large proportion of the POTS population.

On occasion, POTS may be the initial presenting sign of more severe autonomic nervous system disorders such as pure autonomic failure (PAF) or multisystem atrophy (MSA) [62]. In addition, POTS may occur as a paraneoplastic syndrome seen in association with adenocarcinoma of the lung, breast, pancreas, and ovary [63]. Studies have suggested that these tumors may actually produce antibodies against acetylcholine receptors in the autonomic ganglia, similar to those seen in postviral autonomic neuropathies [30].

There is only limited information available on the prognosis of POTS patients. The authors' own experiences have not yet been sufficiently analyzed to provide definite information, and the variable nature of the disorder makes prognostication challenging. Nevertheless, there is a general agreement among investigators that in the postviral onset group of patients approximately one-half will make a good practical recovery over a 2–5-year period. Recovery is defined as "the relative absence of orthostatic symptoms and the ability to perform activities of daily living with no or only minimal restriction" [64]. Symptomatic improvement seems to correlate with falling titers of serum autoantibodies to acetylcholine receptors [30]. In general, the authors have observed much higher recovery rates in younger patients (adolescents and young adult) as compared with those of older individuals. Indeed, there seems to be a "developmental" form of the disorder, principally affecting young women, characterized by an onset of symptoms shortly after menarche, sometime between 10 and 14 years of age [65]. There is then a progressive gradual worsening of symptoms over the ensuing years, which reach their peak of intensity around age 16–17 years, during which time the patient may be nearly incapacitated [22]. This period is then followed by a slow progressive recovery that continues into young adulthood (ages 19–22 years), at which time the majority of symptoms will have abated. While the vast majority of patients who display this "developmental" pattern will enjoy a near complete recovery in young adulthood, there is a significant minority (we estimate approximately 20%) who will remain highly symptomatic. The reason for this pattern is unclear but seems to coincide with an observed period of autonomic imbalance that occurs during the periods of rapid growth and development seen during adolescence, as well as the potential effect of reproductive hormones on autonomic control [65]. It is unclear at present what percentage of these patients may also have the joint hypermobility syndrome; however, studies are currently underway to help clarify this issue.

It is hoped that as time goes on and subgroups of POTS patients are better defined, more accurate prognostic data will become available. The prognosis of patients with the secondary POTS syndromes are usually determined by the prognosis of the underlying disorder.

POTS and pregnancy

POTS patients tend to tolerate pregnancy reasonably well; however, they require close follow-up during the course of their pregnancies. A number of significant adaptations in the cardiovascular system occur during pregnancy, principal among which is a major increase in circulating blood volume [66]. Most investigators have reported that there is an increase in blood volume during pregnancy to approximately 50% higher than in the non-pregnant state [67]. The increase in circulating volume is accompanied by a significant fall in systemic vascular resistance. This causes an overall fall in blood pressure (mostly diastolic) with a widening in the pulse pressure [68]. Blood flow thorough the extremities increases significantly during pregnancy. The mechanisms by which this occurs are not well understood; however, both estrogen and progesterone have been shown to have significant effects on peripheral vascular resistance [66].

We usually ask that the POTS patient contemplating pregnancy should have been stable for approximately 1 year. During that time, medications should be reduced to a minimum with agents that are felt to be relatively safe to use during pregnancy. The fall in vascular resistance occurs during the first trimester of pregnancy and the volume increase mainly during the second. As a consequence, the pregnant POTS patient may experience an increase in symptoms during the first trimester with a subsequent improvement during the second. The severity of symptoms during the third trimester of pregnancy are variable and seem to be dependent on the degree to which the uterus compresses the inferior vena cava [66]. In some patients symptoms may be severe enough to require bed rest during the first month of pregnancy. While delivery seems potentially daunting, in practice there have been few problems. The patient should be monitored closely during the delivery process and kept well hydrated. We have not noted a significant difference in outcome between women who had vaginal births and those who underwent cesarean sections. Therefore, we advise the obstetrician to pursue whatever options they feel are in the best interests of the mother and child.

The postpartum period is characterized by a fairly rapid return to the non-pregnant state. While the reduction in circulating volume occurs fairly promptly, the alterations in peripheral blood flow may present up to 6 weeks postpartum [67]. This reduction in circulating volume combined with a persistence of low vascular resistance may result in an increase in symptoms during this period. Nursing appears to attenuate this effect, possibly by reducing this sudden shift in volume and hormonal status. Thus, we have not noted an increased incidence of problems in either mother or child in POTS patients compared with normal controls (other than the previously mentioned periods of maternal hypotension). Some patients will enjoy a dramatic reduction in symptoms following pregnancy, while others will worsen. The majority seem to return to their prepregnancy symptom level.

Orthostatic intolerance and the chronic fatigue syndrome

In 1995, Rowe *et al.* [69] reported on a series of

seven adolescents with chronic fatigue or CFS and no history of syncope. All seven experienced significant hypotension during head-up tilt, four of whom had an improvement in fatigue in response to therapies aimed at correcting this hypotension. This group then described a larger group of 23 adolescent and adult patients with strictly defined CFS who underwent tilt table testing [70]. Of these, 22 experienced an abnormal hypotensive response, whereas only four of 14 control subjects experienced an abnormal response during head-up tilt, with the most frequent pattern being a neurocardiogenic one. Supine BP in patients with CFS was not significantly different from control subjects prior to testing: 119/72 mmHg in CFS and 118/75 mmHg in controls. However, during tilt table testing the mean BP had declined to 68/38 mmHg in the CFS patients vs. 118/66 mmHg in the control group (P < 0.001).

A subsequent study by Freeman and Komaroff [71], which looked at a series of 20 CFS patients, found that only 25% had an abnormal response to tilt table testing. However, Chung et al. [72], in evaluating 40 CFS patients with tilt table testing (HUTT), found a 95% abnormal response rate (28% orthostatic hypotension, 25% neurocardiogenic syncope, and 43% POTS). Schondorf et al. [73] later evaluated 75 CFS patients with HUTT and reported 40% abnormal response rate. A detailed series of observations was then made by Stewart et al. [74], who compared 26 adolescents with CFS with 26 patients with suspected NCS and 13 healthy controls using HUTT. A total of four of 13 controls and 18 of 26 NCS patients demonstrated an abrupt fall in BP and heart rate associated with loss of consciousness, as opposed to 25 of 26 CFS patients who experienced severe orthostatic symptoms associated with syncope in seven of 25, orthostatic tachycardia with hypotension in 15 of 25, and orthostatic tachycardia without significant hypotension in three of 25. Interestingly, 18 of 25 CFS patients developed acrocyanosis, cool extremities, and edema (indicative of venous pooling), whereas none of the controls or NCS patients had similar responses.

Streeten and Anderson [75] have demonstrated evidence for delayed orthostatic hypotension and/or tachycardia among 15 CFS patients, caused by excessive gravitational venous pooling (which was correctable with external lower body compression), together with a suboptimal circulating erythrocyte volume.

Although not all investigations have identified a higher rate of orthostatic intolerance among those with CFS, we believe that the weight of evidence supports the concept that orthostatic intolerance is an important component of CFS in a subset of patients [76–81]. The proportion of CFS patients with POTS or neurally mediated hypotension may depend on the duration of tilt testing, the age of the subjects, the type of patients selected for study, and other factors. The largest study of tilt testing among adults with CFS thus far was the Florinef trial, in which 171 patients had a two-stage upright tilt test, the first stage consisting of 45 min at a 70° angle, and the second stage involving 15 min at the same angle during 2 µg min^{-1} isoproterenol infusion [82]. Of the 171, hypotension developed during tilt in 106, 39 of whom met criteria for the diagnosis of POTS in the first 10 min of tilt. Another seven subjects had POTS alone. Overall, 66% had defined hemodynamic abnormalities during tilt, and the remaining patients had symptoms of CFS provoked by the orthostatic stress. Conversely, Kenny and Graham [83] have reported that CFS-like symptoms are common in those being evaluated for vasovagal syncope. While a number of causes of CFS have been proposed, including enteroviral or other infections, immune dysfunction, a psychiatric disorder, hypothalamic-pituitary-adrenal insufficiency or a disorder of serotonin metabolism, orthostatic intolerance may be a final common pathway for symptoms in CFS, providing a framework in which many of the clinical features can be understood. Further studies are necessary to better elaborate this relationship.

Differential diagnosis and management

The first and most important step is to obtain a detailed history followed by a thorough physical examination, which should include a complete neurologic examination [84]. It is paramount that conditions that may produce orthostatic intolerance (such as dehydration, anemia, or chronic debilitating illness) be identified. In addition, any medications that could cause or exacerbate the

Table 13.3 Pharmacologic agents that may cause or worsen orthostatic intolerance.

Angiotensin-converting enzyme inhibitors
α-Receptor blockers
Calcium-channel blockers
Beta-blockers
Phenothiazines
Tricyclic antidepressants
Bromocriptine
Ethanol
Opiates
Diuretics
Hydralazine
Ganglionic-blocking agents
Nitrates
Sildenafil citrate
Monoamine oxidase (MAO) inhibitors

condition (e.g., any vasodilator, alcohol, tricyclic antidepressants, or monoamine oxidase inhibitors) should be noted (Table 13.3). Blood pressure and heart rate need to be measured in the supine, sitting, and standing positions. The latter should be taken not only immediately after standing but also at 2 and 5 min. Electrocardiograms are obtained for almost all patients. Other evaluations, such as echocardiography, are performed when the evaluator deems them appropriate. Tachycardias that are abrupt in onset and termination, and that have no relation to position, suggest a possible cardiac re-entrant arrhythmia and may require electrophysiologic study for proper identification. In addition, we check patients for the presence of the joint hypermobility syndrome using the Brighton revised criteria (Table 13.4; Fig. 13.2).

In addition to orthostatic measurements, the authors frequently use head-up tilt table testing as a standardized measure of an individual's response to postural change [1,84]. The patient is positioned on a standard tilt table and following baseline measurements of blood pressure and heart rate are gradually inclined to a 70° head-up angle. Blood pressure and heart rate are measured every 1–2 min thereafter. A sustained heart rate increase > 30 b min^{-1} or a sustained rate of 120 b min^{-1} in the first 10 min of passive upright tilt is considered diagnostic. In select patients, the authors also measure plasma catecholamine levels in the supine and upright positions, and measure the supine heart

Table 13.4 The Brighton revised criteria for diagnosis of the joint hypermobility syndrome.

Major criteria
Brighton score of 4/9 or greater (either currently or historically)
Arthralgia for longer than 3 months in four or more joints

Minor criteria
Brighton score of 1–3/9 (0–3 if aged 50 years or older)
Arthralgia (≥ 3 months) in one to three joints, or back pain (≥ or equal to 3 months), spondylosis, spondylolysis/spondylolisthesis
Dislocation/subluxation in more than one joint, or in one or more joints on more than one occasion
Soft tissue rheumatism three or more lesions (e.g., epicondylitis, tenosynovitis, bursitis)
Marfanoid habitus (tall, slim, span : height ratio > 1.03, upper segment : lower segment ratio < 0.89, arachnodactyly [+ Steinberg/wrist sign])
Abnormal skin: striae, hyperextensibility, thin skin, or papyraceous scarring
Eye signs: drooping eyelids or myopia or antimongoloid slant
Varicose veins or hernia or uterine/rectal prolapse

Joint hypermobility syndrome diagnosis requires:
Two major criteria, or one major + two minor criteria, or four minor criteria, or two minor criteria and unequivocally affected first-degree relative

Joint hypermobility syndrome is excluded by presence of Marfan or Ehlers–Danlos syndromes (as defined by the Berlin nosology)

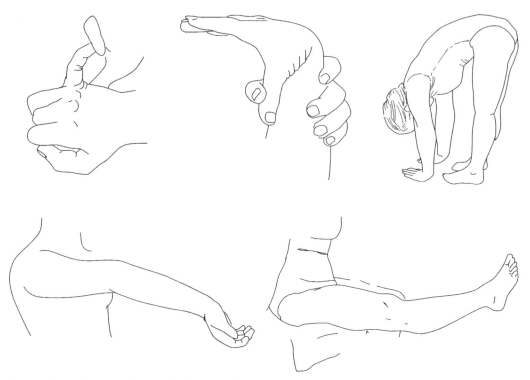

Fig. 13.2 The Brighton Revised Criteria for diagnosis of joint hypermobility syndrome.

rate response to an intravenous infusion of 1 μg min^{-1} isoproterenol. An increase of > 30 b min^{-1} is considered abnormal. Many of the POTS patients, if they are kept upright during head-up tilt for a sufficient period of time, can demonstrate a neurocardiogenic-like decompensation with hypotension and syncope.

During upright tilt or standing, many patients report the development of an intense coldness of the extremities. With continued standing, there may be excessive venous prominence that produces a deep blue discoloration of the lower extremities and hands. Sometimes, swelling of the feet is seen.

Some investigators use red cell isotope labeling techniques followed by gamma camera scanning techniques to determine the extent of peripheral blood pooling [85]. Other potential tests that may be used include thermoregulatory sweat testing, Valsalva maneuver, and sudomotor axion testing, the details of which can be found elsewhere [86,87].

The differential diagnosis is with panic or somatization disorder, extreme deconditioning, and autonomic causes of true orthostatic hypotension. Panic and somatization disorders can be distin-

guished from POTS by the fact that in the latter symptoms are usually precipitated by upright posture, reduction in systems with recumbency, and the laboratory findings of a dysautonomia [64]. Panic and somatization disorders are not associated with autonomic laboratory abnormalities, nor are symptoms confined to the upright posture. Interestingly, patients with POTS report relatively little psychologic distress, in contrast to patients with recurrent NGS where psychosocial impairment is reported to be greater than physical impairment [36].

The differentiation of POTS from autonomic causes of orthostatic hypotension (PAF, MSA) is reasonably straightforward (Table 13.5) [88]. The symptoms of orthostatic hypotension are comparable but the symptoms of sympathetic overactivity (e.g., postural anxiety, tremor, nausea, palpitations, and sweating) that are so characteristic of POTS are absent in autonomic orthostatic hypotension. In addition, patients with autonomic orthostatic hypotension demonstrate evidence of a state of generalized autonomic failure involving cardiovagal, sudomotor, urinary, adrenergic, and

Table 13.5 Comparison between generalized autonomic neuropathy patients and patients with postural orthostatic tachycardia syndrome (POTS). (Adapted from [49].)

Parameter	Autonomic orthostatic hypotension	POTS
Orthostatic dizziness	Variably absent	Present
Orthostatic tremulousness	Absent	Common
Orthostatic palpitations	Absent	Common
Orthostatic hypotension	Consistent	Usually absent
Orthostatic tachycardia	Reduced	Exaggerated
Supine norepinephrine	Usually reduced	Normal or increased
Standing norepinephrine	Reduced	Increased or normal
HR response to deep breathing	Reduced	Normal
Valsalva ratio	Reduced	Normal or increased
BP_{BB} to VM:		
Early phase II	Markedly increased	Increased
Late phase II	Absent	Normal or reduced
Phase IV	Absent	Increased

BP_{BB}, beat-to-beat blood pressure; HR, heart rate; VM, Valsalva maneuver.

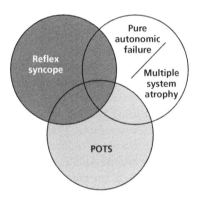

Fig. 13.3 A graphic representation of the overlap between various autonomic disorders associated with orthostatic intolerance. POTS, postural orthostatic tachycardia syndrome. From Kanjwal *et al.* The postural orthostatic tachycardia syndrome: definitions, diagnosis, and management. *PACE* 2003;**26**:1754, with permission.

gastrointestinal systems. However, there can be considerable overlap between these disorders that can make determinations of subgroups difficult (Fig. 13.3).

Another differential diagnosis is with inappropriate sinus tachycardia. There are several similarities between inappropriate sinus tachycardia and POTS, in particular with the hyperadrenergic form [89]. Clinical presentations are much the same and inappropriate sinus tachycardia is seen more frequently in women. Increased heart rate responsiveness to isoproterenol is seen in both conditions, suggesting that they represent different points on

the spectrum of the same disease process [90]. The major differences are that POTS patients seem to display a greater degree of postural change in heart rate and the resting (supine) heart rates infrequently exceed 100 b min^{-1} (as opposed to inappropriate sinus tachycardia where resting heart rates > 100 b min^{-1} are more common).

It should also be kept in mind that POTS may occur secondary to another disorder. These patients present with POTS symptoms and with signs and symptoms of the primary disorder. While some degree of weight loss may be seen in POTS patients, extreme cachexia is uncommon and should prompt the search for other disorders (such as a malignancy or diabetes). In some patients with secondary POTS, the underlying disorder may not be evident at first and will only become apparent over time.

Management

Treatment of patients with POTS can present unique challenges as no single approach is uniformly effective [91]. Initially, one must identify any potentially reversible cause that may require special treatments. These may include prolonged immobilization, significant weight loss, chronic debilitating diseases, malignancy, and diabetes mellitus. Any medications that could be producing or contributing to the problem should be identified (and in some cases one should consider the potential for illicit drug use). Once a diagnosis has been established, the patient and their family must be educated as to the nature of the disorder and to avoid any aggravating factors such as dehydration, extreme heat, and consumption of alcohol. Thereafter, the patient is asked to increase his or her fluid and sodium intake, and to sleep with the head of the bed slightly elevated (the authors usually ask the patient to place a brick under each of the bed's back bedposts) to help condition the patient to orthostatic stress. Aerobic exercise is also encouraged, asking the patient to slowly work up to doing a minimum of 20 min of continuous aerobic activity at least three times per week. Many patients, especially those who are very deconditioned, have found that water exercises are better tolerated and a good place to begin reconditioning. Some of us have found that manual physical therapists can identify movement restrictions in patients with CFS and orthostatic disorders, and that manual physical therapy techniques (as opposed to exercise-based treatments) provide a bridge between reduced activity and the benefits of exercise rehabilitation. When tolerated, resistance training of the lower extremities should also be encouraged. In some patients, elastic support hose are helpful in minimizing the degree of peripheral venous pooling [92]. They are most helpful if they are waist high and provide at least 30 mm of mercury counter-pressure.

In reference to medical therapy, one should keep in mind that a particular agent that is effective in one patient will have little effect in another, and that there is no way to predict the utility of any medication other than by trying it. As there is no medication approved by the US Food and Drug Administration for the treatment of POTS, all agents are used "off label." A variety of different pharmacologic agents have been found to be useful in the management of these patients. The approach to the patient with the partial dysautonomic form of POTS is different than to those with the hyperadrenergic form.

In the partial dysautonomic patient, the mineralocorticoid agent fludrocortisone is often used [93]. It not only expands plasma volume but also appears to sensitize peripheral α-adrenergic receptors to the patient's own catecholamines [94]. Side-effects include hypokalemia and hypomagnesemia. A recent, controlled trial of fludrocortisone in the

treatment of adult patients with CFS did not produce a significant reduction in symptoms [82]. Another volume expanding agent that may be helpful is oral vasopressin (or DDAVP), especially in those patients who complain of nocturnal polyuria. However, vasopressin may sometimes cause headaches and hyponatremia [95].

Because much of the problem occurs as a result of a failure of vascular resistance to increase properly, vasoconstrictors have proven useful in treatment [96,97]. A particularly helpful agent is the peripheral α_1-receptor stimulating agent midodrine hydrochloride. It frequently improves orthostatic tolerance and diminishes the degree of postural tachycardia. It is absorbed rapidly after oral administration, reaching peak concentrations in 20–40 min, with a serum half-life of approximately 30 min. It may produce an unpleasant sensation of "goosebumps" and a sensation of scalp tingling. Some patients may experience extreme nausea from the drug as well as supine hypertension and mild chest discomfort.

Alternative agents are the amphetamine class agents, including methylphenidate and dexamfetamine, also vasoconstrictors, both of which have the advantage of being available in a number of long-acting once-a-day forms [98]. Side-effects include headache, insomnia, tremor, and dependence. Recently, the drug modafinil has been successfully employed to help ameliorate the oppressive sense of fatigue and daytime hypersomnolence that these patients experience. Yohimbine is a centrally active, selective α_2-antagonist that increases central nervous system sympathetic outflow [99]. While helpful in some patients, many cannot tolerate it because of the side-effects of anxiety, tremor, and palpitations. Octreotide (a potent vasoconstrictor) has also been reported to be useful in management of select patients with POTS [100]. Erythropoietin has proven extremely useful in patients refractory to other forms of therapy. Erythropoietin appears not only to augment intravascular volume via its increase in red cell mass, but also appears to have a direct vasoconstrictive effect [101–103]. The drawbacks of treatment with erythropoietin are its extreme expense and the fact that it must be administered by subcutaneous injection and red cell counts monitored closely. In those patients with postviral POTS, the finding of autoantibodies to acetylcholine receptors has prompted evaluation of the acetylcholinesterase inhibitor pyridostigmine as a potential therapy [104].

In patients with the hyperadrenergic form of POTS, therapies are used that compensate for the high catecholamine levels. β-Adrenergic blocking agents are useful; whereas they tend to make patients with the partial dysautonomic form worse [95]. The combined alpha- and beta-blocking agent labetalol is often particularly effective. Agents with central sympatholytic activity can be helpful in the treatment of select patients; however, they should be used carefully as some patients can be quite sensitive to their effects. Clonidine is an α_2-agonist that has a central sympatholytic effect and has been one of the most effective agents in this group of patients [105]. The authors often prefer the patch form because of its more consistent effect and its greater degree of compliance. Clonidine can stabilize heart rate and blood pressure in patients with a large amount of postganglionic sympathetic involvement in whom postjunctional α_2-receptors (which are abundant in the venous system) are hypersensitive. Some groups have reported similar success with methyldopa, while other groups have suggested that phenobarbital may also be useful [95].

The serotonin reuptake inhibitors may be useful in the treatment of select patients with POTS. Several studies have suggested that in some patients with syndromes of autonomic dysfunction there may be a disturbance in central serotonin production and regulation leading to an increase in sympathetic nervous system activity [106]. The serotonin reuptake inhibitors have been shown to reduce sympathetic nervous system activity [107]. While any of the serotonin reuptake inhibitors can be used, some prefer venlafaxine as the most effective (perhaps because of its effects on norepinephrine and serotonin). Side-effects may include nausea, tremor, agitation, and disturbed sleep. Pediatric patients in particular should be monitored for signs of agitation or paradoxical depression. Some investigators have suggested that fluoxetine be used in this age group as it has been the best studied.

Often, POTS patients will do best with a combination of different agents and the authors have often seen that low-dose combination therapy is often more effective and better tolerated than high-dose monotherapy [108]. As with any disorder, some patients will respond to therapy better than others (Table 13.6).

Table 13.6 Potentially useful therapies in postural orthostatic tachycardia syndrome (POTS).

Therapy	Usual usage	Drawbacks
Hydration and increased salt	Fluid intake of 2–2.5 L/day Na intake of 150–250 mEq q.d.	Weight gain, peripheral edema
Exercise	30 min of aerobic exercise three times a week	Too vigorous exercise may worsen symptoms
Elastic support hose	30 mmHg ankle counter-pressure	Hot, uncomfortable
Fludrocortisone	0.1–0.4 mg p.o. q.d.	Peripheral edema, hypokalemia, hypomagnesemia
Midodrine hydrochloride	2.5–10 mg p.o. t.i.d.	Nausea, scalp tingling, supine hypertension
Labetalol	100–200 mg p.o. b.i.d.	Hypotension, fatigue
Yohimbine	5.4 mg p.o. b.i.d. or t.i.d.	Nausea, flushing
Erythropoietin	8000 IU q week	Flu-like syndrome, expensive
Venlafaxine	75 mg XR form b.i.d.	Nausea, insomnia, tremor
Methylphenidate	5–10 mg p.o. t.i.d.	Headache, insomnia, dependence
Pyridostigmine	60–120 mg p.o. t.i.d.	Nausea, constipation, weakness
Phenobarbital	60–100 mg p.o. at bedtime	Sedation, dependence
Vasopressin (DDAVP)	0.1–0.2 mg p.o. at bedtime	Headache, hyponatremia
Clonidine	0.1–0.4 mg p.o. b.i.d. or TTS 1–3 patch q week	Dry mouth, constipation, blurred vision
Octreotide	25 µg b.i.d., may titrate to 100–200 µg t.i.d.	Nausea, abdominal pain, muscle cramps, hypertension

B.i.d., twice daily; p.o., by mouth; q.d., every day; t.i.d., three times a day; XR, extended release.

It should be kept in mind by anyone treating patients with POTS that there may be significant involvement of other systems under autonomic regulation (e.g., sweating, thermoregulation, bowel and bladder control, and sexual function) that may be equally as limiting as the heart rate and blood pressure aspects of the disorder [109,110]. Thus, physicians should be comfortable managing these problems or be able to work together with other specialists in a "team-like" approach. Fragmented and uncoordinated care by a variety of poorly communicating specialists does not serve the best needs of the patient. As time passes, the nature and severity of the disorder may potentially worsen and treatments may require periodic adjustments. Many of the postviral POTS patients seem to improve slowly over a 2–5-year period, and thus may be able to be gradually weaned off therapy [64].

One of the most important components of managing POTS (and often the most neglected) is the significant disruption that can occur in a patient's personal and social life leading to occupational, psychological, marital, legal, and financial problems. Even though many physicians are uncomfortable in helping the patient deal with these issues, these are often the areas that have the greatest impact on a patient's life and the lives of their families. The physician should be prepared to assist in helping the patient gain access to social workers, occupational therapy, psychological, and legal counseling. A biopsychosocial treatment approach including cognitive–behavioral intervention, as well as gradual physical therapy and pharmacotherapy is often needed to restore function and improve the patient's quality of life [36].

The attitude that the physician brings to bear in managing patients with severe POTS cannot be overemphasized. A positive, yet realistic approach by a sympathetic and knowledgeable staff has a significant impact on a patient's sense of well-being. Hope is a powerful medicine that should be encouraged by all who deal with these patients. A support group for adults with POTS is the National Dysautonomia Research Foundation (www.ndrf.org). For children and adolescents, there is the Dysautonomia Youth Network of America in the USA (www.dynakids.org) and the Syncope Trust and Anoxic Reflex Seizure group in the UK (www.stars.org.uk).

Conclusions

POTS is a recognizable and treatable disorder of the autonomic nervous system that is manifested by orthostatic intolerance associated with postural tachycardia, palpitations, fatigue, weakness, and exercise intolerance. The significance of the disorder may be greater than initially apparent as it can produce substantial disability among otherwise healthy people and may be a potential cause of the CFS. At tilt table testing, these patients demonstrate a heart rate increase of > 30 b min^{-1} (or a peak rate of > 120 b min^{-1}) within the first 10 min of upright posture that reproduces a patient's symptoms. Some patients also have high plasma norepinephrine levels and display an exaggerated response to isoproterenol. Other patients may develop POTS because of other underlying conditions. Therapies aimed at correcting the autonomic imbalance may help to relieve the severity of the symptoms. These disorders are not new; what has changed is our ability to recognize them. It has been noted that, "The world undergoes change in the human consciousness. As this consciousness changes, so does the world" [111]. Continued research is necessary to improve understanding of the disease and to differentiate its various subtypes, while at the same time elucidating therapies that will help profoundly symptomatic patients return to a normal life.

References

1 Grubb BP, Kosinski D, Boehm K, *et al.* The postural tachycardia syndrome: a neurocardiogenic variant identified during head upright tilt table testing. *PACE* 1997;**20**:2205–12.

2 Joyner MJ, Shepard JT. Autonomic control of the circulation. In: Low P, ed. *Clinical Autonomic Disorders.* Boston, MA: Little, Brown Co, 1993: 57–67.

3 Streeten DH. Orthostatic intolerance: a historical introduction to the pathophysiological mechanisms. *Am J Med Sci* 1999;**317**(2):78–87.

4 DaCosta JM. An irritable heart. *Am J Med Sci* 1871;**27**:145–63.

5 Lewis T. *The Soldier's Heart and the Effort Syndrome.* London, UK: Shaw & Sons, 1919.

6 Sewall H. On the clinical significance of postural changes in the blood pressures, and the secondary waves of arterial blood pressure. *Am J Med Sci* 1919;**158**:786–816.

7 Nylin G. Relationship between heart volume and stroke

volume in recumbent and erect positions. *Skand Arch Physiol* 1934;**69**:237–46.

8 Bjure A, Laurell H. Om abnormal statiska cirkulationsfenomen och darmed sammanhanganda skukliga symptom: den arterilla orthostatiska animan en forsummad sjukdomsbild. *Upsala Lakareforen Forh* 1927;**33**:1–23.

9 Laurell H. Die "orthostatische arterielle Anamie," eine gewohnliches, aber aft fehlgedeutetes Krankheitsbild. *Fortschr Geb Rontgenstr* 1936;**53**:501–9.

10 MacLean AR, Allen EV, Magath TB. Orthostatic tachycardia and orthostatic hypotension: defects in the return of venous blood to the heart. *Am Heart J* 1944;**27**: 145–63.

11 MacLean AR, Allen EV. Orthostatic hypotension and orthostatic tachycardia: treatment with the "head-up" bed. *JAMA* 1940;**115**:2162–7.

12 Frolich ED, Dustin HP, Page IH. Hyperdynamic beta-adrenergic circulatory state. *Arch Intern Med* 1966;**117**:614–9.

13 Rosen SG, Cryer PE. Postural tachycardia syndrome. *Am J Med* 1982;**72**:847–50.

14 Fouad FM, Tadena-Thoma L, Bravo EL, *et al.* Idiopathic hypovolemia. *Ann Intern Med* 1986;**104**:298–303.

15 Streeten DHP, Anderson GH Jr, Richardson R, *et al.* Abnormal orthostatic changes in blood pressure and heart rate in subjects with intact sympathetic nervous system function: evidence for excessive venous pooling. *J Lab Clin Med* 1988;**111**:326–35.

16 Streeten DHP. Pathogenesis of hyperadrenergic orthostatic hypotension: evidence of disordered venous innervation exclusively in the lower limbs. *J Clin Invest* 1990;**86**:1582–8.

17 Hoeldtke RD, Dworkin GE, Gaspar SR, *et al.* Sympathotonic orthostatic hypotension: a report of four cases. *Neurology* 1989;**39**:34–40.

18 Hoeldtke RD, David KM. The orthostatic tachycardia syndrome: evaluation of autonomic function and treatment with octreotide and ergot alkaloids. *J Clin Endocrinol Metab* 1991;**73**:132–9.

19 Schondorf R, Low P. Idiopathic postural orthostatic tachycardia syndrome: an attenuated form of acute pandysautonomia? *Neurology* 1993;**43**:132–7.

20 Low P, Opfer-Gehrking T, Textor S, *et al.* Postural tachycardia syndrome. *Neurology* 1995;**45**:519–25.

21 Khurana RK. Orthostatic intolerance and orthostatic tachycardia: a heterogenous disorder. *Clin Auton Res* 1995;**5**:12–8.

22 Karas B, Grubb B, Boehm K, *et al.* The postural orthostatic tachycardia syndrome: a potentially treatable cause of chronic fatigue, exercise intolerance, and cognitive impairment in adolescents. *PACE* 2000;**23**:344–51.

23 Shannon JR, Flatten NL, Jordan J, *et al.* Orthostatic intolerance and tachycardia associated with norepinephrine-transporter deficiency. *N Engl J Med* 2000;**342**:541–9.

24 Nankiewicz K, Somers V. Chronic orthostatic intolerance: part of a spectrum of dysfunction in orthostatic cardiovascular homeostasis? *Circulation* 1998;**98**:2105–7.

25 Rowe PC, Barron DF, Calkins H, *et al.* Orthostatic intolerance and chronic fatigue syndrome associated with Ehlers–Danlos syndrome. *J Pediatrics* 1999;**135**:494–9.

26 Vernino S, Low P, Fealey RD, *et al.* Autoantibodies to ganglionic acetylcholine receptors in autoimmune autonomic neuropathies. *N Engl J Med* 2000;**343**:847–55.

27 Singer W, Shen WK, Opfer-Gehrking T, *et al.* Evidence of an intrinsic sinus node abnormality in patients with postural tachycardia syndrome. *Mayo Clin Proc* 2002;**77**:246–52.

28 Shen WK, Low PA, Jehangir A, *et al.* Is sinus node modification appropriate for inappropriate sinus tachycardia with features of postural orthostatic tachycardia syndrome? *PACE* 2001;**242**:217–30.

29 Grubb BP, Kosinski D, Samoil D, *et al.* Postpartum syncope. *PACE* 1995;**18**(I):1028–31.

30 Klein CM, Verino S, Lennon VR, *et al.* The spectrum of autoimmune autonomic neuropathies. *Ann Neurol* 2003;**53**:752–8.

31 Jacob G, Biaggioni I. Idiopathic orthostatic intolerance and postural tachycardia syndromes. *Am J Med Sci* 1999;**317**:88–101.

32 Jacob G, Ertl AC, Costa F, *et al.* The neuropathic postural tachycardia syndrome. *N Engl J Med* 2000;**343**: 1008–14.

33 Low P, Opfer-Gehrking TL, Textor SC, *et al.* Comparison of the postural tachycardia syndrome (POTS) with orthostatic hypotension due to autonomic failure. *J Auton Nerv Syst* 1994;**50**:181–8.

34 Low P, Schondorf R, Novak V, *et al.* Postural tachycardia syndrome. In: Low P, ed. *Clinical Autonomic Disorders*, 2nd edn. Philadelphia, PA: Lippincott Raven, 1997: 681–97.

35 Benrud-Larson LM, Dewar M, Sandroni P, Haythornthwaite JA, Low PA. Quality of life in patients with postural tachycardia syndrome. *Mayo Clin Proc* 2002;**77**:531–7.

36 Benrud-Larson LM, Sandroni P, Haythornthwaite JA, Rummins TA, Low PA. Correlates of functional disability in patients with postural tachycardia syndrome: preliminary cross-sectional findings. *Health Psychology* 2003;**22**:643–8.

37 Robertson D. The epidemic of orthostatic tachycardia and orthostatic intolerance. *Am J Med Sci* 1999;**317**:75–7.

38 Weir B, Donat K. Arterielle hypotonic. *Fortschr Med* 1982;**30**:1396–9.

39 Critchley HD, Mathias CJ. Blood pressure, attention and cognition: drivers and air traffic controllers. *Clin Auton Res* 2003;**13**:399–401.

40 Goldstein DS, Holmes C, Frank SM, Dendi R, *et al.* Cardiac sympathetic dysautonomia in chronic orthostatic intolerance syndromes. *Circulation* 2002;**106**(18): 2358–65.

41 Stewart JM. Pooling in chronic orthostatic intolerance: arterial vasoconstrictive but not venous compliance defects. *Circulation* 2002;**105**(19):2274–81.

42 Tani H, Singer W, McPhee BR, *et al.* Splanchnic-mesenteric capacitance bed in the postural tachycardia syndrome. *Auton Neurosci* 2000;**86**:107–13.

43 Low P, Novak V, Spies J, *et al.* Cerebrovascular regulation in the postural orthostatic tachycardia syndrome (POTS). *Am J Med Sci* 1999;**317**:124–233.

44 Hermosillo AG, Jauregui-Renaud K, Kostine A, Marquez MF, Lara JL, Cardenas M. Comparative study of cerebral blood flow between postural tachycardia and neurocardiogenic syncope during head up tilt test. *Europace* 2002;**4**: 369–74.

45 Ali YS, Daamen N, Jacob G, *et al.* Orthostatic intolerance: a disorder of young women. *Obstet Gynecol Surv* 2000;**55**(4):251–9.

46 Robertson D, Shannon JR, Biaggioni I, *et al.* Orthostatic intolerance and the postural tachycardia syndrome: genetic and environmental pathophysiologies. *Pflugers Arch* 2000;**441**:R48–51.

47 Duschek S, Weisz N, Schandry R. Reduced cognitive performance and prolonged reaction time accompany moderate hypotension. *Clin Auton Res* 2003;**13**:427–32.

48 Low P, Schondorf R. Postural tachycardia syndrome. In: Robertson D, Low P, Polinsky R, eds. *Primer on the Autonomic Nervous System*. San Diego, CA: Academic Press, 1996: 279–83.

49 Low PA, Schondorf R, Rummans TA. Why do patients have orthostatic systems in POTS? *Clin Auton Res* 2001;**11**:223–4.

50 Pilgram JR, Stanfield S, Marmot M. Low blood pressure, low mood? *BMJ* 1992;**304**:75–8.

51 Mann A. Psychiatric symptoms and low blood pressure; more evidence for an association. *BMJ* 1992;**304**:64–5.

52 Pilgram JA. Psychological aspects of high and low blood pressure. *Psychol Med* 1994;**24**:9–24.

53 Stewart JM. Orthostatic intolerance in pediatrics. *J Pediatr* 2002;**140**:404–11.

54 Cohen BH, Gold DR. Mitochondrial cytopathy in adults: what we know so far. *Cleve Clin J Med* 2001; **68**(7):625–42.

55 Furlan R, Jacob G, Snell M, *et al.* Chronic orthostatic intolerance: a disorder with discordant cardiac and vascular control. *Circulation* 1998;**98**:2154–9.

56 Polinsky RJ, Kapin IJ, Ebert MH, *et al.* Pharmacological distinction of different orthostatic hypotension syndromes. *Neurology* 1981;**31**:1–7.

57 Jordan J, Shannon JR, Diedrich A, *et al.* Increased sympathetic activation in idiopathic orthostatic intolerance: role of sympathetic adrenoreceptors sensitivity. *Hypertension* 2002;**39**(1):173–8.

58 Jacob G, Shannon JR, Costa F, *et al.* Abnorman norepinephrine clearance and adrenergic receptor sensitivity in idiopathic orthostatic intolerance. *Circulation* 1999;**99**(13):1706–12.

59 Schroeder C, Tank J, Luft FC, Jordan J. Norepinephrine transporter function and orthostatic syndromes. *J Funtional Synd* 2002;**2**:3–8.

60 Barron DF, Cohen BA, Geraghty MT, Violand R, Rowe P. Joint hypermobility is more common in children with chronic fatigue syndrome than in healthy controls. *J Pediatr* 2002;**141**:421–5.

61 Gazit Y, Nahir AM, Grahme R, Jacob G. Dysautonomia in the joint hypermobility syndrome. *Am J Med* 2003;**115**:33–40.

62 Grubb BP, Karas B. Clinical disorders of the autonomic nervous system associated with orthostatic intolerance: an overview of classification, clinical evaluation and management. *PACE* 1999;**22**:798–809.

63 Khurana R. Paraneoplastic autonomic dysfunction. In: Robertson D, Low P, Polinsky R, eds. *Primer on the Autonomic Nervous System*. San Diego, CA: Academic Press, 1996: 260–4.

64 Sandroni P, Opfer-Gehrking TL, McPhee BR, Low PA. Postural tachycardia syndrome: clinical features and follow-up study. *Mayo Clinic Proc* 1999;**74**:1106–10.

65 Stewart JM. Autonomic nervous system dysfunction in adolescents with postural tachycardia syndrome is characterized by attenuated vagal baroreflex and potentiated sympathetic vasomotion. *Pediatr Res* 2000;**48**: 218–26.

66 Elkayam U, Gleicher N. Cardiovascular physiology of pregnancy. In: Elkayam U, Gleicher N, eds. *Cardiac Problems in Pregnancy*. New York, NY: Alan R Liss, 1982: 5–26.

67 Uleland K. Maternal cardiovascular dynamics: interpartum blood volume changes. *Am J Obst Gynecol* 1972;**126**:671–7.

68 Metcalfe J, Uleland K. Maternal cardiovascular adjustments to pregnancy. *Prog Cardiovasc Dis* 1974;**16**: 363–74.

69 Rowe PC, Bov-Holaigah I, Kan JS, *et al.* Is neurally mediated hypotension an unrecognized cause of chronic fatigue? *Lancet* 1995;**345**:623–4.

70 Bov-Holaigah I, Rowe PC, Kan J, Calkins H. Relationship between neurally mediated hypotension and the chronic fatigue syndrome. *JAMA* 1995;**274**:961–7.

71 Freeman R, Komaroff AL. Does the chronic fatigue syndrome involve the autonomic nervous system? *Am J Med* 1997;**102**:357–64.

72 Chung J, Cash J, Calabrese L, Wilke W. Mechanisms of abnormal response to head-up tilt in chronic fatigue syndrome [Abstact]. *PACE* 1997;**20**:1058.

73 Schondorf R, Benoit J, Wein T, Phaneuf D. Orthostatic intolerance in the chronic fatigue syndrome. *J Auton Nerv System* 1999;**75**(2–3):192–201.

74 Stewart JM, Gewitz MA, Weldon A, Arlievsky N, Li K, Munoz J. Orthostatic intolerance in adolescent chronic fatigue syndrome. *Pediatrics* 1999;**103**:116–21.

75 Streeten DH, Anderson GH Jr. The role of delayed orthostatic hypotension in the pathogenesis of chronic fatigue. *Clin Auton Res* 1998;**8**(2):119–24.

76 DeLorenzo F, Hargreaves J, Kakkar VV. Pathogenesis and management of delayed orthostatic hypotension in patients with chronic fatigue syndrome. *Clin Auton Res* 1997;**5**:185–90.

77 LaManca JJ, Peckerman A, Walker J, *et al.* Cardiovascular response during head-up tilt in chronic fatigue syndrome. *Clin Physiol* 1999;**19**:111–20.

78 Soetekouw PMMB, Lenders JWM, Bleijenberg G, Thien Th, van der Meer JWM. Autonomic function in patients with chronic fatigue syndrome. *Clin Auton Res* 1999;**9**:334–40.

79 Naschitz JE, Sabo E, Naschitz S, *et al.* Fractal analysis and recurrence quantification analysis of heart rate and pulse transit time for diagnosing chronic fatigue syndrome. *Clin Auton Res* 2002;**12**:264–72.

80 Timmers HJLM, Weiling W, Soetekouw P, Bleijenberg G, van der Meer J, Lenders J. Hemodynamic and neurohumoral responses to head-up tilt in patients with chronic fatigue syndrome. *Clin Auton Res* 2002;**12**:273–80.

81 Poole J, Herrell R, Ashton S, Goldberg J, Buchwald D. Results of isoproterenol tilt table testing in monozygotic twins discordant for chronic fatigue syndrome. *Ann Intern Med* 2000;**160**:3461–8.

82 Rowe PC, Calkins H, DeBusk K, *et al.* Fludrocortisone acetate to treat neurally mediated hypotension in chronic fatigue syndrome: a randomized controlled trial. *JAMA* 2001;**285**:52–9.

83 Kenny R, Graham C. Chronic fatigue symptoms are common in patients with vasovagal syncope. *Am J Med* 2001;**110**:242–3.

84 Novak V, Novak P, Opfer-Gehrking TL, O'Brien PL, Low PA. Clinical and laboratory indices that enhance the diagnosis of postural tachycardia syndrome. *Mayo Clinic Proc* 1988;**73**:1141–50.

85 Streeten DH. *Orthostatic Disorders of the Circulation: Mechanisms, Manifestations and Management.* New York, NY: Plenum Press, 1987.

86 Robertson D. Clinical assessment of autonomic failure. In: Robertson D, Low P, Polinsky R, eds. *Primer on the Autonomic Nervous System.* San Diego, CA: Academic Press, 1996: 111–5.

87 Malik M, ed. *Clinical Guide to Autonomic Tests.* Dordrecht, the Netherlands: Kluwer Academic, 1998.

88 Low P, Opfer-Gehrking TL, Textor SC, *et al.* Comparison of the postural tachycardia syndrome (POTS) with orthostatic hypotension due to autonomic failure. *J Auton Nerv Syst* 1994;**50**:181–8.

89 Morillo C, Klein G, Thakur R, *et al.* Mechanism of "inappropriate" sinus tachycardia: role of sympathovagal balance. *Circulation* 1994;**90**:873–7.

90 Krahn AD, Yee R, Klein GJ, *et al.* Inappropriate sinus tachycardia: evaluation and therapy. *J Cardiovasc Electrophysiol* 1995;**6**:1124–8.

91 Bloomfield DM, Sheldon R, Grubb BP, *et al.* Putting it together: a new treatment algorithm for vasovagal syncope and related disorders. *Am J Cardiol* 1999; **84**(8A):33Q–9Q.

92 Sheps SG. Use of an elastic garment in the treatment of orthostatic hypotension. *Cardiology* 1976;**61**(Suppl 1): 271–9.

93 Hickler RB. Successful treatment of orthostatic hypotension with 9-alpha-flurohydrocortisone. *N Engl J Med* 1959;**261**:788–90.

94 Freitas J, Santos R, Azevedo E, *et al.* Clinical improvement in patients with orthostatic intolerance after treatment with bisoprolol and fludrocortisone. *Clin Auton Res* 2000;**10**(5):293–9.

95 Kanjwal MY, Kosinski DJ, Grubb BP. Treatment of postural orthostatic tachycardia syndrome and inappropriate sinus tachycardia. *Curr Cardiol Rep* 2003; **5**(5):402–6.

96 Stewart JM, Munoz J, Weldon A. Clinical and physiological effects of an acute α_1-adrenergic agonist and a β_1-adrenergic agonist in chronic orthostatic intolerance. *Circulation* 2002;**106**(23):2946–54.

97 Grubb BP, Karas B, Kosinski D, Boehm K. Preliminary observations on the use of midodrine hydrochloride in the treatment of refractory neurocardiogenic syncope. *J Interv Card Electrophysiol* 1993;**3**:139–43.

98 Grubb BP, Kosinski D, Mouhaffel A, *et al.* The use of methylphenidate in the treatment of refractory neurocardiogenic syncope. *PACE* 1996;**19**:836–40.

99 Mosqueda-Garcia R, Fernandez-Violante R, Tank T, *et al.* Yohimbine in neurally mediated syncope: pathophysiological implications. *J Clin Invest* 1998;**102**:1824–30.

100 Hoeldtke RD, Davis KM. The orthostatic tachycardia syndrome: evaluation of autonomic function and treatment with octreotide and ergot alkaloids. *J Clin Endocrinol Metab* 1991;**73**:132–9.

101 Biaggioni I, Robertson D, Kranz S, *et al.* The anemia of primary autonomic failure and its reversal with recombinant erythropoietin. *Ann Intern Med* 1994;**121**: 181–6.

102 Hoeldtke RD, Streeten DHP. Treatment of orthostatic hypotension with erythropoietin. *N Engl J Med* 1993;**329**:611–5.

103 Grubb BP, Karas B. Preliminary observations on the use of erythropoietin in the treatment of refractory postural tachycardia syndrome. *Clin Auton Res* 1999; **9**(4):228.

104 Singer W, Opfer-Gehrking TL, McPhee BR, Hilz MJ, Bharucha AE, Low PR. Acetylcholinesterase inhibition: a novel approach in the treatment of neurogenic orthostatic hypotension. *J Neurol Neurosurg Psychiatry* 2003;**74**:1294–8.

105 Gaffney FA, Lane LB, Pettinger W, *et al.* Effects of long-term clonidine administration on the hemodynamic and neuroendocrine postural responses of patients with dysautonomia. *Chest* 1983;**83**:436–8.

106 Grubb BP, Karas BJ. The potential role of serotonin in the pathogenesis of neurocardiogenic syncope and related autonomic disturbances. *J Interv Card Electrophysiol* 1998;**2**:325–32.

107 Shores MM, Pascualy M, Lewis NL, Flatness D, Veith RC. Short-term sertraline treatment suppresses sympathetic nervous system activity in healthy human subjects. *Psychoneuroendocrinology* 2001;**26**:433–9.

108 Grubb BP, Kanjwal Y, Kosinski D. The postural orthostatic tachycardia syndrome: current concepts in pathophysiology, diagnosis and management. *J Interv Card Electrophysiol* 2001;**5**:9–16.

109 Fealy R, Robertson D. Management of orthostatic hypotension. In: Low P, ed. *Clinical Autonomic Disorders*, 2nd edn. Philadelphia PA: Lippincott-Raven, 1997: 763–75.

110 Bannister R, Mathias C. Management of postural hypotension. In: Mathias C, Bannister R, eds. *Autonomic Failure: A Textbook of Clinical Disorders of the Autonomic Nervous System*, 4th edn. Oxford, UK: Oxford University Press, 1999: 342–56.

111 Cowan J. *A Mapmaker's Dream: The Meditations of Fra Mauro, Cartographer to the Court of Venice.* New York, NY: Warner Books, 1996: xvi.

CHAPTER 14

Carotid sinus hypersensitivity

Steve W. Parry, MD*, & Rose Anne Kenny,* MD

Introduction

"In patients, whose hearts have been beating with undue quickness and force, I have often, in a few seconds, retarded their motions many pulsations in a minute, by strong pressure on one of the carotid arteries" [1].

So wrote the Welsh physician Caleb Hillier Parry in 1799, writing primarily on "ossification" and obstruction of the coronary arteries but mentioning as an aside his observations on carotid sinus massage (CSM; Figs 14.1 and 14.2) [1]. Although clearly referring to cardioinhibition following carotid stimulation, Parry made no clinicopathologic association with his findings, and it was not until Roskam [2] published his seminal case report in 1930 that syncope came to be associated with carotid sinus hypersensitivity (CSH).* Roskam was also the first to use the term "hypersensitivity" (*"hyperréflectivité"*) when describing a 53-year-old man with recurrent syncope first elicited by stretching of the skin while shaving. During clinical examination, compression of the carotid sinus caused > 15 s asystole with loss of consciousness and "convulsions," as graphically described by Roskam:

"... Pendant cette syncope que se prologea plus de quinze secondes apres la fin de l'attouchement, j'auscultai avec la plus grande attention la region precordiale: silence absolu. Finalement, survinrent des convulsions epileptiformes generalisees.

Puis brusquement, le coeur se remit a battre sur un rythme accelere, a 120 pulsations environ a la minute, des extrasystoles venant frequemment entrecouper la succession precipitee des systoles regulieres [2]."†

Repeated light carotid sinus pressure resulted in 16 s asystole, again with syncope and convulsions. The patient was treated successfully with atropine and remained symptom-free at follow-up [2]. The stage was thus set for Soma Weiss and James Baker's [3] landmark case series in CSH published later in 1933, describing "the carotid sinus reflex in health and disease" and "its role in the causation of fainting and convulsions."

Fifteen subjects with CSH, all with symptom reproduction during carotid sinus pressure of variable degrees and duration, were described in detail, with the division of responses to carotid stimulation designated "vagal" where marked bradycardia or asystole occurred, "depressor" where arterial pressure fell independently of cardiac slowing, and "cerebral" where syncope occurred with no hemodynamic changes. The cerebral subtype was the subject of much controversy over the ensuing 15 years. Daneilopolu [4] felt that CSH was intimately involved in the causation of convulsions in epilepsy, while later reports from Ferris *et al.* [5] and Weiss *et al.* [6] further promulgated the

---

* Where CSH is thought to be the attributable cause of symptoms, the term carotid sinus syndrome is used, but for the sake of uniformity, CSH is used throughout this chapter.

---

† "... As syncope occurred for more than 15 s following discontinuation of pressure, I auscultated attentively over the praecordium: absolute silence. Finally, generalized epileptiform convulsions ensued. Then, abruptly, the heart began to beat with an accelerated rhythm, at around 120 b min⁻¹, with initial frequent extrasystoles interrupting the succession to normal sinus rhythm."

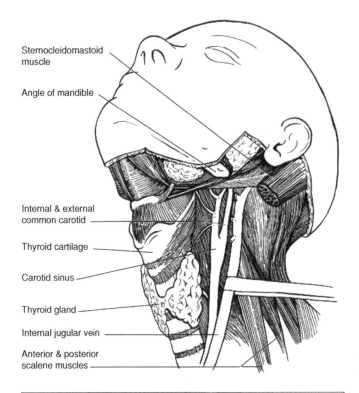

Sternocleidomastoid muscle

Angle of mandible

Internal & external common carotid

Thyroid cartilage

Carotid sinus

Thyroid gland

Internal jugular vein

Anterior & posterior scalene muscles

Fig. 14.1 The carotid sinus and associated structures.

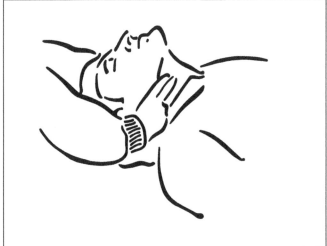

Fig. 14.2 Carotid sinus massage: head in the neutral position.

cerebral CSH cause. Other authors reported similar findings [7], sometimes in tandem with abnormal electroencephalography [8]. However, later cerebral angiographic studies showed conclusively that the so-called cerebral type of CSH was actually a result of cerebral anterior circulatory compromise secondary to carotid artery obliteration during CSM in the presence of hemodynamically significant contralateral carotid sinus stenosis [9,10].

Although not appreciated by Weiss *et al.* at the time, they nevertheless assumed that fainting was caused by "sudden changes in the cerebral vessels as a result of stimulation of the carotid sinus . . . probably constriction, followed by dilatation" [3].

While the lack of standardization of carotid sinus stimulation, *ad hoc* subject selection, and absence of diagnostic definitions hamper Weiss and Baker's original paper, their contribution, in terms of drawing attention to the pathologic role of the carotid sinus and making some sense of the presentation, natural history, and management of the condition, is unique.

Diagnosis of carotid sinus hypersensitivity

Defining carotid sinus hypersensitivity

Carotid sinus hypersensitivity is currently diagnosed when CSM elicits 3 s asystole (cardioinhibitory subtype, CICSH; Fig. 14.3), a fall in systolic blood pressure of ≥ 50 mmHg (vasodepressor subtype, VDCSH), or both (mixed subtype, MxCSH) in a patient with otherwise unexplained dizziness or syncope [11,12]. A recent study found that the three subtypes occur with equal frequency in an unselected population attending a falls and syncope facility [13]. While these diagnostic criteria are widely accepted [14,15], their basis is in arbitrary clinical observation rather than experimental method. The early clinical descriptions of CSH in the 1930s were models of clinical observation and case reporting, but offered no standard definitions to guide diagnosis of the condition [2,3,5,6]. In 1942, Engel and Engel [16] arbitrarily chose 3 s of asystole determined by precordial auscultation as the diagnostic standard for the "hypersensitive carotid sinus reflexes" they found in association with biliary disease, while Galdston *et al.* [7] stated that a "bradycardia, and often asystole of 3–7 s duration . . . constituted evidence of the circulatory effects of carotid sinus stimulation." Later work by Nathanson [17], who reviewed his experience with 115 patients over the preceding 12 years, concluded that cardiac standstill of more than 5 s constituted a hyperactive response to carotid sinus pressure; 20 years later, Peretz *et al.* [18] agreed, although with

no explanation offered. Case series described by Sigler [19,20] and Franke [21], and two review articles by Thomas [22,23], provide the foundation upon which the currently accepted diagnostic criteria for CSH are based. Franke's monograph detailed his clinical and experimental observations over a 20-year period with some 3900 patients [21]. He concluded that there were four types of response to CSM. In 70% of subjects there was virtually no change in heart rate (HR) or systolic blood pressure (SBP) (Group I). In 10%, HR falls by approximately 20 b min^{-1} and SBP by 10–20 mmHg; asystole did not exceed 2 s (Group II). A further 10% exhibit a 30–50% fall in HR, with or without asystole of 2 s duration, and a fall in SBP of 30–50 mmHg (Group III). The final 10% had 3–5 s asystole, and a fall in SBP of more than 50 mmHg (Group IV) [21]. These findings were virtually identical to Sigler's experience with 1,886 patients who were grouped in exactly the same fashion as Franke's, but labeled + to + + + + (Groups I–IV respectively) [19]. Both authors labeled Groups III and IV as having pathologically hypersensitive carotid sinus reflexes. Thomas' oft-quoted reviews mention the lack of "agreement as to where the physiologic response ends and the pathologic response begins" [23] but suggests that experimentally induced asystole of more than 2–3 s is diagnostic of cardioinhibitory carotid sinus syndrome (CICSS) [22,23]. The only physiologic rationale to date on the subject supports a diagnosis of CICSH or MxCSH in excess of 2 s. Heidorn and McNamara [24] noted asystole of 2–5.7 s duration in the subjects they described with CSH, all of whom had symptoms during massage, and concluded that the absence of ventricular contraction for more than 2 s was likely to be pathologic because the sinus node rarely discharges at less than 30 min^{-1} in

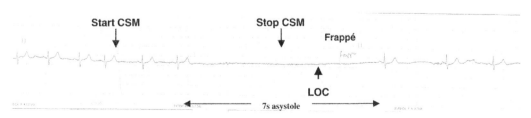

Fig. 14.3 Cardioinhibitory carotid sinus hypersensitivity. CSM, carotid sinus massage; Frappé, precordial thump; LOC, loss of consciousness; s, seconds; SBP, systolic blood pressure.

physiologic conditions [24]. As sinus arrest is the most common cause of asystole in CSH [25], this would indeed seem logical.

Thus, while the rationale for the definition of CSH is somewhat imperfect, the use of 3 s asystole with or without a 50 mmHg fall in SBP during CSM is now a widely accepted standard [11–15,26–33] sanctioned by both the British Pacing and Electrophysiology Group [29] and the American College of Cardiology/American Heart Association taskforce in their recommendations for permanent pacemaker implantation [28], and will be used throughout this chapter.

Technique of carotid sinus massage

Carotid sinus massage was initially a non-standardized procedure, of varying duration from a few seconds up to a minute. In recent years, a consensus has been arrived at for the technique of CSM, and is widely adhered to [11,12,33]. Following a detailed history, clinical examination (including carotid auscultation), and explanation of the procedure, the patient should lie supine for a minimum of 5 min with continuous surface electrocardiogram (ECG) and blood pressure monitoring[‡] on a footplate-type tilt table. Baseline blood pressure and heart rate are recorded. Firm, longitudinal massage should then be performed for 5 s over the site of maximal pulsation of the right carotid sinus [11], which is located between the superior border of the thyroid cartilage and the angle of the mandible (see Figs 14.1 and 14.2). Some authors recommend continuing CSM for 10 s if there is no asystole after 5 s [34,35], but this is not our current practice. Simple light pressure over the carotid sinus will not reliably produce a hypersensitive response. CSM is performed initially on the right side when supine, as up to 66% of subjects with CSH have a positive response on the right side [22], potentially avoiding the need for repeated CSM. Massage should be discontinued if asystole > 3 s occurs, while prolonged

asystole should result in prompt frappe. Symptoms, including symptom reproduction, BP, and R-R interval should be recorded.

If right-sided massage is non-diagnostic, the procedure should be repeated, consecutively, in the left supine position, and the right and left 70° head-up tilt position, following hemodynamic re-equilibration in all cases. In up to 30% of subjects the response cannot be elicited in the supine position and is only present during massage in the head-upright tilt position [14,32,36–38]. At the end of the procedure the patient should remain supine for at least 10 min, which in our experience has reduced neurologic complication rates. CSM should only be performed by a clinician skilled in the management of its potential complications.

The reliance on digital stimulation for CSM is the source of much criticism [39,40], because of its subjectivity and the lack of a standardized stimulus to the baroreflex pathway. Several authors have tried to surmount this problem through the development of a neck suction chamber that allows graded negative suction over the carotid region [41,42]. The technique requires a bespoke suction device, is cumbersome, and may be poorly tolerated in older subjects [40], while reference ranges for hemodynamic responses to neck suction in healthy subjects is lacking. Thus, the technique has not been well evaluated in the diagnosis of CSH, with only one report evaluating the device in subjects with CSH, two of whom had asystole > 3 s with the neck suction chamber compared with all 10 with conventional digital CSM [43].

Symptom reproduction and the diagnosis of carotid sinus hypersensitivity

The issue of whether the reproduction of symptoms during positive carotid sinus massage is a necessary facet of the diagnosis of CSH has attracted much debate. Early reports did not mention the requirement of symptoms during CSM-induced asystole, although reports frequently mentioned the presence of syncope during massage [3,20,21]. Some authors specifically mention the necessity of symptom reproduction during CSM [17,22], but later authorities felt that symptoms during massage were not an essential part of the diagnosis [11,25]. Current guidance emphasizes the need for symptom

---

[‡] Where possible, phasic, non-invasive, beat-to-beat, blood pressure (BP) monitoring (e.g., Finapres, Ohmeda, Wisconsin) is to be preferred because the BP nadir occurs at approximately 18 s, returning to baseline at 30 s. Conventional automated systems will thus be insufficiently sensitive to track this rapid response. Of course, this is of most import where the vasodepressor response is of particular interest.

reproduction during CSM-induced hemodynamic changes [35], although the association between falls and syncope may cloud the issue somewhat (see below).

Contraindications to carotid sinus massage

Myocardial infarction, transient ischaemic attack (TIA), or stroke in the 3 months prior to attendance are absolute contraindications, as is any previous adverse reaction to CSM. Previous ventricular fibrillation (VF) or tachycardia (VT) are relative contraindications. If carotid bruits are present, carotid Doppler ultrasonography should precede CSM. Our practice is to avoid CSM in those with a > 70% stenosis and perform the test supine only in those with a 50–70% stenosis. It is noteworthy that the presence of a carotid bruit is a poor indicator of the presence or severity of carotid artery stenosis [44] but, in the absence of prospective studies on the predictive value of carotid Doppler studies, our unit's current practice reflects a safe and pragmatic approach to this test.

Complications of carotid sinus massage

Stroke and TIA following CSM are rare [45–51]. A recent series by Richardson et al. [47] demonstrated the safety of the procedure, with only transient neurologic signs and symptoms in 0.8% of more than 1000 patients subjected to CSM. Stroke or TIA may be more likely during CSM in the upright position; the vasodepressor component may be more pronounced, and the likelihood of watershed events increased [46]. Where neurologic signs ensue, the procedure should be abandoned, the patient placed in the supine position, and measures taken to ensure that the blood pressure is returned rapidly to normotensive levels. Consideration should be given to the administration of 300 mg aspirin if not contraindicated, although there is no evidence base to this. Stroke should be managed as per local guidelines. Cardiac complications, including ventricular [52–58] and atrial arrhythmias [59] have been reported rarely, almost invariably during prolonged CSM. The majority of ventricular dysrrhythmic complications have been reported during massage for supraventricular tachycardia termination, and not for the investigation of syncope. In more than 16,000 episodes of CSM at our unit, we have never encountered VT or VF, although advanced resuscitation facilities should be immediately to hand.

Carotid sinus hypersensitivity: pathophysiologic disease entity or age-related epiphenomenon?

Incidence of *symptomatic* carotid sinus hypersensitivity

The incidence of CSH associated with the traditional symptoms of dizziness and syncope is not known with certainty, although the Westminster group estimated that 35 patients per million per year would be affected. There are no other incidence data in the literature, although the rates of permanent pacemaker implantation for CSH may provide some clues. For example, in centers with an interest in the disorder (in this case, our facility in Newcastle-upon-Tyne, UK), CSH can account for up to 24% of all new implants [60]. With 416 new implants per million population this extrapolates to 100 per million cases of symptomatic CICSH and MxCSH.

Hemodynamic responses to carotid stimulation in asymptomatic subjects

The true incidence and prevalence of CSH are unknown. Attempts to provide estimates of these parameters are hampered by the varying diagnostic criteria used to define the response until consensus was reached in the 1970s and 1980s, and by the lack of standardization regarding the methodology for carotid stimulation and recording of its consequences. Early observations in healthy subjects found exaggerated vasodepressor responses in older patients, and those with coexistent hypertension and arteriosclerotic disease, but no significant hemodynamic changes in young healthy subjects [61–63]. Bradycardic and asystolic consequences of carotid sinus stimulation were not documented. Weiss and Baker [3] found essentially similar results in 50 healthy subjects, with no significant bradycardia and a minor fall in both systolic and diastolic blood pressures of < 10 mmHg. Several studies since have attempted to address this issue, with estimates of CICSH prevalence in asymptomatic individuals ranging between 0% and 38% (Table 14.1). Several of the more relatively recent

Table 14.1 Summary of studies of incidence of cardioinhibitory carotid sinus hypersensitivity in asymptomatic individuals.

References	n (M)	Mean age (range) (years)	Number (%) with CICSH	Duration CSM (s)	% CVS disease	Definition CICSH (asystole s)
Purks [71]*	67 (20)	42.4 (12–69)	3 (4.4%)	12	67	U
Nathanson [17]†	115 (98)	58.9 (30–81)	All 71 (62%) aSx	Up to 30	None	≥ 5
Heidorn & McNamara [24]	40 (40)	39.3 (25–85)	5 (13%) 4 (10%)	30	None	2–3 ≥ 3
Franke [21]‡	3507 (1662)	U (15–92)	315 (9%)	10	U	≥ 3
Smiddy et al. [173]§	58 (58)	> 65 ?	Group 1,0% Group 2,20%	5	None	"Prolonged asystole"
Mankikar & Clark [72]¶	386 (71)	? (62–104)	6 (2%)	U	50	≥ 2
Hudson et al. [65]	333 (209)	66 (50–?)	14 (4%)	5	36	≥ 3
Murphy et al. [64]	100 (14)	80 (6–97)	14 (14%)	10	48	≥ 3 or > 50% fall HR
Volkmann et al. [66]**	163 (88)	57.9 (35–80)	32 (20%)	5–10	None	≥ 3
McIntosh et al. [67]	25 (U)	69 (61–87)	0 (0%)	5	None	≥ 3
Jeffreys et al. [68]	95 (51)	74 (65–95)	4 (4.2%)	5	U	≥ 3
Ward et al. [70]	31 (13) 35 (9) ≥ 330 (12)	74 ± 7 82 ± 8 79 ± 7	0 (0%) EHS 7 (17%) FEC 4 (13%) MIC	5	U	≥ 3
Davies et al. [69]	54 (11)	77 ?	7 (13%)	5	U	≥ 3
Seifer et al. (2002) [personal communication]	55 (33)	70.6	17 (38%)	5	None	≥ 3

aSx, asymptomatic; CICSH, cardioinhibitory carotid sinus hypersensitivity; CSM, carotid sinus massage; CVS, cardiovascular; EHS, elective hip surgery controls; FEC, well, frail, elderly controls; HR, heart rate; (M), number of male subjects; MIC, medically ill inpatients; n, number; s, seconds; U, unspecified; ?, not stated.
* 42% of those with CVS disease had unspecified "significant bradycardia."
† 115 subjects with CICSH; 71 (62%) were asymptomatic.
‡ 28% of hypertensives and 28% of diabetics had CICSH.
§ Mean age unspecified; Group 1, normal ECG; Group 2, abnormal ECG.
¶ Asystole diagnosed on auscultation.
** 41% of older males had CICSH.

studies deserve more detailed mention. Murphy et al. [64] found that 14 of 100 (14%) consecutive subjects had CSH (defined as asystole > 3 s on CSM, or a fall in heart rate by > 50% of the baseline), although unfortunately there is no indication in the study of the numbers with an asystolic response to CSM [64]. Interestingly, there were no differences in the mean age (80 years), sex, medications, or comorbid conditions of the CSH positive and negative groups [64]. Hudson et al. [65] found that 14 of 333 (4%) subjects over 50 years of age attending for "routine" ECG had > 3 s asystole on 5 s of sequential bilateral supine CSM, with a hypersensitive response being more common in those with antecedent symptoms suggestive of bradycardia, such as dizziness, near-syncope, and syncope [65]. As in other series, massage was more likely to be positive on the right, and in male subjects [65]. Volkmann *et al.* [66] found that 20% of 163 asymptomatic subjects had a conventionally defined cardioinhibitory response to 5–10 s CSM, versus 41% of 210 subjects with syncope and dizziness undergoing electrophysiologic studies, although unfortunately their sampling methods for the asymptomatic group were not disclosed [66]. Again, there was a much higher incidence of CICSH in asymptomatic males (28%) than in females (10%), and in older (27% over 60 years) than in younger subjects [66]. Fully 41% of older asymptomatic males demonstrated a cardioinhibitory response to CSM [66].

McIntosh *et al.* [67] found no significant cardioinhibitory responses to 5 s of sequential, bilateral, supine, and upright CSM in 25 healthy, elderly subjects (age range 61–87 years, 11 male), although three (12%) subjects had a vasodepressor response to CSM in the head-up tilt position, while Jeffreys *et al.* [68] found CICSH in only 4.2% of 95 healthy, older subjects (mean age 74 years) drawn randomly from a general practice population. More recently, Davies *et al.* [69] found a cardioinhibitory response to CSM in 13% of a group of 54 controls, compared with 46% of 26 patients with unexplained falls presenting to the accident and emergency department. Ward *et al.* [70] compared the responses to CSM in 55 patients with femoral neck fracture, 33 controls admitted for elective hip surgery, 39 frail elderly outpatients, and 35 consecutive elderly acutely medically ill in patients. None of the hip surgery controls had CSH, but 13% of the medically ill inpatients, and 17% of the frail outpatients had CSH. However, recent, prospective, unpublished data have found a much higher proportion of cardioinhibitory responses in 55 elderly subjects without falls or syncope, with 17 (38%) exhibiting CICSH (Seifer and Kenny, personal communication). The Jeffreys study does not report on whether CSM was performed both supine and upright [68], while Davies *et al.* [69], and Ward *et al.*'s [70] data are derived from both supine and erect CSM. Positivity rates have been shown to

increase by over one-third where upright massage follows an initial non-diagnostic supine test [14]. Furthermore, several of the studies showing a lower prevalence of CSH in asymptomatic subjects have a much lower proportion of males, which may skew the number of positive responses considerably, given the much greater male predominance of CSH.

The true prevalence of CSH in healthy subjects thus remains uncertain. The data from many of the studies reported are hampered by vague or inadequate definitions of CSH [3,61–64,71], prolonged, ill-defined, or non-standardized CSM techniques [3,17,24,64,66,71,72], and poorly defined subject selection [3,6,17,20,21,65]. Overall, CICSH is reported as being present in between 0% and 42% of asymptomatic subjects; a true mean figure for the studies listed in Table 14.1 is difficult (and potentially misleading) to calculate because of the variability in techniques and diagnostic criteria applied, although advancing age and male sex are uniformly reported as independent predictors of a higher incidence rate. Whether CSH is a pathologic disease entity or not thus remains open to question. Symptoms traditionally associated with CSH, along with intervention studies improving symptoms in the absence of other causes for them, strongly suggest a pathologic disease entity. The prevalence data in healthy and asymptomatic subjects suggests a different interpretation: is CSH a disease or an age- and cardiovascular comorbidity related epiphenomenon, a clinical syndrome or simply a clinical sign? Further work is clearly needed to disentangle these issues, not only for the sake of scientific interest but also to prevent overtreatment of those with CSH not truly related to symptoms. A large community prevalence study currently underway in Newcastle will go some way towards answering these questions more comprehensively.

Pathophysiology of carotid sinus hypersensitivity

Neurophysiology of carotid sinus hypersensitivity

The pathophysiology of CSH has yet to be elucidated. Indeed, the dearth of published work on the etiology of the hypersensitive response is remarkable, and may be partly a result of the lack of a

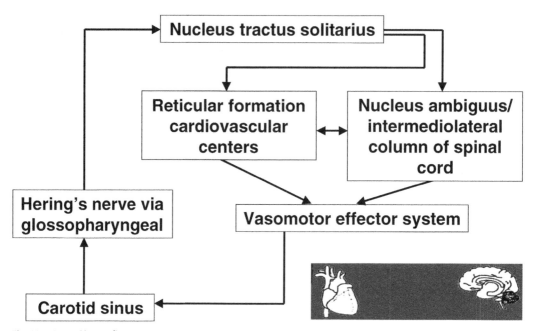

Fig. 14.4 Carotid baroreflex neuroanatomy.

suitable animal model for the disease. What *is* known is that the afferent part of the reflex is via neuronal projections from the carotid sinus to the brainstem (in particular the nucleus tractus solitarius [73,74]) via Hering's nerve and the glossopharyneagal nerve, while the efferent manifestations of CSH are mediated by the vagus nerve in CICSH [25,30,75] and by sympathetic withdrawal, with subsequent vasodilatation and arterial hypotension in MxCSH and VDCSH [75–78] (Fig. 14.4). The nature of the primary abnormality is less well understood. An abnormality of the afferent limb of the baroreflex arc was suggested following the association of CSH with both treated and untreated neck tumors [79–82], although these comprise a small minority of cases of CSH. Others have suggested that atherosclerotic disease of the carotid sinus and resultant carotid ischemia induced by CSM causes the hypersensitive response [83], although the absence of cerebral ischemic symptoms during CSM and the presence of CSH in subjects with no carotid atheroma makes this unlikely [67,84]. Neck tumors notwithstanding, the carotid sinus and its projections are unlikely sources of the primary defect in CSH given the essentially normal histology of the intima and nerve terminals in CSH

[73,85], the continuation of both vasodepressor and cardioinhibitory effects of CSM despite the termination of carotid stimulation (and carotid sinus neural output) [25,76], and the initiation of the hyperactive reflex by other vagal stimuli, such as defecation and micturition [25]. Furthermore, denervation of the carotid sinus is not always a successful intervention in the management of CSH [86,87]. Although the sinus itself may be an unlikely primary source of the hypersensitive response, intriguing work from Tea *et al.* [15] and later expanded on by Blanc *et al.* [88] found a powerful (and unexpected) association between skeletal muscle denervation and CSH [15,88]. Subjects with CSH and healthy controls underwent a battery of central and peripheral neurophysiologic tests [15] along with electromyography of the sternocleidomastoid muscles [15,88] during CSM, with resulting clear evidence of severe sternocleidomastoid denervation in subjects with CSH. The authors postulate that chronic loss of innervation of the sternocleidomastoid muscles causes increased sensitivity of the baroreflex arc and hence CSH, although they agree that the link is tenous [15]. Furthermore, causality in the opposite direction must be considered: there is no evidence to refute

the possibility of sternocleidomastoid denervation as a *consequence* of CSH.

The efferent limb of the carotid baroreflex arc appears to be intact given the exaggerated vasodepression and normal bradycardic response to muscarinic stimulation with edrophonium seen in CSH [11,84]. By exclusion, a central, brainstem level abnormality in modulation of central baroreflex gain is therefore likely, and indeed was suggested more than a decade ago [11], although interestingly Tea *et al.*'s [15] study found no abnormalities of central neurophysiologic parameters in subjects with CSH. One recent hypothesis suggests that central α_2-adrenoceptor up-regulation provides the substrate for this baroreflex gain, resulting in the phenomenon of CSH [84]. We recently tested this hypothesis in a randomized, placebo-controlled, crossover study of the effects of a centrally active, α_2-adrenoceptor antagonist (yohimbine) on vasodepressor responses to CSM in subjects with CSH [89]. If α_2-adrenoceptor hypersensitivity was the major pathophysiologic defect in CSH, yohimbine should abolish or attenuate the effects of CSM in patients with documented CSH. Similar responses were seen in patients and controls, with similar degrees of vasodepression during CSM with both yohimbine and placebo. The only attempt to investigate the role of central α_2-adrenoceptors in CSH to date thus offers no support for the hypothesis whatsoever.

Carotid sinus hypersensitivity and dementia

There is an emerging body of data for a particularly high prevalence of CSH in dementia. It is present in one-third of Alzheimer dementia patients with falls [90] and 41% of Lewy body dementia patients [91–93]. Furthermore, hypotension induced by CSH may contribute to microvascular pathology. We have recently shown that the severity of CSH-induced hypotension correlates with the severity of cognitive impairment in addition to the density of deep white matter and basal ganglia lesions [92]. These associations are independent of other vascular risk factors such as hypertension [93]. It is now well recognized that such microvascular pathology underpins the neurodegenerative process in dementia [94–96]. Although this recently recognized high prevalence for CSH in established

dementias is striking, it is not known whether the converse is true – that patients with CSH are more likely to develop dementia. Similarly, the possibility of neurodegenerative disease causing CSH cannot be ruled out. Ongoing neuropsychologic and neuropathophysiologic studies in patients with CSH will help disentangle these exciting developments further.

Clinical characteristics and symptoms associated with carotid sinus hypersensitivity

Clinical characteristics

Carotid sinus hypersensitivity is a disorder associated with older males, particularly where there is comorbid coronary artery disease and hypertension, with right-sided CSH being more common than left. These findings are universal in the CSH literature. The prevalence of CSH rises considerably with increasing age [11,97,98], again particularly in males [98]. Historically, maneuvers associated with pressure on the carotid sinus, including tight collars [3], shaving [2], head turning [13], and even orthodontic appliances [99] were the traditional precipitants of syncope, but a recent study found that only 28 of 64 (44%) subjects associated head turning with their symptoms [13]. Prolonged standing, meals, and vagotonic maneuvers including coughing, micturition, and defecation were also noted as precipitants, although nine subjects (14%) could not recall any particular predisposing factor [13]. However, Schellack *et al.* [100] found that cervical pressure and motion precipitated symptoms in 40% of their series of 82 subjects with CSH. Various drugs have been implicated as either causative agents in CSH, or exacerbators of an underlying tendency to CSH. Digoxin [61,23,101–103] and beta-blockers [101,104] have long been known to exacerbate CSH, in particular the cardioinhibitory subtypes, but others (including α-methyldopa, physostigmine, morphine, nicotine, and methacholine) have also been implicated as sensitizers of the carotid sinus reflex. Brignole *et al.* [105] found no difference in the hemodynamic responses to CSM in subjects with CSH on long-term vasodilator therapy, although there was a trend towards more prolonged vasodepressor responses in the vasodilator-treated group.

"Traditional" symptoms: syncope and dizziness

From Roskam's [2] early case report to the present, syncope and dizziness are the cardinal symptoms associated with CSH. Dizzy symptoms range from transient lightheadedness to presyncope, although true vertigo should prompt investigation for vestibular causes of dizziness. Syncope tends to be sudden, of short duration, with spontaneous and complete recovery, although persistent dizziness and lightheadedness can occur, particularly with VDCSH and MxCSH. The frequent absence of premonitory symptoms predisposes to (often serious) injury. Collapse secondary to CSH was associated with fractures (particularly fractured neck of femur) in 25% of 64 subjects with CSH in a recent report [13], while CSH was found in 36% of 40 consecutive admissions with femoral neck fracture, compared with none of a control group admitted for elective hip surgery [70]. Seventy per cent of 175 subjects enrolled in a recent, randomized, controlled trial of permanent pacing intervention in CSH presenting with unexplained falls suffered injuries during their falls, with 30% sustaining fractures [106].

Rarely, tonic–clonic movements cause confusion with epileptiform disorders [107,108], although the absence of postevent confusion and incontinence should raise clinical suspicion of a cardiovascular cause of collapse with loss of consciousness [107]. Solti et al. [109] noted TIAs in several patients with severe internal carotid artery stenosis and concomitant CSH. This is an extremely rare presentation and it is difficult to ascribe CSH as causal in the presence of such severe carotid disease.

The overlap between falls and syncope

Syncope has traditionally been considered a separate symptom from the phenomenon of unexplained falls in the elderly, but recent publications provide compelling evidence for considerable overlap between these two entities [13,26,32,64,70,106,110–120]. The conventional distinction between falls and syncope in the elderly is confounded by the frequent absence of witness accounts of falls: nearly half of falls in elderly patients go unwitnessed, thus making a corroborative history of loss of consciousness less likely [26,117]. In one study, a witness account for falls was available in only 40–60% of elderly patients attending outpatient clinics [26]. Accurate recall of the index fall (or falls) may be limited in some older subjects, whether overt cognitive impairment is present or not [26,117,121]. In Cummings et al.'s [117] prospective study, 179 of 304 community dwelling, elderly people over the age of 60 years fell over a 12-month period, but only 32% recalled their falls 3 months after the event, despite normal cognition as assessed by the Mini Mental State Examination [122]. Furthermore, amnesia for loss of consciousness in elderly fallers has been observed during laboratory testing in up to 80% patients with witnessed loss of consciousness during CSM-induced asystole [32,69,106,113,118], and one-quarter of all patients with CSS irrespective of presentation [13]. The association between falls and cardiovascular syncope is well described. One series found that more than half of 40 older subjects with orthostatic hypotension (OH) as their attributable cause of symptoms had unexplained falls in addition to dizziness and syncope [111]. This powerful association is now well documented in subjects with CSH as their attributable cause of symptoms. Kenny and Traynor [32] found CSH to be the attributable cause of symptoms in 33 of 130 (25%) consecutive patients referred for the investigation of falls and dizziness, with 13 (40%) of these presenting with varying combinations of falls, syncope, and dizziness. In contrast, McIntosh et al. [26], in a later series of 65 subjects, referred to a dedicated syncope facility, found considerable overlap between falls and dizziness, and syncope and dizziness, but no relation between falls and syncope (Fig. 14.5).

Carotid sinus hypersensitivity was found to be the cause of symptoms in 45% of these patients, with the majority of the remainder having other cardiovascular disorders, including OH, vasovagal syncope, and cardiac dysrrhythmias [26]. A later study of 132 subjects with unexplained falls and syncope showed that 64 (48%) had CSH as the attributable cause of symptoms (63% cardioinhibitory or mixed), although falls, syncope, and dizziness were the presenting symptom complex in only three of these [13]. Davies et al. [69] showed that 12 of 26 (46%) patients presenting to the accident and emergency department with unexplained falls had a cardioinhibitory response to CSM versus only seven of 54 (13%) control subjects, with

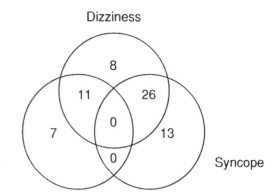

Fig. 14.5 Number of patients presenting to a dedicated facility with dizziness falls or syncope in presenting symptoms (From [26].)

significantly more patients reporting syncope than controls. Dey *et al.* [118] found CSH to be the attributable cause of symptoms in 18 of 35 elderly subjects with drop attacks (episodes of sudden collapse, often with injury, often with difficulty in rising, but with no overt loss of consciousness [123]), 15 with the cardioinhibitory subtype who benefitted from permanent pacemaker implantation. Other neurocardiovascular causes were documented in a further six of these subjects (Table 14.2) [118]. Furthermore, Ward *et al.* [70] found a high incidence of CSH (36%) in 55 consecutive elderly patients admitted with fracture of the femoral neck compared with controls undergoing elective hip surgery (none of 33).

Thus, not only has the traditional distinction between falls and syncope become somewhat blurred in recent years, the evidence for a causal relationship between falls and CICSH has also emerged, in the guise of intervention studies. Permanent pacemaker therapy is the treatment of choice in the cardioinhibitory subtypes of CSH associated with syncope (see below) [28,29,124–129], but the treatment of CICSH and MxCSH associated with falls is more controversial. Anecdotal accounts of benefit have been reported over the last decade [13,32,118], while a recent retrospective study found a reduction in the number of falls in older subjects with cardioinhibitory forms of CSH following dual-chamber pacemaker implantation [114]. More importantly, a randomized, controlled study of permanent pacing in the treatment of CICSH associated with recurrent and unexplained falls has recently been reported [106]. Kenny *et al.* [106] demonstrated a 70% reduction in the number of falls post-pacemaker implantation in the intervention group over the 1-year follow-up period (216 falls versus 699 in controls, odds ratio [OR] 0.42, 95% confidence intervals [CI] 0.23–0.75), although interestingly the adjusted number of falls in both groups increased overall, the paced group less so. These studies will be discussed in more detail below.

Table 14.2 Associated and attributable diagnoses in 35 patients with drop attacks. (From [118].)

	Associated diagnosis	Attributable diagnosis	Intervention	
Carotid sinus syndrome	24	18	Pacemaker	15
			Fludrocortisone and/or midodrine	2
			Atenolol withdrawal	1
Orthostatic hypotension	10	5	Fludrocortisone and/or midodrine, withdrawal of culprit drug	
Vasovagal syncope	4	1	Midodrine	
Gait/visual defect	1	1	Gait retraining	
Unexplained	3			

Natural history of carotid sinus hypersensitivity

Mortality and symptom recurrence

Studies on long-term outcome in patients with CSH are few, with most of the work coming from one Italian group [126,130,131]. Brignole et al. [131] followed 262 subjects with carotid sinus syncope and 55 controls with unexplained syncope over a 6-year period, and found that mortality was similar in both groups. Furthermore, syncopal subjects had the same mortality as that expected for the general population [131]. Brignole et al. [130] had previously reported the results of a randomized, controlled trial of pacing versus no pacing in 35 subjects with CICSH and MxCSH. At 16 months, the 16 paced patients remained 100% free of syncope, while syncope recurrence occurred in 64% of the 19 non-paced patients [130]. Similar results were reported in Brignole et al.'s [126] later randomized study of pacing versus no pacing in 60 subjects with CSH and syncope. Syncope recurred in 16 (57%) of the 28 non-paced patients, but in only three (9%) of the paced group at 36 ± 10 months' follow-up ($P = 0.002$) [126]. In contrast, others found a much lower incidence of syncope recurrence (Table 14.3) [132,133]. Sugrue et al. [133] reviewed their experience in 56 patients with CSH and syncope, 13 of whom underwent no treatment, 23 were treated with permanent pacing, and 20 were treated with anticholinergic drugs. At 6–120 (median 40) months' follow-up, syncope recurred in none of the paced group, only one of the untreated group, and in four of the group managed pharmacologically [133]. Huang et al. [132] implanted pacemakers in 13 of 21 patients with CSH and syncope, none of whom reported syncope at 42 ± 19 months' follow-up, versus only one of the eight patients who did not receive a pacemaker.

Thus, while the available studies are small and predominantly retrospective in nature, it is clear that syncope recurrence is likely with symptomatic CSH, although the presence of CSH does not appear to confer a mortality risk. Symptoms certainly appear to wax and wane in this condition, as in the other neurocardiovascular disorders (e.g., vasovagal syncope, OH), although a common group of provocateurs of symptoms, as seen in vasovagal syncope for example [134], is not a prominent feature of CSH. None of the above studies were designed to assess significant morbidity. Similarly, the natural history of CSH associated with falls has yet to be described.

Treatment strategies in carotid sinus hypersensitivity

Culprit medications and precipitating factors (e.g., removal of tight collars, minimizing neck movements, avoidance of constipation, treatment of chronic bronchitis to avoid cough) should be identified and addressed before further specific therapies are considered. Where symptoms persist, the treatment modality depends upon the subtype of CSH, clinician preference, and the individual patient's needs. Treatment of symptomatic CSH can be divided into denervation of the carotid sinus, medical treatments, and permanent pacemaker implantation.

Denervation of the carotid sinus

Surgical denervation of the carotid sinus has been used as a successful treatment of symptomatic CSH for almost six decades. Weiss et al.'s [3] original paper reported curative removal of a mass compressing the sinus in one of their patients, with intentional section of the carotid sinus nerve. In later series they report successful and uncomplicated carotid sinus denervation in 17 of 71 patients with different types of CSH [5,6]. Others soon reported favorable results [135,136], but one case report of fatal hypertensive crisis following carotid sinus denervation in 1957 [137] and a later report of unsuccessful denervation therapy with an eventually fatal outcome in 1965 [138] dampened enthusiasm for the technique somewhat. Coupled to this were Nathanson's [17] and Sigler's [20] cautions regarding the lack of knowledge regarding the pathophysiology of the disease.

Interest was rekindled in the technique when Cheng and Norris [139] reported a favorable outcome, with no symptom recurrence at 19 months, in a patient with MxCSH. Soon afterwards, Cohen et al. [140] reported benefit in three subjects who underwent carotid sinus denervation, while Trout et al. [87] reported on 19 patients with CSH (the subtypes were not clearly defined) who underwent surgical denervation of the sinus with impressive results. Fourteen patients had complete symptom

Table 14.3 Pacing intervention studies in cardioinhibitory carotid sinus hypersensitivity.

Reference (S/F Study) [X]	n	Study design	Patients with no syncope at F-U	Mean F-U (months)
Peretz et al. [18]	10	Retro	10 (100%)	30
Morley et al. [128] (S)*	70	Retro		18
AAI pacing	8		0 (0%)	
VVI pacing	54		48 (89%)	
DVI pacing	13		12 (92%)	
DDD pacing	3		2 (66%)	
Sugrue et al. [133] (S)	56	Retro		Median 40
No treatment	13		10 (77%)	
Pacing	23		21 (91%)	
VVI pacing	11			
DVI pacing	15			
Anticholinergics	20		16 (80%)	
Stryjer et al. [161] (S)	20	Retro	20 (100%)	
VVI pacing	20			
Huang et al. [132] (S)	21	Retro		42
No treatment	8		7 (88%)	
VVI pacing	9		9 (100%)	
DDD pacing	4		4 (100%)	
Brignole et al. [130] (S)	35	RCT		
No treatment	19		10 (53%)	8.4
VVI pacing	11		11 (100%)	7.2
DDD pacing	5		5 (100%)	7.2
Brignole et al. [165] (S)		RCT		
No treatment	24		15 (62%)	14
VVI/DDD pacing	22		22 (100%)	7.2
Brignole et al. [164] (S) [X]		RCT		
VVI pacing			20 (87%)	2
DDD/DVI pacing			23 (100%)	2
Brignole et al. [127] (S)†		RCT		12
VVI pacing	16		16 (100%)	
DVI/DDD pacing	23		23 (100%)	
Brignole et al. [174] (S) [X]‡	26	RCT		
VVI pacing			24 (92%)	2
DDD pacing			26 (100%)	2
Crilley et al. [114] (S/F)	42	Retro		10
DDI pacing				
falls	30		19 (63%)	
syncope	24		20 (83%)	
Kenny et al. [106] (S/F)	175	RCT		12
No treatment	88		669 falls	
DDDR pacing	87		216 falls§	

F, falls; F-U, follow-up; n, number of patients; RCT, randomized controlled trial; Retro, retrospective study; S, syncope; X, crossover study.

* All eight AAI patients converted to ventricular-based systems (5 DDD, 3 VVI) because of persistent symptoms and appearance of AV block during CSM at F-U.

† Early VVI crossover to DDD because of syncope recurrence. Mixed CSH most likely to experience recurrent symptoms.

‡ 69% of patients had pacemaker syndrome symptoms in VVI mode.

§ Outcome measure was number of falls rather than fallers; OR 0.42, 95% CI: 0.23, 0.75.

resolution at 76 months' follow-up, four had substantial improvement, and only one was unchanged [87]. In the same year, Arenberg *et al.* [86] reported their experience of denervation therapy in 32 of 64 patients with CSH associated with dizziness and syncope. In common with Craig and Smith [135] some 40 years previously, glossopharyngeal nerve section was used, with a novel technique, intracranial section of the glossopharyngeal nerve via suboccipital craniectomy. Both Trout *et al.* [87] and Arenberg *et al.* [86] reported no complications associated with the procedure apart from transient hypertension, and similarly beneficial outcomes. None of their group had recurrence of symptoms at 24 months' follow-up [86]. Interestingly, Kodama *et al.* [141] published a case report 13 years later showing resolution of symptoms following glossopharyngeal nerve block in a patient with MxCSH secondary to laryngeal lymphoma.

Intermittent interest in denervation therapy for CSH has continued since then. Two case reports [142,143] showing cure of CSH-related symptoms have been published, along with three series reporting on a total of 25 patients with symptomatic CSH [100,144,145]. Ninety-two percent of subjects had no evidence of symptom recurrence over a mean of 31.3 months' follow-up [100,144,145].

Effective denervation of the carotid has also been accomplished via radiotherapeutic means [146–148]. Stevenson and Moreton [147] reported complete remission of symptoms in 10 of the 24 patients subjected to radiotherapy, while Greeley *et al.* [148] found complete symptom resolution in 58% of their 52 subjects with carotid sinus syncope, and "slight to moderate" remission in a further 30%. No side-effects or complications were noted in either report.

While denervation of the carotid sinus has thus proved a successful treatment in selected cases, none of the studies mentioned above were prospective or even controlled in any way, patient selection criteria were not disclosed, and the method of recording of follow-up was unclear. The duration of CSM and the definitions of CSH were also variable, while in many cases, the subtype of CSH being treated was not specified. Surgical or radiotherapeutic denervation of the carotid sinus has therefore yet to withstand methodologic scrutiny, and cannot be currently recommended.

Medical treatment

Medical therapy in CSH has proved limited and unsatisfactory, particularly for the cardioinhibitory subtypes. Early series reported good results with oral atropine sulfate in uncontrolled observations, with ephedrine reserved for vasodepressor CSH [3,23]. Side-effects, particularly in older subjects, limited the usefulness of these agents, with later case reports favoring other anticholinergics: for example, propantheline bromide [133,149]; combination therapy with ephedrine, propranolol, and permanent pacing [150]; aminophylline [151]; and sympathotonics including isoprenaline and amphetamines [11]. Dan *et al.* [152] and Grubb *et al.* [153] recently reported remission of symptoms with selective serotonin reuptake inhibitors (SSRIs) in five subjects with troublesome vasodepressor symptoms of CSH. There is no clear pathophysiologic rationale for their use, and no robust evidence of benefit. Fludrocortisone has proved useful in the management of VDCSH, with a substantial fall in the vasodepressor response to CSM [154]. None of 11 patients complained of syncope and only two reported dizziness at 6 months' follow-up in one series [155].

The medical treatment of CSH thus remains unsatisfactory, in part because of a poor understanding of the pathophysiology of the disorder. There are no randomized, controlled trials to guide therapy, which remains difficult and, of necessity, tailored to the individual. Permanent pacing therapy revolutionized the management of the cardioinhibitory subtypes of CSH, and will be discussed next.

Permanent pacemaker therapy

Permanent pacemaker therapy for CSH was first described by Voss and Magnin in 1970 [156–159]. Subsequent studies reporting case series and randomized trials are summarized in Table 14.3. Peretz *et al.* [18] reported the first case series of 10 subjects with CICSH treated with permanent ventricular pacing therapy, with no recurrence of syncope or dizziness during the 30-month follow-up period. The Westminster group were the first to use dual-chamber pacemakers in the treatment of CSH, with the publication of a large, although retrospective and uncontrolled, series of 70 patients paced for symptomatic CSH over the 4-year period to 1982 [128]. Forty-eight (89%) of the 54 patients treated with ventricular pacing (VVI) were free of symptoms at 30 months' follow-up, while in the dual-chamber group, 12 (92%) of the 13 patients treated with DVI and two (66%) of the DDD-treated patients remained asymptomatic. All of the eight patients who were initially treated with atrial pacing (AAI) were changed to other modes (three to VVI, five to dual chamber) because of persistent symptoms and the appearance of retrograde conduction during CSM on sequential testing. Furthermore, persistent symptoms in those with VVI pacing was associated with a high incidence of pacemaker syndrome [128]. The authors thus strongly recommended dual-chamber pacing in CSH in particular DVI mode (because of the theoretical risks of pacemaker-mediated tachycardia with DDD-programmed devices), advice consonant with Probst *et al.*'s [160] findings of a high incidence of retrograde conduction block in patients with CSH undergoing electrophysiology studies. Stryjer *et al.* [161] disagreed, however, because none of their group of 20 subjects with pure cardioinhibitory carotid sinus syncope treated with VVI pacing experienced symptom recurrence at 20 months' follow-up, although again the data are retrospective and uncontrolled.

Soon afterwards, Sugrue *et al.* [133] reported retrospectively on 56 subjects with CSH, 11 of whom underwent VVI and 15 DVI pacing. Twenty-one (92%) of the permanent pacing group remained free of symptoms at 23 months' follow-up, although interestingly 10 (69%) of 77 untreated patients had no syncopal recurrence at 39 months [133]. Huang *et al.* [132], again retrospectively, found that 100% of the nine patients with VVI and four patients with DDD pacemakers implanted for symptomatic CSH were symptom free at 42 months, although again a high proportion of the untreated group also remained asymptomatic (seven of eight subjects, 88%).

The few randomized, controlled trials of pacing therapy in CSH patients presenting with the traditional symptoms of syncope and dizziness were published in a series of articles by Brignole *et al.* [130,162–164]. In the only randomized, controlled trial of pacing versus no pacing to date, Brignole *et al.* [130] found that 100% of the 16 subjects randomized to permanent pacing therapy had no

symptom recurrence, while 10 (53%) of the 19 untreated patients remained well at 8.4 months' follow-up. In an abstracted update, the number of asymptomatic, untreated patients increased to 15 of 24 (62%), while all of the 22 paced subjects had no further syncope [165]. Later studies compared single- with dual-chamber pacing, and the factors associated with each pacing mode likely to lead to symptom recurrence. One crossover study of VVI versus DVI/DDD pacing in 23 subjects showed that although syncope recurrence rates were similar (8% versus 0%), eight patients crossed over to dual-chamber pacing early because of more frequent pacemaker syndrome-related symptoms [164]. The following year, Brignole *et al.* [127] studied 39 subjects with CICSH or MxCSH, 16 of whom underwent VVI pacing, with the remaining 23 having DVI/DDD pacemakers. None of the subjects had syncope recurrence at 12 months' follow-up, although eight patients and a VVI pacemaker patient with MxCSH had persistent nonsyncopal symptoms, compared with none of the dual-chamber group. An initial crossover part of the study found that 14 of 23 patients preferred dual-chamber pacing because of the lower incidence of other symptoms, including dizziness and palpitations [127]. A further crossover comparison from the same group 2 years later again found a similar syncope recurrence rate (none in DDD mode versus 8% in VVI mode) but higher incidence of pacemaker syndrome-related symptoms during ventricular pacing [162].

While there have been no further controlled studies on the efficacy of permanent pacing in CSH patients presenting with syncope, two studies provide compelling evidence of the appropriateness of pacing in this patient group. Graux *et al.* [166] implanted a dual-chamber pacemaker with an intrinsic bradycardia detection algorithm in 10 syncopal patients with CICSH and MxCSH. All patients achieved complete resolution of symptoms, and at a mean of 14 months the bradycardia algorithm was activated, allowing ventricular pauses of up to 2 s and recording the date and time of all pauses. During the subsequent mean 8.25 months' follow-up, recurrence of asystolic episodes occurred in 90% of subjects, with a marked propensity for nocturnal pauses, although symptoms (of dizziness, lightheadedness, and malaise) could not be correlated with rhythm disturbances. As the authors point out, the pacemaker could not detect tach-yarrhythmias, but strong circumstantial evidence thus exists for the appropriateness of pacing in this condition [166]. Menozzi *et al.* [167] found similar results almost a decade earlier, with recurrence of asystole in 74% of subjects paced for CSH.

Thus, while permanent pacing has become the treatment of choice in CSH associated with syncope, the evidence, by today's standards, is far from overwhelming. The few randomized trials all originated from the same unit, with only one of these being a paced versus non-paced study. Even this trial suffers from small numbers and the absence of blinding or placebo control [130]. Nevertheless, pacing is recommended by the American College of Cardiology [28] and the British Pacing and Electrophysiology Group [29] and certainly appears to offer a largely curative therapy in everyday clinical practice.

Choice of pacing mode

The studies presented in the last section provide robust evidence for the pre-eminence of dual-chamber pacing over ventricular pacing. While syncope resolution rates are similar with both pacing modalities, dual-chamber pacing is associated with fewer pacemaker syndrome-related and other hypotension-related symptoms, while the higher incidence of retrograde conduction in subjects with CSH makes ventricular pacing even less desirable. Several studies have since shown a substantial and significant fall in arterial blood pressure during CSM that is more prominent during VVI pacing than DVI [168], DDI [124], or DDD [27,169] pacing modalities. Latterly, a rate drop responsive DDD program (Kappa DR, Medtronic Inc, Minneapolis [170]) developed for use in the malignant vasovagal syndrome [171] has been used successfully in CSH [129]. The algorithm is complex, but in essence allows preprogrammable detection not only of asystole, but a rapid fall in heart rate, with a rapid intervention rate which then has a slow fallback to the intrinsic heart rate [170]. These parameters are attractive in providing rapid pacing at intrinsic heart rates not usually associated with intervention in more conventional bradyarrhythmia pacing algorithms (including DDI with hysteresis), and have theoretical advantages in MxCSH, where a

rapid intervention rate may help counter (to a degree) vasodepression. To date, there have been no head-to-head randomized trials of the various dual-chamber pacing modalities, with pacing prescription largely at the whim of physician preference.

Does pacing intervention benefit patients with CSH and unexplained falls?

More recently, permanent pacing therapy has also been shown to be of benefit in the management of patients with unexplained falls associated with the cardioinhibitory subtypes of CSH, with several uncontrolled reports noting a reduction in the number of falls following permanent pacing [26,32,114,118]. Crilley *et al.*'s [114] series of 42 patients paced for CICSH and MxCSH showed a reduction in the number of patients experiencing falls from 30 to 11, again in an uncontrolled and retrospective study. Close *et al.* [172] studied the impact of the multidisciplinary management of falls in older subjects, and although not powered as a trial of pacing in CSH, benefit was seen in the small subgroup paced for CSH.

The first, large-scale, prospective evaluation of the role of permanent pacing in the treatment of recurrent unexplained falls is Kenny *et al.*'s [106] recently reported, randomized, controlled trial of rate drop response, dual-chamber pacing versus no pacing. Not only is the reduction in the number of falls dramatic in this study, it is the largest trial of pacing in CSH (whatever the presenting symptom complex) ever performed. However, the study suffers from the absence of blinding and the potential for a placebo response, given the invasive intervention versus none at all, and although the overall number of falls was less in the intervention group, the actual number of falls per patient increased slightly in both intervention and control groups. In addition, the number of subjects who fell was similar in both intervention and control groups. Furthermore, the inclusion of a substantial number of subjects with syncope as part of their presenting complaint clouds the issue further, although numbers of syncopal episodes were similar in both groups. We have recently completed a small, double-blind, randomized, placebo-controlled, cross-over study of dual-chamber pacing therapy in highly symptomatic patients with CSH presenting with unexplained falls (Parry and Kenny, unpublished data). Twenty-five patients underwent dual-chamber pacemaker implantation and were randomized to pacemaker on (DDDR pacing mode) or off (ODO mode) for 6 months in randomized, double-blind fashion. Fall rates were the same whether pacing intervention was active or not, and time to first fall and number of patients falling in both limbs of the study were similar. The multicenter SAFE-PACE 2 study of pacing versus implantable loop recorder in patients with CSH-related unexplained falls will report soon and provide clarification on this important issue.

Challenges in carotid sinus hypersensitivity

> "Ignorance is a like rare, exotic fruit; touch it and the bloom has gone." Oscar Wilde, *The Importance of Being Earnest*

While the CSH bloom of ignorance is long gone, the fruit remains ready to harvest. From pathophysiology and prevalence through clinical characteristics and intervention studies, challenges abound in this fascinating condition. Important first steps will include teasing out the differences between a pathologic and physiologic hypersensitive response, using epidemiologic techniques and neuroanatomical and neurohistochemical studies on postmortem studies. This approach, with long-term neuropsychologic follow-up antemortem will help to discern the putative role of CSH as a risk factor for the dementias. The results of such studies would also have the advantage of informing more sound intervention studies, possibly allowing medical management rather than pacing intervention for the cardioinhibitory subtypes and a more rational and effective treatment approach for the enigmatic vasodepressor subtype. Even without basic scientific evidence, the time is ripe for further pacing intervention studies using double-blind, placebo controlled designs in both falls and syncope associated with CSH. Much preliminary work is underway, but much more has yet to be done.

References

1 Parry CH. *An Inquiry into the Symptoms and Causes of Syncope Anginosa, Commonly Called Angina Pectoris*. Bath, UK: R Cuttwell, 1799.

2 Roskam J. Un syndrome noveau: syncopes cardiaques gràves et syncopes répétées par hyperréflectivité sino-carotidienne. *Presse Med* 1930;**38**:590–1.

3 Weiss S, Baker JP. Carotid sinus reflex in health and disease: its role in the causation of fainting and convulsions. *Medicine* 1933;**12**:297–354.

4 Danielopolu D. Sur la pathogenie de l'epilepsie et sur son traitment chirurgical. *Presse Med* 1933;**41**:170.

5 Ferris EB, Capps RB, Weiss S. Carotid sinus syncope and its bearing on the mechanism of the unconscious state and convulsions: a study of 32 additional cases. *Medicine* 1935;**14**:377–456.

6 Weiss S, Capps RB, Ferris EB, Munro D. Syncope and convulsions due to a hyperactive carotid sinus reflex. *Arch Intern Med* 1936;**58**:407–17.

7 Galdston M, Goldstein G, Steele JM. Studies of the variation in circulatory and respiratory responses to carotid sinus stimulation in man. *Am Heart J* 1943;**26**:213–31.

8 Galdston M, Govons S, Wortis SB, Steele JM, Taylor HK. Thrombosis of the common, internal and external carotid arteries: a report of two cases with a review of the literature. *Arch Intern Med* 1941;**67**:1162–5.

9 Gurdjian ES, Webster JE, Martin FA, Hardy WG. Carotid compression in the neck: results and significance in carotid ligation. *JAMA* 1957;**163**:1030–6.

10 Gurdjian ES, Webster JE, Hardy WG, Lindner DW. Non-existence of the so-called cerebral form of carotid sinus syncope. *Neurology* 1958;**8**:818–26.

11 Morley CA, Sutton R. Carotid sinus syncope. *Int J Cardiol* 1984;**6**:287–93.

12 Kenny RA, O'Shea D, Parry SW. The Newcastle protocols for head-up tilt table testing in the diagnosis of vasovagal syncope, carotid sinus hypersensitivity, and related disorders. *Heart* 2000;**83**:564–9.

13 McIntosh SJ, Lawson J, Kenny RA. Clinical characteristics of vasodepressor, cardioinhibitory, and mixed carotid sinus syndrome in the elderly. *Am J Med* 1993;**95**:203–8.

14 Parry SW, Richardson DA, O'Shea D, Sen B, Kenny RA. Diagnosis of carotid sinus hypersensitivity in older adults: carotid sinus massage in the upright position is essential. *Heart* 2000;**83**:22–3.

15 Tea SH, Mansourati J, L'Heveder G, Mabin D, Blanc JJ. New insights into the pathophysiology of carotid sinus syndrome. *Circulation* 1996;**93**:1411–6.

16 Engel GL, Engel FL. The significance of the carotid-sinus reflex in biliary-tract disease. *N Engl J Med* 1942;**227**(13):470–4.

17 Nathanson MH. Hyperactive cardioinhibitory carotid sinus reflex. *Arch Intern Med* 1946;**77**:491–502.

18 Peretz DI, Gerein AN, Miyagishima RT. Permanent demand pacing for hypersensitive carotid sinus syndrome. *CMAJ* 1973;**108**:1131–4.

19 Sigler LH. Hyperactive caridoinhibitory carotid sinus reflex: a possible aid in the diagnosis of coronary disease. *Arch Intern Med* 1941;**67**:177–93.

20 Sigler LH. The cardioinhibitory carotid sinus reflex: its importance as a vagocardiosensitivity test. *Am J Cardiol* 1963;**12**:175–83.

21 Franke J. *Über das Karotissinus-Syndrome und den Sogenannten Hyperaktiven*. Stuttgart: Friedrich-Karl Schattauer-Verlag, 1963: 149.

22 Thomas JE. Hyperactive carotid sinus reflex and carotid sinus syncope. *Mayo Clin Proc* 1969;**44**:127–39.

23 Thomas JE. Diseases of the carotid sinus: syncope. In: Vinken PJ, Bruyn GW, eds. *Handbook of Clinical Neurology*, Amsterdam, the Netherlands: North-Holland Publishing, 1972: 532–51.

24 Heidorn GH, McNamara AP. Effect of carotid sinus stimulation on the electrocardiograms of clinically normal individuals. *Circulation* 1956;**14**:1104–13.

25 Strasberg B, Sagie A, Erdman S, Kusniec J, Sclarovsky S, Agmon J. Carotid sinus hypersensitivity and the carotid sinus syndrome. *Prog Cardiovasc Dis* 1989;**31**:379–91.

26 McIntosh S, da Costa D, Kenny RA. Outcome of an integrated approach to the investigation of dizziness, falls and syncope in elderly patients referred to a "syncope." *Age Ageing* 1993;**22**:53–8.

27 Blanc JJ, Cazeau S, Ritter P, *et al*. Carotid sinus syndrome: acute hemodynamic evaluation of a dual chamber pacing mode. *Pacing Clin Electrophysiol* 1995;**18**:1902–8.

28 Cheitlin MD, Conill A, Epstein AE, *et al*. ACC/AHA Guidelines for Implantation of Cardiac Pacemakers and Antiarrhythmia Devices. Report of the American College of Cardiology/American Heart Association Task Force on Practice Guidelines (Committee on Pacemaker Implantation). *J Am Coll Cardiol* 1998;**31**(5):1175–209.

29 Recommendations for pacemaker prescription for symptomatic bradycardia. Report of a working party of the British Pacing and Electrophysiology Group. *Br Heart J* 1991;**66**:185–91.

30 Walter PF, Crawley IS, Dorney ER. Carotid sinus hypersensitivity and syncope. *Am J Cardiol* 1978;**42**:396–403.

31 Brignole M, Barra M, Prato R, Sartore B, Bertulla A. Carotid sinus syndrome: evaluation of the cardio-inhibitor and vasodepressive components and of the association with orthostatic hypotension. *Cardiologia* 1985;**30**:601–3.

32 Kenny RA, Traynor G. Carotid sinus syndrome: clinical characteristics in elderly patients. *Age Ageing* 1991;**20**:449–54.

33 Parry SW. How to do it: carotid sinus massage. *CME Bull Geriatr Med* 1997;**1**:7.

34 Brignole M, Menozzi C, Gianfranchi L, Oddone D, Lolli G, Bertulla A. Neurally mediated syncope detected by carotid sinus massage and head-up tilt test in sick sinus syndrome. *Am J Cardiol* 1991;**68**:1032–6.

35 Brignole M, Alboni P, Benditt DG, *et al*. Guidelines on management (diagnosis and treatment) of syncope. *Eur Heart J* 2001;**22**:1256–306.

36 Hammill SC, Holmes DRJ, Wood DL, *et al*. Electrophysiologic testing in the upright position: improved evaluation of patients with rhythm disturbances using a tilt table. *J Am Coll Cardiol* 1984;**4**:65–71.

37 Morillo CA, Camacho ME, Wood MA, Gilligan DM, Ellenbogen KA. Diagnostic utility of mechanical, pharmacological and orthostatic stimulation of the carotid sinus in patients with unexplained syncope. *J Am Coll Cardiol* 1999;**34**:1587–94.

38 Bocchiardo M, Alciati M, Buscemi A, Cravetto A, Richiardi E, Gaita F. Usefulness of a protocol for carotid sinus massage in supine and erect postures in patients with syncope without other cardiovascular or neurological diseases. *G Ital Cardiol* 1995;**25**:553–60.

39 Landau WM. Clinical neuromythology. XIII. Neuro-skepticism: sovereign remedy for the carotid sinus syndrome. *Neurology* 1994;**44**:1570–6.

40 O'Mahony D. Carotid sinus hypersensitivity in old age: clinical syndrome or physical sign? *Age Ageing* 2001;**30**:273–4.

41 Eckberg DL, Cavanaugh MS, Mark AL, Abboud FM. A simplified neck suction device for activation of carotid baroreceptors. *J Lab Clin Med* 1975;**85**:167–73.

42 Hainsworth R, al-Shamma YM. Cardiovascular responses to stimulation of carotid baroreceptors in healthy subjects. *Clin Sci* 1988;**75**:159–65.

43 Dehn TC, Morley CA, Sutton R. A scientific evaluation of the carotid sinus syndrome. *Cardiovasc Res* 1984;**18**:746–51.

44 Hankey GJ, Warlow CP. Symptomatic carotid ischaemic events: safest and most cost effective way of selecting patients for angiography, before carotid endarterectomy. *BMJ* 1990;**300**:1485–91.

45 Munro NC, McIntosh S, Lawson J, Morley CA, Sutton R, Kenny RA. Incidence of complications after carotid sinus massage in older patients with syncope. *J Am Geriatr Soc* 1994;**42**:1248–51.

46 Davies AJ, Kenny RA. Frequency of neurologic complications following carotid sinus massage. *Am J Cardiol* 1998;**81**:1256–7.

47 Richardson DA, Bexton RS, Shaw FE, Steen N, Bond J, Kenny RA. Complications of carotid sinus massage: a prospective series of older patients. *Age Ageing* 2001;**29**:413–7.

48 Askey J. Hemiplegia following carotid sinus stimulation. *Am Heart J* 1946;**31**:131–7.

49 Bastulli JA, Orlowski JP. Stroke as a complication of carotid sinus massage. *Crit Care Med* 1985;**13**:869.

50 Beal MF, Park TS, Fisher CM. Cerebral atheromatous embolism following carotid sinus pressure. *Arch Neurol* 1981;**38**:310–2.

51 Ferguson S, Ellis CJ. Monoplegia following carotid sinus massage. *J Intern Med* 1994;**235**:379–81.

52 Alexander S, Ping WC. Fatal ventricular fibrillation during carotid sinus stimulation. *Am J Cardiol* 1966;**18**:289–91.

53 Bohm A, Pinter A, Preda I. Non-sustained ventricular tachycardia during carotid massage. *Heart* 2001;**86**:6.

54 Matthews OA. Ventricular tachycardia induced by carotid sinus stimulation. *J Maine Med Assoc* 1969;**60**: 135–6.

55 Porus RL, Marcus FI. Ventricular fibrilation during carotid-sinus stimulation. *N Engl J Med* 1963;**268**: 1338–42.

56 Cohen MV. Ventricular fibrillation precipitated by carotid sinus pressure: case report and review of the literature. *Am Heart J* 1972;**84**:681–6.

57 Greenwood RJ, Dupler DA. Death following carotid sinus pressure. *JAMA* 1962;**181**:605–9.

58 Hilal H, Massumi R. Fatal ventricular fibrillation after carotid-sinus stimulation. *N Engl J Med* 1966;**275**:157–8.

59 Blumenfeld S, Schaeffeler KT, Zullo RJ. An unusual response to carotid sinus pressure. *Am Heart J* 1950; **40**:319–22.

60 Dey AB, Bexton RS, Tynan MM, Charles RG, Kenny RA. The impact of a dedicated "syncope and falls" clinic on pacing practice in northeastern England. *Pacing Clin Electrophysiol* 1997;**20**:815–7.

61 Koch E. Über den depressorischen gefässereflex beim karotisdruckverusche am menschen. *Münch Med Wochenschr* 1924;**71**:704.

62 Mehrmann K. *Der Heringsche Karotisdruckversuch am Menschen.* Bonn: Inaug Diss, 1925.

63 Mandelstamm M, Lifschitz S. Die wirkung der karotissinusreflexe auf den blutdruck beim menschen. *Klin Wochenschr* 1928;**22**:321.

64 Murphy AL, Rowbotham BJ, Boyle RS, Thew CM, Fardoulys JA, Wilson K. Carotid sinus hypersensitivity in elderly nursing home patients. *Aust N Z J Med* 1986;**16**:24–7.

65 Hudson WM, Morley CA, Perrins EJ, Chan SL, Sutton R. Is a hypersensitive carotid sinus reflex relevant? *Clin Prog* 1985;**3**:155–9.

66 Volkmann H, Schnerch B, Kuhnert H. Diagnostic value of carotid sinus hypersensitivity. *Pacing Clin Electrophysiol* 1990;**13**:2065–70.

67 McIntosh SJ, Lawson J, Kenny RA. Heart rate and blood pressure responses to carotid sinus massage in healthy elderly subjects. *Age Ageing* 1994;**23**:57–61.

68 Jeffreys M, Wood DA, Lampe F, Walker F, Dewhurst G. The heart rate response to carotid artery massage in a sample of healthy elderly people. *Pacing Clin Electrophysiol* 1996;**19**:1488–92.

69 Davies AJ, Steen N, Kenny RA. Carotid sinus hypersensitivity is common in older patients presenting to an accident and emergency department with unexplained falls. *Age Ageing* 2001;**30**:289–94.

70 Ward CR, McIntosh S, Kenny RA. Carotid sinus hypersensitivity: a modifiable risk factor for fractured neck of femur. *Age Ageing* 1999;**28**:127–33.

71 Purks WK. Electrocardiographic findings following carotid sinus stimulation. *Ann Intern Med* 1939;**13**:270–9.

72 Mankikar GD, Clark AN. Cardiac effects of carotid sinus massage in old age. *Age Ageing* 1975;**4**:86–94.

73 Baig MW, Kaye GC, Perrins EJ. Can central neuropeptides be implicated in carotid sinus reflex hypersensitivity? *Med Hypotheses* 1989;**28**:255–9.

74 Talman WT. Glutamatergic transmission in the nucleus tractus solitarii: from server to peripherals in the cardiovascular information superhighway. *Braz J Med Biol Res* 1997;**30**:1–7.

75 Jaeger F, Fouad-Tarazi FM, Castle LW. Carotid sinus hypersensitivity and neurally mediated syncope. In: Ellenbogen KA, Kay GN, Wilkoff BL, eds. *Clinical Cardiac Pacing*, Philadelphia, PA: W.B. Saunders, 1995: 333–52.

76 Luck JC, Hoover RJ, Biederman RW, *et al.* Observations on carotid sinus hypersensitivity from direct intraneural recordings of sympathetic nerve traffic. *Am J Cardiol* 1996;**77**:1362–5.

77 Costa F, Biaggioni I. Microneurographic evidence of sudden sympathetic withdrawal in carotid sinus syncope: treatment with ergotamine. *Chest* 1994;**106**:617–20.

78 Smith ML, Ellenbogen KA, Eckberg DL. Sympathoinhibition and hypotension in carotid sinus hypersensitivity. *Clin Auton Res* 1992;**2**:389–92.

79 Patel AK, Yap VU, Fields J, Thomsen JH. Carotid sinus syncope induced by malignant tumors in the neck: emergence of vasodepressor manifestations following pacemaker therapy. *Arch Intern Med* 1979;**139**:1281–4.

80 Muntz HR, Smith PG. Carotid sinus hypersensitivity: a cause of syncope in patients with tumors of the head and neck. *Laryngoscope* 1983;**93**:1290–3.

81 Fourquet N, Genet L, Davy-Chedaute F, Jezequel J, Blanc JJ. Carotid sinus hypersensitivity associated with a treated otorhinolaryngologic cancer: study of 103 patients. *Presse Med* 1991;**20**:1713–6.

82 Cicogna R, Bonomi FG, Curnis A, *et al.* Parapharyngeal space lesions syncope syndrome: a newly proposed reflexogenic cardiovascular syndrome. *Eur Heart J* 1993;**14**:1476–83.

83 Wiedemann G, Grotz J, Bewermeyer H, Hossmann V, Heiss WD. High-resolution real-time ultrasound of the carotid bifurcation in patients with hyperactive carotid sinus syndrome. *J Neurol* 1985;**232**:318–25.

84 O'Mahony D. Pathophysiology of carotid sinus hypersensitivity in elderly patients. *Lancet* 1995;**346**:950–2.

85 Smith HL, Moerrsch FD. Further study on the hypersensitive carotid reflex. *Mayo Clin Proc* 1935;**11**:380–3.

86 Arenberg IK, Cummins GMJ, Bucy PC, Oberhill HR. Symptomatic hyperirritable carotid sinus mechanism. *Laryngoscope* 1979;**81**:253–63.

87 Trout HH, Brown LL, Thompson JE. Carotid sinus syndrome: treatment by carotid sinus denervation. *Ann Surg* 1979;**189**:575–80.

88 Blanc JJ, L'Heveder G, Mansourati J, Tea SH, Guillo P, Mabin D. Assessment of a newly recognized association: carotid sinus hypersensitivity and denervation of sternocleidomastoid muscles. *Circulation* 1997;**95**:2548–51.

89 Parry SW, Baptist M, Gilroy JJ, Steen N, Kenny RA. Central α_2-adrenoceptors and the pathogenesis of carotid sinus hypersensitivity. *Heart* 2004;**90**:935–6.

90 Shaw FE, Bond J, Richardson DA, *et al.* Multifactorial intervention after a fall in older people with cognitive impairment and dementia presenting to the accident and emergency department: randomised controlled trial. *BMJ* 2003;**326**(7380):73.

91 Ballard C, Shaw F, McKeith I, Kenny R. High prevalence of neurocardiovascular instability in neurodegenerative dementias. *Neurology* 1998;**51**(6):1760–2.

92 Kenny RA, Shaw FE, O'Brien JT, Scheltens PH, Kalaria R, Ballard C. Carotid sinus syndrome is common in dementia with Lewy body and correlates with deep white matter lesions. *J Neurol Neurosurg Psychiatry* 2004;**75**:966–7.

93 Kenny RA. Kalaria R. Ballard C. Neurocardiovascular instability in cognitive impairment and dementia. *Ann N Y Acad Sci* 2002;**977**:183–95.

94 Ross GW, Petrovitch H, White LR, *et al.* Characterization of risk factors for vascular dementia: the Honolulu–Asia Aging Study. *Neurology* 1999;**53**(2):337–43.

95 Breteler MM, van Swieten JC, Bots ML, *et al.* Cerebral white matter lesions, vascular risk factors, and cognitive function in a population-based study: the Rotterdam Study. *Neurology* 1994;**44**(7):1246–52.

96 de Groot JC, de Leeuw FE, Oudkerk M, Hofman A, Jolles J, Breteler MM. Cerebral white matter lesions and subjective cognitive dysfunction: the Rotterdam Scan Study. *Neurology* 2001;**56**(11):1539–45.

97 Hartzler GO, Maloney JD. Cardioinhibitory carotid sinus hypersensitivity: intracardiac recordings and clinical assessment. *Arch Intern Med* 1977;**137**:727–31.

98 Richardson DA, Shaw FE, Kenny RA. The prevalence of carotid sinus hypersensitivity is high in patients with atrial fibrillation and unexplained falls [Abstract]. *Age Ageing* 1999;**28**(Suppl. 2):A128.

99 Achiron A, Regev A. Carotid sinus syncope induced by an orthodontic appliance. *Lancet* 1989;**2**:1339.

100 Schellack J, Fulenwider JT, Olson RA, Smith RB, Mansour K. The carotid sinus syndrome: a frequently overlooked cause of syncope in the elderly. *J Vasc Surg* 1986;**4**:376–83.

101 Nathanson MH. Effects of drugs on cardiac standstill induced by pressure on the carotid sinus. *Arch Intern Med* 1933;**51**:387.

102 Lown B, Levine A. The carotid sinus: clinical value of its stimulation. *Circulation* 1961;**23**:766–89.

103 Nichol AD, Strauss H. Effects of digitalis, urginin, congestive cardiac failure and atropine on hyperactive carotid sinus. *Am Heart J* 1943;**25**:746–54.

104 Mulcahy R, Allcock L, O'Shea D. Timolol, carotid sinus hypersensitivity, and elderly patients. *Lancet* 1998;**352**:1147–8.

105 Brignole M, Menozzi C, Gaggioli G, *et al.* Effects of long-term vasodilator therapy in patients with carotid sinus hypersensitivity. *Am Heart J* 1998;**136**:264–8.

106 Kenny RA, Richardson DA, Bexton RS, Steen N, Bond J. Cardiac pacing reduces falls in carotid sinus hypersensitivity: the SAFE-PACE trial. *J Am Coll Cardiol* 2001;**38**:1491–6.

107 Parry SW, Kenny RA. Carotid sinus syndrome masquerading as epilepsy in an older patient. *Postgrad Med J* 2000;**76**:656–7.

108 McCrea W, Findley LJ. Carotid sinus hypersensitivity in patients referred with possible epilepsy. *Br J Clin Pract* 1994;**48**:22–4.

109 Solti F, Mogan ST, Renyi-Vamos F, Moravcsik A. The association of carotid artery stenosis with carotid sinus hypersensitivity: transitory cerebral ischaemic attack provoked by carotid sinus reflex. *J Cardiovasc Surg* 1990;**31**:693–6.

110 Ward C, McIntosh SJ, Kenny RA. The prevalence of carotid sinus syndrome in elderly patients with fractured neck of femur [Abstract]. *Age Ageing* 1994;**23**(Suppl 1):A16.

111 Ward C, Kenny RA. Reproducibility of orthostatic hypotension in symptomatic elderly. *Am J Med* 1996;**100**:418–22.

112 Kenny RA, Davies A, Bexton RS. Benefits of pacing in older patients with carotid sinus syndrome: reduction in the frequency of falls, injury rates and in hospital service utilisation. 2000;(UnPub).

113 Davies AJ, Kenny RA. Falls presenting to the accident and emergency department: types of presentation and risk factor profile. *Age Ageing* 1996;**25**:362–6.

114 Crilley JG, Herd B, Khurana CS, *et al.* Permanent cardiac pacing in elderly patients with recurrent falls, dizziness and syncope, and a hypersensitive cardioinhibitory reflex. *Postgrad Med J* 1997;**73**:415–8.

115 Richardson DA, Bexton RS, Shaw FE, Kenny RA. Prevalence of cardioinhibitory carotid sinus hyper-

sensitivity in patients 50 years or over presenting to the accident and emergency department with "unexplained" or "recurrent" falls. *Pacing Clin Electrophysiol* 1997;**20**:820–3.

116 Lipsitz LA. Abnormalities in blood pressure homeostasis that contribute to falls in the elderly. *Clin Geriatr Med* 1985;**1**:637–48.

117 Cummings SR, Nevitt MC, Kidd S. Forgetting falls: the limited accuracy of recall of falls in the elderly. *J Am Geriatr Soc* 1988;**36**:613–6.

118 Dey AB, Stout NR, Kenny RA. Cardiovascular syncope is the most common cause of drop attacks in the elderly. *Pacing Clin Electrophysiol* 1997;**20**:818–9.

119 Shaw FE, Kenny RA. The overlap between syncope and falls in the elderly. *Postgrad Med J* 1997;**73**:635–9.

120 Gordon M. Occult cardiac arrhythmias associated with falls and dizziness in the elderly: detection by Holter monitoring. *J Am Geriatr Soc* 1978;**26**:418–23.

121 Shaw FE, Richardson DA, Steen IN, McKeith IG, Bond J, Kenny RA. Clinical characteristics of fallers with cognitive impairment and dementia who comply with multidisciplinary post-fall intervention. *Age Ageing* 2000;**29**(Suppl. 2):22.

122 Folstein MF, Folstein SE, McHugh PR. "Mini mental state": a practical method for grading the cognitive state of patients for the clinician. *J Psychiatr Res* 1975;**12**:189–98.

123 Sheldon JH. On the natural history of falls in old age. *BMJ* 1960;**2**:1685–90.

124 McIntosh SJ, Lawson J, Bexton RS, Gold RG, Tynan MM, Kenny RA. A study comparing VVI and DDI pacing in elderly patients with carotid sinus syndrome. *Heart* 1997;**77**:553–7.

125 Brignole M, Menozzi C, Lolli G, Oddone D, Gianfranchi L, Bertulla A. Pacing for carotid sinus syndrome and sick sinus syndrome. *Pacing Clin Electrophysiol* 1990; **13**:2071–5.

126 Brignole M, Menozzi C, Lolli G, Bottoni N, Gaggioli G. Long-term outcome of paced and non-paced patients with severe carotid sinus syndrome. *Am J Cardiol* 1992;**69**:1039–43.

127 Brignole M, Sartore B, Barra M, Menozzi C, Lolli G. Ventricular and dual chamber pacing for treatment of carotid sinus syndrome. *Pacing Clin Electrophysiol* 1989;**12**:582–90.

128 Morley CA, Perrins EJ, Grant P, Chan SL, McBrien DJ, Sutton R. Carotid sinus syncope treated by pacing: analysis of persistent symptoms and role of atrioventricular sequential pacing. *Br Heart J* 1982;**47**:411–8.

129 Bexton RS, Davies A, Kenny RA. The rate-drop response in carotid sinus syndrome: the Newcastle experience. *Pacing Clin Electrophysiol* 1997;**20**:840.

130 Brignole M, Menozzi C, Lolli G, Sartore B, Barra M. Natural and unnatural history of patients with severe carotid sinus hypersensitivity: a preliminary study. *Pacing Clin Electrophysiol* 1988;**11**:1628–35.

131 Brignole M, Oddone D, Cogorno S, Menozzi C, Gianfranchi L, Bertulla A. Long-term outcome in symptomatic carotid sinus hypersensitivity. *Am Heart J* 1992;**123**:687–92.

132 Huang SK, Ezri MD, Hauser RG, Denes P. Carotid sinus hypersensitivity in patients with unexplained syncope: clinical, electrophysiologic, and long-term follow-up observations. *Am Heart J* 1988;**116**:989–96.

133 Sugrue DD, Gersh BJ, Holmes DRJ, Wood DL, Osborn MJ, Hammill SC. Symptomatic "isolated" carotid sinus hypersensitivity: natural history and results of treatment with anticholinergic drugs or pacemaker. *J Am Coll Cardiol* 1986;**7**:158–62.

134 Parry SW, Kenny RA. The management of vasovagal syncope. *Q J Med* 1999;**92**:697–705.

135 Craig WM, Smith HL. The surgical treatment of hypersensitive carotid sinus reflexes: a report of 12 cases. *Yale J Biol Med* 1939;**11**:415–22.

136 Ray BS, Stewart HJ. Role of the glossopharyngeal nerve in the carotid sinus reflex in man: relief of carotid sinus syndrome by intracranial section of the glossopharyngeal nerve. *Surgery* 1948;**23**:411–24.

137 Ford FR. Fatal hypertensive crisis following denervation of the carotid sinus for the relief of repeated attacks of syncope: case history. *Bull Johns Hopkins Hosp* 1957;**100**:14–6.

138 Heron JR, Anderson EG, Noble IM. Cardiac abnormalities associated with carotid-sinus syndrome. *Lancet* 1965:**1**(7428):214–6.

139 Cheng LH, Norris CW. Surgical management of the carotid sinus syndrome. *Arch Otolaryngol Head Neck Surg* 1973;**97**:395–8.

140 Cohen FL, Fruehan CT, King BB. Carotid sinus syndrome: report of five cases and review of the literature. *J Neurosurg* 1976;**45**:78–84.

141 Kodama K, Seo N, Murayama T, Yoshizawa Y, Terasako K, Yaginuma T. Glossopharyngeal nerve block for carotid sinus syndrome. *Anesth Analg* 1992;**75**:1036–7.

142 Fahmy RN, Cohen BJ, Summers ST, Baker JD, Heng MK. Revisiting carotid sinus denervation in carotid sinus hypersensitivity. *Am Heart J* 1994;**128**: 1257–9.

143 Mathias CJ, Armstrong E, Browse N, Chaudhuri KR, Enevoldson P, Russell RW. Value of non-invasive continuous blood pressure monitoring in the detection of carotid sinus hypersensitivity. *Clin Auton Res* 1991;**1**:157–9.

144 Streian C, Huditeanu D. Glomectomy in carotid sinus syncope. *Med Interne* 1988;**26**:47–52.

145 Fachinetti P, Bellocchi S, Dorizzi A, Forgione FN. Carotid sinus syndrome: a review of the literature and

our experience using carotid sinus denervation. *J Neurosurg Sci* 1998;**42**:189–93.

146 Stevenson CA. The use of roentgen therapy in the carotid sinus syndrome. *Radiology* 1939;**32**:209–14.

147 Stevenson CA, Moreton RD. A subsequent report on roentgen therapy in the carotid sinus syndrome. *Radiology* 1948;**50**:207–10.

148 Greeley HP, Smedal MI, Most W. The treatment of the carotid sinus syndrome by irradiation. *N Engl J Med* 1955;**252**:91–4.

149 Palmer RA. The treatment of carotid sinus syncope with propantheline. *CMAJ* 1971;**104**:923–5.

150 Keating EC, Burks JM, Calder JRJ. Mixed carotid sinus hypersensitivity: successful therapy with pacing, ephedrine, and propranolol. *Pacing Clin Electrophysiol* 1985;**8**: 356–9.

151 Tomcsanyi J, Papp L, Naszlady A. Carotid sinus hypersensitivity abolished by aminophylline. *Int J Cardiol* 1993;**38**:299–301.

152 Dan D, Grubb BP, Mouhaffel AH, Kosinski DJ. Use of serotonin reuptake inhibitors as primary therapy for carotid sinus hypersensitivity. *Pacing Clin Electrophysiol* 1997;**20**:1633–5.

153 Grubb BP, Samoil D, Kosinski D, Temesy-Armos P, Akpunonu B. The use of serotonin reuptake inhibitors for the treatment of recurrent syncope due to carotid sinus hypersensitivity unresponsive to dual chamber cardiac pacing. *Pacing Clin Electrophysiol* 1994;**17**: 1434–6.

154 Hussain RM, McIntosh SJ, Lawson J, Kenny RA. Fludrocortisone in the treatment of hypotensive disorders in the elderly. *Heart* 1996;**76**:507–9. [Published erratum appears in *Heart* 1997;**77**:294.]

155 da Costa D, McIntosh S, Kenny RA. Benefits of fludrocortisone in the treatment of symptomatic vasodepressor carotid sinus syndrome. *Br Heart J* 1993;**69**:308–10.

156 Voss DM, Magnin GE. Demand pacing and carotid sinus syncope. *Am Heart J* 1970;**79**:544–7.

157 Bahl OP, Ferguson TB, Oliver GC, Parker BM. Treatment of carotid sinus syncope with demand pacemaker. *Chest* 1971;**59**:262–5.

158 Von Maur K, Nelson EW, Holsinger JWJ, Eliot RS. Hypersensitive carotid sinus syncope treated by implantable demand cardiac pacemaker. *Am J Cardiol* 1972;**29**:109–10.

159 Ramirez A. Demand pacemaker for the treatment of carotid sinus syncope. *J Thorac Cardiovasc Surg* 1973;**66**:287–9.

160 Probst P, Muhlberger V, Lederbauer M, Pachinger O, Kaliman J, Steinbach K. Electrophysiologic findings in carotid sinus massage. *Pacing Clin Electrophysiol* 1983;**6**:689–96.

161 Stryjer D, Friedensohn A, Schlesinger Z. Ventricular

pacing as the preferable mode for long-term pacing in patients with carotid sinus syncope of the cardioinhibitory type. *Pacing Clin Electrophysiol* 1986;**9**:705–9.

162 Brignole M, Menozzi C, Lolli G, Oddone D, Gianfranchi L, Bertulla A. Validation of a method for choice of pacing mode in carotid sinus syndrome with or without sinus bradycardia. *Pacing Clin Electrophysiol* 1991;**14**:196–203.

163 Menozzi C, Brignole M, Pagani P, Lolli G, Casali G. Assessment of VVI diagnostic pacing mode in patients with cardioinhibitory carotid sinus syndrome. *Pacing Clin Electrophysiol* 1988;**11**:1641–6.

164 Brignole M, Sartore B, Barra M, Menozzi C, Lolli G. Is DDD superior to VVI pacing in mixed carotid sinus syndrome? An acute and medium-term study. *Pacing Clin Electrophysiol* 1988;**11**:1902–10.

165 Brignole M, Menozzi C, Lolli G, Sartore B, Barra M. Natural and unnatural history of severe carotid sinus hypersensitivity [Abstract]. 4th European Symposium on Cardiac Pacing, Stockholm 1989.

166 Graux P, Guyomar Y, Lejeune C, Carlioz R, Durieu C, Dutoit A. Contribution of a pacemaker bradycardia detection algorithm in the study of patients with carotid sinus syndrome. *Pacing Clin Electrophysiol* 2001;**24**:921–4.

167 Menozzi C, Brignole M, Lolli G, *et al.* Follow-up of asystolic episodes in patients with cardioinhibitory, neurally mediated syncope and VVI pacemaker. *Am J Cardiol* 1993;**72**:1152–5.

168 Madigan NP, Flaker GC, Curtis JJ, Reid J, Mueller KJ, Murphy TJ. Carotid sinus hypersensitivity: beneficial effects of dual-chamber pacing. *Am J Cardiol* 1984;**53**:1034–40.

169 Mabo P, Druelles P, Kermarrec A, Bedossa M, Le Breton H, Daubert C. Haemodynamic mechanisms of arterial hypotension in carotid sinus syndrome and of prevention by dual chamber pacing. *Eur J Clin P E* 1992;**2**:129–38.

170 Medtronic Inc. Kappa DR. Dual chamber rate responsive pacemaker (DDDR). Minneapolis, MN: 1996.

171 Gammage MD. Rate-drop response programming. *Pacing Clin Electrophysiol* 1997;**20**:841–3.

172 Close J, Ellis M, Hooper R, Glucksman E, Jackson S, Swift C. Prevention of falls in the elderly trial (PROFET): a randomised controlled trial. *Lancet* 1999;**353**:93–7.

173 Smiddy J, Lewis HD Jr, Dunn M. The effect of carotid massage in older men. *J Gerontol* 1972;**27**:209–11.

174 Brignole M, Menozzi C, Bottoni N, *et al.* Mechanisms of syncope caused by transient bradycardia and the diagnostic value of electrophysiologic testing and cardiovascular reflexity maneuvers. *Am J Cardiol* 1995;**76**: 273–8.

CHAPTER 15

Miscellaneous causes of syncope

Daniel J. Kosinski, MD, *& Blair P. Grubb,* MD

Introduction

There are several unique etiologies of syncope that are not readily classified into the discussion in previous chapters. The purpose of this chapter is to review several of these etiologies of syncope.

Situational syncope

Situational syncope is defined as syncope related to a particular circumstance (Table 15.1). The various entities comprised in this condition have in common a mechanism that generally involves a combination of decreased preload, increased vagal activity, and/or decreased sympathetic activity. The afferent stimulus varies clinically, but the efferent response is varying degrees of cardioinhibitory and vasodepressor effects. In addition, some of these situations also involve a component of decreased cardiac filling.

Several of these situations deserve special mention, as the mechanisms involved are somewhat unusual. *Glossopharyngeal syncope* is generally precipitated by intense pain in the external auditory canal or posterior pharynx and is thought to occur

as a result of vagal stimulation by way of afferent impulses originating in the glossopharyngeal nerve [1]. *Hot tub syncope* occurs generally upon abrupt exit from a hot tub or jacuzzi. When an individual is immersed in such an environment, vasodilation occurs as part of the normal compensation to heat. Abrupt standing to exit the tub leads to a normal displacement of volume with upright posture. However, this volume displacement in the face of vasodilation can lead to excessive peripheral vascular pooling with a decrease in blood pressure that is sufficient to produce syncope. Defecation syncope refers to sudden hypotension and/or bradycardia that occurs during sudden evacuation of the rectum or during removal of an impaction.

Breath holding, particularly a problem in children, can lead to syncope via a vagal reflex [2,3] (see Chapter 16). On occasion these episodes may be mistaken for epilepsy [4]. *Airway stimulation* may also provoke syncope or cardiac arrest via a vagal mechanism [5].

Syncopal episodes may also occur during or immediately following ingestion of a bolus of food. Patients who experience this type of syncope are often found to have an abnormality of the esophagus such as a diverticulum, stricture, or cancer. Thus, the patient with recurrent *swallow syncope* should be examined for these disorders. A similar situation is sometimes seen when a person who is quite hot takes a cold drink. In this situation it is thought that the cold liquid induces esophageal or gastric spasm (and pain) enough to produce a vagal reflex-mediated period of hypotension and bradycardia. Swallowing cold liquid while in an overheated state is reported to have resulted in death in otherwise healthy soldiers and athletes. A poem in the *Lancet* warns:

Table 15.1 Causes of situational syncope.

Micturition	Occulovagal
Glossopharyngeal	Instrumentation
Deglutition	Hot tub
Defecation	Post-phlebotomy
Tussive	Sneeze
Postprandial	Trumpet/horn playing
Valsalva	(Valsalva maneuver)

Full many a man, both young and old
Has gone to his sarcophagus
Through pouring water, ice cold, down
His too hot oesophagus [6].

Syncope caused by increased intrathoracic pressure

Increased intrathoracic pressure may lead to a decrease in venous return to the heart. The autonomic nervous system is generally able to compensate for this. However, in some instances compensatory mechanisms are overcome and syncope occurs. Such situations include but are not limited to trumpet playing, cough, or deliberate Valsalva maneuver [6,7]. *Cough syncope* is particularly interesting in that a single cough may cause only a brief increase in intrathoracic pressure. Severe paroxysms of cough, however, can severely elevate intrathoracic pressure. Syncope may occur as a consequence of decreased venous return or a vagal reaction triggered by a reflex overshoot of arterial pressure when coughing stops. Sneeze syncope is thought to be produced by a similar mechanism [6].

Hair-grooming syncope seizures

This is an unusual cause of syncope that is generally seen in young females [8]. It involves convulsive syncope that occurs in relation to hair grooming. The convulsive syncope is almost invariably preceded by a prodrome of presyncope, nausea, lightheadedness, diaphoresis, and visual disturbance. The reaction is thought to be a variant of neurocardiogenic (vasovagal) syncope that is triggered by hair pulling or scalp stimulation activating the trigeminal nerve.

Syncope caused by the use of therapeutic or recreational drugs

Many therapeutic agents have "prosyncopal" effects. The major culprit drugs are, in general, agents designed to lower heart rate or promote vasodilation (primarily antihypertensive agents). These types of drugs may inhibit the body's ability to make proper adjustments for the maintenance of adequate cerebral perfusion.

Several other therapeutic agents can be responsible for syncope. Phenothiazine agents can cause syncope secondary to cardiac arrhythmia or sudden hypotension [9]. Tricyclic antidepressants can cause cardiac arrhythmias and can also cause hypotension through α-receptor blockage [10]. Antiarrhythmic agents can cause syncope via multiple effects including proarrhythmia phenomena, hypotension, and myocardial depression.

Several recreational drugs are also associated with syncope. Alcohol ingestion is associated with cardiac arrhythmias (the "holiday heart" syndrome), particularly atrial fibrillation [11]. However, more serious arrhythmias may occur from alcohol ingestion. Cocaine may cause syncope secondary to arrhythmia resulting from myocarditis, ischemia, sympathomimetic effects, or direct electrophysiologic effects, leading to ventricular tachycardia and fibrillation. Interestingly, these effects may be seen days or weeks after exposure to the drug.

Syncope in pacemaker patients

When patients with pacemakers experience syncope, it is frequently assumed to represent either pacemaker dysfunction or pacemaker syndrome. However, Pavlovic *et al.* [12] found that this is not necessarily so. They evaluated 46 patients who experienced syncope after pacemaker implantation. Extensive evaluation was performed on each patient. The etiology of syncope was found to be exit block in 4.5% of patients and failed sensing in 2.1%. The majority of the patients (36.9%) were found to have tilt table-induced syncope. In 30.4% of patients, no cause was assigned to syncope despite extensive evaluation. They concluded that pacemaker dysfunction is not a major cause of syncope in pacemaker patients, and that other causes, in particular neurally mediated syncope, should be considered.

Syncope during sexual activity

Sexual activity is quite naturally associated with sympathetic activation. Such activity can cause tachycardia, tachypnea, and transient hypertension. These changes return to baseline shortly after orgasm [13]. In individuals without heart disease, the oxygen consumption of the heart is not substantially increased during sexual activity, and electrocardiographic abnormalities are not noted. In patients with ischemic heart disease, the situation may be quite different and either symptomatic or silent ischemia may be generated [14]. In such instances, the combination of ischemia and sympathetic activation may lead to arrhythmia [15].

In addition, in select patients without ischemic heart disease, sympathetic stimulation during sexual activity can lead to syncope. Such patients include those with long QT syndrome or neurocardiogenic syncope. Also, a variety of agents used in the treatment of erectile dysfunction (sildenafil, vardenafil, and tadalafil) may lower blood pressure and contribute to syncope in susceptible individuals.

Narcolepsy and cataplexy

Narcolepsy is a potentially disabling disorder of sleep regulation that may affect as many as 1 in 2,000 Americans [16]. The condition is felt to represent an intrusion of the dream cycle of sleep (also referred to as REM or rapid eye movement) into normal wakefulness. The disorder usually appears somewhere between the age of 15 and 30 years [17]. There are four characteristic symptoms of narcolepsy:

1 Excessive daytime sleepiness, with sleep coming on suddenly in inappropriate settings.

2 Hypnogonic hallucinations (vivid dream-like images or smells that come on with sleep).

3 Sleep paralysis (a sense of paralysis upon waking or falling asleep).

4 Cataplexy (the sudden loss of skeletal muscle tone without loss of consciousness, brought on by emotions such as anger, surprise, or even laughter) [18].

Excessive daytime sleepiness is often the earliest symptom, later followed by "sleep attacks," lasting anywhere between 30 s and 30 min [19]. These can occur at any time even while eating or talking. During attacks of cataplexy, patients may fall suddenly unable to speak or move, during which injury may occur. The etiology is unclear; current research has focused on a potential genetic and autoimmune etiology [17]. The majority of patients are not diagnosed and therefore not treated, sometimes with

devastating results (e.g., motor vehicle accidents). Stimulant drugs such as methylphenidates have been employed in the past. In 1999, the US FDA approved the drug modafinil for relief of excessive daytime sleepiness resulting from narcolepsy [20].

Mastocytosis

Mastocytosis is a relatively uncommon disorder caused by episodes of mast cell activation [21]. This may occur either because of excessive production or enhanced responsiveness of mast cells. Episodes are triggered by heavy exercise, extreme heat, strong emotions, or narcotics. The skin becomes red and flushed, followed by nausea, vomiting, diarrhea, headaches, and chest pain [22]. Some patients may experience extreme hypotension, requiring treatment with intravenous pressor agents. The patient's mental status may be disproportionately affected. The diagnosis is made by finding extreme elevation in urinary methylhistamine and prostaglandin D_2 levels. Treatment with a combination of H1 and H2 blockers is often helpful, often used in combination with aspirin [23].

Subclavian steal syndrome

Steal syndromes occur when either a stenosis or obstruction of an artery creates a low pressure area beyond the site of obstruction, such that blood from another artery is redirected to the low pressure area [24]. The best described of these conditions occurs because of a stenosis of the subclavian artery that results in a loss of flow in that side's vertebral artery, which is redirected to the post-stenotic subclavian artery. Basilar artery insufficiency results, often brought on by exertion of the affected arm (usually the left) [25]. Symptoms include syncope and near-syncope, headache, vertigo, diplopia, and loss of vision. Syncope occurring during arm exertion, associated with claudication and blood pressure differences between both arms, should prompt consideration of the diagnosis [26].

Pheochromocytoma

Pheochromocytoma is an uncommon neuroendocrine disorder caused by a catecholamine-producing tumor of chromaffin cells of the adrenal medulla [27]. Less commonly, it arises from the parachromaffin cells of sympathetic nerves in the neck, abdomen, pelvis, and chest. The majority of patients display periodic episodes of hypertension, associated with palpitations, headache, anxiety, tremor, and nausea. A small number of patients may present with only orthostatic hypotension and syncope (especially in those tumors that secrete only epinephrine) [28]. Pheochromocytomas are associated with conditions such as Hippel–Lindau disease, neurofibromatosis, acromegaly, and Cushing's syndrome [29]. Measurement of plasma catecholamines or 24-h urinary metanephrines are often diagnostic. Some patients with neurogenic or essential hypertension may have elevated serum catecholamines. To distinguish these from pheochromocytoma, the clonidine suppression test is useful as it suppresses plasma norepinephrine levels in patients without tumors but not in those with tumors [27].

Baroreflex failure

Normally, the baroreflex arc does not allow the blood pressure to rise or fall excessively. Baroreflex failure is an incompletely understood condition with multiple etiologies that all lead to impairment of afferent baroreceptive nerves or their central components [30]. This leads to a loss in buffering ability, which results in wide fluctuations in both blood pressure and heart rate. Etiologies include trauma, tumors, and surgery, or radiation to the brainstem, neck, or upper chest. Periods of extreme hypertension may alternate with hypotensive episodes [31]. Baroreflex failure may occur in the face of preserved parasympathetic function, in which case hypertension alternates with extreme drops in blood pressure associated with bradycardia or asystole. The hypertensive events tend to lessen in severity over time (unlike the hypertension with pheochromocytoma). The classic finding of baroreflex failure is the ability of patients to augment their heart rate during stress and lower it at rest, yet show bradycardic response to pressor agents or tachycardic response to vasodilators [30]. Plasma norepinephrine levels are markedly elevated during hypertensive episodes [31].

Syncope caused by metabolic or endocrine abnormalities

Although certain metabolic abnormalities have been noted as etiologies of syncope, the proportion of episodes resulting from metabolic causes is likely to be low. In a study by Racco et al. [32], only 5% of episodes of syncope could be identified as being of metabolic cause. In general, the most common metabolic causes of syncope are thought to be hypoglycemia, hypoxia, and forced or voluntary hyperventilation [23].

Hypoglycemia is perhaps the most traditional metabolic abnormality associated with syncope. Accompanying symptoms are generally dizziness, diaphoresis, and altered behavior. To assign hypoglycemia as a cause of syncope, it is necessary to actually demonstrate hypoglycemia during the time of symptoms. This can be very difficult. Hypoglycemia may be spontaneous because of a number of endocrine abnormalities such as insulinoma or autoimmune hypoglycemia. Hypoglycemia, however, is often iatrogenic as a result of the use of insulin or oral hypoglycemic agents in diabetic patients. This is particularly a problem in elderly patients.

Hypoxemia has also been recognized as a cause of syncope. One study identified hypoxemia as a cause of syncope in 3% of the patients studied [33].

It has traditionally been viewed that hyperventilation can produce syncope through a reduction in cerebral blood flow. However, in a study of young subjects, forced hyperventilation alone could not induce syncope. Therefore it is reasonable to hypothesize that syncope resulting from hyperventilation may have a psychological as well as a physical component [33].

One cause of syncope that deserves mention is hypoadrenalism, which is a failure in the body's capacity to mount an adequate glucocorticoid response to stress. The disorder may either be primary in nature resulting from disordered adrenal gland function (Addison's disease), or may occur secondary to dysfunction of the anterior pituitary or because of failure of the hypothalmo-pituitary-adrenal axis (most frequently as a result of exogenous steroids) [34,35].

The clinical features of Addison's disease are somewhat non-specific, consisting principally of

Table 15.2 Metabolic causes of syncope and endocrine disorders.

Metabolic causes of syncope	
Hypo- and hyperkalemia	Hypoxia
Hypo- and hypercalcemia	Hypoglycemia
Hypo- and hypermagnesemia	Hyperventilation

Endocrine disorders

Hypoadrenalism – may be caused by hypopituitarism, Addison's disease, adrenal suppression

Endocrine disorders in which vasoactive substances are produced – carcinoid syndrome, pheochromocytoma, mastocystosis

extreme fatigue, nausea, and vomiting. Primary adrenal failure results not only in glucocorticoid loss, but also mineral corticoid deficiency, giving rise to orthostatic hypotension and syncope [36]. Syncope is the presenting complaint in up to 10% of patients with Addison's disease. Most often, the disease becomes evident when an apparently minor illness provokes a life-threatening sequence of abdominal pain, syncope, and death. One of the classic (and often forgotten) signs of Addison's disease is a pigmentation of non-exposed areas (e.g., the buccal mucosa) that occur as a result of the melanotrophic actions of elevations in corticotropin (ACTH). While reductions in serum sodium along with elevations in serum potassium are common, serum electrolytes are just as likely to be normal. The time of onset is usually in middle age, and it is often autoimmune in nature. The diagnosis is made through the measurement of cortisol levels as well as administration of the short tetracosactrin test [35,36].

There are numerous other metabolic or endocrine causes of syncope that are much less common. Such causes are listed in Table 15.2.

Summary

There are several unique and unusual causes of syncope. While uncommon, they may nevertheless be encountered in clinical practice. The diagnosis of these unique instances of syncope can often be established by a thorough history and appropriately directed evaluations.

References

1 Kong Y. Glossopharyngeal neuralgia associated with bradycardia, syncope, and seizure. *Circulation* 1964;**3**: 109–13.

2 Bridge E, Livingston S, Tietze E. Breath holding spells. *J Pediatr* 1943;**23**:539–61.

3 Lombroso C, Lerman P. Breath holding spells. *Pediatrics* 1967;**39**:563–81.

4 Stephenson J. Reflex anoxic seizures while breath holding: non-epileptic vagal attacks. *Arch Dis Child* 1978;**53**: 193–200.

5 Johnson R, Lambie D, Spalding J. *Neurocardiology*. London: W.B. Saunders, 1984: 167–8.

6 Johnson R, Lambie D, Spalding J. *Neurocardiology*. London; W.B. Saunders, 1984: 174–6.

7 Faulkner M, Sharper-Schaefer E. Circulatory effects of trumpet playing. *BMJ* 1959;**1**:685–6.

8 Lewis P, Frank L. Hair grooming syncope seizures. *Pediatrics* 1993;**91**(4):836–7.

9 Leestma J, Koenig K. Sudden death and phenothiazines. *Arch Gen Psychiatry* 1988;**18**:137–48.

10 Hackel D, Reimer K. Role of recreational and therapeutic drugs in occurrence of sudden death. *Cardiovasc Rev Rep* 1994;**7**:321.

11 Ettinger P, Wu CF, De La Cruz L, *et al*. Arrhythmias and the "holiday heart": alcohol-associated cardiac rhythm disorders. *Am Heart J* 1978;**95**:555–62.

12 Pavlovic S, Kocovic D, Djordjevic M, *et al*. The etiology of syncope in pacemaker patients. *Pacing Clin Electrophysiol* 1991;**14**(12):2086–91.

13 Hellerstein H, Friedman E. Sexual activity and the post coronary patient. *Arch Intern Med* 1970;**125**:987–99.

14 Dory Y, Shapira I, Fisman EZ, Pines A. Myocardial ischemia during sexual activity in patients with coronary artery disease. *Am J Cardiol* 1995;**75**:835–7.

15 Marwick TH. Safe sex for men with coronary artery disease: exercise, sildenafil and risk of coronary events. *JAMA* 2002;**287**:766–7.

16 Nauman A, Daum I. Narcolepsy: pathophysiology and neuropsychological changes. *Behav Neurol* 2003;**14**:89–98.

17 Guilleminault C. Investigations into the neurologic basis of narcolepsy. *Neurology* 1998;**50**(Suppl.1):S8–15.

18 Aldrich MS. Diagnostic aspects of narcolepsy. *Neurology* 1998;**50**(Suppl. 1):S2–7.

19 Siegel JM. Narcolepsy. *Sci Am* 2000;**282**:76–81.

20 US Modafinil in Narcolepsy Study Group. Randomized trial of modafinil for the treatment of pathologic hypersomnolence in narcolepsy. *Ann Neurol* 1998;**43**:88–97.

21 Roberts LJ II. Recurrent syncope due to systemic mastocytosis. *Hypertension* 1984;**6**:285–94.

22 Karnam U, Rodgers A. Systemic mastocytosis. *Dig Dis* 1999;**17**:299–307.

23 Worobec AS. Treatment of systemic mast cell disorders. *Hematol Oncol Clin North Am* 2000;**14**:659–87.

24 Fisher CM. A new vascular syndrome, "the subclavian steal". *N Engl J Med* 1961;**265**:912–3.

25 Taylor CL, Selman WR, Ratcheson RA. Steal affecting the central nervous system. *Neurosurg* 2002;**50**:679–89.

26 Gosselin C, Walker PM. Subclavian steal syndrome: existence, clinical features, diagnosis, and management. *Semin Vasc Surg* 1996;**9**:93–7.

27 Bravo EL, Gifford RW Jr. Pheochromocytoma. *Endocrinol Metab Clin North Am* 1993;**22**:329–41.

28 Bravo EL, Gifford RW Jr. Current concepts: pheocyromocytoma: diagnosis, localization and management. *N Engl J Med* 1984;**311**(20):1298–303.

29 Sheps SG, Jiang NS, Kice GG. Recent developments in the diagnosis and treatment of pheochromotytoma. *Mayo Clin Proc* 1990;**61**(1):88–95.

30 Robertson D, Hollister AS, Biaggioni I, *et al.* The diagnosis and treatment of baroreflex failure. *N Eng J Med* 1993;**329**:1449–55.

31 Ketch T, Biaggioni I, Robertson RM, Robertson D. Four faces of baroreflex failure. *Circulation* 2002;**105**:2158–523.

32 Racco F, Sconocchini C, Reginelli R. La sincope in una popolazone generale: diagnosi ezilogoca e follow-up. *Minerva Med* 1993;**84**:249–61.

33 Wayne H. Clinical differentiation between hypoxia and hyperventilation. *J Aviation Med* 1958;**29**:307–15.

34 Robertson D, Taylor R. Metabolic and endocrine causes of syncope. In: Kenny R, ed. *Syncope in the Older Patient.* London, UK: Chapman and Hall Medical, 1995: 249–65.

35 Wincert TD, Mulrow PJ. Chronic adrenal insufficiency. In: Carr RB, ed. *Current Diagnosis.* Philadelphia, PA: Saunders, 1985: 860–3.

36 Loriaux DL, Cutler GB. Diseases of the adrenal glands. In: Kohler PO, ed. *Clinical Endocrinology.* New York, NY: John Wiley & Sons, 1986: 208–15.

CHAPTER 16

Syncope in the child and adolescent

Blair P. Grubb, MD, *& Richard Friedman,* MD

Introduction

Syncope is a relatively common complaint among both children and adolescents. The term is derived from the Greek *synkoptein*, meaning "to cut short" or "cessation" as it refers to a transient loss of consciousness and postural tone with spontaneous recovery without neurologic sequelae. Both a sign and a syndrome, syncope can result from a variety of different causes, some of which may ultimately culminate in death. The incidence of syncope has been variously reported to account for 1 of every 2,000 pediatric emergency room visits to 47% of surveyed college students [1,2]. Driscoll *et al.* [3] reported that syncope was the chief complaint in 125 of 100,000 (or 0.125%) pediatric medical visits. Syncope was reported to be more frequent in girls than in boys, with the highest frequency between the ages of 15 and 19 years. The frequency of the problem is compounded by the fact that syncope produces a tremendous amount of anxiety among patients, parents, coaches, teachers, and physicians [4]. Indeed, the social repercussions of syncope may have a more dramatic impact on a child than the syncope itself. As children differ from adults, so too do the causes of syncope. In this chapter some of the common causes of syncope in children and adolescents are discussed. When these causes are covered in detail elsewhere, a brief summary is given and the differences between pediatric and adult patients is emphasized.

Classification and approach

The causes of syncope in children and adolescents can be classified in a variety of different ways. One simple, yet useful way of organizing the various potential etiologies is found in Table 16.1, which divides these into cardiac, autonomic, and non-cardiac. While in the child or adolescent the majority of syncopal episodes are a result of benign causes such as neurocardiogenic (reflex) syncope, the aim of any evaluation is the careful determination of those, albeit uncommon, patients with potentially serious or life-threatening conditions for which syncope may be the principal symptom.

As with the adult patient, the history and physical examination is key. When available, descriptions of the episode by bystanders are particularly helpful, as the child may have difficulty remembering and may be frightened by the questioning process. It is important to find out if there is any history of unexplained sudden death among family members, and to learn the circumstances surrounding these deaths. One should endeavor to determine the frequency of episodes, the conditions under which the episodes occurred, whether there was a prodrome, the duration of loss of consciousness, and whether injury resulted from the fall. Was there tonic–clonic activity? Incontinence? A postictal state?

As in adults, one of the principal determinations to be made in children and adolescents is whether the heart is structurally normal. Aspects of the history may provide a clue to the potential for cardiac etiologies. For example, occurrence of syncope in the supine position suggests a cardiac source. In addition, the absence of any prodrome prior to loss of consciousness is more common in cardiac syncope.

Cardiovascular syncope

Cardiovascular syncope occurs as a consequence of conditions that result in either an obstruction to

Table 16.1 Causes of syncope in children and adolescents.

Cardiac syncope

Obstructive lesions
Hypertrophic cardiomyopathy
Aortic valve stenosis
Primary pulmonary hypertension
Eisenmenger's syndrome

Myocardial dysfunction
Primary
   Neuromuscular disorders
   Dilated cardiomyopathy
Secondary
   Ischemic
      Anomalous coronary arteries
      Kawasaki's disease

Dysrhythmias
Normal heart
   Supraventricular tachycardia
   Long QT syndrome
   Brugada syndrome
   Arrhythmogenic right ventricular dysplasia
Repaired or palliated structural disease
   Sick sinus syndrome
   Atrial flutter/fibrillation
   AV block
   Ventricular tachycardia

Autonomic syncope

Neurocardiogenic syncope

Dysautonomic syncope
Primary
Familial dysautonomia

Non-cardiac syncope

Breath-holding spells
Cyanotic
Pallid

Seizures

Psychogenic

Child abuse/Munchausen's by proxy

Drug related

Migraine/cerebral syncope

Metabolic

Situational

blood flow, dysfunction of myocardial function, or disturbances in heart rhythm.

The obstructive causes may be further divided into two groups: those occurring because of a structural cardiac lesion leading to either a fixed or dynamic obstruction, and those occurring because of disturbances in the pulmonary vasculature.

Obstructive lesions
Hypertrophic cardiomyopathy

Hypertrophic cardiomyopathy (HCM) can produce a combination of both a dynamic as well as fixed obstruction to the outflow of blood from the heart, and represents the single most common cause of sudden death in otherwise healthy young people. While it appears that a significant number of cases may be caused by spontaneous genetic mutations, it has also been recognized that an autosomal dominant pattern of inheritance exists that involves at least four distinct gene foci [5]. The incidence of HCM has been reported to range from 1 in 1000 to 1 in 500 of the general population (or approximately up to 0.2% of the population) [6]. Usually, the disorder develops during adolescence with progressive myocardial hypertrophy during periods of rapid growth and development (although it may be seen in childhood or, on rare occasions, before birth). HCM is characterized by hypertrophy and hyperplasia of several cell types, which include cardiac myocytes, smooth muscle cells, fibroblasts as well as excessive collagen deposition within the extracellular space; thus, the normal parallel arrangement of myocytes is disrupted [7]. The excessive hypertrophy may produce a dynamic left ventricular outflow tract obstruction, diastolic abnormalities, and myocardial ischemia. In keeping with the genetic basis of the disorder, HCM is seen more commonly in clinical disorders such as Friedreich's ataxia, LEOPARD syndrome and Noonan's syndrome. Typical symptoms include dyspnea, lightheadedness, chest discomfort, fatigue, exercise intolerance, palpitations, near-syncope, syncope, and sudden death.

While syncope is reported to occur in approximately 15–20% of adult patients with HCM, it appears less frequently in pediatric patients. However, when syncope is present in pediatric HCM patients it indicates a more dire prognosis [8]. The syncope itself often occurs because of either fixed or dynamic obstruction to left ventricular outflow, and is often provoked by exertion [6]. Dynamic obstruction of left ventricular outflow is reported to occur in one-third of HCM patients [7]. The hyperdynamic left ventricle and narrowed outflow tract increase the systolic blood velocity. The high velocity flow displaces the mitral valve leaflet anteriorly toward the interventricular septum with resultant outflow obstruction and mitral regurgitation. However, syncope may also occur because of atrial fibrillation that occurs in the face of severe diastolic dysfunction as well as short periods of ventricular tachycardia [9]. In obstructive HCM, neural reflex mechanisms involving mechanoreceptor-mediated bradycardia and dilation may also be a factor.

In children with HCM, an important risk factor for death is the age at which symptoms begin, with infants having the worst prognosis. Maron *et al.* [10] reported that nine out of 11 symptomatic infants had died by the age of 1 year.

Pediatric patients may have somewhat different presentations than their older counterparts. Infants frequently present with prominent cyanosis and heart failure [4]. Infants and young children often have significant right ventricular outflow obstruction as well as subaortic obstruction. The subpulmonic obstruction is usually fixed and may have gradient equal to (or exceeding) the subaortic obstruction [10].

Therapy is directed at two problems: severe symptoms and sudden death (in HCM the two may not always be well correlated). First-line treatment is usually pharmacologic with negative inotropes such as beta-blockers, calcium-channel blockers, and disopyramide (however, calcium-channel blockers must be used with extreme caution in children less than 1 year of age) [11]. Surgical myotomy and myomectomy (Morrow procedure) may relieve symptoms, with an operative mortality of between 1 and 2%; however, long-term mortality rates do not appear to be altered by the procedure [12]. Dual-chamber pacing may lessen the degree of outflow tract gradient. Implantable cardioverter defibrillators (ICDs) are an increasingly popular and effective form of therapy, especially in patients with recurrent syncope, suspected or documented arrhythmias, or a family history of sudden death [13]. Patients with recurrent atrial fibrillation require anticoagulation either with coumarin or patients with severe refractory heart failure may ultimately require heart transplantation [9].

Aortic valvular stenosis

Another example of an obstructive (in this instance, fixed) lesion is aortic valvular stenosis. Congenital aortic stenosis accounts for approximately 5% of cardiac malformations diagnosed in childhood [14]. Bicuspid aortic valves may be present in up to 1–2% of the population [15]. The more severe (and, with respect to pediatric patients, the more important) form of the disorder presents as a unicommissural or severely dysplastic valve. These may first manifest with signs of heart failure in a newborn [4.] Nearly one-quarter of these patients will have other cardiac abnormalities (such as the coarctation of the aorta seen with Turner's syndrome) [16]. The malformed aortic valves usually thicken over time, which can result in an increasing obstructive gradient. As opposed to their adult counterparts, children rarely exhibit valvular calcification [17]. Many children with severe aortic stenosis will be asymptomatic and display a normal growth and development pattern, and are often discovered by detection of a murmur during physical examination. As the disorder progresses, children with critical aortic stenosis may first present with exertional syncope, resulting as a consequence of reduction of cardiac output and its resultant decrease in cerebral blood flow [15]. Indeed, those individuals who develop exertional symptoms (such as syncope) may be at the highest risk of sudden death. Death is felt to occur following a sudden rise in intraventricular pressure that provokes a reflex-mediated period of hypotension with resultant diffuse myocardial ischemia and ventricular fibrillation [18].

Primary pulmonary hypertension

Primary pulmonary hypertension may result in syncope because of a reduction in cardiac output despite a structurally normal heart. While most frequently a disease of young adults, it may present in adolescence. Primary pulmonary hypertension is said to be present when there is no other explanation for the increase in pulmonary arterial pressure, which exceeds 25 mmHg at rest and 30 mmHg on exercise [19]. On the Indian Subcontinent, children have a particularly aggressive and devastating form of the illness; however, the reason for this is unclear [20]. While most cases are sporadic in nature in children, there is a tendency for the disease to be familial, where it is inherited in an autosomal dominant manner with incomplete penetrance [21].

Over half of children with primary pulmonary hypertension will experience syncope, not only because of the obstruction of pulmonary flow, but also because of an increased incidence of both supraventricular and ventricular dysrhythmias [20]. The pulmonary arterial pressure, vascular resistance, and cardiac index of children presenting with primary pulmonary hypertension tend to be higher than those of adults [19].

Therapy is directed at reducing pulmonary artery pressure, treatment of right heart failure (if present), vasodilators, and anticoagulation. Currently employed vasodilators include calcium-channel blockers and prostacyclin, a vasodilatory prostaglandin.

Other causes

Eisenmenger's syndrome is the development of pulmonary hypertension in association with a cardiac shunt. Initially the shunt is left-to-right, which decreases and then becomes right-to-left as the pulmonary vascular resistance increases over time. The rate at which the pulmonary hypertension develops is largely dependent on the type of cardiac shunt present, (ventricular septal defect, atrial septal defect, or patent ductus arteriosus) [22]. As many as 50% of patients with Eisenmenger's syndrome may experience syncope (as well as chest pain, dyspnea, and hemoptysis) [23]. Patients with right ventricular outflow tract obstruction may experience what is referred to as a hypercyanotic spell. These spells may be seen in association with tetralogy of Fallot, transposition of the great arteries with left ventricular outflow tract obstruction (either subpulmonary or pulmonary stenosis), and tricuspid atresia. Severe hypercyanotic episodes are also referred to as "tetralogy spells" [22]. The spell often begins with crying and then progresses to rapid deep breathing. Crying results in the prolonged forced expiration of air, leading to an increase in intrathoracic pressure, which in turn leads

to a further reduction in pulmonary blood flow and right-to-left shunting. The resultant decrease in oxygen saturation and pH of blood produces more cyanosis and leads to a compensatory increase in respirations and/or crying, causing the cycle to repeat itself. When the hypoxia is severe enough, loss of consciousness may ensue. The episode may be ended in a variety of fashions, the most frequent of which occurs by calming the child and bringing their knees to their chest. Older, unoperated patients may actually squat, with a resultant increase in systemic vascular resistance, thus an increase in pulmonary blood flow.

Syncope occurs either from these hypercyanotic spells or from a significant abrupt increase in pulmonary vascular resistance which causes a rapid reduction in cardiac output and precipitates acute right ventricular failure [22]. It is felt that the cessation of blood flow that occurs from the sudden increase in pulmonary resistance leads to both syncope and sudden death in Eisenmenger's syndrome [23].

Myocardial dysfunction

While rarely a direct cause of syncope, myocardial dysfunction in children may be seen in conjunction with a number of different conditions, often related to a specific ischemic or inflammatory event or as part of a generalized myopathy [4]. Several neuromuscular diseases such as Emery–Dreifuss and Becker and Duchenne muscular dystrophies can be accompanied by myocardial dysfunction as well as arrhythmias (such as AV block). Myocardial inflammation is seen in the setting of viral myocarditis with the subsequent development of a dilated cardiomyopathy. Unrecognized myocarditis is also a leading cause of unexpected sudden death in young patients.

A somewhat uncommon, but nevertheless important, cause of syncope in children may be myocardial ischemia and infarction. The most frequent cause in pediatric patients is anomalous origin of the coronary arteries, most often when the left coronary artery arises from the pulmonary artery. Alternatively, the left coronary artery may take an anomalous course between the trunks of the aorta and pulmonary arteries, leaving it vulnerable to compression during exercise. Myocardial infarction may also be seen as a sequela of coronary artery narrowing or aneurysm thrombosis resulting from Kawasaki's disease.

Arrhythmias: normal heart

Disturbances of the heart rhythm that are severe enough to result in syncope are relatively rare in the patient with a structurally normal heart. These disturbances are essentially similar to those problems seen in older patients which are discussed in more detail elsewhere in this text.

As with their adult counterparts, children rarely experience syncope caused by supraventricular tachycardia. The two most common forms of supraventricular tachycardia in children, AV re-entry via an accessory AV connection and AV nodal re-entry, are essentially the same in children as in adults, and the interested reader is directed to the chapter of this text that deal with supraventricular tachycardia (see Chapter 5).

Syncope associated with exercise or emotion in a patient with a structurally normal heart should raise suspicion of the long QT syndrome [24]. The syncope that occurs in the long QT syndrome is brought about by the hemodynamic compromise caused by a polymorphic "torsade de pointes" ventricular tachycardia. Episodes of sudden loss of consciousness have been associated with fright or being awakened by a loud noise. Most patients first exhibit symptoms sometime in the first two decades of life, and there may be several tragic sudden deaths among members of the same family. This disorder may be misdiagnosed as seizures. Mortality in the syndrome can be high (approximately 71%) in untreated patients [25]. Mortality rates fall to 7% if patients are treated with beta-blocking agents (with implantable defibrillators or ganglionectomy reserved for refractory cases) [26,27]. Recently, a short QT syndrome has also been described [28].

A similar condition exists in Brugada syndrome, a hereditary disease characterized by an electrocardiogram (ECG) pattern consisting of right bundle branch block pattern as a result of ST segment elevation in leads V_1–V_3 [29]. As in long QT syndrome, patients may experience syncope resulting from potentially lethal episodes of a polymorphic ventricular tachycardia. Some patients with Brugada syndrome may have a normal resting ECG and will only demonstrate the typical QRS-ST segment changes following administration of a type I antiarrhythmic agent (e.g., procainamide) [30]. Antiarrhythmic agents have not been shown to be useful in preventing recurrences in these patients; therefore, symptomatic patients or those with a strong family history of sudden death may be treated with an ICD placement [31]. Unfortunately, risk stratification in this group is not well defined.

Arrhythmogenic right ventricular dysplasia (ARVD) can result in ventricular tachycardia and syncope [32]. The disorder seems more common in parts of Europe than in North America. ARVD should be suspected in any patient with exercise-induced ventricular tachycardia with a left bundle branch pattern [33]. The ventricular tachycardia occurs secondary to a patchy right ventricular cardiomyopathy (although the left ventricle may also be involved) [34]. Usually, structural changes do not become manifest until the third to fourth decade of life, although in some cases changes can be seen earlier.

Dysrhythmias: repaired or palliated structural disease

In the pediatric population, congenital heart disease is the single most common cause of arrhythmias that lead to syncope. More often than not, these patients have undergone a prior correction or palliation of a congenital cardiac defect, with the arrhythmia presenting at a later time. The type and anatomic location of the arrhythmia are usually related to the site of the surgical intervention.

For example, some atrial repairs will produce sick sinus syndrome, which, if severe enough, may lead to syncope or even death. Although there are a number of definitions of what constitutes sick sinus syndrome, the most common is that of sinus bradycardia or arrest either with or without supraventricular tachycardia [35]. Interestingly, there is evidence to suggest that the tachycardias are the more important cause of syncope, as patients continue to experience syncope after pacemaker implantation. The actual syncopal episode is of sudden onset and usually of a brief duration. Treatment for these problems often involves antiarrhythmic therapy combined with permanent pacemaker implantation, or radiofrequency catheter ablation.

In a similar manner, those patients who have undergone atrial surgery are more prone to intra-atrial re-entry tachycardia (IART) or, less commonly, atrial fibrillation. These disorders seem particularly common in those patients who have undergone atrial baffling repairs such as the Senning and Mustard operations, which were the standard repairs for transposition of the great arteries for over 20 years [36]. These patients often have an atrial tachycardia with a rapid ventricular response combined with sinus node dysfunction, which may produce hemodynamic compromise and syncope [35]. These problems may also be seen in atrial septal defect repairs, mitral valve annuloplasties or replacements, tricuspid valve annuloplasty for Ebstein's anomaly, and AV canal repairs and single ventricle surgery (Fontan procedure). Syncope in these patients must be taken seriously, as it can foretell impending sudden death [37].

AV block in the pediatric population can either be congenital or acquired (usually following cardiac surgery) [38]. Congenital complete AV block (often associated with maternal lupus) in the presence of a normal heart may not require pacing. One study found that syncope in this group was associated with a heart rate during exercise of < 50 b min^{-1} [39]. Pacing should be recommended in patients with congenital AV block with rates lower than 50 b min^{-1} who have experienced syncope or heart failure. In addition, the development of mitral valve regurgitation portends a poor prognosis. Thus, significant left ventricular dilation should be addressed with pacing early in adolescence. A Stokes–Adams (or drop) attack may be the first symptom in otherwise unrecognized "asymptomatic" patients. L-transposition of the great vessels (or "anatomically corrected" transposition) has a more superiorly and superficially placed AV node and is associated with an increased risk for the development of AV block [36]. Acquired heart block may be seen in pediatric patients in association with systemic infections such as diphtheria, endocarditis, Lyme disease, Rocky Mountain spotted fever, acute rheumatic fever, and viral myocarditis.

Ventricular tachycardia and ventricular fibrillation are seen in children with either damaged ventricles or in those whose repairs produce large amounts of ventricular scarring [40]. A classic example of the latter is seen following repair of tetra-logy of Fallot [37]. The ventricular arrhythmias can originate from the right ventricular outflow tract as well as from the ventricular septum proximate to the ventricular septal patch. Patients with significant residual obstruction or poor ventricular function and severe pulmonary insufficiency with high ventricular end diastolic pressures appear to be at increased risk, as are those who undergo the repair later in life [41]. Arrhythmias usually appear years after surgery.

Autonomic syncope

Over the last few years, a large body of research has demonstrated that transient alterations in the autonomic nervous system's control of heart rate and blood pressure may lead to hypotension and loss of consciousness. This type of syncope is quite common in pediatric patients, particularly in adolescents. Rather than a single entity, this type of syncope represents a group of different disorders, each of which occurs because of a disturbance in autonomic control. Although it is dealt with in more detail in other chapters, a brief description of each of these entities with regard to the pediatric population is provided.

Neurocardiogenic syncope (see Chapter 3)
Also referred to as the "common faint" or vasovagal syncope, this disturbance in neuroregulatory control of vascular tone is by far the most common cause of syncope in otherwise healthy children and adolescents [42–47]. The episodes themselves are characterized by a sudden fall in blood pressure that is associated with lightheadedness, dizziness, and loss of consciousness, frequently accompanied by signs of autonomic nervous system hyperactivity such as diaphoresis, nausea, pallor, hyperventilation, and tachycardia followed by bradycardia. The pathophysiologic aspects of this disorder are dealt with in detail elsewhere in this text; however, a brief description is appropriate. Current thought holds that a sudden increase in peripheral vascular pooling results in a sudden reduction in venous return to the heart, allowing for overvigorous ventricular contractions [7]. These hyperdynamic beats activate myocardial C-fibers (which usually only respond to stretching of the myocardial wall during periods of increased blood pressure), sending a sudden surge

in neural traffic to the brainstem, thus activating a reflex that "signals" that the patient is hypertensive. The brainstem then responds with an apparent "paradoxic" lowering of blood pressure by sympathetic withdrawal, leading to vasodilation and bradycardia. Thus, these patients demonstrate a sudden profound drop in blood pressure followed by a fall in heart rate. As opposed to adults, we have found that children often panic at the onset of prodromal signs, and begin to hyperventilate because of anxiety, an act that may further reduce cerebral perfusion by producing systemic hypocapnia.

The clinical presentation may take a variety of forms in the pediatric patient. Classically, these episodes are often provoked by environmental stimuli such as anxiety, blood drawing (or just the sight of a needle), pain, or even the sight of blood [48]. However, it is just as common to hear that the patient had been engaged in normal activities (such as playing, shopping, or walking outside), when he or she suddenly turned pale, appeared sweaty, and then lost consciousness [46]. Interestingly, in 33% of children with tilt-confirmed neurocardiogenic syncope, there is a family history of syncope. In adolescents there is often a history of a period of rapid growth that precedes the onset of symptoms. In young women there is a trend for episodes to be more frequent at the time just preceding menses. We have also noted an increased frequency of episodes among adolescents who lose a large amount of weight quickly during crash dieting.

Tilt table testing can be used to confirm the diagnosis (see Chapters 2 and 7) [42–47]. It should be kept in mind that classic tilt table testing, which produces an orthostatic stress on the autonomic nervous system's ability to maintain blood pressure, may not be an adequate stress for smaller children, given their shorter stature and smaller body surface area. A more prolonged upright time or other increase in orthostatic stress (such as the use of isoproterenol as a provocative agent) may be necessary [49]. Often a good history from both parent and child with typical descriptors of the event in the absence of demonstrable heart disease is sufficient to make the diagnosis.

Heart rate variability studies using power spectral analysis have shown abnormal responses to orthostatic stress in children with recurrent syncope [50]. Interestingly, these abnormal findings

occurred while the mean heart rate and blood pressure were still normal and the patient was asymptomatic. These findings preceded the eventual syncopal event by 5 min or more.

Therapeutic options for pediatric and adolescent patients are discussed in detail elsewhere in this text (see Chapter 2), and tend to be somewhat different from those for adults. Treatment of this condition with fludrocortisone has been an option for a number of years. Adult patients, however, have had problems with side-effects, most notably hypertension. This may be much less of a problem for pediatric or adolescent patients. We have used fludrocortisone as our first treatment option, and in over 10 years we have had only two episodes of hypertension that required discontinuation of the medication. In one of those two patients, after continued treatment failures with other medical regimens, the medication was restarted at the family's request, and with reinstitution there was no recurrence of hypertension. If serotonin reuptake inhibitors are employed in the treatment of young people with neurocardiogenic syncope, it is probably best to use fluoxetine, as it has been the best studied of these agents in this age group. As opposed to their adult counterparts, methylphenidate and its analogs are sometimes easier to use when a vasoconstrictor is desired (especially in a patient intolerant of, unresponsive to, or non-compliant with midodrine), mainly because these agents come in sustained released preparations with regimens designed for pediatric use. However, we often try midodrine first, mainly because it is not a controlled substance and to avoid the misconception that the patient has attention deficit disorder.

Permanent pacing has been used as a treatment for this condition, especially in those children with prolonged asystole associated with a positive tilt table test. Although the most effective and appropriate treatment is unclear, it has been our experience that almost all of our pediatric-aged patients have opted for treatment medically without the need for permanent pacing. We have had several patients who have had asystole for 20–30 s during testing and were treated medically (with various agents) without pacing. These patients are now asymptomatic and are off all therapy up to 5 years later.

We generally treat children and adolescents

medically until they have been without symptoms for 12 months. Based on our experience over the last 15 years, we have found that the majority require only 12–24 months of therapy, while a small number need therapy for up to several years. Similarly, a significant majority of patients, as they mature, have no or few further episodes, although a minority (usually those most severely affected) continue to have symptoms but at differing frequencies.

Dysautonomic syncope (see Chapter 4)

Upon assumption of an upright posture, there is usually a gravity-mediated downward displacement of up to 500 cc of blood to the more dependent areas of the body. This is compensated for by a reflex-mediated increase in both heart rate and force of contraction and peripheral vasoconstriction. In dysautonomic syncope, one or more of the compensatory mechanisms for orthostatic stress fails, with a resultant fall in blood pressure and cerebral perfusion which leads to syncope. In contrast to classic neurocardiogenic syncope, there is less of a prodrome and an absence of bradycardia or diaphoresis. Often there are other signs and symptoms of autonomic failure present. While these disorders are often felt to occur in adults, we have observed the condition in adolescents and occasionally in young children [51]. Symptoms usually begin in early adolescence, often following a period of rapid growth and development. Some researchers have reported that there is an increase in parasympathetic tone over sympathetic tone during this period of time, resulting in a tendency toward vasodilation and hypotension in predisposed individuals [48]. Patients not only complain of lightheadedness upon standing, but may also experience a sense of severe, unremitting fatigue as well as exercise intolerance and cognitive impairment. Some of these patients may initially be diagnosed as having chronic fatigue syndrome [52]. Patients often exhibit a > 20 mmHg fall in systolic pressure upon standing and/or a 10 mmHg fall in diastolic pressure. Because blood pressures while standing are often quite low, averaging 70–80 mmHg systolic, these patients may experience frequent syncopal and near-syncopal episodes. Many of these adolescents display acral cyanosis caused by excessive pooling of blood in the lower extremities.

Recently, several groups of investigators have noted an association between dysautonomic hypotension and the joint hypermobility syndrome (also referred to as type III Ehlers–Danlos syndrome) [53,54]. This is a genetically heterogeneous type of connective tissue disorder, the severity of which varies considerably with mild or incomplete forms of the disease. The condition results from a defect in the major structural protein of the body (collagen). Collagen is a tough, fibrous type of protein that serves to hold together, strengthen, and provide elasticity to the cells and tissues of the body [55]. Because of a defect in collagen, these individuals manifest abnormally flexible loose joints (articular hypermobility), which are prone to frequent dislocations and/or subluxations; soft velvety and fragile skin that bruises easily, as well as a fragile and abnormally lax vasculature. When either sitting or standing, these patients' excessively compliant vasculature permits an increased distensibility of the dependent veins in response to ordinary degrees of orthostatic stress, thus leading to excessive peripheral pooling of blood with subsequent orthostatic intolerance, progressive hypotension, and ultimately syncope. Many of these patients are quite hypotensive all the time, with blood pressures barely sufficient to maintain cerebral perfusion. Others may demonstrate normal resting pressures, but during head-up tilt table testing display a progressive steady decline in pressure, which may or may not be accompanied by a compensatory tachycardia. When fully expressed the condition may be quite disabling as, in addition to hypotensive symptoms, patients may also experience varying degrees of joint pain and bowel problems (most often hypomotility syndromes).

Many of the young people with these disorders are at their worst in mid-adolescence and improve as they enter young adulthood. The reason for this is unclear but may represent a return of the adolescent increase in parasympathetic tone to more normal levels. Unfortunately, a small group of patients exhibit symptoms for the remainder of their lives. Treatment of young patients with dysautonomic syndromes can be challenging; however, they seem to respond best to a combination of volume expanding and vasoconstrictive agents.

Another important but much less common form of pediatric dysautonomia is the condition referred to as familial dysautonomia or Riley–Day syndrome [56]. The disorder is inherited in an autosomal recessive pattern, most notably in children of Ashkenazic Jewish ancestry. In this population the carrier rate has been estimated to be 1 in 30, with a disease frequency of 1 in 3600 live births. It is currently thought that familial dysautonomia (FD) is one of a group of rare disorders referred to as hereditary and sensory autonomic neuropathies (HSAN), of which FD patients are listed as HSAN type III. These disorders are caused by a failure of migration and maturation of neural-crest-derived cells, in particular those that evolve into sensory and autonomic nerves. In FD, the gene has been mapped to the distal long arm of chromosome 9 (q31). While penetrance is felt to be complete, the clinical expression of the disorder varies greatly even among siblings, which suggests that modifying genes are also present. The features of FD are often noted in infancy and often include failure to thrive, poor suck and swallow ability, alacrima (loss of tears), thermoregulatory disturbances, breath-holding spells, sleep apnea, and seizures. Syncope and near-syncope resulting from postural (dysautonomic) hypotension increase in frequency as the child grows older and can be a significant limiting factor in late adolescence and young adulthood. Approximately 63% of children with FD exhibit breath-holding spells sometime during the first 5 years of life. Some FD patients may experience a "dysautonomic crisis" associated with hypertension, tachycardia, excessive sweating, erythematous skin blotching, irritability, and nausea. With good medical care, current statistics indicate that a child born with FD has a 50% probability of reaching 30 years of age.

Non-cardiac syncope

Breath-holding spells

Breath-holding spells can be a frightening experience for parents, who often bring their children for evaluation. These can be divided into two forms: cyanotic and pallid [57,58].

The cyanotic form is the more common [59]. The typical episode occurs after the child becomes upset or startled. The clinical presentation begins with a loud cry followed by a forced expiration then apnea (noiseless expiration). The child quickly becomes pale or cyanotic and loses consciousness, and there may be associated generalized myoclonic jerks and rigidity (opisthotonos) followed by limpness. The entire event is usually brief, lasting less than 1 min. The episode usually ends with the child taking gasping breaths, followed by a sudden deep inspiration resulting in the return of normal color and consciousness. In severe episodes, the child may be somewhat drowsy for a few moments prior to recovery. The onset of these events is uncommon prior to 6 months of age, peak at around 2 years, and usually disappear by age 5 years [60].

Pallid breath-holding spells (also referred to as "reflex anoxic seizures") are similar in nature, but nevertheless unique. Usually, these spells are brought on by injury or pain, such as falling, head trauma, or being suddenly startled. Here the child suddenly stops breathing without crying and quickly loses consciousness. The child becomes pallid and hypotonic, often followed by rhythmic muscular contractions [61]. Bradycardia or asystole may be seen on monitor during a pallid breath-holding spell. The age of onset is between 12 and 24 months [58]. Spells can occur as frequently as several times a day or as rarely as once a year. Approximately 20–30% of these children have a family history of similar spells [62]. In addition, between 10 and 20% of these children experience neurocardiogenic syncope later in life, suggesting that pallid breath-holding spells may be a form of reflex syncope [59].

Neither cyanotic nor pallid breath-holding spells require any specific therapy other than reassuring parents that the episodes are not dangerous. By the age of 4 years, half of cases have spontaneously resolved, and by age 7 or 8 virtually all have resolved. There are rare patients with pallid breath holding with severe symptoms associated with prolonged asystole who have undergone permanent pacemaker implantation.

Seizures

Although seizures are not syncope *per se*, they nevertheless represent an important part of the differential diagnosis. Most seizures can be fairly easily distinguished from syncope; however, in some cases it may be less clear. Neonatal seizures and complex partial seizures present a particular challenge [63]. In the latter, the patient may faint, stop moving and stare, followed by a series of inappropriate actions. Indeed, in some cases it may be difficult to tell if the patient actually lost consciousness; rather, all that can be determined is that there was some type of episode during which consciousness appeared to be lost [64]. In general, seizures are usually associated with tonic–clonic movements, incontinence, and prolonged loss of consciousness [65]. This is followed by a postictal period of confusion and lethargy. Stephenson has written that epileptic tonic–clonic seizures differ from syncope in the following ways:

1 They are not usually provoked by the stimuli that provoke syncope.

2 The convulsion is usually long – often 1 min or more.

3 The convulsion is always rhythmic – fast generalized twitching that slows down [66].

Other indications of seizures rather than syncope are supine rather than upright posture, convulsive activity that precedes rather than follows the loss of consciousness, and a flushed, warm, or cyanotic skin color rather than a pale and diaphoretic appearance. However, in some patients the myoclonic jerks and clonic extensions of the body can be difficult to distinguish from epilepsy, a phenomenon often referred to as convulsive syncope. Lempert et al. [67] induced syncopal events in 59 healthy subjects and found that as many as 71% exhibited movements suggestive of seizures. They felt that this occurred because of transient global hypoxia resulting in cortical suppression with subsequent disinhibition of subcortical and limbic areas.

In a similar fashion, some seizures may mimic syncope [65]. An akinetic seizure (also called atonic seizure) is manifested by a sudden fall to the ground. The episode may be so dramatic that onlookers describe the patient as "having been thrown to the ground," an event that may be accompanied by head or facial trauma. This type of seizure occurs most often between the ages of 2 and 8 years, and rarely in adolescence. The differentiation is made with the electroencephalogram, which is abnormal, demonstrating generalized or multifocal epileptiform discharges. These seizures are often quite challenging to treat, with the highest success rates seen with valproic acid or clonazepam. Some patients have responded to use of the medium-chain triglyceride (MCT) variant of the ketogenic diet.

Other non-cardiac causes

One of the most important causes of syncope in pediatric patients (especially in adolescents) is psychogenic (or hysteric) syncope (see Chapter 9). Psychogenic causes of syncope are often distinguished by the extreme frequency of the episodes (sometimes two to three per day) and the fact that episodes are usually not associated with injury [68]. In those individuals, the loss of consciousness may be quite prolonged (occasionally as long as an hour), during which time heart rate and blood pressure are normal, and assumption of a recumbent position does not terminate the event. These patients may seem to display a remarkable indifference to their syncope. During tilt table testing these patients may suddenly faint without observable changes in heart rate, blood pressure, transcranial Doppler blood flow, or electroencephalographic recording [69]. After detailed psychiatric evaluations, many of these individuals are found to have conversion reactions, most frequently resulting from sexual abuse. It is important to realize that patients who experience conversion reactions are not consciously aware of their actions [70]. Indeed, these events may be the only way an abused child or adolescent is able to "cry for help."

We have also seen parents who claim that their child has experienced multiple syncopal episodes and, in order to hide evidence of physical abuse, claim that the child injured him or herself during the falls associated with these events. A close history will often reveal inconsistencies, and a physical examination will reveal wounds of such a nature and location that they are unlikely to have occurred during a fall. Any such suspicions must be reported to the proper authorities. In addition, we have seen cases of Munchausen's by proxy, where a parent will secretly administer a diuretic or vasodilator to a child so as to produce hypotension syncope. One such case was uncovered only after a toxicology screen was obtained in the emergency department after the mother brought the child following a syncopal event. Only later was it discovered that the mother was deeply emotionally disturbed.

Another group of patients who seem to display a high degree of indifference (as well as open hostility to the physician) is the group of patients whose syncope may result from illicit drug use. Unfortunately, substance abuse is occurring in increasingly younger age groups. Toxicology screens often provide important clues to the diagnosis, as patients rarely volunteer this information (particularly when their parents are present). The presence of needle marks ("tracks") may be revealing, as may evidence of nasal septal damage.

Occasionally, patients may have hyperventilation syndrome. Often associated with panic attacks, hyperventilation syndrome is manifested by rapid and frequently deep breathing, tightness in the chest, palpitations, and a feeling of dyspnea [71]. If it is sufficient to produce hypocapnia, hyperventilation is associated with circumoral hand numbness and tingling. Episodes may last up to half an hour, and the patient is able to reproduce his or her symptoms by hyperventilation. However, it should be kept in mind that some children may begin to hyperventilate as a result of the anxiety provoked during an episode of neurocardiogenic syncope. We have found that biofeedback training may be helpful for hyperventilation.

Migraine headaches have long been associated with the development of syncope, either directly or as an atypical presentation (cerebral syncope) [72]. A typical attack begins with premonitory aura followed by loss of consciousness. Upon awakening the patient experiences a severe headache that is biooccipital and throbbing in nature. Syncope may also be seen in the absence of headache. For example, basilar artery migraines account for up to 24% of childhood migraines (often in adolescent girls) [73]. Inflammation and intense vasoconstriction of the vertebrobasilar arteries may produce visual disturbances (especially in the temporal and nasal fields), vertigo, confusion, dysarthria, and ultimately syncope. Many of these patients also have Raynaud's phenomenon, suggesting that a general state of vasomotor dysregulation may be present. In addition, there are some patients who seem to develop syncope diffuse cerebral vasoconstriction alone, a condition referred to as cerebral syncope [74]. While most reports of this disorder have been in adults, Rodriguez-Nunez *et al.* [75] have reported that it may occur in children.

Metabolic abnormalities can occasionally cause syncope in children. Hypoglycemia can accompany several disorders in children, such as diabetes mellitus, ketotic hypoglycemia, as well as several hepatic enzyme deficiency syndromes. In these instances, the child or parent reports that the loss of consciousness is gradual in nature and often associated with weakness, diaphoresis, hunger, and confusion. Loss of consciousness may be prolonged and may require administration of glucose for termination. There are some metabolic syndromes (e.g., hyperammonemia) that can produce loss of consciousness because of direct cytotoxic actions on the central nervous system.

There are several forms of situational syncope that are of importance in pediatrics. One is cough syncope, which in children occurs most frequently in the setting of obstructive lung disease, especially cystic fibrosis. Coughing produces high intrathoracic pressures resulting in a marked Valsalva response. Stretch syncope can be seen (mainly in adolescent boys) and occurs during stretching with the neck hyperextended when standing. It has been attributed to the effects of an exaggerated Valsalva maneuver in combination with a reduction in cerebral blood flow resulting from mechanical compression of the craniocervical arteries. Therapy consists of avoidance of neck hyperextension. The disorder usually subsides in adulthood.

Evaluation

As with adult patients, a complete history is of paramount importance. However, unlike their older counterparts, a young child may not be capable of providing a detailed or totally accurate history. Frequently, the physician must depend on parents, teachers, or other adults to provide important information as to the nature of the event. Many of the diagnoses discussed can be uncovered via the history. The family history is important and should include questions about syncope, sudden death, sudden infant death syndrome (SIDS), apparent life-threatening episodes (ALTEs), congenital heart disease, deafness, and seizures.

The examination of the pediatric syncope patient is essentially similar to that of the adult patient, save that in younger children the usual order may be modified to reassure an overly anxious or frightened child. Heart rate, blood pressure, and respiratory rate should be noted. Blood pressures should be obtained in the supine, sitting, and standing positions. In addition, blood pressures should be taken in the standing position after 2, 5, and 10 min

Table 16.2 Conditions that warrant more detailed evaluation of syncope.

---

1 Syncope that occurs during peak exertion
2 Seizure/convulsive activity
3 Recurrent syncope (more than two to three times)
4 Chest pain that precedes syncope
5 Syncope resulting in significant injury
6 Abnormal cardiac examination
7 Repaired or palliated structural disease
8 Abnormal cardiovascular examination
9 Family history of sudden death

---

upright. During the physical examination, special attention should be paid to the cardiovascular and neurologic examination. Close attention should be paid for features such as murmur, clicks, gallops, or rhythm disturbances, as well as for focal neurologic signs that may indicate a possible diagnosis.

An electrocardiogram should be included as a standard in the evaluation of syncope in all children, in particular those with exercise-induced syncope. Particular care is given to the possible prolongation of the corrected QT interval, the presence of delta waves, bundle branch block pattern, and evidence of left ventricular hypertrophy or complete AV block. Qualities of syncope in children and adolescents that may merit more extensive evaluation are listed in Table 16.2. If there is any question as to whether the heart is normal an echocardiogram should be performed. If there is any concern about the origin or course of the coronary arteries and routine transthoracic echocardiography is suboptimal in visualization, consideration for a cardiac magnetic resonance imaging scan should be given. The exact course and sequence of evaluation and testing should be determined by the information obtained from the history, physical examination, and ECG. The details of other testing modalities are discussed in other chapters.

Summary

Recurrent syncope in the pediatric patient can be an important symptom of a variety of disorders that range from a simple faint to potentially lethal ventricular arrhythmias. Episodes must be taken seriously, with the history and physical examination serving as the basis for subsequent laboratory investigations. Syncope in patients with congenital heart disease should be cause for particular concern.

References

1 Pratt JL, Fleisher GR. Syncope in children and adolescents. *Pediatr Emerg Care* 1989;**5**:80.
2 Murdoch BB. Loss of consciousness in healthy South African men. *S Afr Med J* 1980;**57**:771.
3 Driscoll DJ, Jacobsen SJ, Porter CJ. Syncope in children and adolescents: a population-based study of incidence and outcome. *Circulation* 1996;**94**:1–54.
4 Janel R, Walsh EP. Syncope in the pediatric patient. *Cardiol Clin* 1997:**15**:277–94.
5 Solomon SD, Jarcho JA, McKenna WJ, *et al.* Familial hypertrophic cardiomyopathy is a genetically heterogenous disease. *J Clin Invest* 1990;**86**:993–6.
6 Nishimura RA, Holmes DR. Hypertrophic obstructive cardiomyopathy. *N Engl J Med* 2004;**350**:1320–7.
7 Maron BJ. Hypertrophic cardiomyopathy: a systematic review. *JAMA* 2002;**287**:1308–20.
8 McKenna WJ, Deanfield JE. Hypertrophic cardiomyopathy: an important cause of sudden death. *Arch Dis Child* 1984;**59**:971–4.
9 Braunwald E, Seidman CE, Sigwart U. Contemporary evaluation and management of hypertrophic cardiomyopathy. *Circulation* 2002;**106**:1312–6.
10 Maron BJ, Tajik AJ, Ruttenberg HD, *et al.* Hypertrophic cardiomyopathy in infants: clinical features and natural history. *Circulation* 1982;**65**:7–12.
11 Spirto P, Seidman CE, McKenna WJ, Maron BJ. The management of hypertrophic cardiomyopathy. *N Engl J Med* 1997;**336**:775–85.
12 Schulta HD, Brisov K, Gams E, Gramsch-Zabel H, Losse B, Schwartzkoff B. Management of hypertrophic obstructive cardiomyopathy: long-term results after surgical therapy. *Thorac Cardiovasc Surg* 1999;**47**:213–8.
13 Maron BJ, Shen WK, Link MS, *et al.* Efficacy of implantable cardioverter-defibrillator for the prevention of sudden death in patients with hypertrophic cardiomyopathy. *N Engl J Med* 2000;**342**:365–73.
14 Moller JH, Nakib A, Elliott RS, Edwards JE. Symptomatic congenital aortic stenosis in the first year of life. *J Pediatr* 1966;**69**:728–34.
15 Braunwald E, Goldblatt A, Aygen MM, *et al.* Congenital aortic stenosis: clinical and hemodynamic findings in 100 patients. *Circulation* 1963;**27**:426–31.
16 Tawes RJ Jr, Berry CL, Aberdeen E. Congenital bicuspid aortic valve associated with coarctation of the aorta in children. *Br Heart J* 1969;**31**:127–30.

17 Beppu S, Suzuki S, Matsuda H, *et al.* Rapidity of progression of aortic stenosis in patients with congenital bicuspid aortic valves. *Am J Cardiol* 1993;**71**:322–5.

18 Johnson AM. Aortic stenosis, sudden death, and the left ventricular baroreceptors. *Br Heart J* 1971;**33**:1–6.

19 Haworth SG. Primary pulmonary hypertension in childhood. *Arch Dis Child* 1998;**79**:452–5.

20 Barst RJ. Primary pulmonary hypertension in children. In: Rubin LJ, Rich S, eds. *Primary Pulmonary Hypertension.* New York, NY: Marcel Dekker, 1987: 179–225.

21 Langleben D. Familial primary pulmonary hypertension. *Chest* 1994;**105**:135–65.

22 Brammell, HL, Vogel JHK, Pryor R, *et al.* The Eisenmenger syndrome: a clinical and physiological reappraisal. *Am J Cardiol* 1971;**28**:679–92.

23 Young D, Mark H. Fate of the patient with Eisenmenger syndrome. *Am J Cardiol* 1971;**28**:658–61.

24 Schwartz PJ, Moss AJ. Prolonged QT interval: what does it mean? *J Cardiovasc Med* 1982;**7**:1317.

25 Priori SG, Schwartz PJ, Napolitano C, *et al.* Risk stratification in the long QT syndrome. *N Engl J Med* 2003;**348**:19.

26 Vincent GM. The long QT syndrome: bedside to bench to bedside. *N Engl J Med* 2003;**348**:19.

27 Moss AJ, Zereba W, Hall WJ, *et al.* Effectiveness and limitations of beta-blocker therapy in congenital long QT syndrome. *Circulation* 2000;**101**:616–23.

28 Gaita F, Giustetto C, Bianchi F, *et al.* Short QT syndrome: a familial cause of sudden death. *Circulation* 2003; **108**:965–70.

29 Brugada P, Brugada J. Right bundle branch block, persistent ST segment elevation and sudden cardiac death: a distinct clinical and electrocardiographic syndrome – a multicenter report. *J Am Coll Cardiol* 1992;**20**:1392–6.

30 Brugada J, Brugada R, Brugada P. Right bundle branch block and ST segment elevation in leads V_1 through V_3: a marker for sudden death in patients without demonstrable structural heart disease. *Circulation* 1998;**97**:457–60.

31 Brugada J, Brugada R, Brugada P. Determinates of sudden cardiac death in individuals with the electrocardiographic pattern of Brugada syndrome and no previous cardiac arrest. *Circulation* 2003;**108**:3092–6.

32 Thiene G, Nava A, Corrado D, *et al.* Right ventricular cardiomyopathy and sudden death in young people. *N Engl J Med* 1988;**318**:129–33.

33 Molinari G, Sardinelli F, Garta F, *et al.* Right ventricular dysplasia as a generalized cardiomyopathy: findings on magnetic resonance imaging. *Eur Heart J* 1995;**16**:1619.

34 Fontaine G, Fontaliran F, Rosas-Andrada F, *et al.* The arrhythmogenic right ventricle: dysplasia vs. cardiomyopathy. *Heart Vessels* 1995;**10**:227–35.

35 Porter CJ, Battiste CE, Humes RA, *et al.* Risk factors for supraventricular tachycardia after Fenton procedure for tricuspid atresia. *Am Heart J* 1986;**112**:645–9.

36 Tressler GR, Castaneda AR, Rosenthal A, *et al.* Current results of management in transposition of the great arteries, with special emphasis on patients with associated ventricular septal defect. *J Am Coll Cardiol* 1987;**10**:1061–71.

37 Vaksmann G, Fournier A, Davignon A, *et al.* Frequency and prognosis of arrhythmias after operative "correction" of tetralogy of Fallot. *Am J Cardiol* 1990;**66**:346–9.

38 Michaels M, Engle MA. Congenital complete heart block: an international study of the natural history. *Cardiovasc Clin* 1972;**4**:85–7.

39 Ross RA, Trippel DL. Atrioventricular block. In: Garson A, Bricker JT, Fisher DJ, Neish SR, eds. *The Science and Practice of Pediatric Cardiology.* Baltimore, MD: Williams and Wilkins, 1995.

40 Rocchini AP, Chun PO, Dick M. Ventricular tachycardia in children. *Am J Cardiol* 1981;**47**:1091–7.

41 Garson A, Randall DC, Gillette PC, *et al.* Prevention of sudden death after repair of tetralogy of Fallot: treatment of ventricular arrhythmias. *J Am Coll Cardiol* 1985;**6**:221–7.

42 Ross BA, Hughes A, Anderson E, *et al.* Orthostatic versus electrophysiologic testing in unexplained syncope in children and adolescents. *J Cardiovasc Electrophysiol* 1992;**3**:418–22.

43 Samoil D, Grubb BP, Kip K, Kosinski D. Head upright tilt table testing in children with unexplained syncope. *Pediatrics* 1993;**92**:426–30.

44 Thilenius OG, Quinones JA, Husayni TS, Novak J. Tilt table test for diagnosis of unexplained syncope in pediatric patients. *Pediatrics* 1991;**87**:334–8.

45 Hannon D, Ross BA. Head up tilt testing in children who faint. *J Pediatr* 1991;**118**:731–2.

46 Lerman-Sagie T, Recharia E, Strausborg B. Head up tilt for the evaluation of syncope of unknown origin in children. *J Pediatr* 1991;**118**:676–9.

47 Grubb BP, Temesy-Armos P, Moore J, *et al.* The use of head up tilt table testing in the evaluation and management of syncope in children and adolescents. *Pacing Clin Electrophysiol* 1992;**15**:742–8.

48 Kosinski D, Grubb BP. Pathophysiologic aspects of neurocardiogenic syncope. *Pacing Clin Electrophysiol* 1995;**18**:716–21.

49 Thilanius OG, Ryd KJ, Husanyi J. Variations in the expression and treatment of transient neurocardiogenic syncope. *Am J Cardiol* 1992;**69**:1193–5.

50 Ross BA, Aknan AA, Schneider DS, *et al.* Abnormal heart rate variability responses to head upright tilt table testing in children and adolescents with recurrent unexplained syncope. *Circulation* 1993;**88**(Suppl):4841–51.

51 McLeod KA. Dysautonomia and neurocardiogenic syncope. *Curr Opin Cardiol* 2001;**16**:92–6.

52 Stewart JM, Gewitz MH, Weldon A, *et al.* Orthostatic intolerance in adolescent chronic fatigue syndrome. *Pediatrics* 1999;**103**:116–21.

53 Rowe PL, Barron DF, Calkins H, *et al.* Orthostatic intolerance and chronic fatigue syndrome associated with Ehlers–Danlos syndrome. *J Pediatr* 1999;**135**:494–9.

54 Gazit Y, Nahir M, Grahame R, Jacob G. Dysautonomia in the joint hypermobility syndrome. *Am J Med* 2003; **115**:33–40.

55 Grahame R. Joint hypermobility and genetic collagen disorders: are they related? *Arch Dis Child* 1999;**80**:188–91.

56 Axelrod F. Familial dysautonomia. In: Mathias C, Bannister R, eds. *Autonomic Failure: A Textbook of Clinical Disorders of the Autonomic Nervous System.* Oxford, UK: Oxford University Press, 1999: 402–9.

57 Lombroso CJ, Lerman P. Breath-holding spells (cyanotic and pallid infantile syncope). *Pediatrics* 1967;**39**:563–5.

58 Stephenson JBP. Reflex anoxic seizures ("white breath holding"): non-epileptic vagal attacks. *Arch Dis Child* 1978;**53**:193–6.

59 Stephenson JBP. Anoxic seizures or syncopes. In: Stephenson JBP, ed. *Fits and Faints.* London, UK: MacKeith Press, 1990: 41–58.

60 Breningstall G. Breath-holding spells. *Pediatr Neurol* 1996;**14**:91–4.

61 Livingston S. Breath-holding spells in children: differentiation from epileptic attacks. *JAMA* 1970;**212**:2231–5.

62 DiMario F, Chee C, Berman P. Pallid breath-holding spells: evaluation of the autonomic nervous system. *Clin Pediatr* 1990;**29**:17–22.

63 Stephenson JBP. Epileptic seizures and epileptic syndromes. In: Stephenson JBP, ed. *Fits and Faints.* London, UK: MacKeith Press, 1990: 37–40.

64 van Dijk G. Conditions that mimic syncope. In: Benditt D, Blanc JJ, Brignole M, Sutton R, eds. *The Evaluation*

and Treatment of Syncope. Elmsford, NY: Blackwell-Futura, 2003: 186.

65 Wiederholt WG. Seizure disorders. In: Wiederholt WG, ed. *Neurology for Non-neurologists.* Philadelphia, PA: W.B. Saunders, 1995: 211–31.

66 Stephenson JBP. Non-epileptic seizures, anoxic–epileptic seizures and epileptic–anoxic seizures. In: Wallace SJ, ed. *Epilepsy in Children.* London UK: Chapman and Hall, 1996: 5–26.

67 Lempert T, Bauer M, Schmidt D. The clinical phenomenology of induced syncope. *Neurology* 1991;**41**:127–9.

68 Linzer M, Varia I, Pontinem M, *et al.* Medically unexplained syncope: relationship to psychiatric illness. *Am J Med* 1992;**92**:185–245.

69 Grubb BP, Gerard G, Wolfe D, *et al.* Syncope and seizures of psychogenic origin: identification with upright tilt table testing. *Clin Cardiol* 1992;**15**:839–42.

70 Shihabuddin L, Shehadeh A, Agla D. Syncope as a conversion mechanism. *Psychosomatics* 1994;**35**:496–8.

71 O'Laughlin MP. Syncope. In: Gillette P, Garson A, eds. *Pediatric Arrhythmias: Electrophysiology and Pacing.* Philadelphia, PA: W.B. Saunders, 1990: 600–15.

72 Bickerstaff ER. Impairment of consciousness in migraine. *Lancet* 1961;**2**:1057.

73 Hockaday JM, Barlow CF. Headache in children. In: Olson J, Tfelt-Hansen P, Welsch KMA, eds. *The Headache.* New York, NY: Raven Press, 1993: 795.

74 Grubb BP, Samoil D, Kosinski D, *et al.* Cerebral syncope, loss of consciousness associated with cerebral vasoconstriction in the absence of systemic hypotension. *Pacing Clin Electrophysiol* 1997;**20**:1667–72.

75 Rodriguez-Nunez A, Fernandez-Cebrian S, Perez-Munuzuri A, *et al.* Cerebral syncope in children. *J Pediatr* 2000;**136**:348–53.

CHAPTER 17

Syncope in the athlete

Olaf Hedrich, MD, Mark S. Link, MD, Munther K. Homoud, MD, & N.A. Mark Estes III, MD

Introduction

Syncope in athletes presents a unique challenge to the physician. Causes of syncope in these individuals vary from benign neurocardiogenic episodes to life-threatening conditions such as ventricular tachycardia [1]. Considerations in this population include, among others, discrimination of cardiac pathology from normal physiologic adaptation to physical training (the "athlete's heart"); identifying etiologies of syncope particular to a generally young, healthy patient population; implications of the syncopal event with regard to prognosis, recurrence, and possible sudden cardiac death; impact on the individual's subsequent athletic participation and livelihood in the current era of sport as a competitive and lucrative business; and legal implications of "clearance" for athletic activity after a syncopal episode.

Epidemiology

Syncope is extremely common in the general population, constituting a significant proportion of emergency department visits and hospital admissions [2]. In the Framingham study [3], 3% of men and 3.5% of women experienced one or more syncopal events during a 26-year period. The prevalence in the elderly (5.6%) was significantly greater than in the youngest subjects (0.7%). There is very little known about the prevalence and incidence of syncope specifically among athletes.

The need for evaluation

Through several high profile cases of sudden car-diac death (SCD) in professional athletes [4,5], public awareness of the potential for acute, catastrophic events has been heightened. Although these events are not common [6], they elicit a profound emotional responses from both the lay public and professional circles, largely because athletes are intuitively thought of as representing the healthiest segment of the population. While syncopal events occurring during or after athletic pursuits usually engender less intense interest, their importance should not be underemphasized. Furthermore, a real concern of athletes and their families is that an important diagnosis will be missed in the work-up of syncope. There is also the risk of misdiagnosing a benign cardiovascular condition as one that is more serious, thereby unnecessarily restricting athletic activity.

Syncope in the setting of exercise may be predictive of an impending adverse outcome, particularly SCD, especially in those with underlying heart disease. In a restrospective study of all sudden, non-traumatic deaths occurring over a period of 12 years in young Israeli soldiers (n = 44, age range 17–22 years), it was found that 23% had experienced at least one episode of syncope prior to death [7]. The syncopal event(s) occurred between 1 h and 4 years before death. In 16%, the syncopal episode had occurred during exercise. Maron *et al.* [8] reported an incidence of syncope or presyncope of 17% in a cohort of 29 young athletes who died suddenly.

Evaluation of syncope occurring in the athlete is therefore required for several reasons:

1 to diagnose underlying heart disease, either structural or electrophysiologic;

2 to determine safety of resumption of athletic activities;

3 to reassure the athlete in whom the syncopal event is likely to be benign;

4 to institute appropriate therapy when needed.

Exertional syncope in this group could be considered the equivalent of an episode of aborted SCD until an etiology is identified or a satisfactory explanation can be offered.

Definitions

Syncope refers to the transient loss of consciousness with spontaneous recovery. There is loss of postural tone, varying degrees of recall of events surrounding the syncopal spell, and absence of neurologic sequelae [9]. These episodes are typically brief, but may be prolonged. Occasionally, cardiopulmonary resuscitation (CPR) may be initiated. Spontaneous recovery of consciousness supports the diagnosis of syncope, because it is unlikely that CPR alone would abort lethal arrhythmias resulting in loss of consciousness, or reverse other, non-cardiac causes of syncope [10].

Aborted sudden death may initially appear to be a syncopal episode, but typically requires initiation of life-saving intervention such as CPR and defibrillation [1]. The differentiation of syncope from aborted sudden death is important, because the latter carries a poor prognosis and has important therapeutic and lifestyle implications.

To simply extend the definition of an *athlete* to anyone participating in sport is fraught with difficulty, because a wide range of people of varying fitness levels, ages, and engaging in different athletic activities can be considered athletes. A *competitive athlete* is defined as one who participates in a sport requiring systematic training and regular competition against others, either on an individual basis or in an organized team [11]. It has been noted that an important facet of this group of individuals is the low likelihood of termination of exercise in the face of warning symptoms, either because of the pressure of organized athletic competition, or because of an inability to distinguish these symptoms from the normal sensation of intense physical exertion [12]. *Recreational athletes* encompass a wide array of people of different fitness levels and may include people who, because of their profession, face physical challenges requiring exertion. The heterogeneity of these individuals

and their activities make it difficult to quantify their physical exertion accurately.

Type of exercise: it is helpful to make the differentiation between the two broad types of exercise any given athletic activity may require [13]. *Dynamic exercise* (e.g., cross-country skiing, soccer, squash, and distance running) causes an increase in cardiac output, heart rate, stroke volume, and systolic blood pressure, and a decrease in diastolic blood pressure, end systolic volume, and total peripheral resistance. *Static exercise* (e.g., weight lifting and field events involving throwing) causes a marked increase in systolic, diastolic, and mean arterial blood pressure, and only a small increase in oxygen consumption, cardiac output, and heart rate. Overall, dynamic exercise causes a volume load on the left ventricle, while static exercise causes a pressure load on the cardiovascular system [13]. Although most physical activity has both static and dynamic components, an appreciation of the differences in cardiovascular compensation that result is useful when interpreting results of non-invasive testing, particularly electrocardiography (ECG) and echocardiography.

The classification of sports into dynamic and static categories has limitations and is to a large degree theoretical, as most athletic activities have some component of each. Emotional involvement during the competition can markedly increase cardiovascular sympathetic stimulation, and environmental factors (such as temperature extremes and altitudinal stress) can add additional burden to the stressed cardiovascular system [13].

The "athlete's heart"

Many athletes engaged in competitive sports undergo cardiac structural changes in response to the chronic stresses placed on the cardiovascular system, which do not appear to have adverse consequences, and are associated with preservation of systolic and diastolic function. These may include physiologic myocardial hypertrophy, with increased volume of the ventricles and cavitary enlargement, and increased left ventricular wall thickness [14]. Isometric training associated with static exercise may result in relative or absolute increases in left ventricular wall thickness resulting from pressure loading, while dynamic exercise with its associated volume loading tends to result in more significant changes in cavity dimensions [14].

The concept of a "gray area" of overlap between the adaptive changes evident in the athlete's heart and pathologic cardiomyopathies (including myocarditis, hypertrophic cardiomyopathy, and arrhythmogenic right ventricular dysplasia) has been described by Maron *et al.* [15], highlighting the possibility that overdiagnosis of pathology may be a pitfall in the non-invasive evaluation of trained athletes experiencing syncope. On the other hand, it is conceivable that not all changes caused by exercise are necessarily benign, especially at the extremes of hypertrophy and chamber enlargement, and may have adverse implications over time. One longitudinal study of retired athletes demonstrated echocardiographic evidence of residual chamber dilation in 20% of the study population, even after prolonged deconditioning [16]. The significance of these residual abnormalities in relation to the risk of developing syncope and sudden death is not known.

ECG manifestations of athletic conditioning may resemble those found in cardiac disease. In one large cohort of athletes, the ECG was normal in only 60% of cases [17]. Forty percent of athletes in the cohort had ECG changes consistent with physiologic cardiac remodeling, and changes were more prevalent in the disciplines requiring dynamic exercise. This number included a small subgroup with more striking ECG changes that could indicate cardiac pathology, including increased voltage, repolarization abnormalities, and pathologic Q waves. Overall, it is felt that the increase in vagal tone associated with physical conditioning is primarily responsible for ECG manifestations in athletes which do not necessarily have major significance, including sinus bradycardia, junctional rhythm, first-degree or Möbitz type I AV block, and others [11,18].

Etiology of syncope in the athlete

Syncope has a wide range of etiologies, spanning the spectrum of conditions from the benign to the life-threatening (Table 17.1) [9,19,20]. In athletes, the etiologies of syncope are generally the same as in the wider population. Of note, however, is that retrospective analyses of cases of SCD in young

Table 17.1 Etiologies of syncope. (After [20].)

Vascular

Anatomical
Subclavian steal

Orthostatic
Drug-induced
Hypovolemia
Primary disorders of autonomic failure
    Pure autonomic failure (Bradbury–Eggleston syndrome)
    Multiple system atrophy (Shy–Drager syndrome)
    Parkinson's disease with autonomic failure
Secondary neurogenic
Postprandial (in the elderly)
Postural orthostatic tachycardia syndrome (POTS)

Reflex-mediated
Neurally mediated syncope/vasovagal syncope
Carotid sinus hypersensitivity
Situational (cough, defecation, micturition, swallow)
Glossopharyngeal syncope
Trigeminal neuralgia

Cardiac

Anatomical
Aortic dissection
Aortic stenosis
Atrial myxoma
Cardiac tamponade
Hypertrophic cardiomyopathy
Mitral stenosis
Myocardial ischemia/infarction
Pulmonary embolism
Pulmonary hypertension

Arrhythmias
Bradyarrhythmias
  AV block
  Pacemaker malfunction
  Sinus node dysfunction/bradycardia
Tachyarrhythmias
  Supraventricular tachycardia
  Ventricular tachycardia
  Torsade de pointes/long QT syndrome

Neurological/cerebrovascular
Arnold–Chiari malformation
Migraine
Seizures (partial complex, temporal lobe)
Transient ischemic attack/vertebrobasilar
   insufficiency/cerebrovascular accident

(continued)

Table 17.1 (cont'd)

Metabolic/miscellaneous

Metabolic
Hyperventilation (hypocapnea)
Hypoglycemia
Hypoxemia
Drugs/alcohol

Miscellaneous
Psychogenic syncope
  Hysterical
  Panic disorder
  Anxiety disorder
Cerebral syncope
Hemorrhage

Unknown

---

individuals and athletes have uncovered a significant number who experience at least one syncopal event prior to death [7,8]. Discussion of conditions causing syncope is therefore inherently linked with a consideration of the causes of SCD in this patient population. A large majority of studied individuals had organic heart disease, among which hypertrophic cardiomyopathy was the largest single contributor in those younger than 35 years [21–24]. Other organic cardiac diseases implicated in SCD in this population included anomalous coronary arteries (24%) [25], dilated cardiomyopathy, acute myocarditis, arrhythmogenic right ventricular dysplasia (ARVD), and Marfan's syndrome [20,23]. Of interest is that in an Italian series [26], ARVD was the most common structural heart disease found.

In those over 35 years, atherosclerotic coronary disease accounts for the majority of identifiable causes of sudden death in this population [21,22,27]. Electrophysiologic anomalies such as long QT syndrome or bypass tract pathology (e.g., Wolff–Parkinson–White syndrome) may be relatively under-recognized as causes of sudden death because of either lack of pathologic manifestations at autopsy or low clinical suspicion. Commotio cordis, sudden death, or transient arrhythmias caused by chest wall impact may be confused with or linked to a syncopal event [25].

In athletes without structural heart disease, neurally mediated hypotension is the most common

cardiac cause of syncope. Ventricular arrhythmias, supraventricular arrhythmias, bradyarrhythmias, and low cardiac output states are less common causes of syncope in the absence of structural heart disease. Table 17.2 relates the mechanisms of syncope to the type of underlying cardiac pathology.

Non-cardiac causes of syncope in athletes include neurocardiogenic syndromes, Valsalva maneuver (as may occur in weight-lifters), dehydration, hyperventilation, circulating mediators (histamine, serotonin), dietary supplements (Ma-huang [28], ephedra, androgens, creatine), seizures, hypoglycemia, and psychogenic causes (conversion disorder).

Evaluation of syncope in the athlete

Evaluation of the syncopal athlete is a potentially complex endeavor. While many diagnostic modalities are available, the cost, practicality, and risk of each must be carefully weighed against their potential benefit and diagnostic yield. Not all athletes experiencing a syncopal event will require complex diagnostic work-ups to arrive at a diagnosis; similarly, not all causes of syncope will be uncovered simply by the indiscriminate application of complicated diagnostic procedures. There is no "gold" standard against which other diagnostic tests may be measured. A schema for evaluating and managing the athlete with syncope is suggested in Fig. 17.1, with details presented below.

History

Central to the diagnosis of the cause of syncope in the athlete is the *history* [29,30]. A thorough personal and family history must be obtained, with meticulous attention to the details surrounding the syncopal spell. Of additional use are any observations made by witnesses of the episode, but such information is not always available. A carefully obtained history may also be valuable in excluding seizures as an alternative diagnosis to syncope. Several useful historical points that may be elicited to differentiate arrhythmic from non-arrhythmic syncope are summarized in Table 17.3.

Factors favoring a benign diagnosis (such as dehydration or neurally mediated syncope) include occurrence only after cessation of activity (vaso-

Table 17.2 Mechanisms of syncope and underlying structural heart disease. (After [1].)

Mechanisms	Associated cardiovascular conditions
Neurally mediated syncope	Generally no structural heart disease
Ventricular arrhythmias	Hypertrophic cardiomyopathy
	Arrhythmogenic right ventricular dysplasia
	Long QT syndrome
	Dilated cardiomyopathy
	Myocarditis
	Valvular heart disease
	Congenital malformations
	Drug abuse
	No structural heart disease
Supraventricular arrhythmias (including atrial flutter and fibrillation)	Wolff–Parkinson–White syndrome
	Hypertrophic cardiomyopathy
	Aortic stenosis
	Pulmonary hypertension
	Congenital malformations
	No structural heart disease
Bradycardia	Physiologic response to training
	Congenital complete heart block
	Congenital malformations
	Conduction system disease
Reduced cardiac output	Aortic stenosis
	Hypertrophic cardiomyopathy
	Left atrial myxoma
	Pulmonary hypertension
	Severe volume and salt depletion

dilation and hypotension); occurrence only with upright posture; occurrence in the setting of a clear "trigger" such as extreme excitement or fear; presence of premonitory symptoms; and frequent recurrence of syncope without injury [31]. Avoidance of the trigger or modification of the exercise may be all that is required, without much further evaluation.

However, in athletes in whom symptoms occur that are consistent with a ventricular arrhythmia, full evaluation should be pursued, primarily because of the increased subsequent risk of sudden death [31]. These clinical factors include syncope of sudden onset, occurring without premonition; exertional syncope; injury; and knowledge of underlying structural heart disease.

Athletes with a family history of unexplained or sudden death, especially at a young age, or familial congenital heart disease, should be extensively evaluated regardless of their presenting symptoms, because several of the described organic causes of sudden death (including hypertrophic cardiomyopathy, long QT syndrome, coronary artery disease, the Brugada syndrome, and some types of arrhythmogenic right ventricular dysplasia and idiopathic cardiomyopathy) may have genetic predispositions [32].

As in all cases of syncope, the possibility of drug and alcohol abuse should be considered, and a careful medication history should be obtained, including dietary supplements and performance enhancing drugs.

Physical examination

A thorough history should be complemented by a directed physical examination, which may uncover evidence for structural heart disease. Together, a well-performed history and physical examination can be diagnostic in 75–85% of cases [19]. These data may be broadly applicable but are derived

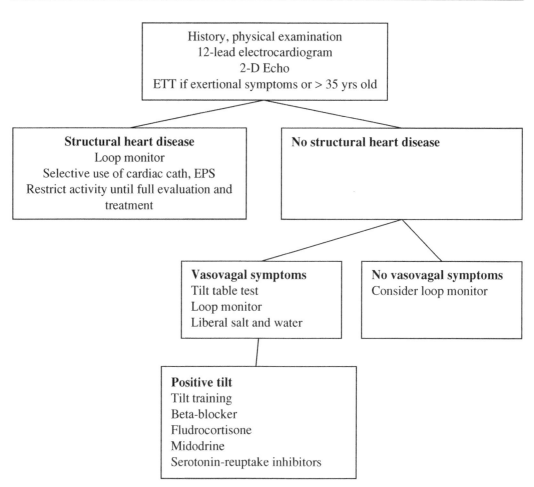

Fig. 17.1 An algorithm for the evaluation and treatment of the athlete with syncope. EPS, electrophysiologic studies; ETT, exercise treadmill test. (After [1].)

Table 17.3 Clinical characteristics helpful in differentiating arrhythmic from non-arrhythmic syncope. (After [31].)

	Neurocardiogenic or non-arrhythmic	*Arrhythmic*
Prodrome	Lightheadedness, warmth, nausea	None, or brief lightheadedness
Number of episodes	Multiple	Few or none
Situational factors	Fear, fright, upright posture	Exertional, unrelated to posture
Postsyncopal symptoms	Frequently fatigue	Usually none
Injury	Unusual	Common
Underlying heart disease	Unusual	Common

from series in non-athletes, and so may not be reproducible in this population.

Efforts should be made to uncover obstructive murmurs, using methods such as auscultating during the Valsalva maneuver, squatting, and sitting. Hypertrophic obstructive cardiomyopathy with left ventricular outflow obstruction, aortic stenosis and, rarely, atrial myxoma may occasionally be diagnosed clinically in this manner. Attention should also be paid to the presence of orthostatic hypotension, features of dehydration, and neurologic deficits.

Determining the presence or absence of structural heart disease

This is essential not only to further define the etiology of syncope, but also to stratify the patient in terms of subsequent risk of sudden death. In general, the presence of structural heart disease increases the risk of SCD, whereas its absence denotes a low risk. Specifically, it appears that young patients (under 35 years) are at highest risk of sudden death if they have hypertrophic cardiomyopathy, arrhythmogenic right ventricular dysplasia, or anomalous origin of the coronary arteries [33,34]. It would seem feasible therefore to concentrate initial efforts on uncovering these pathologic processes. Congenital heart diseases associated with ventricular arrhythmias also indicate a higher risk of sudden death in the athlete [35], although these occur with less frequency. Over the age of 35 years, coronary artery disease is the chief risk factor for sudden death in these patients [27], mandating an approach focused on eliciting ischemic pathology as part of the work-up.

In a recent series of 33 competitive athletes with recurrent, unexplained, exercise-induced syncope, without any identifiable structural heart disease, no adverse events were noted during long-term follow-up (33.5 ± 17.2 months) [36]. In the absence of structural heart disease, concern for increased risk for sudden death should be raised in only a few circumstances:

1 patients with a history of resuscitated/aborted sudden death;
2 patients with a history of syncope and a family history of sudden death; and
3 those with syncope occurring at peak exercise [37].

Fortunately, ECG and echocardiography are readily available modalities, and should form the basis of investigation of syncope in all athletes.

Electrocardiography

ECG may be useful in the initial work-up of syncope, recognizing that ECG changes mimicking disease states may occur in athletes [38]. These include resting bradycardia and other resting bradyarrhythmias (disappearing with exercise); resting AV block (again, disappearing with exercise); high chest lead voltage; intraventricular conduction defects; and repolarization abnormalities, includ-ing ST segment deviation and T-wave inversion. Nevertheless, thorough evaluation of the 12-lead ECG may show evidence of pre-excitation, long QT syndrome, ventricular hypertrophy, and right ventricular dysplasia [10,39]. Table 17.4 highlights ECG abnormalities found in various disease states.

In patients with frequent or reproducible symptoms, long-term Holter ECG monitoring may be helpful, whereas intermittent symptoms may be best evaluated with the aid of a continuous loop monitor [10].

Echocardiography

Echocardiography can uncover physiologic changes that may mimic myocardial hypertrophy. Wall thickness ≥ 13 mm is only rarely seen in athletes (1.7%), with a preponderance in rowers [40]. Maximal wall thickness ≥ 16 mm has not been de-scribed in athletes, and should raise concern about hypertrophic cardiomyopathy [40]. Wall thickness between 12 and 15 mm falls into the "gray" zone as some rare athletes may have physiologic hypertrophy in this range. Diastolic function can be used as a surrogate for differentiating physiologic changes from hypertrophic cardiomyopathy; impaired diastolic function is present in this condition, whereas the "athlete's heart" consistently retains normal diastolic function [40,41]. A period of deconditioning (usually 3 months), during which regression of physiologic hypertrophy should occur, may be useful in separating physiologic hypertrophy from pathology [9].

In addition to hypertrophy, a complete echocardiographic evaluation for syncope in the young athlete should involve assessment for dilated cardiomyopathy, myocarditis, right ventricular dysplasia, congenital anomalies, and valvular disorders. Visualization of the coronary ostia can assist in defining those with anomalous origin of the coronary arteries. As the sensitivity of stress testing is not high in individuals with anomalous origin of the coronary arteries, transesophageal echocardiography should be considered to visualize the coronary ostia and bifurcation of the left main coronary artery in athletes in whom this diagnosis is considered as a cause for their syncope [42,43].

Exercise testing

Exercise testing should be considered if the events

Heart disease diagnosis	Electrocardiographic abnormalities
Arrhythmogenic right ventricular dysplasia	T-wave inversions anteriorly Epsilon wave RBBB (complete or incomplete) Rarely normal
Hypertrophic cardiomyopathy	Left ventricular hypertrophy Pseudoinfarct with q waves anteriorly Rarely normal
Idiopathic dilated cardiomyopathy	LBBB Prolonged QT Can be normal
Long QT syndrome	Prolonged QT Abnormal appearance of ST segment
Brugada syndrome	RBBB (complete or incomplete) ST elevation anteriorly Changes can vary with time
Anomalous coronary artery	Typically no abnormalities
Coronary artery disease	Typically no abnormalities Q waves ST segment abnormalities
Wolff–Parkinson–White	Short PR interval Delta waves Pseudoinfarct patterns

Table 17.4 Electrocardiographic abnormalities found in various disease states. (After [31].)

LBBB, left bundle branch block; RBBB, right bundle branch block.

are exercise induced or if there is suspicion of ischemic heart disease. It is reasonable to begin at a high level of exercise, such as Bruce stage 4, to stimulate the abrupt exertional demands of athletics [11]. Rarely, an exercise test will elicit exercise-induced syncope, but should probably be performed in athletes over age 30 years, in whom the incidence of coronary disease rises significantly, or in those in whom there is clear clinical suspicion based on history or non-invasive testing [1]. In a series of athletes who had exercise-related sudden deaths, those dying from severe atherosclerosis (26%) had a mean age of 32 years [44]. In the absence of occult coronary disease, exercise testing may still elicit exercise-induced tachyarrhythmias, as well as exercise-induced neurally mediated syncope [45]. Asymptomatic athletes with anomalous coronary arteries should also undergo maximal stress testing but, because sudden death often occurs without preceding symptoms in this group,

a normal test does not necessarily confer low risk. Transesophageal echocardiography should be considered in such patients [42,43].

Tilt table testing

While tilt table testing may not specifically identify an underlying pathology, this modality may determine an exaggerated susceptibility to normal reflex events leading to syncope [46]. There is general agreement that tilt testing is indicated in athletes, given their "high-risk" status for injury, provided the cause is presumed to be vasovagal or neurocardiogenic in origin [47]. However, controversy remains regarding the sensitivity and specificity of tilt table testing, with particular unease surrounding its use in athletes. Estimates of the accuracy of tilt testing have ranged between 30 and 80% [46]. In persons with neurocardiogenic syncope, up to 80% may have an abnormal result [48]; a significant proportion of those tested may have a positive result without preceding history of syncope, suggesting that an abnormal response could be elicited from normal individuals. Additionally, the trade-off between sensitivity and specificity may be further altered by increasing the period in the upright position as well as by provocative agents (e.g., isoproterenol): the longer the duration of the test, the steeper the angle of incline, and the use of provocative agents all increase sensitivity at the expense of specificity.

Concern over the broader use of tilt testing in athletes with an undefined cause for their syncope has centered on the observation that orthostatic stress can cause a positive result in athletes with no clinical history of syncope [48]. By extrapolation, these "false positives" may conceal other, more serious causes of syncope if no further testing is performed, with potentially adverse consequences [49], prompting mixed recommendations. These range from advocating avoidance of tilt table testing in athletes [49], to warning that the diagnostic ability of tilt testing is limited [10], to endorsing the use of this modality if the diagnosis of neurocardiogenic syncope is likely [39,47]. Recent data suggest that the sensitivity and specificity of tilt table testing is similar in both the athletic and general populations [45], leaving the debate open for future input. For purposes of current practice, it seems a reasonable approach to employ tilt table testing within recent recognized guidelines [47], acknowledging that these may change in time. However, results of tilt table testing should not be solely relied upon to make a diagnosis.

Electrophysiologic testing

Selected athletes presenting with syncope should undergo electrophysiologic testing. Testing should be performed if there is concern about ventricular or supraventricular tachyarrhythmias [50]. In patients with bradycardias, electrophysiologic evaluation is of limited value because of the poor sensitivity and specificity of the test. In athletes, high vagal tone may influence the specificity.

Comprehensive electrophysiologic testing includes evaluation of the sinus node, AV node, and His–Purkinje system; assessment for AV bypass tracts and dual AV–nodal pathways; and attempts to induce atrial and ventricular arrhythmias [37]. As with tilt table testing, the goal of electrophysiologic testing is to provoke symptoms, under controlled conditions, to arrive at a diagnosis. However, caution must be applied in the interpretation of the results, as reproducing an arrhythmia using invasive means remains a surrogate for the spontaneous event [33].

Bradyarrhythmias

Normal athletes with high vagal tone at rest may have resting heart rates as low as 30 b min^{-1} during sleep [51]. Resting bradycardia is therefore usually of no concern and requires no elaborate work-up. The resting vagal tone does not affect heart rates during exercise, unless chronotropic incompetence occurs. In young athletes, although unusual, chronotropic incompetence may be caused by a genetic predisposition to sinus node dysfunction. In older athletes, especially over the age of 35 years, the inability to appropriately augment heart rate during exercise becomes more common. Sinus node dysfunction may occasionally necessitate permanent pacing in these individuals if symptoms such as significant exercise limitation, presyncope or syncope occur [52]. Electrophysiologic studies are neither specific nor sensitive for sinus bradyarrhythmias [50].

Möbitz type I heart block (Wenckebach) appears to be related to the high vagal tone in athletes, and is common at rest. As with sinus bradycardia, Wenckebach resolves with activity. If it occurs during exertion or is related to symptoms of fatigue, presyncope, or syncope, then a permanent pacemaker may be indicated [52]. Möbitz type II or complete heart block is usually treated with a permanent pacemaker [52]. In those athletes in whom the level of block cannot be determined, an electrophysiologic study may assist in determining the level and need for therapy: if the block is in the AV node and there are no symptoms, there is usually no role for pacing; if the level of the block is in the His–Purkinje system, the athlete is usually treated as a Möbitz II patient [37].

Supraventricular tachyarrhythmias

The treatment of supraventricular tachycardias (including atrial fibrillation and flutter, AV reentrant tachycardia, and AV nodal re-entrant tachycardia) has been revolutionized by the advent of radiofrequency ablation. It is against this background, the fact that rate-controlling agents such as beta-blockers are banned in many sports, as well as the relatively young age of this patient population (with resulting concern for intolerance or potential long-term toxicity of pharmaceutical agents) that radiofrequency ablation may present a viable first-line treatment option [37].

Patients with Wolff–Parkinson–White (WPW) syndrome who present with symptoms of palpitations, presyncope, or syncope may be at risk for sudden death on the basis of fatal ventricular tachyarrhythmias. Radiofrequency ablation offers cure rates in excess of 95% in AV re-entrant and AV nodal re-entrant tachycardias [53] and should be considered early, particularly if heart rates of ≥ 240 b min^{-1} (refractory period of 250 ms) are demonstrated [54]. Asymptomatic individuals with WPW syndrome are usually not restricted from athletic activities. However, whether they should undergo electrophysiologic testing is debatable. While athletic conditions these individuals experience may be extreme (especially in the competitive athlete), some recommendations fall in favor of not performing electrophysiologic evaluation, because the life-long risk of developing arrhythmia is felt to be low, as is the perceived risk of experiencing a fatal arrhythmia [55]. If an electrophysiologic study is performed, and the bypass tract is shown to be able to sustain a rapid arrhythmia (especially one that causes hemodynamic compromise), then an ablation should be performed [56]. Inducibility of AV tachycardia during invasive electrophysiologic study in patients younger than 35 years and refractory times of the bypass tract ≤ 250 ms with asymptomatic WPW identifies a subgroup of patients who are at risk for arrhythmic events. It has been determined in a prospective, randomized, controlled trial that prophylactic catheter ablation provides meaningful and durable benefits with respect to freedom from arrhythmic events at follow-up [57]. Antegrade refractory period and location of the bypass tracts were not characteristics found to be helpful for predicting future arrhythmias.

Ventricular arrhythmias

In the absence of structural heart disease, ventricular arrhythmias rarely lead to sudden death, with the exception of primary electrical diseases such as the long QT or Brugada syndromes. The presence

Table 17.5 Value of programmed stimulation in patients with spontaneous sustained ventricular tachycardia. (After [58].)

Condition	Sensitivity	Specificity
Normal heart	+	+++
HCM	+	+
CAD	++++	++++
Anomalous CAD	No utility	No utility
ARVD	+++	+++
LQTS	No utility	No utility
IDCM	+	+
Idiopathic LV VT	+++	+++
Idiopathic RV VT	+++	+++

+ Poor utility; + + fair utility; + + + good utility; + + + + excellent utility.
ARVD, arrhythmogenic right ventricular dysplasia; CAD, coronary artery disease; HCM, hypertrophic cardiomyopathy; IDCM, idiopathic cardiomyopathy; LQTS, long QT syndrome; LV, left ventricle; RV, right ventricle; VT, ventricular tachycardia.

of an underlying cardiac abnormality greatly increases the risk of SCD. Indeed, as demonstrated in a large series (n = 134) of athletes suffering sudden death, 97% had a defined underlying cardiac abnormality [24]. This is most commonly hypertrophic cardiomyopathy, followed by coronary artery anomalies, and less common causes such as aortic stenosis, dilated cardiomyopathy, myocarditis, arrhythmogenic right ventricular dysplasia, coronary artery disease, and congenital heart disease.

In the work-up of a spontaneous sustained ventricular tachycardia, the sensitivity and specificity of invasive electrophysiologic evaluation vary with the underlying etiology (Table 17.5). In coronary disease, invasive electrophysiologic testing has high sensitivity (90–95%) [59] and specificity (95% for the induction of monomorphic ventricular tachycardia) [59]. In patients with arrhythmogenic right ventricular dysplasia, sensitivity ranges from 70 to 80% [60,61]. Diagnosis, prognosis, and treatment of spontaneous sustained ventricular tachycardia may therefore be guided effectively with electrophysiologic testing in these two conditions. It is less clear whether induced, non-sustained, ventricular tachycardia and ventricular fibrillation are of significance [62].

The sensitivity and specificity of invasive electrophysiologic evaluation is low in other diseases causing sudden death in young athletes, including hypertrophic cardiomyopathy, idiopathic dilated cardiomyopathy, long QT syndrome, and congenital heart disease.

Whereas the yield from electrophysiologic testing in instances where there is neither underlying structural heart disease nor a primary conduction abnormality appears low, such testing may be indicated in those with recurrent syncope; family history of syncope or sudden death; professional athletes; those participating in vigorous competitive sports or sports with a high potential for injury; and contact sports [39].

Coronary angiography and myocardial biopsy

The lack of substantive data to assess utility of these more invasive modalities in the management of younger individuals with syncope hinders recommendations regarding their use in athletes. Atherosclerotic coronary artery disease is more prevalent in older athletes (> 35 years), in whom it is associated with sudden death. Other potentially dangerous "ischemic" causes of syncope (usually in younger individuals) include anomalies of the coronary arteries, hypoplastic coronary arteries, and "tunnel" coronary arteries (caused by myocardial bridging) [22]. In most cases, non-invasive screening with stress testing (with radionuclide agent) can assist in defining those individuals who may benefit from coronary angiography [39], which should be reserved for cases in which a high level of suspicion exists or in whom exclusion of this condition is essential [11].

Endomyocardial biopsy in this patient population serves primarily to diagnose suspected myocarditis or intrinsic myocardial disease, such as amyloid or sarcoid. These conditions are sufficiently rare to prohibit the use of biopsy as a routine diagnostic modality unless clinical suspicion is extremely high and other diagnostic tools have failed to arrive at a diagnosis [39].

Treatment of syncope in the athlete

Therapy of syncope is directed by the specific cause. A full discussion of therapy of all potential causes of syncope in the athlete is beyond the scope of this chapter, but several important points can be made. What follows is a synopsis of treatment strategies for several of the important causes of syncope discussed above. Treatment guidelines have also been promulgated to assist the physician in making recommendations regarding resumption of athletic activity, in the form of the Bethesda Conference guidelines [63 and in press]. The rationale for prohibition from competitive athletics includes the possibility of exacerbation of an arrhythmia with physical exertion, the concern over the integrity of the ICD or pacemaker and the lead system (especially where the potential for body contact exists), and the possibility that defibrillation may be ineffective in the presence of a heightened adrenergic state.

Neurally mediated causes of syncope

Initial management includes conservative measures such as maintaining adequate hydration and salt intake, and tilt training [64], in which patients "retrain" their heightened neurologic reflex by maintaining upright posture for varying periods of time. Concomitant medical disorders that may cause a dysautonomic response, and medications that may promote syncope should be identified. Pharmacologic options include fludrocortisone, midodrine, beta-blockers, and serotonin-reuptake inhibitors [46]. Pacing may occasionally be of benefit in cases of syncope with a marked chronotropic component [10].

Bradyarrhythmias

Resting sinus bradycardia is physiologic and does not require specific therapy. According to the Bethesda guidelines, first-degree or Möbitz I heart block does not require treatment or activity restrictions, provided there is no worsening with activity. Reassessment should occur periodically to determine that the bradycardia is not being aggravated by training. Möbitz II or complete heart block generally requires pacing. Precautions regarding pacemakers are detailed below.

Supraventricular arrhythmias

Beta-blockers and antiarrhythmic agents present a complex problem for the physician treating the athlete. The former are often banned in competition, and untoward side-effects can impair the athlete's quality of life. The latter cause concern regarding long-term side-effects in young patients, as well as proarrhythmia. Radiofrequency ablation presents a viable treatment option in these patients, particularly considering that the common causes for syncope in this category (AV nodal re-entrant tachycardia and WPW syndrome) are readily amenable to this treatment modality. Athletes who have experienced significant palpitations, presyncope, or syncope should not engage in any competitive sports until they have been adequately treated and have no recurrence for at least 3–6 months [63].

Ventricular arrhythmias

In the absence of structural heart disease (idiopathic left ventricular tachycardia or right ventricular outflow tract ventricular tachycardia), cure rates of up to 95% may be achieved by radiofrequency ablation [65,66]. These athletes may participate in competitive athletics after 6 months of non-recurrence [63]. In contrast, athletes with structurally abnormal hearts do not benefit from radiofrequency ablation in terms of sudden death prevention, and consequently the Bethesda guidelines permit only low-intensity sports, regardless of whether the arrhythmia has been suppressed [63]. Ventricular arrhythmias and even undiagnosed syncope in the presence of conditions such as hypertrophic cardiomyopathy, idiopathic dilated cardiomyopathy, arrhythmogenic right ventricular dysplasia, and congenital heart disease should raise concern for SCD, and in most cases an ICD may be required [67].

Structical heart disease

In athletes with no documentation or symptoms (presyncope or syncope) of ventricular arrhythmia, the presence of structural heart disease may preclude the athlete from being permitted to resume any activity except low-intensity sports. Such conditions include hypertrophic cardiomyopathy, idiopathic dilated cardiomyopathy, arrhythmogenic right ventricular dysplasia, and congenital heart disease.

Conclusions

The evaluation and appropriate treatment of syncope in the athlete often presents a considerable challenge, in which clinical judgment has a significant role. Although benign causes predominate, accurate diagnosis is important to allow for effective management. The aim is to protect individual athletes from recurrent syncopal events and potentially serious sequelae, including sudden death. Central to the issue is the differentiation of those athletes with structurally abnormal hearts from those with normal (or conditioned) anatomy. Non-invasive evaluation is often sufficient in making a diagnosis, and should be performed in all cases. Where structural abnormality is discovered, invasive testing may be required, including coronary angiography, electrophysiologic assessment, and potentially endomyocardial biopsy. Treatment recommendations must include prescriptions for physical activity, and thorough guidelines in this regard are available. The role and potential of newer diagnostic and therapeutic modalities are still being defined.

References

1 Michaud GF, Wang PJ, Estes NAM. Syncope in the athlete. In: Estes NAM, Salem DN, Wang PJ, eds. *Sudden Cardiac Death in the Athlete*. Armonk, NY: Futura, 1998: 419–40.

2 Day SC, Cook EF, Funkenstein H, Goldman L. Evaluation and outcomes of emergency room patients with transient loss of consciousness. *Am J Med* 1982;**73**:15–23.

3 Savage D, Corwin L, McGee D, Kannel WB, Wolf PA. Epidemiologic features of isolated syncope: the Framingham Study. *Stroke* 1985;**16**:626–9.

4 Maron BJ. Sudden death in young athletes: lessons from the Hank Gathers affair. *N Engl J Med* 1993;**329**:55–7.

5 Maron BJ, Mitten MJ, Quandt EK, Zipes DP. Competitive athletes with cardiovascular disease: the case of Nicholas Knapp. *N Engl J Med* 1998;**339**:1632–5.

6 Maron BJ, Gohman TE, Aeppli D. Prevalence of sudden cardiac death during competitive sports activities in Minnesota high school athletes. *J Am Coll Cardiol* 1998;**32**:1881–4.

7 Kramer MR, Drori Y, Lev B. Sudden death in young soldiers: high incidence of syncope prior to death. *Chest* 1988;**93**:345–7.

8 Maron BJ, Roberts WC, McCallister WA, *et al.* Sudden death in young athletes. *Circulation* 1980;**62**:218–29.

9 Goldschlager N, Epstein AE, Grubb BP, *et al.* Etiologic considerations in the patient with syncope and an apparently normal heart. *Arch Intern Med* 2003;**163**:151–62.

10 Link MS, Homoud MK, Wang PJ, Estes NAM. Syncope in athletes. *Cardiovasc Rev Rep* 2002;**23**:625–32.

11 Estes NAM, Link MS, Cannom D, *et al.* Report of the NASPE policy conference on arrhythmias and the athlete. *J Cardiovasc Electrophysiol* 2001;**12**:1208–19.

12 Maron BJ, Mitchel JH. Revised eligibility recommendations for competitive athletes with cardiovascular abnormalities. *J Am Coll Cardiol* 1994;**24**:848–50.

13 Mitchell JH, Haskell WH, Raven PB. Classification of sports. *J Am Coll Cardiol* 1994;**24**:864–6.

14 Pluim BM, Zwinderman AH, van der Laarse A, van der Wall EE. The athlete's heart: a meta-analysis of cardiac structure and function. *Circulation* 2000;**101**:336–44.

15 Maron BJ, Pelliccia A, Spirito P. Cardiac disease in young trained athletes: insights into methods for distinguishing athlete's heart from structural heart disease with particular emphasis on hypertrophic cardiomyopathy. *Circulation* 1995;**91**:1596–601.

16 Pelliccia A, Maron BJ, De Luca R, Di Paolo FM, Spataro A, Culasso F. Remodeling of left ventricular hypertrophy in elite athletes after long-term deconditioning. *Circulation* 2002;**105**:944–9.

17 Pelliccia A, Maron BJ, Culasso F, *et al.* Clinical significance of abnormal electrocardiographic patterns in trained athletes. *Circulation* 2000;**102**:278–84.

18 Estes NAM, Link ML, Homoud M, Wang PJ. Electrocardiographic variants and cardiac rhythm and conduction distribution in the athlete. In: Thompson PW, ed. *Textbook of Sports Physiology*. New York: McGraw Hill, 2001.

19 Olshansky B. Syncope: Overview and approach to management. In Grubb BP, Olshansky B, eds. *Syncope: Mechanisms and Management*. Armonk, NY: Futura, 1998: 15–71.

20 Calkins H, Zipes DP. Hypotension and syncope. In: Braunwald E, Zipes DP, Libby P, eds. *Heart Disease: A Textbook of Cardiovascular Medicine*, 6th edn. Philadelphia, PA: W.B. Saunders, 2001: 932–40.

21 Maron BJ. Sudden death in young athletes. *N Engl J Med* 2003;**349**:1064–75.

22 Burke AP, Farb A, Virmani R. Causes of sudden death in athletes. *Cardiol Clin* 1992;**10**:303–17.

23 Maron BJ. Cardiovascular risks to young persons on the athletic field. *Ann Intern Med* 1998;**129**:379–86.

24 Maron BJ, Shirani J, Poliac LC, *et al.* Sudden death in young competitive athletes: clinical, demographic, and pathologic profiles. *JAMA* 1996;**276**:199–204.

25 Maron BJ, Gohman T, Kyle SB, Estes NAM, Link MS. Clinical profile and spectrum of commotio cordis. *JAMA* 2002;**287**:114–26.

26 Corrado D, Thiene G, Nava A, *et al.* Sudden death in young competitive athletes: clinicopathologic correlations in 22 cases. *Am J Med* 1990;**89**:588–96.

27 Thompson PD. Sudden death in the athlete: atherosclerotic coronary disease. In: Estes NAM, Salem DN, Wang PJ, eds. *Sudden Cardiac Death in the Athlete*. Armonk, NY: Futura, 1998: 588–96.

28 Samenuk D, Link MS, Homoud MK, *et al.* Adverse cardiovascular events temporally associated with ma huang, an herbal source of ephedrine. *Mayo Clin Proc* 2002;**77**:12–6.

29 Calkins H, Shyr Y, Frumin H, Schork A, Morady F. The value of the clinical history in the differentiation of syncope due to ventricular tachycardia, atrioventricular block, and neurocardiogenic syncope. *Am J Med* 1995;**98**:365–73.

30 Alboni P, Brignole M, Menozzie C, *et al.* Diagnostic value of history in patients with syncope with or without heart disease. *J Am Coll Cardiol* 2001;**37**:1921–8.

31 Link MS, Wang PJ, Estes NAM. Ventricular arrhythmias in the athlete. *Curr Opin Cardiol* 2001;**16**:30–9.

32 Maron BJ, Moller JH, Seidman CE, *et al.* Impact of laboratory molecular diagnosis on contemporary diagnostic criteria for genetically transmitted cardiovascular diseases: hypertrophic cardiomyopathy, long QT syndrome, and Marfan syndrome. *Circulation* 1998;**98**:1460–71.

33 Klein GJ, Gersh BJ, Yee R. Electrophysiologic testing: the final court of appeal for diagnosis of syncope? *Circulation* 1995;**92**:1332–3.

34 Graham TP Jr., Bricker JT, James FW, Strong WB. 26th Bethesda conference: recommendations for determining eligibility for competition in athletes with cardiovascular abnormalities. Task Force 1: congenital heart disease. *J Am Coll Cardiol* 1994;**24**:867–73.

35 Pelliccia A, Maron BJ, Spataro A, Proschan MA, Spirito P. The upper limit of physiologic cardiac hypertrophy in highly trained elite athletes. *N Engl J Med* 1991;**324**: 295–301.

36 Colivicchi F, Ammirati F, Biffi A, Verdile L, Pelliccia A, Santini M. Exercise-related syncope in young competitive athletes without evidence of structural heart disease: clinical presentation and long-term outcome. *Eur Heart J* 2002;**23**:1125–30.

37 Link MS, Homoud MS, Wang PJ, Estes NAM. Cardiac arrhythmias in the athlete: the evolving role of electrophysiology. *Curr Sports Med Rep* 2002;**1**:75–85.

38 Oakley C. The electrocardiogram in the highly trained athlete. *Cardiol Clin* 1992;**10**:295–302.

39 Kosinski DJ. Syncope in the athlete. In: Grubb BP, Olshansky B, eds. *Syncope: Mechanisms and Management*. Armonk, NY: Futura, 1998: 317–35.

40 Pellicia A, Maron B, Spataro A, *et al.* The upper limit of physiologic cardiac hypertrophy in highly trained athletes. *N Engl J Med* 1991;**324**:295–301.

41 Maron BJ. Structural features of the athlete's heart: as defined by echocardiography. *J Am Coll Cardiol* 1986;**7**:190–203.

42 Basso C, Maron BJ, Corrado D, Thiene G. Clinical profile of congenital coronary artery anomalies with origin from the wrong aortic sinus leading to sudden death in

young competitive athletes. *J Am Coll Cardiol* 2000;**35:** 1493–501.

43 Frescura C, Basso C, Thiene G, *et al.* Anomalous origin of coronary arteries and risk of sudden death: a study based on an autopsy population of congenital heart disease. *Hum Pathol* 1998;**29:**689–95.

44 Burke A, Farb A, Virmani R, *et al.* Sports-related and non-sports-related sudden cardiac death in young adults. *Am Heart J* 1991;**121:**568–75.

45 Sneddon J, Scalia G, Ward D, *et al.* Exercise-induced vasodepressor syncope. *Br Heart J* 1994;**71:**554–7.

46 Grubb BP. Neurocardiogenic syncope. In: Grubb BP, Olshansky B, eds. *Syncope: Mechanisms and Management.* Armonk, NY: Futura, 1998: 73–106.

47 Benditt D, Ferguson D, Grubb BP, *et al.* Tilt table testing for assessing syncope: an American College of Cardiology Consensus document. *J Am Coll Cardiol* 1996;**28:**263–75.

48 Grubb BP, Temsey-Armos PN, Samoil D, Wolfe DA, Hahn H, Elliott L. Tilt table testing in the evaluation and management of athletes with recurrent exercise-induced syncope. *Med Sci Sports Exerc* 1993;**25:**24–8.

49 O'Connor FG, Oriscello RG, Levine BD. Exercise-related syncope in the young athlete: reassurance, restruction or referral? *Am Fam Physician* 1999;**60:**2001–8.

50 Link MS, Wang PJ, Estes NAM. Cardiac arrhythmias and electrophysiologic observations in the athlete. In: Richard A, Williams M, eds. *The Athlete and Heart Disease.* Philadelphia, PA: Lippincott, Williams & Wilkins; 1998: 197–216.

51 Smith ML, Hudson DL, Graitzer HM, *et al.* Exercise training bradycardia: the role of autonomic balance. *Med Sci Sports Exerc* 1989;**21:**40–44.

52 Gregoratos G, Cheitlin MD, Conill A, *et al.* ACC/AHA guidelines for implantation of cardiac pacemakers and antiarrhythmic devices. *J Am Coll Cardiol* 1998;**31:**1175–209.

53 Jackman WM, Wang X, Friday KJ, *et al.* Catheter ablation of accessory atrioventricular pathways (Wolff–Parkinson–White syndrome) by radiofrequency current. *N Engl J Med* 1991;**324:**1605–11.

54 Sharma AD, Yee R, Guiraudon G, *et al.* Sensitivity and specificity of invasive and non-invasive testing for risk of sudden death in Wolff–Parkinson–White syndrome. *J Am Coll Cardiol* 1987;**10:**373–81.

55 Zardini M, Yee R, Thakur RK, *et al.* Risk of sudden arrhythmic death in the Wolff–Parkinson–White syndrome: current perspectives. *PACE* 1994;**17:**966–75.

56 Link MS, Homoud MK, Wang PJ, Estes NAM. Cardiac arrhythmias in the athlete. *Cardiol Rev* 2001;**9:**21–30.

57 Pappone C, Santinelli V, Manguso F, *et al.* A randomized study of prophylactic catheter ablation in asymptomatic patients with Wolff–Parkinson–White syndrome. *N Engl J Med* 2003;**349:** 1803–11.

58 Link MS, Estes NAM. Ventricular arrhythmias. In: Estes NAM, Salem DN, Wang PJ, eds. *Sudden Cardiac Death in the Athlete.* Armonk, NY: Futura, 1998: 253–75.

59 Bigger JT, Reiffel JA, Livelli FD, *et al.* Sensitivity, specificity, and reproducibility of programmed ventricular stimulation. *Circulation* 1986;**73**(Suppl. 2):73–8.

60 Peters S, Reil GH. Risk factors of cardiac arrest in arrhythmogenic right ventricular dysplasia. *Eur Heart J* 1995;**16:** 77–80.

61 Wichter T, Martinez-Rubio A, Kottkamp H, *et al.* Reproducibility of programmed ventricular stimulation in arrhythmogenic right ventricular dysplasia/cardiomyopathy [Abstract]. *Circulation* 1996;**94**(Suppl. 1):626.

62 Prystowsky EN. Electrophysiologic–electropharmacologic testing in patients with ventricular arrhythmias. *PACE* 1988;**11:**225–51.

63 Zipes DP, Garson A Jr. 26th Bethesda conference: recommendations for determining eligibility for competition in athletes with cardiovascular abnormalities. Task Force 6: arrhythmias. *J Am Coll Cardiol* 1994;**24:**892–9.

64 DiGirolamo E, Di Iorio C, Leeonzio L, *et al.* Usefulness of a tilt training program for the prevention of refractory neurocardiogenic syncope in adolescents: a controlled study. *Circulation* 1999;**100:**1798–801.

65 Klein LS, Miles WM. Ablative therapy for ventricular arrhythmias. *Prog Cardiovasc Dis* 1995;**37:**225–42.

66 Calkins H, Kalbfleisch SJ, El-Atassi R, *et al.* Relation between efficacy of radiofrequency catheter ablation and site of origin of idiopathic ventricular tachycardia. *Am J Cardiol* 1993;**71:**827–33.

67 Corrado D, Leoni L, Link, MS, *et al.* Implantable cardioverter-defibrillator therapy for prevention of sudden death in patients with arrhythmogenic right ventricular cardiomyopathy/dysplasia. *Circulation* 2003;**108:**3084–91.

CHAPTER 18

Syncope in the elderly

Lewis Lipsitz, MD, *& Blair P. Grubb,* MD

Introduction

Syncope, defined as the transient loss of consciousness and postural tone with spontaneous recovery, is a common clinical problem. While syncope can be seen in all age groups, the elderly seem particularly prone to it [1]. The fastest growing segment of the population in most Western countries is those individuals aged 65 or older. The percentage of people over 65 years of age in the USA is expected to increase from 12.6% in 1990 to approximately 17% by the year 2020 [2]. Today, an individual aged 65 years can expect to live 16.9 years more, while an average 75-year-old can anticipate an additional 10.7 years of life [3]. It is presently estimated that approximately two-thirds of all the money spent on heart disease goes to care of older patients [4].

The epidemiology of syncope in the general elderly population has not been well studied. Part of the problem lies in the poor availability of good eyewitness accounts of syncopal events, and the close association (and overlap) that these episodes have with falls [5]. Syncope accounts for approximately 3% of all emergency department visits and between 2 and 6% of hospital admissions (80% of which are people aged over 65 years) [6–8]. In one study of the institutionalized elderly (over 70 years of age), the annual incidence of syncope was 6% with a 10% prevalence [9]. The annual recurrence rate over a 2-year follow-up was 30%.

Both a sign and a symptom, syncope can result from a wide variety of different causes, some of which may ultimately culminate in death. Thus, syncope in the older patient often provokes a deep sense of anxiety among patients, their families, physicians, and the staff of nursing homes and extended care facilities. Even if the cause of the patient's syncope is relatively benign, the conse-quences of the resultant fall may not be. Injuries from syncope have been reported to result in 17–53% of events, with bone fractures in as many as 5–7% (most of whom are elderly) [10–15], and subsequent traffic accidents in 1–5% of syncopal events [16,17]. Recurrent, unpredictable episodes of syncope may create a level of functional impairment similar to that seen in patients with chronic debilitating diseases such as rheumatoid arthritis [18]. The morbidity associated with syncope is often greater in the geriatric population, where falls are more likely to be complicated by fractures, subdural hematomas, and other serious injuries [19]. In one study of elderly patients with syncope resulting from carotid sinus hypersensitivity, over half had sustained a serious injury during syncope (either a fracture or an injury sufficiently severe so as to require hospitalization) [20,21]. Therefore, a simple syncopal episode could potentially convert a functional, independent, older person into a patient who requires permanent nursing home placement at great cost to the individual, their family, and society at large.

While syncope in younger patients is often caused by a single pathologic process, in older adults syncope is often multifactorial in origin. The elderly seem particularly prone to syncope because of age-related changes in the cardiovascular system with respect to control of the circulation as well as the concurrence of multiple illnesses combined with the use of numerous medications.

Pathophysiology of syncope in the older patient

The mechanisms by which the autonomic nervous system regulates normal control of blood pressure and heart rate have already been outlined in detail in Chapters 2 and 3. These autonomic control mechanisms are responsible for maintaining adequate blood flow to the areas of the brain responsible for maintaining consciousness (in particular the area known as the reticular activating system). Failure to maintain adequate cerebral blood flow causes a reduction in the amount of oxygen and glucose delivered to the brain, thus compromising consciousness. Because cerebral perfusion pressure is, for the most part, determined by the systemic arterial pressure, any process resulting in a reduction in either cardiac output or in total peripheral vascular resistance may result in a decline in systemic blood pressure and thereby diminish cerebral blood flow sufficiently to cause syncope [22].

A number of different diseases, either by themselves or combined, may increase the risk of syncope by their effects on systemic arterial pressure and oxygen delivery. The average adult over the age of 65 years suffers from an average of 3.5 chronic illnesses [23]. These often include conditions such as chronic obstructive pulmonary disease, coronary artery disease, carotid artery disease, congestive heart failure, and renal failure. At the same time, the pharmacotherapies employed in their management may further complicate the situation and add substantially to the risk of syncope. Current estimates are that up to 11% of syncopal events in the institutionalized elderly are caused by medication-related hypotension, with three-quarters of these associated with nitrate use [24]. The use of multiple medications further clouds the picture.

While in younger individuals cerebral autoregulation maintains cerebral blood flow at a constant level over a wide range of arterial blood pressures, age-related changes in autonomic control of blood pressure and heart rate may compromise the process [25,26]. Additionally, cerebral blood flow often declines by as much as 25% in older individuals, particularly those with hypertension, because of a combination of reduced cardiac output and increased cerebral vascular stiffness [27–30].

Age-related changes in cardiovascular control

The sympathetic nervous system undergoes a series of changes as a person ages. Plasma norepinephrine levels have been observed to increase, because of an increase in spillover from sympathetic nerve terminals as well as a reduced rate of clearance [31–33]. There is a reduction in the β-adrenergic-related cardioacceleratory response to sympathetic activation that occurs even though circulating norepinephrine levels are increased [34]. In addition, there is a reduction in β-adrenergic vasodilatory responses and α-adrenergic vasoconstrictive responses [35,36]. This may occur because of a reduced number of adrenergic receptors which result from high circulating plasma norepinephrine levels [37]. The diminished β-adrenergic vasodilatory response may account in part for the increased peripheral vascular resistance seen in elderly people [38–40].

While the mechanisms involved remain elusive, the aging process is also associated with a reduction in parasympathetic tone. This has been determined from observations of heart rate variability in elderly subjects and a reduced parasympathetic response to the Valsalva maneuver, respiration, and cough [41–46]. In addition, older patients experiencing syncope have been noted to have a lower degree of heart rate variability in response to deep breathing as compared with matched control subjects [45].

Reflex changes in heart rate that occur in response to sudden alterations in blood pressure are mediated by the baroreflex [47,48]. The baroreflex has been noted to lose its sensitivity with age as demonstrated by a blunted increase in heart rate in response to hypotension (possibly because of the reduction in β-receptor responsiveness) [49,50]. Most older patients can easily compensate for this through an increase in vascular resistance; this effect can be diminished by the effects of vasodilatory drugs or dehydration. As a consequence, older patients display an increased susceptibility to the hypotensive effects of diuretics, vasodilatory agents, or volume contraction. Compounding the risk of volume contraction is an age-related reduction in renal salt and water conservation (resulting from decreased renin and aldosterone production), and diminished thirst [51].

The reduction in parasympathetic tone seen with aging may be protective from the vagally mediated fall in heart rate and blood pressure seen with neurocardiogenic (or reflex) syncope [52–55]. This may account for the observed lower incidence of classic neurocardiogenic syncope in elderly as opposed to younger individuals.

In addition to changes in autonomic control of the heart, there is also a significant reduction in the absolute number of pacemaker cells in the sinus nodal region associated with aging, as well as a more general increase in collagenous and elastic tissue which affects the entire cardiac conduction system. It has been observed that by the age of 75 years there are less than 10% of the sinoatrial cells that were once present in young adulthood [22]. These changes predispose elderly patients to brady-cardia and heart block, two common causes of syncope. Furthermore, they make elderly people more susceptible to the bradyarrhythmic effects of beta-blockers, certain calcium-channel blockers, digoxin, and cardiac ischemia [20].

Another important physiologic change is the age-related reduction in left ventricular, early diastolic filling which makes elderly people quite sensitive to reductions in cardiac preload. The same changes in collagenous and elastic tissue that affect the conduction system increase myocardial stiff-ness. Also, age-related impairments in calcium re-uptake by the sarcoplasmic reticulum significantly lengthen the stage of isometric relaxation. As a result, a reduction in preload or marked increase in heart rate can decrease ventricular filling, reduce cardiac output, and cause syncope [56–60]. These changes also make the heart more dependent on atrial contraction to generate a normal cardiac out-put. Therefore, the loss of atrial contraction that may occur during atrial fibrillation (a common problem in the elderly) may diminish cardiac out-put by half in some individuals. For these reasons, syncope is particularly common in elderly patients in response to standing up, eating a meal, or taking nitrate medications, which all reduce preload, or at the onset of atrial fibrillation.

In addition to the autonomic and cardiac changes thus far described, the aging process affects the vasculature. In elderly people, the blood vessels go through a process of both elongation and dilation, as well as an increase in intimal thickness as a result of migration of smooth muscle cells into the lumen [61]. The type of tissue most important in the com-pliance of vasculature is elastin. In aging, elastin begins to fragment in the intima and media, and then later calcifies, resulting in increased vessel wall stiffness [62]. Vasodilatory dysfunction may also be seen because of a variety of different mechanisms

[63]. Both reduced nitric oxide release combined with increased endothelin release favor a state of vasoconstriction [64]. Compounding these changes is the common finding of atherosclerosis in the elderly, brought on by prior cigarette use, high levels of low-density lipoprotein, increased homocysteine levels, and reduced levels of physical activity.

Contributing factors to syncope in older patients

One of the more challenging aspects of evaluating syncope in older patients is that often more than one potential cause of syncope may be present in a particular individual. At the same time, the number of medications the average older person consumes (both prescribed and over-the-counter) is increas-ing all the time. Indeed, current estimates are that at least one-third of individuals over the age of 65 years are routinely taking at least three or more prescribed medications [2]. While no exact figures are available, use of herbal supplements (such as gingko) have also been increasing. One frequently encounters a situation in which multiple potential conditions that could cause syncope are present, none of which may be sufficiently severe to result in syncope by itself, but in combination may be more than enough to result in episodic loss of consciousness.

A number of conditions may have a major role in contributing to syncope, some of which are dis-cussed in detail elsewhere in this book. The follow-ing conditions are outlined in regard to their effects in older patients.

Hypertension

It is estimated that at least 30% of people older than 75 years suffer from hypertension, to a large extent because of the age-related changes already reviewed [65]. Interestingly, the presence of systolic hyper-tension seems to be a significant risk factor for the development of both orthostatic and postprandial hypotension [66–68]. Consequently, the elderly patients at greatest risk for orthostatic hypoten-sion are those with supine systolic hypertension [69]. The reasons for this are not completely un-derstood but are probably related to the effects of hypertension on further reducing baroreflex sensitivity and increasing vascular and ventricular stiffness. At the same time, hypertension is thought to shift the threshold of the cerebral autoregulatory curve to higher levels of blood pressure [70]. Thus, cerebral perfusion may decline at higher blood pressures in chronic hypertensive individuals, producing cerebral ischemia and potentially syncope at blood pressure levels that would otherwise be considered normal.

In some older patients the arteries become quite thickened and calcified. As a result, compression of the brachial artery with a sphygmomanometer requires a cuff pressure greater than that which is present in the artery. The net effect of this is termed pseudohypertension; the systolic and diastolic blood pressures measured from the sphygmomanometer are higher than the directly measured intra-arterial pressures [71,72]. Pseudohypertension should be suspected if there is severe hypertension in the absence of end-organ damage, if there is severe calcification of the brachial arteries on radiologic examination, and if antihypertensive therapy induces symptoms compatible with cerebral hypoperfusion (such as dizziness and weakness) in the absence of an excessive reduction in blood pressure. Some studies have reported that when one or more of these findings are present that the incidence of true pseudohypertension may be between 25 and 50%. Unfortunately, the diagnosis of pseudohypertension can only be definitively confirmed by direct measurement of intra-arterial pressure; however, some have suggested that Osler's maneuver may sometimes suggest the diagnosis. This is performed by inflating the sphygmomanometer to a level above the systolic blood pressure, which should collapse the brachial artery. In this setting, the radial artery will only be palpable as the arterial wall is markedly stiffened and thick. Unfortunately, the results of Osler's maneuver are poorly reproducible and demonstrate significant intra-observer variability.

Hypotension

The physiologic changes induced by aging combined with the effects of chronic or acute illness, dehydration, poor physical tone, prolonged bed rest, and the effect of medications (and sometimes alcohol), may work together to produce significant hypotension that may lead to syncope. Two conditions causing hypotension require specific mention because of their high prevalence in the elderly: orthostatic hypotension and postprandial hypotension.

Orthostatic hypotension

Orthostatic hypotension (OH) is defined as a fall in systolic blood pressure of 20–30 mmHg systolic and ≥ 10–15 mmHg diastolic upon standing. Approximately 30% of community dwelling adults over the age of 75 years have orthostatic hypotension (with rates rising with both age and increasing supine systolic hypertension) [71,73]. Studies have demonstrated that OH is a significant risk factor for recurrent falls, difficulty walking, and syncope [74,75]. However, Liu *et al.* [76] found no significant relationship between OH and falls, possibly because the frequency of OH is so high in the elderly population it may not have appeared as significant risk factor on multifactorial analysis. It should also be kept in mind that elderly people can display considerable variation in postural blood pressure change throughout the course of any particular day [77]. OH may accompany disease states such as Parkinson's disease, pure autonomic failure, and multisystem atrophy (see Chapter 3).

Postprandial hypotension

An important cause of syncope in the elderly and in those suffering from autonomic insufficiency syndromes is postprandial hypotension [78–81]. Indeed, postprandial hypotension may actually be more frequent in the elderly population than OH (and both may often coexist in the same patient) [82]. Postprandial hypotension is defined as ≥ 20 mmHg fall in systolic blood pressure within 75 min after a meal (some investigators have used a 90-min cut-off) [78]. Studies of nursing home residents have shown that between 24 and 30% demonstrate postprandial hypotension, which in most cases is asymptomatic [79,83]. However, among nursing home residents with syncope, 8% were felt to have postprandial hypotension as the likely cause [75]. In one study, nearly half of cases of unexplained syncope had postprandial hypotension as a likely cause [19]. The exact pathophysiologic mechanisms that cause postprandial hypotension are still not well understood. Most studies have demonstrated an inability to maintain systemic vascular resistance following a meal during the period of maximal splanchnic blood pooling

[84]. This concept is supported by the observation that somatostatin can prevent postprandial hypotension by decreasing splanchnic blood flow and increasing forearm vascular resistance [85–87].

Recent studies have focused on a variety of vasoactive gastrointestinal peptides (especially neurotensin and insulin). Among these, only insulin appears to be related to postprandial hypotension. Elevations in insulin after a meal can decrease vascular resistance and cause hypotension if counterregulatory adaptive mechanisms are impaired. Postprandial hypotension is frequently not recognized because symptoms are subtle (often only dizziness or weakness). Nevertheless, the resultant hypotension can be sufficiently profound to contribute to syncope, falls, angina, and cerebrovascular accidents, all of which may happen within 60–90 min of a meal.

Reflex syncopes

These are a group of disorders that appear mediated by stimulation of the medullary vasodepressor areas of the brainstem, with subsequent withdrawal of sympathetic tone. Vasodilation and bradycardia with subsequent hypotension and loss of consciousness may then occur [88].

Reflex syncopes include neurocardiogenic syncope, carotid sinus hypersensitivity (CSH), and other situational syncopes (see Chapters 2, 14, and 15) [89]. In contrast to younger patients, CSH and medication-related triggers are much more common in older adults; indeed, it is estimated that over half of episodes may occur because of the effects of cardiovascular medications [90]. CSH is rarely seen before the age of 50 years and increases in prevalence with age [91]. Recent studies have demonstrated that the cardioinhibitory form of CSH may be responsible for up to 20% of syncopal episodes in older patients (see Chapter 14). Syncope may also occur in any condition that provokes a Valsalva-like maneuver, thereby reducing venous return to the heart. These situations include defecation, urination, coughing, and other similar stresses [92,93].

Cardiovascular syncope

Syncope in elderly patients is precipitated by a cardiac cause in 21–34% of cases. Amongst all causes of syncope, various cardiac arrhythmias comprise 16%; sick sinus syndrome 3–6%; aortic stenosis 4–5%; myocardial infarction 2–6%; and heart block 1–3% [75,94]. Aortic stenosis is by far the most common structural lesion associated with syncope in the elderly. The prevalence of aortic stenosis increases with age: 75% of community-dwelling elderly people over the age of 85 have mild calcification of the aortic valve on echocardiography, and 6% have critical aortic stenosis [95]. Syncope affects approximately 25% of patients with symptomatic aortic stenosis. The patients who experience syncope have an increased incidence of sudden cardiac death [96–98]. Typically, syncope in a patient with aortic stenosis occurs with exercise, but it can also occur in response to directly acting vasodilators or even vasodilation induced by a hot bath.

Another underrecognized cause of cardiovascular syncope in the elderly is hypertrophic cardiomyopathy. Approximately 5–25% of patients with hypertrophic cardiomyopathy experience syncope at rest or on exercise [20]. Although there are no current demographic data on the incidence of hypertrophic cardiomyopathy in community-dwelling elderly, one study [99] shows that 83% of patients were over 50 years of age at the time of diagnosis.

An important cause of postoperative syncope in the elderly is pulmonary embolism. Pulmonary embolism should be included in the differential diagnosis of syncope in all patients, as it is common and often overlooked. In one study [100], 18% of elderly patients who were admitted to an acute geriatric ward had pulmonary embolism. Other, less common cardiovascular causes of syncope include cardiac tamponade, aortic dissection, obstructive cardiac tumors, and thrombotic occlusion of a prosthetic cardiac valve.

Asymptomatic arrhythmias are common in healthy elderly individuals, and it is difficult to determine if an arrhythmia is responsible for syncope unless there is electrocardiographic (ECG) confirmation during the episode. Because syncopal episodes are unpredictable and infrequent, even prolonged ECG monitoring may yield a low diagnostic rate. Bass *et al.* [101] performed Holter monitoring in 95 patients with unexplained syncope and discovered major ECG abnormalities in 15% of patients within the first 24 h. Of the remaining patients, 11% showed ECG abnormalities when monitored for another 24 h. Beyond 48 h, the yield of Holter monitoring was poor. However, in this study, as in a number of previous studies, there was no significant correlation between ECG abnormalities and symptoms of syncope.

An advancement in technique is the use of patient-activated loop recorders, which can retroactively record up to 4 min of ECG prior to the syncopal episode. These are useful for patients with frequent episodes of syncope and for those individuals who have sufficient understanding to be able to activate them at the time of an episode. Implantable loop recorders have further enhanced monitoring capabilities (see Chapter 19).

Endocrine diseases

Diabetes mellitus, its complications, and its treatment can produce syncope via different mechanisms. Diabetic autonomic neuropathy can produce orthostatic hypotension and syncope. Hypoglycemia can occur in any illness in which the patient is not eating well. One should be aware of interactions between sulphonylureas and high-dose salicylates, phenylbutazone, sulphonamides, chloramphenicol, and dicoumarol, all of which reduce clearance of sulphonylureas and enhance their hypoglycemic effects. Reduced creatinine clearance because of renal impairment will increase the circulating levels of insulin and oral hypoglycemics, resulting in hypoglycemia. Uncontrolled diabetes mellitus can cause an osmotic diuresis and dehydration, resulting in syncope.

Other endocrine causes of hypotension and syncope include Addison's disease, chronic adrenal suppression from steroid use, and hypopituitarism, all of which can produce hypoglycemia and hypovolemia. Conditions that are associated specifically with fluid loss are diabetes insipidus and salt-losing nephropathies. Other rarer entities, such as systemic mastocytosis, carcinoid, and pheochromocytoma, produce syncope via release of vasoactive substances such as histamine, epinephrine, and serotonin, respectively.

Evaluation and management of syncope in the elderly

History

Among cases of syncope for which an explanation can be found, approximately 70–80% can be diagnosed by a good history and physical examination [102]. It is important to obtain a detailed account of the situation in which syncope occurred, because many common, everyday activities can impose significant stress on an elderly individual and produce hypotension (see above). Antihypertensives, especially the directly acting vasodilators, and psychoactive medications can produce orthostatic hypotension and syncope. Although a recent study of nursing home residents suggests that long-term use of cardiovascular medications has no significant effect on orthostatic or postprandial blood pressure [82], the acute administration of any hypotensive drug may produce syncope. Caution must be exercised in elderly patients who may be more susceptible to adverse drug effects because of autonomic dysfunction or impairments in renal or hepatic clearance of hypotensive medications. Many over-the-counter cold or antimotility bowel medications have anticholinergic side-effects that can induce tachyarrhythmias and syncope. Ophthalmic beta-blockers have been implicated in bradyarrhythmias and cardiac conduction blocks. Medications therefore need to be reviewed diligently in the elderly patient with syncope.

Syncope associated with exercise is usually secondary to left or right ventricular outflow tract obstruction from aortic stenosis, hypertrophic cardiomyopathy, pulmonary hypertension, or pulmonary embolus. Patients who experience prodromal nausea, dizziness, or diaphoresis may have vasovagal syncope. Sudden onset of syncope without warning is usually associated with arrhythmias or conduction blocks [102]. Strokes and seizure activity usually have accompanying neurologic signs and symptoms [103]. Because approximately 6% of myocardial infarctions present as syncope, the history should also elicit risk factors and symptoms of coronary artery disease [102]. While the history is of paramount importance, it should be kept in mind that approximately 30% of elderly patients cannot remember documented falls 3 months later [104]. Additionally, approximately half of syncopal episodes are unwitnessed [9]. Amnesia of the syncope is seen in approximately 50% of patients with carotid sinus syndrome who present with falls [105].

Physical examination

A detailed physical examination should include blood pressure and pulse measurements in the supine position, then after 1 min of standing, and after 3 min of standing. Postural hypotension is frequently asymptomatic in the elderly, but a drop in systolic blood pressure of more than 20 mmHg should be regarded as a potentially dangerous finding that may predispose to syncope. If post-prandial hypotension is suspected, blood pressure and pulse should be measured before a meal as well as at least 30 min and 60 min after the meal. The cardiovascular examination should include auscultation of the heart for murmurs of aortic stenosis, hypertrophic cardiomyopathy, mitral stenosis, and regurgitation.

There are differences in the examination of the geriatric patient that are helpful to remember. The carotid upstroke may not be reduced in aortic stenosis because of stiffening of the vessel wall and consequent rapid rate of rise of the upstroke. The murmur of aortic stenosis may be displaced and better heard at the apex rather than the base of the heart. As the aortic valve becomes calcified, the intensity of the aortic component of the second heart sound diminishes. The gap between the aortic and the pulmonary component of the second heart sound shortens with increasing severity of aortic stenosis until A2 may follow P2; this is called paradoxical splitting. The systolic murmur of hypertrophic cardiomyopathy may be difficult to differentiate from that of aortic stenosis or mitral regurgitation. Therefore, to adequately evaluate a murmur, echocardiography may be required. The salient features that distinguish hypertrophic obstructive cardiomyopathy from other causes of systolic murmurs are a decrease in the intensity of the murmur with squatting and an increase in the murmur with standing and the performance of the Valsalva maneuver [45]. The intensity of the murmur is directly proportional to the gradient of the blood flow from the left ventricle to the sub-aortic region.

Autonomic dysfunction can be assessed by simple tests of heart rate responses to deep breathing and Valsalva [45]. Deep breathing is done with simultaneous recording of the ECG. The patient is asked to take slow deep breaths with 5 s for inspira-tion and 5 s for expiration, for a total of 3 min. The ratio of the R-R interval during expiration to the R-R interval during inspiration in the elderly should be > 1 : 15 [95]. This test provides an estimate of the integrity of the efferent vagal neural pathway to the heart.

The Valsalva maneuver tests heart rate responses to the changes in blood pressure that occur with straining maneuvers. The patient is asked to strain as if moving their bowels without holding their breath for 10 s. Another method is to blow into a tube attached to a mercury sphygmomanometer to maintain a pressure of 30–40 mmHg for 10 s. The ratio of the longest R-R interval after the release of the Valsalva to the shortest R-R interval during the procedure should be > 1 : 2 [43]. This ratio indicates normal vagal withdrawal in response to a decrease in cardiac output during straining, and vagal activation resulting from the blood pressure overshoot following release of the Valsalva.

Carotid sinus massage should be performed under ECG monitoring in patients who have no evidence of cerebrovascular disease, carotid bruits, cardiac conduction disease, or a recent myocardial infarction. One carotid sinus is massaged for 5 s, and the blood pressure is measured immediately before and after the procedure. If there is no response, massage should be repeated on the other side. Three types of responses may be produced: a reduction in heart rate, a drop in blood pressure, or both. Carotid sinus syndrome is diagnosed if there is a sinus pause of > 3 s, a drop in systolic blood pressure of > 50 mmHg (or 30 mmHg in the presence of symptoms), or occurrence of both responses simultaneously.

Tilt testing is occasionally helpful to detect neuro-cardiogenic syncope and orthostatic hypotension [106–109], and it can also be used to evaluate the effectiveness of treatment for these conditions. Although there is no standard protocol for tilt, an angle of 60° for 45 min has been found to be useful for eliciting symptoms. Shorter duration of tilt may give false-negative results. If the tilt test is negative, isoproterenol is sometimes used to provoke neurally mediated syncope by mimicking the intense sympathetic response that precedes loss of consciousness. This is generally avoided in elderly patients because it may produce myocardial ischemia.

Some studies show that vasovagal syncope and presyncope in response to tilt is less common in old age [110]. However, several recent studies suggest that neurocardiogenic syncope is underrecognized in elderly individuals, because they are less likely to report prodromal symptoms [109]. Therefore, tilt table testing is often recommended for diagnosis. However, 10–30% of healthy subjects without a history of syncope can have a positive test. Hence, a positive test does not necessarily mean that a vasovagal reaction was the cause of the patient's syncopal event.

Echocardiographic evaluation and Holter monitoring are recommended in patients with suspected cardiac causes of syncope. It is important for heart rate to be monitored during activities similar to those that were associated with syncope, and not only during bed rest in the hospital. Loop recorders may be used in patients with frequent episodes of syncope, but they require activation at the time of symptoms, which might not be possible for elderly patients with impaired cognition. Implantable loop recorders are becoming increasingly useful in evaluation of unexplained syncope (see Chapter 19).

Electrophysiologic studies may be used in the diagnosis of unexplained syncope in elderly patients. Kapoor et al. [94] studied 400 patients with syncope who underwent electrophysiologic studies; electrophysiologic testing was diagnostic in 1% of younger patients and in 2% of elderly patients. The role of electrophysiologic studies for the diagnosis and management of syncope in the elderly is controversial. Wagshal et al. [111] performed electrophysiologic studies on 45 octogenarians, 53% of whom had syncopal episodes. In this group, electrophysiologic studies were negative in 75% of patients; however, 8% of the patients had induced ventricular tachycardia and 17% had conduction abnormalities that required pacemaker implantation. The overall incidence of complications was between 2% and 3%, and not significantly different from other age groups.

Electrophysiologic studies are of low yield in patients without organic heart disease. Patients with coronary or structural heart disease with an ejection fraction < 40%, an abnormal resting ECG, and a history of injury caused by syncope have a > 95% chance of significant electrophysiologic abnormalities [112]. However, unless symptoms of near-syncope or syncope are reproduced, it is difficult to determine if the abnormalities on electrophysiologic testing are the cause of syncope. The greatest value of electrophysiologic testing lies in the management of ventricular tachycardia and fibrillation, in determining the efficacy of anti-arrhythmic therapy, and in the placement of pacemakers. In very elderly patients where mortality is not an issue, electrophysiologic testing may not be necessary for the work-up of syncope. Detailed discussion of the role of electrophysiologic studies in syncope is covered in other chapters. A suggested algorithm for the evaluation of the elderly patient with syncope is shown in Fig. 18.1.

Treatment

The management of elderly patients with syncope requires an understanding of their vulnerability to hypotension because of age- and disease-related physiologic changes that impair compensation for hypotensive stress. Patients should be educated about preventive measures; for example, elderly patients should be advised to avoid dehydration, prolonged inactivity, or bed rest after an illness. Waist-high support stockings can be worn, or low-dose fludrocortisone (0.1 mg to 1 mg) can be prescribed for hypotensive syndromes, provided there is careful monitoring for hypertension, congestive heart failure, and hypokalemia. Patients with postprandial hypotension should take a brief walk or rest in the supine position after a meal. Large carbohydrate meals and alcoholic drinks should be avoided. Antihypertensives should not be given to coincide with meals, as they may exacerbate postprandial hypotension. As a general rule, the number of medications should be minimized to avoid additive side-effects. Venodilators such as nitrates should be avoided if possible in patients with diastolic dysfunction and cardiac outflow tract obstruction, as they can precipitate syncope.

Structural heart disease is generally amenable to surgical treatment, even in the very elderly. Syncope associated with aortic stenosis may be the harbinger of sudden death, and it requires urgent attention. The operative mortality of aortic valve surgery in selected elderly patients over the age of 80 has been shown to be < 6% in one series [113]. However, mortality is much higher (24–35%) if coronary artery bypass graft (CABG) or mitral valve surgery is performed. Percutaneous balloon dilation of the aortic

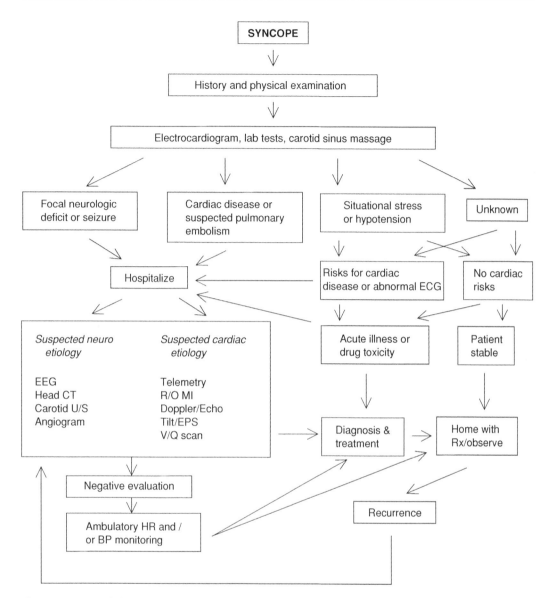

Fig. 18.1 A suggested algorithm for the evaluation of the elderly patient with syncope. BP, blood pressure; CT, computed tomography; ECG, electrocardiogram; EEG, electroencephalogram; EPS, electrophysiologic studies; HR, heart rate; U/S, ultrasound.

valve has a high restenosis rate, but it may significantly improve the quality of life in patients who are at high risk for major operative procedures [114].

Age is not a contraindication to pacemaker therapy. VVI pacing should generally be reserved for chronic atrial fibrillation; in every other case in which the atria are functioning an AV sequential or DDD mode is preferable in order to preserve the atrial contribution to cardiac output. VVI pacing in the elderly can cause retrograde conduction through the AV node. This can produce atrial con-

traction during ventricular systole, resulting in presyncope or syncope. The constellation of signs and symptoms associated with asynchronous atrioventricular contraction with VVI pacing is termed the "pacemaker syndrome." It may vary from simple fatigue to facial edema, dyspnea, chest pain, palpitations, and syncope. There may be associated cannon "A" waves in the neck and retrograde P waves on ECG. Treatment of the pacemaker syndrome involves conversion to a more physiologic mode of pacing.

The elderly have a narrower margin for drug toxicity than do younger individuals, primarily because of their reduced renal and hepatic clearance of drugs. Drugs such as lidocaine, procainamide, quinidine, and digoxin may accumulate to toxic levels at usual doses. As with all medications in the elderly, the axiom should be "start low and go slow," and the first dose of any vasodilator should be given in the supine position with blood pressure monitoring, if possible.

A detailed account of treatment for specific causes of syncope is covered in other chapters. General and specific modalities for the treatment of syncope in the elderly are described in Table 18.1.

Table 18.1 General principles of treatment for the elderly patient with syncope.

Non-pharmacologic treatment

Avoid hypotensive stresses
Prolonged standing or sitting; particularly after meals
Nitrates and vasodilators
Diuretics during acute illnesses
Excessive heat
Large meals with alcohol

Maximize venous returns
Exercise
Support hose
Volume – if no history of hypertension or congestive heart failure
Avoid sudden assumption of upright position, straining maneuvers (e.g., at defecation)

Driving precautions
Advise not to drive if frequent syncopal episodes. Driving-free period postsyncope until evaluation of syncope is completed and appropriate treatment/precautions prescribed

Pharmacologic treatment

Adjust medication doses for altered pharmacokinetics
Decreased hepatic oxidation, e.g., quinidine, procainamide, lidocaine, amiodarone
Decreased renal clearance, e.g., digoxin, procainamide

Altered pharmacodynamics
Increased beta-blocker effect
Increased confusion in response to drugs

Monitor drug interactions
Exacerbation of hypoglycemia, enhanced effect of sulfonylurea in combination with alcohol, high-dose salicylates, phenylbutazone, sulphonamides, warfarin
Exacerbation of orthostatic hypotension
1 Beta-blockers with negative chronotropic drugs such as digoxin, diltiazem, verapamil, and negative ionotropes as nifedipine, which can cause congestive heart failure
2 Nitrates with directly acting vasodilators as prazosin and other potent antihypertensives
3 Tricyclics and trazodone with antihypertensives cause hypotension
4 Alpha-blockers for hypertension or urinary outlet obstruction

Medications useful for autonomic failure
1 Mineralocorticoid, e.g., Florinef® (Squibb) (0.1–1.0 mg day^{-1})
  Increased salt and water retention
  Useful in orthostatic hypotension
2 Beta-blockers/calcium-channel blockers (propranolol, atenolol)
  Counteract sympathetic stimulation – useful in vasovagal syncope
  Beta-blockers also prevent vasodilation in orthostasis

(continued)

Table 18.1 (cont'd)

3 Prostaglandin synthetase inhibitors, e.g., indometacin – counteract vasodilation

Caution in elderly subjects – gastrointestinal bleeding and renal insufficiency

4 Serotonin reuptake inhibitors

Fluoxetine

Downregulation of postsynaptic serotonin receptors used in vasovagal/neurocardiogenic

5 Gut peptide release inhibitor

Octreotide (50 mg s.c. 30 min before each meal) vasoconstrictor

In severe orthostatic/postprandial hypotension

Caution – diarrhea

6 Adenosine receptor blocker

Caffeine, 2 cups of coffee (250 mg) before morning meal. Avoid later in the day to prevent tolerance and insomnia

7 Alpha-agonists, e.g., midodrine (2.5–10 mg t.i.d. p.o.), phenylephrine (60 mg b.i.d., q.i.d.) in severe orthostatic hypotension

8 Dopamine agonist

e.g., DOPS – dihydroxphenylserine 25 mg t.i.d. p.o. titrated to blood pressure

In isolated dopamine β-hydroxylase deficiency with orthostatic hypotension

9 Erythropoietin 25–75 U/kg three times a week s.c./i.v.

Increases hematocrit and blood pressure

Useful in autonomic failure with anemia

b.i.d., twice daily; i.v., intravenous; p.o., by mouth (per os); q.i.d., four times a day; s.c., subcutaneous; t.i.d., three times a day.

References

1 Kapoor WN. Evaluation of syncope in the elderly. *J Am Geriatr Soc* 1987;**35**:826–30.

2 Kenny R. Syncope in the elderly: diagnosis, evaluation and treatment. *J Cardiovasc Electrophysiol* 2003;**14**:S74–7.

3 Spencer G. Projections of the population of the United States by age, sex and race: 1988 to 2080. *US Bureau of the Census. Current Population Reports*. Series P-25. No. 1018, Washington DC: US Government Printing Office, 1989: 1–17.

4 Gillium RF. Trends in acute myocardial infarction and coronary heart disease death in the United States. *J Am Coll Cardiol* 1994;**23**:1273–7.

5 Savage DD, Corwin L, McGee CL, *et al.* Epidemiological features of isolated syncope: the Framingham Study. *Stroke* 1985;**16**(4):626–9.

6 Day SC, Cook EF, Funkenstein H, *et al.* Evaluation and outcome of emergency room patients with transient loss of consciousness. *Am J Med* 1982;**73**:15–23.

7 Doherty JU, Pembrook-Rogers D, Grogan EW, *et al.* Electrophysiologic evaluation and follow-up characteristics of patients with recurrent unexplained syncope and pre-syncope. *Am J Cardiol* 1985;**55**:703–8.

8 Lipsitz LA. Syncope in the elderly patient. *Hosp Pract* 1986;**21**:33–44.

9 Lipsitz L, Wei JY, Rowe JW. Syncope in an elderly, institutionalized population: prevalence, incidence, and associated risk. *Q J Med* 1985;**55**:45–54.

10 Campbell AJ, Reinken J, Allan BC, *et al.* Falls in old age: a study of frequency and related clinical factors. *Age Ageing* 1981;**10**:264–70.

11 Nevitt MC, Cummings SR, Hudes ES. Risk factors for injurious falls: a prospective study. *J Gerontol* 1991;**46**:M164–70.

12 Kapoor WN. Evaluation and outcome of patients with syncope. *Medicine* 1990;**69**:160–75.

13 Kapoor WN, Karpf M, Wieand S, *et al.* A prospective evaluation and follow-up of patients with syncope. *N Engl J Med* 1983;**309**:197–208.

14 Eagle KA, Black HR, Cook EF, *et al.* Evaluation of prognostic classifications for patients with syncope. *Am J Med* 1985;**79**:455–60.

15 Kapoor WN, Karpf M, Maher Y, *et al.* Syncope of unknown origin: the need for a cost effective approach to its diagnostic evaluation. *JAMA* 1982;**247**:2687–91.

16 Herner B, Smedby B, Ysander L. Sudden illness as a cause of motor vehicle accidents. *Br J Int Med* 1966;**23**:37–41.

17 Petch MC, prepared on behalf of the ESC Task Force. Driving and heart disease. Task Force Report. *Eur Heart J* 1998;**19**:1165–77.

18 Linzer M, Pontinen M, Gold GT. Impairment of physical and psychosocial function in recurrent syncope. *J Clin Epidemiol* 1991;**44**:1037–43.

19 Lipsitz LA. Syncope in the elderly. *Ann Intern Med* 1983;**99**:92–104.

20 Kenny R. *Syncope in the Older Patient.* London, UK: Chapman and Hall Medical, 1996.

21 Kenny RA, Traynor G. Carotid sinus syndrome: clinical characteristics in elderly patients. *Age Ageing* 1991;**20**: 449–54.

22 Forman DE, Lipsitz LA. Syncope in the elderly. *Cardiol Clin* 1997;**15**:295–311.

23 Besdine RW. Geriatric medicine: an overview. *Ann Rev Gerontol* 1980;**2**:135–41.

24 Liu BA, Topper AK, Reeves RA, *et al.* Falls among older people: relationship to medication use and orthostatic hypotension. *J Am Geriatr Soc* 1995;**43**:1141–6.

25 Strandgaard S. Autoregulation of cerebral flow in hypertensive patients: the modifying influence of prolonged antihypertensive treatment on the tolerance to acute, drug induced hypotension. *Circulation* 1976;**53**:720–7.

26 Strandgaard S, Olesen J, Skinhoj E, *et al.* Autoregulation of brain circulation in severe arterial hypertension. *BMJ* 1973;**1**:507–10.

27 Wollner L, McCarthy ST, Soper NDW, *et al.* Failure of cerebral autoregulation as a cause of brain dysfunction in the elderly. *BMJ* 1979;**1**:1117–8.

28 Mayhan WG, Faraci FM, Baumbach GL, *et al.* Effects of aging on responses of cerebral arterioles. *Am J Physiol* 1990;**27**:H1138–43.

29 Taddei S, Virdia A, Mattei P, *et al.* Aging and endothelial function in normotensive subjects and patients with essential hypertension. *Circulation* 1995;**91**:1981–7.

30 Krajewski A, Freeman R, Ruthazer R, *et al.* Transcranial Doppler assessment of the cerebral circulation during postprandial hypotension in the elderly. *J Am Geriatr Soc* 1993;**141**:19–24.

31 Linares OA, Halter JB. Sympathochromaffin system activity in the elderly. *J Am Geriatr Soc* 1987;**35**:448–53.

32 Morrow LA, Linares OA, Hill TJ, *et al.* Age differences in plasma clearance mechanisms for epinephrine and norepinephrine in humans. *J Clin Endocrinol Metab* 1987;**65**:508–11.

33 Supiano MA, Linares OA, Smith MJ, *et al.* Age related difference in norepinephrine kinetics: effect of posture and sodium-restricted diet. *Am J Physiol* 1990; **259**:E422–31.

34 Rowe JW, Troen BR. Sympathetic nervous system and aging in man. *Endocr Rev* 1980;**1**:167–79.

35 Hogikyan RV, Supiano MA. Arterial α-adrenergic responsiveness is decreased and SNS activity is increased in older humans. *Am J Physiol* 1994;**266**:E717–24.

36 Pan HYM, Blaschke TF. Decline in β-adrenergic receptor-mediated vascular relaxation with aging in man. *J Pharm Exp Ther* 1986;**239**:802–7.

37 Brodde OE, Zerkowski GR, Schranz E, *et al.* Age-dependent changes in the β-adrenoceptor G-protein adenyl cyclase system in human right atrium. *J Cardiovasc Pharmacol* 1995;**26**(1):20–6.

38 Ford GA, Hoffman BB, Vestal RE, *et al.* Age related changes in adenosine and β-adrenoceptor responsiveness of vascular smooth muscle in man. *Br J Clin Pharmacol* 1992;**33**:83–7.

39 Abrass IB, Davis JL, Scarpace PJ, *et al.* Isoproterenol responsiveness and myocardial β-adrenergic receptors in young and old rats. *J Gerontol* 1982;**37**:156–60.

40 Abrass IB, Scarpace PJ. Human lymphocyte β-adrenergic receptors are unaltered with age. *J Gerontol* 1981;**36**: 298–301.

41 Waddington JL, MacCullough MJ, Sambrooks JE, *et al.* Resting heart rate variability in man declines with age. *Experentia* 1979;**35**:1197–8.

42 Jennings JR, Mack ME. Does aging differentially reduce heart rate variability related to respiration? *Exp Aging Res* 1984;**10**:19–23.

43 Gautschy B, Weidmann P. Autonomic function tests as related to age and gender in normal man. *Klin Wochenschr* 1986;**64**:499–505.

44 O'Brien IAD, O'Hare P, Corrall RJM, *et al.* Heart rate variability in healthy subjects: effects of age and derivation of normal ranges for tests of autonomic function. *Br Heart J* 1986;**55**:348–54.

45 Maddens ME, Lipsitz LA, Wei JY, *et al.* Impaired heart rate responses to cough and deep breathing in elderly patients with unexplained syncope. *Am J Cardiol* 1987; **60**:1368–72.

46 Wei JY, Rowe JW, Kestenbaum AD, *et al.* Post-cough heart rate response: influence of age, sex, and basal blood pressure. *Am J Physiol* 1983;**245**:R18–24.

47 Shimada K, Kitazumi T, Ogura H, *et al.* Differences in age-independent effects on blood pressure on baroreflex sensitivity between normal and hypertensive subjects. *Clin Sci* 1986;**70**:489–94.

48 Gribbin B, Pickering TG. Sleight P, *et al.* Effect of age and high blood pressure on baroreflex sensitivity in man. *Circ Res* 1971;**29**:424–31.

49 Smith JJ, Hughes CV, Ptacin MJ, *et al.* The effect of age on hemodynamic response to graded postural stress in normal men. *J Gerontol* 1987;**42**:406–11.

50 Minaker KI, Menielly GS, Young JB, *et al.* Blood pressure, pulse, and neurohumoral responses to nitroprusside-induced hypotension in normative aging in men. *J Gerontol Med Sci* 1991;**46**:M151–4.

51 Taylor JA, Hand GA. Sympathoadrenal circulatory regulation of arterial pressure during orthostatic stress in young and older men. *Am J Physiol* 1992;**263**:R1147–55.

52 Pomeranz B, Macaulay RJB, Caudill MA, *et al.* Assessment of autonomic functions in humans by heart rate spectral analysis. *Am J Physiol* 1985;**248**:H151–3.

53 Billman GE, Dujardin JP. Dynamic changes in cardiac

vagal tone as measured by time-series analysis. *Am J Physiol* 1990;**258**:H869–902.

54 Simpson DM, Wicks R. Spectral analysis of heart rate indicates reduced baroreceptor mediated heart rate variability in elderly persons. *J Gerontol* 1988;**43**(1): M21–4.

55 Lipsitz LA, Mietus J, Moody GB, *et al.* Spectral characteristics of heart rate variability before and during postural tile: relations to aging and risk of syncope. *Circulation* 1990;**81**(6):1803–18.

56 Froelich JP, Lakatta EG, Beard E, *et al.* Studies of sarcoplasmic reticulum function and contraction duration in young and aged rat myocardium. *J Mol Cell Cardiol* 1970;**10**:427–38.

57 Orchard CH, Lakatta EG. Intracellular calcium transients and developed tensions in rat heart muscle: a mechanism for the negative interval–strength relationship. *J Gen Physiol* 1985;**86**:637–51.

58 Wei JY, Spurgeon HA, Lakatta EG, *et al.* Excitation-contraction in rat myocardium: alterations in adult aging. *Am J Physiol* 1984;**246**:H784–91.

59 Bryg RJ, Williams GA, Labovitz AJ. Effect of aging on left ventricular diastolic filling in normal subjects. *Am J Cardiol* 1987;**59**:971–4.

60 Miyatake K, Okamoto M, Kinoshita N, *et al.* Augmentation of atrial contribution to left ventricular inflow with aging as assessed by intracardiac Doppler flowmetry. *Am J Cardiol* 1984;**53**:586–9.

61 Bilato C, Crow MT. Atherosclerosis and the vascular biology of aging. *Aging* 1996;**8**:221–5.

62 Lakatta EG. Cardiovascular regulatory mechanisms in advanced age. *Physiol Rev* 1993;**73**:413–6.

63 Taylor JA, Hand GA. Sympathoadrenal circulatory regulation of arterial pressure during orthostatic stress in younger and older men. *Am J Physiol* 1992;**263**:R1147–9.

64 Taddei S, Virdia A, Mattei P, *et al.* Aging and endothelial function in normotensive subjects and patients with essential hypertension. *Circulation* 1981;**91**:1995.

65 Kannel WE. Hypertension and aging. In: Finch CE, Schneider EL, ed. *Handbook of the Biology of Aging.* New York, NY: Van Nostrand Reinhold, 1985: 859.

66 Harris T, Lipsitz LA, Kleinman JC, *et al.* Postural change in blood pressure associated with age and systolic blood pressure: the national health and nutrition examination survey II. *J Gerontol* 1991;**46**:M159–63.

67 Applegate WB, David BR, Black HR, *et al.* Prevalence of postural hypotension at baseline in the systolic hypertension in the elderly program (SHEP) cohort. *J Am Geriatr Soc* 1991;**39**:1057–64.

68 Valvanne J, Sorva A, Erkinjuntti T, *et al.* The occurrence of postural hypotension in age cohorts of 75, 80, and 85 years: a population study. *Arch Gerontol Geriatr* 1991;**2**:421–4.

69 Lipsitz LA, Ryan SM, Parker JA, *et al.* Hemodynamic and autonomic nervous system responses to mixed meal ingestion in healthy young and old subjects, and dysautonomic patients with postprandial hypotension. *Circulation* 1993;**87**:391–400.

70 Barry DI. Cerebral blood flow in hypertension. *J Cardiovasc Pharmacol* 1985;**7**:594–8.

71 Caird FL, Andrews GR, Kennedy RD, *et al.* Effect of posture on blood pressure in the elderly. *Br Heart J* 1973;**35**:527–30.

72 Stokes G, Duggan K. Comorbid conditions: special considerations. In: Oparil S, Weber M, eds. *Hypertension: A Companion to Brenner and Rector's The Kidney.* Philadelphia, PA: W.B. Saunders, 2000: 515.

73 Harris T, Kleinman J, Lipsitz LA, *et al.* Is age or level of systolic blood pressure related to positional blood pressure change? *Gerontologist* 1986;**26**:59A.

74 Tinetti ME, Williams TF, Mayewski R. Fall risk index for elderly patients based on number of chronic disabilities. *Am J Med* 1986;**80**:429–34.

75 Lipsitz LA, Pluchino FC, Wei JY, *et al.* Syncope in institutionalized elderly: the impact of multiple pathological conditions and situational stress. *J Chronic Dis* 1986; **39**:619–30.

76 Liu BA, Topper AK, Reeves RA, *et al.* Falls among older people: relationship to medication use and orthostatic hypotension. *J Am Geriatr Soc* 1995;**43**:1141–5.

77 Lipsitz LA, Storch HA, Minaker KL, *et al.* Intra-individual variability in postural blood pressure in the elderly. *Clin Sci* 1985;**59**:337–41.

78 Lipsitz LA, Fullerton KJ. Postprandial blood pressure reduction in healthy elderly. *J Am Geriatr Soc* 1986; **34**:267–70.

79 Vaitkevicius PV, Esserwein DM, Maynard AK, *et al.* Frequency and importance of postprandial blood pressure reduction in elderly nursing home patients. *Ann Intern Med* 1991;**115**:865–70.

80 Robertson D, Wade D, Robertson RM. Postprandial alterations in cardiovascular hemodynamics in autonomic dysfunctional states. *Am J Cardiol* 1981;**48**:1048–52.

81 Micieli G, Martignoni E, Cavallini A, *et al.* Postprandial and orthostatic hypotension in Parkinson's disease. *Neurology* 1987;**37**:386–93.

82 Jansen RWMM, Kelley-Gagnon MM, Lipsitz LA. Intra-individual reproducibility of postprandial and orthostatic blood pressure changes in elderly nursing home patients: relationship with chronic use of cardiovascular medications. *J Am Geriatr Soc* 1996;**44**:383–9.

83 Aronow WS, Ahn C. Postprandial alterations in cardiovascular hemodynamics in autonomic dysfunctional states. *Am J Cardiol* 1981;**48**:1048–52.

84 Jansen RWMM, Connelly CM, Kelley-Gagnon MM, *et al.* Postprandial hypotension in elderly patients with

unexplained syncope. *Arch Intern Med* 1995;**155**:945–52.

85 Jansen RWMM, Peeters TL, Lenders JWM, *et al.* Somatostatin analog octreotide (SMS 201-995) prevents the decrease in blood pressure after oral glucose loading in the elderly. *J Clin Endocrinol Metab* 1989;**68**:752–6.

86 Jansen RWMM, de Meijer PHEM, van Lier HJJ, *et al.* Influence of octreotide (SMA 201-995) and insulin administration on the course of blood pressure after an oral glucose load in hypertensive elderly subjects. *J Am Geriatr Soc* 1989;**37**:1135–9.

87 Hoeldtke RD. Postprandial hypotension. In: Low PA, ed. *Clinical Autonomic Disorders, Evaluation and Management.* Boston: Little, Brown and Co, 1993: 701–11.

88 Kosinski D, Grubb BP, Temesy-Armos P. Pathophysiological aspects of neurocardiogenic syncope. *PACE* 1995;**18**:716–21.

89 Sutton R, Petersen M. The clinical spectrum of neurocardiogenic syncope. *J Cardiovasc Electrophysiol* 1995;**6**:569–76.

90 McIntosh SJ, Lawson J, Kenny RA. Clinical characteristics of vasodepressor, cardioinhibitory and mixed carotid sinus syndrome in the elderly. *Am J Med* 1993;**95**:203–8.

91 Morely CA, Sutton R. Carotid sinus syncope. *Int J Cardiol* 1984;**6**:287–93.

92 McIntosh SJ, Lawson J, Kenny RA, *et al.* Heart rate and blood pressure responses to carotid sinus massage in healthy elderly subjects. *Age Ageing* 1994;**23**:57–61.

93 Wenthick JRM, Jansen RWMM, Hoefnagels WHL. The influence of age on the response of blood pressure and heart rate to carotid sinus massage in healthy volunteers. *Cardiology Elderly* 1993;**1**:453–9.

94 Kapoor W, Snustad D, Peterson J, *et al.* Syncope in the elderly. *Am J Med* 1986;**80**:419–28.

95 Lindroos K, Kupari M, Heikkila J, *et al.* Prevalence of aortic valve abnormalities in the elderly: an echocardiographic study of a random population. *J Am Coll Cardiol* 1993;**21**:1220–5.

96 Schwartz LS, Goldfisher J, Sprague GJ, *et al.* Syncope and sudden death in aortic stenosis. *Am J Cardiol* 1969; **23**:647–58.

97 Selzer A. Changing aspects of the natural history of aortic valvular stenosis. *N Engl J Med* 1987;**317**:91–8.

98 Banning AP, Hall RJC. In: Kenny RA, ed. *Syncope in the Older Patient, Causes, Investigation and Consequences of Syncope and Falls.* London, UK: Chapman & Hall Medical, 1996: 201–18.

99 Petrin TJ, Tavel ME. Idiopathic hypertrophic subaortic stenosis as observed in a large community hospital: relation to age and history of hypertension. *J Am Geriatr Soc* 1979;**27**:43–6.

100 Impallomemi MG, Arnot RN, Alexander MS. Incidence of pulmonary embolism in elderly patients newly admitted to an acute geriatric unit: a prospective study. *Clin Nucl Med* 1990;**15**:84–7.

101 Bass EB, Curtiss EI, Arena VC, *et al.* The duration of Holter monitoring in patients with syncope: is 24 hours enough? *Arch Intern Med* 1990;**150**:1073–8.

102 Calkins H, Shyr Y, Frumin H, Schork A, Morady F. The value of the clinical history in the differentiation of syncope due to ventricular tachycardia, atrioventricular block, and neurocardiogenic syncope. *Am J Med* 1995; **98**:365–73.

103 Sheldon R, Rosa S, Ritchie D, *et al.* Historical criteria that distinguish syncope from seizures. *J Am Coll Cardiol* 2002;**40**:142–8.

104 Alboni P, Brignole M, Menozzi C, *et al.* Diagnostic value of history in patients with syncope with or without heart disease. *J Am Coll Cardiol* 2001;**37**:1921–8.

105 Cummings SR, Nevitt MC, Kidd S. Forgetting falls: the limited accuracy of recall of falls in the elderly. *J Am Geriatr Soc* 1988;**36**:613–6.

106 Abi-Samra F, Malony JD, Fouad-Tarazi FM, *et al.* The usefulness of head-up tilt testing and hemodynamic investigations in the work-up of syncope of unknown origin. *Pacing Clin Electrophysiol* 1988;**11**:1202–12.

107 Grubb BP, Kosinski D, Samoil D, *et al.* Recurrent unexplained syncope: the role of head upright tilt table testing. *Heart Lung* 1993;**22**(6):502–8.

108 Hargreaves AD, Hag EO, Boon AN. Head-up tilt testing: the balance of evidence. *Br Heart J* 1994;**72**:216–7.

109 Grubb BP, Wolfe D, Samoil D, *et al.* Recurrent unexplained syncope in the elderly: the use of head-upright tilt table testing in evaluation and management. *J Am Geriatr Soc* 199;**40**:1123–8.

110 Lipsitz LA, Marks ER, Koestner JS, *et al.* Reduced susceptibility to syncope during postural tilt in old age: is beta-blockade protective? *Arch Intern Med* 1989;**149**: 2709–12.

111 Wagshal AB, Scchuger CD, Habbal B, *et al.* Invasive electrophysiologic evaluation in octogenarians: is age a limiting factor? *Am Heart J* 1993;**126**:1142–6.

112 Krol RB, Morady F, Flacker GC, *et al.* Electrophysiologic testing in patients with unexplained syncope: clinical and non-invasive predictors of outcome. *J Am Coll Cardiol* 1987;**10**:358–63.

113 Elayada MA, Hall RJ, Reul RM, *et al.* Aortic valve replacement in patients 80 years and older: operative risks and long-term results. *Circulation* 1993;**88**(2):11–6.

114 Bernard Y, Etievent J, Mourand JL, *et al.* Long-term results of percutaneous aortic valvuloplasty compared with aortic valve replacement in patients more than 75 years old. *J Am Coll Cardiol* 1992;**20**:796–801.

CHAPTER 19

The implantable loop recorder for diagnosis of unexplained syncope

Andrew D. Krahn, MD, *George J. Klein,* MD, *Allan C. Skanes,* MD, *& Raymond Yee,* MD

Introduction

The advent of prolonged monitoring with external and, more recently, implanted loop recorders has enabled the detection of elusive, infrequent arrhythmias causing syncope. Clinicians rely on clinical assessment and abnormal laboratory results to make a diagnosis by inference in most patients. A more direct and accurate diagnosis would result from a prolonged monitoring technology that captures key physiologic data during a spontaneous event. The capability of prolonged monitoring has permitted us to obtain a symptom–rhythm correlation in the majority of patients suspected of having arrhythmia.

The implantable loop recorder

The only currently available implantable loop recorder (ILR: Reveal© Minneapolis, MN) measures 6.1 × 1.9 × 0.8 cm, weighs 17 g, and has a pair of recording electrodes 3.7 cm apart on the shell [1–3] (Fig. 19.1). It has an operating life of approximately 14 months and is inserted in the subcutaneous tissue of the left pectoral region using standard sterile technique and local anesthetic. The battery life is often in the order of 18–24 months, depending on preimplant shelf life and patient variability. It has been implanted in the right parasternal, subcostal, and axillary regions with an adequate, albeit lower amplitude signal. The recorded bipolar electrocardiogram (ECG) signal is stored in a circular buffer capable of storing 21 min of uncompressed signal or 42 min of compressed signal in one or three

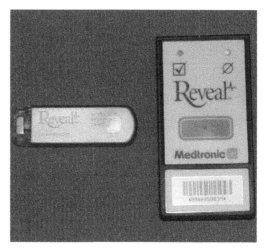

Fig. 19.1 Implantable loop recorder (left) with manual activator (right).

divided parts. Because the compressed signal quality is negligibly different from the uncompressed signal, it is used most often to maximize the memory capacity of the device. The memory buffer is frozen using a hand-held activator provided to the patient at the time of device implant. Events stored by the device are downloaded after interrogation with a standard Medtronic 9790 pacemaker programmer (Fig. 19.2). The current version of the device (Reveal Plus©) has programmable automatic detection of high and low heart rate episodes and pauses (Fig. 19.3). The resultant memory configuration allows for division of multiple 1-min automatic rhythm strips in addition to 1–3 manual recordings. This permits automated event

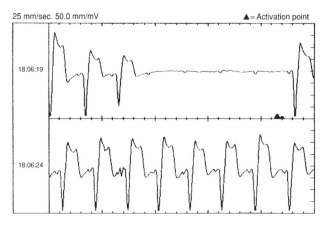

25 mm/sec. 50.0 mm/mV   ▲ = Activation point

18:06:19

18:06:24

Fig. 19.2 Rhythm strip obtained with an implantable loop recorder during presyncope in a 64-year-old woman with three syncopal and two presyncopal episodes in the previous 11 months. An electrophysiology study was negative, and the resting electrocardiogram did not show evidence of bundle branch block. Each line represents 5 s of a single lead rhythm strip in this magnified view. Note bundle branch block with third-degree AV block with an asystolic period lasting just over 3 s. Manual activation took place 90 s later when the patient used the manual activator. Syncope resolved after permanent pacemaker implantation.

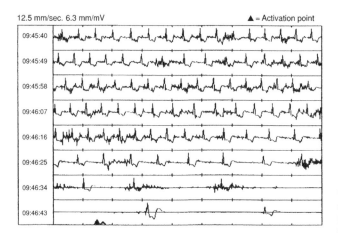

12.5 mm/sec. 6.3 mm/mV   ▲ = Activation point

09:45:40

09:45:49

09:45:58

09:46:07

09:46:16

09:46:25

09:46:34

09:46:43

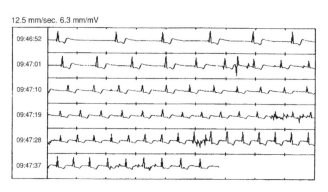

12.5 mm/sec. 6.3 mm/mV

09:46:52

09:47:01

09:47:10

09:47:19

09:47:28

09:47:37

Fig. 19.3 Rhythm strip obtained with an implantable loop recorder during presyncope in a 43-year-old woman with four syncopal episodes in the previous 3 years. Tilt testing and a trial of an external loop recorder were negative. Each line represents 10 s of a single lead rhythm strip. Note gradual slowing of the heart rate with an 8-s pause. In the absence of underlying heart disease in a middle-aged patient, this was interpreted as the cardioinhibitory component of vasovagal syncope. The device was activated automatically when the preprogrammed lower rate autodetection feature was satisfied. Manual activation took place after the patient located the manual activator. P waves are not well seen in this tracing.

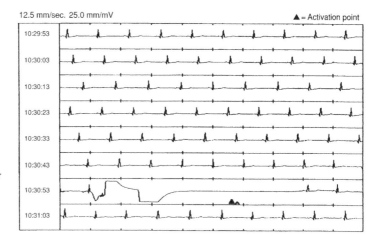

Fig. 19.4 Transient loss of signal felt to be caused by loss of tissue electrode contact within the device pocket. Loss of signal with amplifier saturation and reacquisition of signal is seen during non-physiologic recording, which is detected automatically as a pause.

acquisition to detect prespecified extreme heart rates or pauses (typically < 30 b min^{-1}, > 160 b min^{-1} and pauses > 3 s) in patients incapable of manual activation. Automatic activations are more likely to detect borderline or potentially problematic asymptomatic arrhythmias than conventional patient activation [4]. Automatic detection of asymptomatic arrhythmias may allow diagnosis if the arrhythmia is sufficiently striking and obviate a symptomatic recurrence [5]. Automatic detection has also led to recognition of sensing issues in the current device with transient loss of signal resulting in automatic detection of "pseudo" pauses (Fig. 19.4). Unlike the adjustment of gain and sensitivity that optimizes sensing successfully in most patients, this problem appears to stem from transient loss of contact of the sensing electrodes within the device pocket. This clearly needs to be distinguished from true asystole.

The implant procedure is comparable to creation of a smaller and more superficial pacemaker pocket. Cardiologists and cardiac surgeons have performed the implant in an operating room, in the electrophysiology laboratory, or in the cardiac catheterization laboratory. An adequate signal can be obtained anywhere in the left thorax without the need for cutaneous mapping [2]. Mapping optimizes the sensed signal and is recommended in patients where automatic detection is desirable to prevent oversensing of T waves and double counting leading to automatic detection of high rate episodes. Mapping usually leads to device insertion

in an oblique orientation in the high left parasternal region [5]. Right parasternal sites have been used to optimize P wave amplitude. The patient, together with a spouse, family member, or friend, is instructed in the use of the activator at the time of implant. As with any implanted device, strict sterile technique is necessary and prophylactic antibiotics are recommended to prevent pocket infection.

The prototype of the ILR was implanted in patients with recurrent unexplained syncope after extensive non-invasive and invasive testing was unrewarding [1]. The device proved very successful in establishing a symptom rhythm correlation (85%) in this difficult patient population. These results have been confirmed in a recent study in 184 patients with unexplained syncope and a negative work-up [6,7]. The ILR provided a symptom rhythm correlation in seven of the 15 patients (47%) with negative tilt and electrophysiologic testing in this study. These studies clearly support use of the device as a test of last resort, but also call into question the utility of conventional testing.

Subsequent studies have applied the ILR to less problematic patients with less preimplant testing, lowering the likelihood of recurrence of syncope after implant to 30–70% [8–10]. The utility of the ILR in establishing a symptom rhythm correlation has been established in other populations including pediatric and geriatric patients [3,4,8,11–18]. The largest of these studies combined data from 206 patients from three centers [9]. The majority of patients studied had undergone previous non-invasive testing and selective invasive testing including tilt testing and electrophysiologic studies. Symptoms recurred during follow-up in 69% of patients 93 ± 107 days after device implant. An arrhythmia was detected in 22% of patients; sinus rhythm excluding a primary arrhythmia was seen in 42% of patients; and symptoms resolved without recurrence during prolonged monitoring in 31% of patients. Bradycardia was detected more frequently than tachycardia (17% versus 6%), usually leading to pacemaker implantation. Failed activation of the device after spontaneous symptoms occurred in 4% of patients. In these patients, a symptom rhythm correlation was not obtained during the monitoring period. These patients were implanted with an earlier version of the device that did not include the automatic detection feature. No age group had an incidence of bradycardia requiring pacing greater than 30%, suggesting a limited role for empiric pacing in the unexplained syncope population. Multivariate modeling did not identify any significant preimplant predictors of subsequent arrhythmia detection other than a weak association between advancing age and bradycardia.

The ILR has also proved useful in other circumstances. In a study of atypical epilepsy, Zaidi *et al.* [19,20] studied 74 patients with ongoing seizures despite anticonvulsant therapy or unexplained recurrent seizures. They performed cardiac assessment including tilt testing and carotid sinus massage in all patients, and implantation of the ILR in 10 patients. Tilt testing was positive in 27% of patients, and carotid sinus massage was positive in 10%. Two of the 10 patients who subsequently underwent ILR monitoring demonstrated marked bradycardia preceding seizure activity; one resulting from atrioventricular block and the second because of sinus pauses. This study suggested that seizures that are atypical in presentation or response to therapy might have a cardiovascular cause in as many as 42% of patients, supporting an important role for cardiovascular testing including prolonged ECG monitoring in these circumstances.

The ISSUE investigators (International Study on Syncope of Uncertain Etiology) implanted ILRs in three different groups of syncope patients to obtain ECG correlation with spontaneous syncope after conventional testing [21–23]. The first study performed tilt tests in 111 patients with unexplained syncope suspected to be vasovagal, and implanted loop recorders after the tilt test regardless of result. Syncope recurred in 34% of patients in both the tilt-positive and tilt-negative groups, with marked bradycardia or asystole the most common recorded arrhythmia during follow-up (46% and 62%, respectively). The heart rate response during tilt testing did not predict spontaneous heart rate during episodes, with a much higher incidence of asystole noted than expected based on tilt response, where a marked cardioinhibitory response was uncommon. This study suggests that tilt testing is poorly predictive of rhythm findings during spontaneous syncope, and that bradycardia is more common than previously recognized. This study highlights the limitations of tilt testing and has implications for selection of patients with vasovagal syncope who may benefit from cardiac pacing.

The second part of the ISSUE study performed long-term monitoring in 52 patients with syncope and bundle branch block with negative electrophysiologic testing [22]. Syncope recurred in 22 of the 52 patients. Long-term monitoring demonstrated marked bradycardia mainly attributed to complete AV block in 17 patients, while it excluded AV block in two. This study confirmed the previous view that negative electrophysiologic testing does not exclude intermittent complete AV block, and that syncope may be a clue that conduction system disease is progressive.

The third part of the ISSUE study examined the spontaneous rhythm in 35 patients with syncope and structural heart disease who had negative electrophysiologic testing [23]. The underlying heart disease was predominantly ischemic heart disease or hypertrophic cardiomyopathy with moderate but not severe left ventricular dysfunction. Although previous studies have suggested that patients with negative electrophysiologic testing have a better prognosis, there remains concern about the risk of ventricular tachycardia in this group. Importantly, only two of the 35 patients had an ejection fraction less than 30% that would have made them candidates for primary prevention of sudden death, in keeping with the MADIT 2 Trial [24]. Symptoms recurred in 19 of the 35 patients (54%), with bradycardia in four, supraventricular tachyarrhythmias in five, and ventricular tachycardia in only one patient. There were no sudden deaths during 16 ± 11

months of follow-up. This study supports a monitoring strategy in patients with moderate left ventricular dysfunction related to ischemic heart disease when electrophysiologic testing is negative.

Finally, a single-center, prospective, randomized trial compared primary use of the ILR for prolonged monitoring to traditional testing in patients undergoing a cardiac work-up for unexplained syncope [11,25]. Sixty patients (aged 66 ± 14 years, 33 male) with unexplained syncope were randomized to "conventional" testing with an external loop recorder, tilt and electrophysiologic testing, or immediate prolonged monitoring with an ILR for up to 1 year. Patients were offered crossover to the alternate strategy if they remained undiagnosed after their assigned strategy. Patients were excluded if they had a left ventricular ejection fraction less than 35%.

A diagnosis was obtained in 14 of 30 patients randomized to prolonged monitoring, compared with six of 30 undergoing conventional testing (47 versus 20%, $P = 0.029$). Crossover was associated with a diagnosis in one of six patients undergoing initial monitoring, compared to eight of 21 patients who began with conventional testing (17 versus 38%, $P = 0.44$). Bradycardia was detected in 14 patients undergoing monitoring, compared with three patients with conventional testing (40 versus 8%, $P = 0.005$). These data illustrate the limitations of conventional diagnostic techniques for detection of arrhythmia, particularly bradycardia. Although there is potential selection bias in enrollment of patients referred to an electrophysiologist, this study suggests that tilt testing has a modest yield at best when used as a screening test in all patients undergoing investigation for syncope, and confirms that electrophysiologic testing is of very limited utility in patients with preserved left ventricular function. Cost analysis showed that an initial monitoring strategy with the ILR had a higher initial cost, but was more cost effective because of the higher diagnostic yield, reducing cost per diagnosis by 26% [25].

Loop recorder outcome

All reports using the ILR have suggested a low incidence of life-threatening arrhythmia or significant morbidity during follow-up. This verifies the generally good prognosis of recurrent unexplained syncope in the absence of severe left ventricular dysfunction or when electrophysiologic testing is negative, and supports the safety of a monitoring strategy. Syncope resolves during long-term monitoring in almost one-third of patients despite frequent episodes prior to implantation of the loop recorder. This suggests that syncope is frequently self-limited, or reflects a transient physiologic abnormality.

The literature clearly supports the use of the implantable loop recorder in patients with recurrent unexplained syncope who have failed a noninvasive work-up and continue to have syncope. This represents a select group that has been referred for further testing, where ongoing symptoms are likely and a symptom rhythm correlation is a feasible goal. Widespread early use of the ILR is likely to reduce the diagnostic yield as the probability of recurrent syncope is less in "all comers" [6,7,11]. The optimal patient for prolonged monitoring with an external and implantable loop recorder has recurrent symptoms suspicious for arrhythmia; namely, abrupt onset with minimal prodrome, typically brief loss of consciousness, and complete resolution of symptoms within seconds to minutes of the episode. We have historically used a left ventricular ejection fraction of 35% as a cut-off for performing electrophysiologic testing prior to employing a prolonged monitoring strategy. Primary and secondary prevention trials using implantable defibrillators support this strategy [24,26,27].

A recent study that focused on outcome of prolonged monitoring may help to predict the outcome of prolonged monitoring with the ILR. Assar et al. [18] examined the baseline characteristics in 167 patients who received an ILR, and formulated a risk factor score to predict use of the device (Fig. 19.5). Based on these variables, patients can be advised regarding the likelihood of successful monitoring. Unfortunately, this study also illustrates the difficulty in arriving at a diagnosis in elderly patients with infrequent syncope. The subset of 26 patients who were followed after negative monitoring had a 92% syncope-free survival over 24 ± 16 months of follow-up, suggesting that device replacement at the end of battery life is seldom warranted if syncope has not recurred.

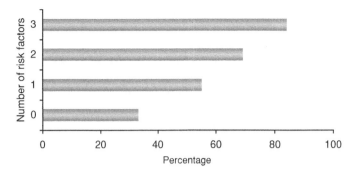

Fig. 19.5 Probability of recurrent symptoms during prolonged monitoring based on a simple risk factor score. Risk factors included age less than 65 years, absence of structural heart disease, and more than three lifetime syncopal episodes. The likelihood of syncope during the implantable loop recorder implant was 33% with no risk factors, 55% with one, 69% with two, and 84% with three. (Adapted from [18].)

Loop recorder use

There may be a low-risk population where an ILR is not warranted. This would include patients without heart disease and with a relatively low burden of syncope, in whom testing has a low yield and the diagnosis is almost certainly benign [7]. A key consideration in this circumstance is the preimplant likelihood of a culprit arrhythmia, balanced with the clinical value of recording sinus rhythm (i.e., a "rule out" result). The previously mentioned clinical trials suggest that the device either rules out arrhythmia or does not yield a diagnosis when symptoms resolve in many patients. Loop recorder skeptics consider this to be the "Achilles heel" of the monitoring approach, but this issue clearly exists for any diagnostic strategy when syncope is not recurrent.

Cost considerations are very relevant in the decision to implant a monitor. Cost modeling and recent cost analysis suggests that the device is cost effective after non-invasive testing has been performed when a diagnosis is aggressively sought, comparing favorably with a conventional work-up [25,28,29]. Cost analysis in the RAST study suggested that a monitoring strategy had a higher initial cost, but was more cost effective because of the higher diagnostic yield, reducing cost per diagnosis by 26% [25]. Cost with a primary monitoring strategy was $5875 ± 1159 per diagnosis, compared with $7891 ± 3193 for a conventional approach first ($P = 0.002$). The diagnostic yield after crossover was comparable between the two arms (50 and 47%).

Other uses of implantable monitors

The current implantable loop recorder is a useful tool in management of patients with syncope but it represents only the beginning in an emerging field of long-term physiologic monitoring [30]. Ideally, the device would include a measure of blood pressure, invaluable in the evaluation of bradycardia and possible vasovagal syncope. Sensor development will bring us commercial products capable of monitoring blood pressure, glucose, oxygen saturation, brain function, and many other physiologic parameters [30]. Long-range telemetry with immediate access to the data will allow implantable monitors to be useful not only in diagnosis, but also in optimal management of many chronic disorders. One example of this is detection of ventricular arrhythmias after myocardial infarction in the pilot study of the CARISMA trial [31].

Conclusions

Prolonged monitoring with an implantable loop recorder has significantly improved our ability to obtain symptom rhythm correlation during infrequent symptoms in patients with unexplained syncope. The implantable loop recorder is most useful and cost-effective in patients with infrequent unexplained syncope when non-invasive testing is negative. Further development will create exciting tools for risk stratification and to manage a variety of chronic disorders.

References

1 Krahn AD, Klein GJ, Norris C, Yee R. The etiology of syncope in patients with negative tilt table and electrophysiological testing. *Circulation* 1995;**92**:1819–24.
2 Krahn AD, Klein GJ, Yee R, Norris C. Maturation of the sensed electrogram amplitude over time in a new

subcutaneous implantable loop recorder. *Pacing Clin Electrophysiol* 1997;**20**:1686–90.

3 Krahn AD, Klein GJ, Yee R, Norris C. Final results from a pilot study with an implantable loop recorder to determine the etiology of syncope in patients with negative non-invasive and invasive testing. *Am J Cardiol* 1998; **82**:117–9.

4 Ermis C, Zhu AX, Pham S, *et al.* Comparison of automatic and patient-activated arrhythmia recordings by implantable loop recorders in the evaluation of syncope. *Am J Cardiol* 2003;**92**:815–9.

5 Krahn AD, Klein GJ, Skanes AC, Yee R. Detection of clinically significant asymptomatic arrhythmias with autodetect loop recorders in syncope patients. *Pacing Clin Electrophysiol* 2003;**26**:1070.

6 Garcia-Civera R, Ruiz-Granell R, Morell-Cabedo S, *et al.* Selective use of diagnostic tests in patients with syncope of unknown cause. *J Am Coll Cardiol* 2003;**41**:787–90.

7 Benditt DG, Brignole M. Syncope: is a diagnosis a diagnosis? *J Am Coll Cardiol* 2003;**41**:791–4.

8 Krahn AD, Klein GJ, Yee R, Takle-Newhouse T, Norris C. Use of an extended monitoring strategy in patients with problematic syncope. Reveal Investigators. *Circulation* 1999;**99**:406–10.

9 Krahn AD, Klein GJ, Fitzpatrick A, *et al.* Predicting the outcome of patients with unexplained syncope undergoing prolonged monitoring. *Pacing Clin Electrophysiol* 2002;**25**:37–41.

10 Nierop PR, van Mechelen R, van Elsacker A, Luijten RH, Elhendy A. Heart rhythm during syncope and presyncope: results of implantable loop recorders. *Pacing Clin Electrophysiol* 2000;**23**:1532–8.

11 Krahn AD, Klein GJ, Yee R, Skanes AC. Randomized assessment of syncope trial: conventional diagnostic testing versus a prolonged monitoring strategy. *Circulation* 2001;**104**:46–51.

12 Kenny RA, Krahn AD. Implantable loop recorder: evaluation of unexplained syncope. *Heart* 1999;**81**:431–3.

13 Alboni P, Brignole M, Menozzi C, *et al.* Diagnostic value of history in patients with syncope with or without heart disease. *J Am Coll Cardiol* 2001;**37**:1921–8.

14 Armstrong VL, Lawson J, Kamper AM, Newton J, Kenny RA. The use of an implantable loop recorder in the investigation of unexplained syncope in older people. *Age Ageing* 2003;**32**:185–8.

15 Donateo P, Brignole M, Menozzi C, *et al.* Mechanism of syncope in patients with positive adenosine triphosphate tests. *J Am Coll Cardiol* 2003;**41**:93–8.

16 Mason PK, Wood MA, Reese DB, Lobban JH, Mitchell MA, DiMarco JP. Usefulness of implantable loop recorders in office-based practice for evaluation of syncope in patients with and without structural heart disease. *Am J Cardiol* 2003;**92**:1127–9.

17 Rossano J, Bloemers B, Sreeram N, Balaji S, Shah MJ. Efficacy of implantable loop recorders in establishing symptom-rhythm correlation in young patients with syncope and palpitations. *Pediatrics* 2003;**112**:E228–33.

18 Assar MD, Krahn AD, Klein GJ, Yee R, Skanes AC. Optimal duration of monitoring in patients with unexplained syncope. *Am J Cardiol* 2003;**92**:1231–3.

19 Zaidi A, Clough P, Cooper P, Scheepers B, Fitzpatrick AP. Misdiagnosis of epilepsy: many seizure-like attacks have a cardiovascular cause. *J Am Coll Cardiol* 2000;**36**:181–4.

20 Zaidi A, Clough P, Mawer G, Fitzpatrick A. Accurate diagnosis of convulsive syncope: role of an implantable subcutaneous ECG monitor. *Seizure* 1999;**8**:184–6.

21 Moya A, Brignole M, Menozzi C, *et al.* Mechanism of syncope in patients with isolated syncope and in patients with tilt-positive syncope. *Circulation* 2001;**104**:1261–7.

22 Brignole M, Menozzi C, Moya A, *et al.* Mechanism of syncope in patients with bundle branch block and negative electrophysiological test. *Circulation* 2001;**104**:2045–50.

23 Menozzi C, Brignole M, Garcia-Civera R, *et al.* Mechanism of syncope in patients with heart disease and negative electrophysiologic test. *Circulation* 2002;**105**:2741–5.

24 Moss AJ, Zareba W, Hall WJ, *et al.* Prophylactic implantation of a defibrillator in patients with myocardial infarction and reduced ejection fraction. *N Engl J Med* 2002;**346**:877–83.

25 Krahn AD, Klein GJ, Yee R, Hoch JS, Skanes AC. Cost implications of testing strategy in patients with syncope: randomized assessment of syncope trial. *J Am Coll Cardiol* 2003;**42**:495–501.

26 Mushlin AI, Hall WJ, Zwanziger J, *et al.* The cost-effectiveness of automatic implantable cardiac defibrillators: results from MADIT. Multicenter Automatic Defibrillator Implantation Trial. *Circulation* 1998;**97**: 2129–35.

27 Buxton AE, Lee KL, Fisher JD, Josephson ME, Prystowsky EN, Hafley G. A randomized study of the prevention of sudden death in patients with coronary artery disease. Multicenter Unsustained Tachycardia Trial Investigators. *N Engl J Med* 1999;**341**:1882–90.

28 Krahn AD, Klein GJ, Yee R, Manda V. The high cost of syncope: cost implications of a new insertable loop recorder in the investigation of recurrent syncope. *Am Heart J* 1999;**137**:870–7.

29 Simpson CS, Krahn AD, Klein GJ, *et al.* A cost effective approach to the investigation of syncope: relative merit of different diagnostic strategies. *Can J Cardiol* 1999;**15**:579–84.

30 Klein GJ, Krahn AD, Yee R, Skanes AC. The implantable loop recorder: the herald of a new age of implantable monitors. *Pacing Clin Electrophysiol* 2000;**23**:1456.

31 Huikuri HV, Mahaux V, Bloch-Thomsen PE. Cardiac arrhythmias and risk stratification after myocardial infarction: results of the CARISMA pilot study. *Pacing Clin Electrophysiol* 2003;**26**:416–9.

CHAPTER 20

Driving and syncope

Brian Olshansky, MD, *& Blair P. Grubb,* MD

"I want to die peacefully in my sleep like my grandfather did, not screaming like the passengers who were in his car."
George Burns

Syncope and driving: the issues

Motor vehicle accidents are a leading cause of death and disability [1]. While it may appear self-evident that syncope and driving do not mix, patients who pass out often want to drive. This can be a source of conflict between physician and patient. The freedom to drive is enjoyed by adults worldwide and, while perceived as a luxury by some, it is felt to be a necessity by others. For those who reside in North America and much of Europe, the inability to drive can be so confining it can be considered a form of complete disability. For many, any driving restrictions may be viewed as barbaric. Amputation may be more acceptable because driving may not be restricted.

Recurrent syncope can be disabling and may produce functional impairment similar to chronic debilitating diseases such as rheumatoid arthritis, which can severely restrict social, educational, and occupational activities [2]. Not infrequently, even if a physician attempts to restrict a patient's driving, the patient will continue to drive or may seek the opinion of another physician [3]. Indeed, the conflict over the "right" to drive may severely compromise the patient–doctor relationship and cause the patient to go "doctor shopping" until he or she finds one willing to place less restrictions on activities. The patient may simply ignore the physician's advice and continue to drive. One of our first implantable cardioverter defibrillator (ICD) patients with recurrent malignant ventricular arrhythmias and syncope had a customized license plate stating plainly: "AICD-1." Another had a plate stating: "I VTACH" (Fig. 20.1).

Individuals who experience recurrent, unpredictable periods of loss of consciousness but who continue to drive, risk not only their own lives but lives of others as well. Even a momentary lapse in orientation while driving even under slow and relatively safe conditions may lead to a disaster

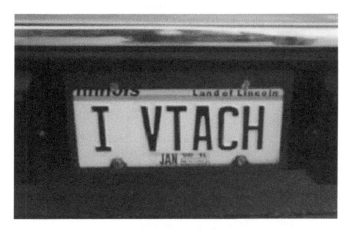

Fig. 20.1 I VTACH.

resulting in injury and death. This unique situation places considerable burden on the physician, who must balance the needs of the patient with those of society and somehow produce recommendations that are appropriate for the patient with syncope.

Arrhythmic conditions that can alter the level of consciousness have been the subject of an organized policy conference. The report was later published as "official" recommendations [4]. These recommendations, not necessarily legally binding, reflect views of a minority with strong opinions on the subject. Subsequent recommendations have been published by the National Transportation and Safety Board [5]. Individuals suffering from advanced congestive heart failure or cardiomyopathy (even if they have not yet passed out) may have a similar risk of cardiac arrest or syncope while driving. This issue has never been considered in a formal way.

Although there is no uniform consensus about syncope, similar conditions that impair driving, such as epilepsy, have been addressed by the creation of legal statutes (see Chapter 21) [6]. These same statutes are often applied to patients with syncope.

Regarding the patient with recurrent syncope who wishes to drive, there are several key issues to the risk the patient has for passing out behind the wheel:

1 What is the likelihood of syncope while driving? What circumstances are related to or precipitate syncope?
2 What is the expected recurrence rate of the syncope? How frequent are the episodes?
3 How much, if any, warning does the patient have before an episode?
4 How long does a typical episode last?
5 How often, how far, and under what circumstances does the patient drive? Is the patient a commercial driver?
6 What are the legal implications of the physician's recommendations?
7 What are the underlying conditions? Do they influence the risk of driving?
8 Is treatment likely to be effective?
9 How likely is the patient to follow the physician's recommendations?

It is important that the treating physician knows the local driving statutes. They are highly variable and continuously subject to change. Some recommendations are shown (Table 20.1). It is likely at the time of publication that restrictions have changed. Updated USA information may be available at: www.aamva.org/Documents/drvSummary OfMedicalAdvisoryBoardPractices.pdf.

This chapter focuses on the problem of syncope and its impact on driving.

Pathophysiology of driving

Although driving is a sedentary activity, operating a motor vehicle can have a major physiologic impact and can exacerbate some underlying medical conditions [7–15]. Mental stress from driving can be substantial [16–19] especially if "road rage" ensues [20]. Like other forms of intense mental stress, driving can provoke ischemia and alter autonomic tone. This is dependent on the driver, driving locale (rush-hour traffic versus driving on an isolated interstate), time of day, abilities and mood of the driver, the use of radar among other factors.

Holter monitors have been applied to drivers to assess heart rate responses [8,17]. Race car driving can increase the heart rate to over 200 b min^{-1}. Heart rates exceeding 140 b min^{-1} can occur even with normal driving. ST segment depression has been observed by continuous Holter recordings in three of 32 normal patients and 13 of 24 patients with known coronary artery disease [8,11,19]. Driving has been associated with extrasystoles but it has not been correlated with sustained tachyarrhythmias or bradyarrhythmias.

For many, driving is one of the most stressful daily activities. The pathophysiologic impact of driving on conditions causing syncope is unknown but driving may conceivably potentiate ischemically mediated or catecholamine-sensitive arrhythmias, among other conditions. The influence of driving on the neurocardiogenic reflex is not well understood.

Epidemiology of driving – causes of crashes

Driving is associated with inherent risk of traffic accidents, crashes, serious injury, and death. This risk continues despite improvements in road safety, innovations in automobile technology, and pristine

Table 20.1 Driving recommendations by state (subject to change [6,158]).

State	Seizure	Syncope	Arrhythmia	Mandatory physician reporting	Physician liable
Alabama	6	6	0	No	No
Alaska	6	6	0	No	Yes
Arizona	3	3	0	No	No
Arkansas	12	0	0	No	Yes
California	3,6,12	Review	Review	Yes	Yes
Colorado	Review	Review	Review	No	No
Connecticut	3	3	0	No	Yes
DC	12	Review	Review	No	Yes
Delaware	Review	0	0	Yes	No
Florida	24	Review	Review	No	No
Georgia	12	12	0	No	No
Hawaii	Review	Review	Review	No	Yes
Idaho	Review	0	0	No	No
Illinois	Review	Review	Review	No	No
Indiana	Review	Review	Review	No	Yes
Iowa[LC]	6	6	6	No	No
Kansas	6	6	Review	No	No
Kentucky	3	3	0	No	No
Louisiana	6	Review	Review	No	No
Maine	3	6	6 (with ICD)	No	No
Maryland	3	3	3	No	No
Massachusetts	6	Review	Review	No	Yes
Michigan[LC]	6	6	0	No	Yes
Minnesota	6	6	0	No	No
Mississippi	12	0	0	No	No
Missouri	6	6	0	No	No
Montana[LC]	Review	Review	0	No	Yes
Nebraska	3	3	0	No	Yes
Nevada	3	3	3	Yes	Yes
New Hampshire	12	Unknown	Unknown	No	Yes
New Jersey	12	12	Review	Yes	No
New Mexico	12	12	0	No	No
New York	12	LC	Review	No	No
North Carolina	6–12	Review	Review	No	No
North Dakota	6	Review	Review	No	No
Ohio	Review	Review	Review	No	No
Oklahoma	12	12	Review	No	No
Oregon	6	6	6–12	Yes	Yes
Pennsylvania	6	Review	Review	Yes	No
Rhode Island	Review	Review	Review	No	No
South Carolina	6	0	0	No	No
South Dakota	12	12	0	No	Yes
Tennessee[LC]	6	0	0	No	Yes
Texas	6	12	6	No	No
Utah	3	3	3	No	No
Vermont	Review	Review	Review	No	Yes
Virginia	6	Review	Review	No	No
Washington	6	6	0	No	Yes
West Virginia	12	12	Review	No	No
Wisconsin	3	Review	Review	No	No
Wyoming	3	3	0	No	Yes

Review, each person is evaluated based on the recommendation of a state medical review board, a non-medical review unit, or the patient's physician.
1991 data. LC, loss of consciousness enacts a specified driving restriction.

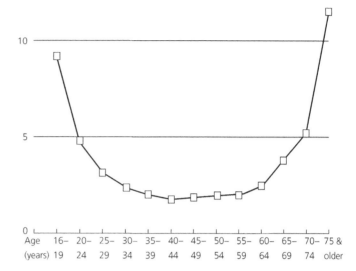

Fig. 20.2 Passenger vehicle driver involvement in fatal crashes per 100 million miles, 1990. Data from The Insurance Institute for Highway Safety. Risks of driving have been positively correlated with young and old age of the driver, previous driving record, time of driving, and conditions of driving. These risks have remained similar over the past few years. Fatal crashes are more related to this than to medical conditions, particularly regarding syncope.

health of drivers. In the USA, each day, 190 million motor vehicles are driven. Nearly 40,000 people die annually from traffic accidents. Many more are injured from the 4000–8000 daily crashes so that 1 of 6800 US drivers dies in an accident each year. In the USA, speeding causes 10,000 accidents a year and, in 2002, 17,419 driving deaths were alcohol-related, costing conservatively $17 billion per year according to the National Highway Traffic Safety Administration. The impaired elderly (often female) and novice (particularly male) drivers are responsible for the greatest share of accidents (Fig. 20.2). These statistics have remained constant over the years.

In a study of driving on the Mexico-Cuernavaca highway, risk of crashes were related to age < 25 years (odds ratio [OR] 3.01), work-related driving (OR 1.74), alcohol intake (OR 4.70), adverse weather (OR 5.70), weekday travel (OR 1.84), daylight driving (OR 4.23), and road direction (OR 2.69) [21]. Medical issues did not contribute to risk.

Drowsiness contributes to 100,000 crashes, 40,000 injuries, and 1550 deaths each year according to the National Sleep Foundation. Crash risk is greater among drivers who felt they were falling asleep (adjusted relative risk [aRR] 14.2) and those who drove longer distances (aRR 2.2 for each additional 100 miles). Crash risk is less for drivers who use highway rest stops (aRR 0.5), drink coffee (aRR 0.5), or play a radio while driving (aRR 0.6) [22].

Distractions cause 25–50% of crashes. In Missouri, driver inattention contributed to 754 accident deaths, 47,064 injuries, and 78,722 instances of property damage in 1998. To document driver distractions and assess the effect of these distractions, inconspicuous video cameras were mounted in 70 volunteers' vehicles. Common distractors are eating and drinking, reaching or looking for an object, manipulating vehicle controls, and activity outside the vehicle [23]. Cell phone use has been linked to crashes. Their use has been curtailed and hand-held phones are now outlawed in several locales [24]. One can only imagine the potential havoc caused by new gadgets such as satellite radios and video players.

The risk of commercial motor vehicle crashes resulting in deaths or serious injury was shown to be double that of passenger vehicles (in Ohio and Pennsylvania). Recently reported data from 200 fatal truck accidents suggests that up to 75% may be caused by careless and erratic driving by other motorists, although this is in dispute (www.general.monash.edu.au/muarc/rptsum/muarc003.pdf). Whether crash rates on toll roads of commercial motor vehicles are higher or lower than those of passenger vehicles appears to depend on the type of crash, specific toll road characteristics, and traffic density [25].

Death behind the wheel

Sudden natural death behind the wheel is unusual and difficult to predict. In a 15-year retrospective German study from 1982 to 1996, 147 drivers died suddenly (13 female, 134 male; mean age 56.8 years; range 20–86 years) out of 34,554 cases of driving deaths. One hundred thirteen had ischemic heart disease. The driver, other passengers, and other road users generally sustained minor injuries otherwise. Minor property damage was the rule. Sudden natural death at the wheel was rare relative to unnatural death at the wheel and not a substantial threat. Screening to exclude high-risk drivers did not prevent sudden natural death at the wheel [26].

Voigt [27] reported 47 cases of death behind the wheel. In 36, the driver stopped the car before dying. Thirty-five deaths resulted in a collision, but injuries were present in only two, and these were minor. These data were corroborated in a report of 871 drivers who died suddenly over 4 years in Baltimore. Over half of drivers stopped their cars before death [28]. Perhaps, even death of a driver is not necessarily a cause for concern. Not all data are consistent.

In a report of 54 individuals who died while driving, 53 of 54 died suddenly [29]. This represents a population of 600 consecutive drivers who died in accidents but had not died before the accident. These data suggest that medical illness leading to death could be the cause of a significant number of car accidents. Nevertheless, intoxicated males aged 20–30 are responsible for the great majority of car accidents, especially causing significant injury.

In another report, 71 of 1348 (5%) coronary deaths occurred while driving [30]. Accidents occurred in 24. In a even larger study, 98 of 9330 (1%) [31] sudden deaths occurred while driving. Based on these and similar data, the actuarial risk of sudden death behind the wheel in the USA has been estimated at 1 in 4.5×10^6 h [32]. The projected net rise in fatal accidents is considered to be 0.001% if *all* individuals were allowed to drive freely.

Medical issues, syncope, and risk of crashes and injury

Medical issues are a minor contributor to overall risk of accidents and crashes. Few cause injury; even fewer accidents are attributable to syncope. It is estimated that < 0.1% of reported accidents are caused by a pre-existing medical condition, the majority of which are cardiac conditions [28,29,33–56]. Fewer than 2% of reported driver sudden deaths or loss of consciousness episodes resulted in injury or death to other road users or bystanders.

Seatbelt usage during, and abstinence from alcohol before, driving has a much greater impact on safety than restricting drivers with syncope. Even so, the cost effectiveness of seatbelts and airbags has been questioned. The cost per life year saved is $69 to $30,000, and with an airbag is $1.6 million [57,58].

Preventing adolescent drivers from driving would reduce a large number of serious accidents but such restriction is considered unfeasible. It is likely that young male and very elderly drivers are not only at higher risk of causing a serious accident than other drivers (Fig. 20.2) but they are more likely to cause an accident than a driver with a history of syncope or one who has a malignant arrhythmia and an ICD.

Many other factors need to be considered [59–88], but syncope is not a major contributor to accidents yet drivers with sporadic loss of consciousness are not treated equally. The risk of driving is dependent on the frequency and the length of the driving. Highway driving and city driving pose different risks [89]. The driving expertise, mood of the individual, and non-cardiac medical conditions have a role in the outcome of driving [16,89].

Rehm and Ross [90,91] prospectively studied drivers involved in road crashes over a 1-year period. Sixty-seven of 84 elderly individuals involved in accidents at a Level I trauma center were deemed at fault. Twelve of the 67 accidents may have been caused by syncope. Fifty-three had significant underlying medical problems; four were intoxicated. Syncope therefore may be a significant cause for serious driving accidents in the elderly but it occurred in the minority.

In 1958, Norman [92] began collecting information on London Transport bus drivers to determine what medical conditions led to accidents [40,93]. Data were subsequently collected to 1972 [93]. In that period, there were 108 incidents of acute illness causing 54 accidents or 1 accident every 115 million miles. This small population is highly select and the accuracy of the data cannot be guaranteed. During that time, syncope of undetermined etiology contributed to 14 of these accidents, of which 10 resulted in a collision. Conditions diagnosed included: vasovagal episodes in 20 causing 12 collisions, transient ischemic attacks in three with one collision, epilepsy in 18 causing 14 collisions. Acute ischemic heart disease was responsible for 32 accidents but only eight resulted in a collision. Most episodes occurred in males over age 50. Regarding drivers of cars, the casualty rates in the 20–29 year age group were 2.5 times that of the 50–59 year age group. This would suggest that acute illness, including syncope, is unlikely to be a major cause of serious accidents.

Assessment of issues surrounding a crash can be difficult. It can be hard to determine if an individual passes out, or simply goes to sleep behind the wheel. Data on the relationship between syncope and driving are difficult to obtain. In the confusion that surrounds an accident, stories are often altered or are confusing. A patient who had a syncopal event may report "falling asleep at the wheel," or vice versa. Amnesia often surrounds the syncopal event. This is especially true if the episode was compounded by associated trauma from the accident. Some drivers, fearful that their license may be revoked, may lie and declare: "I lost control of the car," or "I was trying to beat the red light" in order to hide syncope as the cause. Alternatively, to conceal drug or alcohol use, a driver may claim that an accident was caused by passing out. Reports of transient loss of consciousness may be a ready explanation for other potential, more common, causes for motor vehicle accidents, such as drinking alcohol or clumsiness.

Raffle, in his 1974 paper on bus driving considered risk of driving by following equation:

Risk = hours + route-weight (of the bus) + experience + "unfitness" [93]

While fitness to drive is an important consideration, it appears that unfitness, representing many types of medical conditions, is only a minor aspect and is difficult to quantitate.

The risk of harm to other road users posed by the driver with heart disease has been considered as follows [94]:

Risk of harm = risk by time driving × risk by vehicle type × risk of unconsciousness × risk of a serious accident

The level of risk is relative and for an individual at high risk for sudden cardiac incapacitation, if the driving rates are low enough, it is conceivable that the risk may be less than a truck driver who frequently drives long stretches under adverse circumstances [94].

Grattan and Jeffcoate [95], reviewing 9390 accidents, found that 15 were caused by an acute illness. Six of these were caused by transient loss of consciousness. Herner et al. [41] studied 612 drivers with diabetes, cardiovascular disease, and other problems. Those drivers in the medically ill group had a 4.1% incidence of accidents compared with 7.7% in a "control" group. Forty one of 44,255 road accidents in Sweden were probably caused by illness over a 4-year period but syncope was not a major cause of accidents in these individuals [41]. These results are similar to other European and North American studies, with estimates of 15 in 1000 for non-fatal, and 4 in 1000 for fatal accidents related to medical issues. Similar results were found in other locales [43,96,97].

Hu et al. [98–100] attempted to develop detailed crash prediction models for older drivers and for specific conditions and situations [101]. No attribute explicitly linked the increase in highway crash rates to a medical condition and/or physical limitations. Factors placing female drivers at greater crash risk differed from male drivers. When the analyses controlled for the amount of driving, women living alone or who had back pain had a higher crash risk. Employed men who scored low on word-recall tests, had glaucoma, or used antidepressants had a higher crash risk. Syncope was not even mentioned as a risk.

Stewart et al. [102] evaluated 1431 ambulatory elderly individuals participating in the Florida Geriatric Research Program [103]. A control group consisted of 1289 individuals who were not involved in crashes during the 5-year period. There were 142 individuals involved in crashes. Commonly used drugs, memory loss, age, and gender were not associated with crashes. The most important symptoms associated with an increased likelihood of older drivers being involved in vehicle crashes were cold feeling in the feet and legs, a high level of protein in the urine, and an irregular heart beat [102]. Bursitis was identified as the only chronic disease that contributed to a higher risk of crashing (RR > 2.0).

Marottoli *et al.* [104], studying 283 drivers aged 72 years and older in Connecticut, found 13% reported a crash, a moving violation, or were stopped by police in 1 year. In a multivariable analysis (adjusting for driving frequency and housing type), poor design copying on the Mini-Mental State Examination (RR 2.7; 95% CI 1.5–5.0), fewer blocks walked (RR 2.3; CI 1.3–4.0), and more foot abnormalities (RR 1.9; CI 1.1–3.3) were associated with these preselected outcomes.

In a report from Seattle [105], risk of injury from driving was 2.6-fold higher in older diabetic drivers, especially those treated with insulin (OR 5.8), and those with both diabetes and coronary heart disease (OR 8.0). Increased risk with coronary artery disease (OR 1.4), depression (OR 1.7), alcohol abuse (OR 2.1), or falls (OR 1.4) may have arisen by chance alone.

Koepsell *et al.* [105] found that older diabetic drivers who were treated with insulin were at a sixfold higher crash risk and those treated with oral hypoglycemics were at a threefold increased risk. Drivers with diabetes and coronary heart disease were eight times more likely to be in vehicle crashes than those without. The impact of diabetes has been questioned in other studies [106] and was not considered great enough to warrant further restrictions on driving privileges.

Koepsell *et al.* [105] examined neurologic conditions that can impair sensation, cognition, or motor function including cerebrovascular disease (stroke, transient ischemic attacks, or both), syncope, dizziness, seizures, head injury, dementia, and subdural hematoma. The authors did not find that any of these conditions were associated with significantly larger crash risk.

As part of the Iowa Rural Health Study, 1854 individuals over age 67 formed the basis of a study on vehicle crashes [107,108]. Using a Cox proportional hazards regression model to calculate the age- and gender-adjusted odds ratio for each of the selected risk factors, no chronic disease (myocardial infarction, stroke, diabetes, or arthritis) was significantly correlated with vehicle crashes. Drivers taking non-steroidal anti-inflammatory drugs (but no other medication) were 80% more likely to be involved in crashes. In another report, antidepressants and opioid analgesics taken by older drivers was associated with increased risk for injurious motor vehicle collisions but there was no evidence of a dose-related effect [109]. The issue continues to be a concern and has not been examined fully [63,110,111].

While common sense would dictate that elderly patients with dementia and visual and hearing losses are at greater risk for accidents, ironically, individuals with these conditions are not subject to restrictions [112]. It appears from available evidence that this group does not provide a greater risk on the road than the general cross-section of drivers [49]. Perhaps better screening methods are needed [113]. Another concern is the elderly affluent, who may live longer but with more impairments and disabilities, creating a new danger on the road [114]. This is especially surprising regarding the demented patient. Because cognitive impairment can confound the diagnosis of syncope [115], it is even possible that a demented patient with syncope be allowed to drive simply because the history of syncope was not obtained [116]. There are even those who strongly support the continued driving of demented patients [117].

Causes of syncope while driving

An individual who has a history of syncope (or, in Department of Motor Vehicle vernacular, transient loss of consciousness) may be at increased risk for driving. The cause of loss of consciousness is important. This issue has been most notably addressed regarding epilepsy [35,118–123]. Unfortunately, in many locales, syncope and epilepsy are often considered similarly with respect to driving and driving restrictions. In a patient who has an ICD for malignant ventricular arrhythmias, the risk varies based on the type of arrhythmia or indication for which the ICD was implanted, the underlying cardiac condition, the hemodynamic response to the arrhythmia, and the patient's reaction to a shock [124–130].

Table 20.2 Evaluation of syncope while driving (without syncope history).

Events surrounding the episode
Is it clearly syncope? Is it seizure?
How many episodes?
What were the circumstances?
What are the triggers?
Was there a prodrome?
Are there underlying medical conditions?
Was the patient taking medications? Drugs? Alcohol?
Was there a crash?
Were there injuries?
Was there head trauma?
Were there witnesses?

Physical examination
Cardiac or neurologic findings?
Carotid massage?

Testing
Depends on the history and physical
Tilt table testing
Electrophysiology testing
Monitoring

In a patient who has syncope, estimates of the risk of recurrent syncope behind the wheel may be 0.02% [40]. The Canadian Cardiovascular Society estimated the risk of death and injury to others caused by syncope while driving was acceptable at 0.005% [131,132]. This is partly determined by the type of driving, the length of driving, and the underlying condition.

Based on 2000 road accidents reported by police in the UK, collapse at the wheel was most commonly caused by epilepsy in 38%; heart disease accounted for 8%; and unexplained blackouts accounted for 22%. Approximately one-quarter of those with a cardiac cause for collapse were previously not diagnosed with a cardiac condition [1].

Syncope from any of a long list of causes can occur while driving but some forms of syncope are less likely in the sitting position (e.g., neurocardiogenic syncope and syncope caused by aortic stenosis), while others may be more likely (e.g., carotid hypersensitivity when turning the head to look back, a classic cause for syncope while driving). Any cause for alteration in consciousness during driving, including supraventricular tachycardia, ventricular tachycardia, cough syncope, vasovagal syncope, or any other cause, will increase the risk of motor vehicle accidents [133–135]. Likely, most episodes of syncope that occur with driving will

never be fully or correctly diagnosed. Information gleaned from the history and ancillary testing provides only a presumptive diagnosis, yet it provides important clues. Table 20.2 addresses an evaluation approach.

Neurocardiogenic syncope

Neurocardiogenic syncope tends to occur in an upright position but it can occur while driving. The incidence of arrhythmic and neurocardiogenic syncope while driving was assessed by Blitzer *et al.* [136] in a retrospective analysis of 71 patients. A presumptive diagnosis for impaired consciousness was made in 57 of 71 patients (80%) based on clinical findings and test results. Vasovagal syncope was diagnosed in 21 patients (30%) in whom a suggestive history was supported by a positive tilt-table test result. Eighteen patients (25%) had supraventricular tachycardia induced during electrophysiologic study. Ventricular tachycardia was confirmed in 12 patients (17%). In six patients, ventricular tachycardia was found upon interrogation of their cardiac defibrillators after the accident. In another six patients, ventricular tachycardia was induced at electrophysiologic study. Advanced atrioventricular block was documented in seven patients (10%), vestibular disease in one patient, and a seizure in one patient who had a negative electrophysiologic study result and a positive 24-h ambulatory electro-encephalograph. Three patients had a positive tilt-table test as well as inducible supraventricular tachycardia at electrophysiologic study and were included in both of the previously mentioned categories.

In another report [137], of 245 consecutive patients undergoing tilt table testing, 23 (9%) had syncope during driving. Tilt table testing was positive in 19 and negative in four patients. Most passed out several times before finally passing out with driving. Injury during driving occurred in nine of the 23 patients with one incident causing the driver's death. During follow-up (51 ± 26 months), one patient had another syncope-related driving incident.

Sheldon and Koshman [138] evaluated 217 adult patients with syncope suspected to be caused by a neurocardiogenic mechanism. Seven patients stopped driving after their first syncopal spell. One individual had an estimated 6000 spells but never had a motor vehicle accident! The remaining 209 patients, mean age 42, had a median of four syncopal episodes before being evaluated with tilt table testing. Five of 6988 patients lost consciousness while driving, of whom four had motor vehicle accidents and two caused driver injury. No one was killed and no bystanders were injured. Sheldon and Koshman [138] estimated the risk of syncope was 0.33% per driver per year. The risk of harm from a crash related to neurocardiogenic syncope was even less, 2 per 1534 per year or 0.13% per year. Based on time spent driving, there should have been 280 instead of five syncopal spells, suggesting that driving is a low-risk activity for neurocardiogenic syncope.

Sheldon and Koshman [138] suspected that counseling and proper treatment might reduce the risk of syncope while driving by 90% so that the risk may be low as 0.026%, an acceptable risk. While the risk may be low, they considered that, if there are recurrent symptoms and especially if there is no prodrome for syncope, driving should be restricted for at least 3 months [138]. This number is similar to restrictions placed on driving in several states lasting a mean of 4.3 ± 4.9 months.

Malignant arrhythmias and devices therapy

Brady- and tachyarrhythmias can cause syncope and, if they occur during driving, motor vehicle accidents. With proper treatment, however, the risk of collapse behind the wheel is low.

Sowton [139] reviewed several reports and personnel communications concerning driving in patients with permanent pacemakers for brady-cardia over 30 years ago. Even based on the data of the times, not considering the major advances in pacemakers (and refinements of the indications to implant), it appears that patients with pacemakers are not at substantially increased risk of motor vehicle accidents. Based on the data of the time, it did not appear that pacemakers or conditions for which pacemakers were placed (after placement) were associated with motor vehicle accidents [139,140].

Several studies have addressed the risk of driving in patients with malignant ventricular arrhythmias in the modern era. Kou et al. [141] found that 16 of 180 patients with an ICD from which they had a shock had lost consciousness (13 had syncope and three died). Absence of syncope during one shock did not predict absence of syncope during subsequent shocks. In this population, age, sex, history of syncope, left ventricular function, type of underlying heart disease, electrophysiologic findings, rate of ventricular tachycardia, or antiarrhythmic medications did not predict subsequent syncope. The authors recommended that patients with an ICD who drive should be "extra vigilant" [141].

DiCarlo et al. [142] evaluated driving restrictions in a Midwestern ICD population. Fifty-three percent of responding cardiologists advised only those who had arrhythmia-initiated presyncope or collapse to cease driving. The remainder advised all implanted patients to stop driving. Most cardiologists recommended temporary driving abstinence for 2–12 (mean 6 ± 3) months for these patients.

Bansch et al. [143] evaluated patients with ICDs retrospectively to assess the incidence of syncope and implications regarding driving. Of 421 patients, 62 had syncope and survival free of syncope was 90%, 85% and 81% at 12, 24 and 36 months, respectively. An impaired left ventricular ejection fraction, induction of fast ventricular tachycardia during electrophysiology test, and atrial fibrillation were associated with increased risk for syncope. These parameters may help identify which ICD patients are at higher risk for syncope after ICD implantation and at risk on the road. The problem now is even more complex with prophylactic ICD implantation without even the presence of clinically documented ventricular tachycardia.

Conti *et al.* [129] examined driving patterns of patients at risk for arrhythmic death who underwent an ICD implant. Surveys, distributed to 742 US doctors involved with ICD management, were returned by 452. Twenty-five doctors reported 30 accidents related to ICD shocks over 12 years (1980–92). Nine accidents were fatal, involving eight ICD patients and one passenger. There were 21 non-fatal accidents. The estimated fatality rate, of 7.5 per 100,000 patient-years for patients with an ICD, was markedly lower than that of the general population (18.4 per 100,000 patient-years; $P < 0.05$). The estimated injury rate, 17.6 per 100,000 patient-years, was substantially lower than that for the general public (2224 per 100,000 patient-years; $P < 0.05$).

The AVID (Antiarrhythmic drug Versus Implantable Defibrillator) trial evaluated patients with poorly tolerated, malignant ventricular arrhythmias randomized to medical versus ICD therapy. Of 627 patients who had driven within 1 year before enrollment, 57% reported resuming driving within 3 months and 88% within 12 months [3]. Physicians discussed driving restriction with 403 of the 627 patients and generally recommended 6–11 months restriction. Of 559 who resumed driving, 2% reported syncope while driving, 11% had dizziness or palpitations necessitating stopping the vehicle, and 22% dizziness or palpitations that did not require stopping. Of 295 patients with ICDs, 8% received a shock while driving. No shock caused an accident. Fifty-five accidents occurred (mean follow-up 35 months) for an annual accident risk of 3.4% and an annual risk for an apparent arrhythmia-related accident of 0.4%. In comparison, 6.2% reported having an accident the year before diagnosis versus a 7.1% annual accident rate among all US drivers. Accident rates did not differ by randomization (antiarrhythmic drugs versus ICD) [3].

In another analysis from the same trial [144], younger, college-educated men and those whose arrhythmia was ventricular tachycardia were most likely to resume driving < 6 months after initiation of therapy. Patients with an ICD did not appear to resume driving later than those taking an antiarrhythmic drug alone.

For patients with malignant arrhythmias, whether or not an ICD is placed, the risk of driving and causing an accident is probably similar to a teenage male driver. Ironically, other disease conditions can impact on driving to a greater extent, including bursitis [12,14,76–82,145–148].

Several concerns have been raised about the risks of allowing patients with ICDs to drive and some have suggested long or permanent driving bans for ICD patients [126]. These risks have been incorporated in European guidelines [149] and are considered in American Heart Association/North American Society of Pacing and Electrophysiology (AHA/NASPE) recommendations [4].

Larsen *et al.* [128] found that at 6 months, the incidence of recurrent ICD shocks levels off for patients with malignant arrhythmias and ICD implant. Some patients who have malignant arrhythmias declare early after device implantation that they are at high risk for an ICD shock. Others do not easily fit into this category. As there is always the possibility of loss of consciousness with the development, even transiently, of a ventricular arrhythmia, many physicians restrict patients with ICDs temporarily or even prematurely. Alternatively, many ICD devices are being placed in relatively asymptomatic patients based on their long-term risk. Many patients now enjoy additional longevity with an ICD placed prophylactically with no history of a malignant arrhythmia. Such a patient may not require any driving restriction at all. If ICD shocks do occur, it may be prudent at that point to restrict activity but, even in this situation, syncope might or, more likely, might not occur.

Case 1
A 67-year-old man driving down the road found himself in his car in a stream alongside the road. The patient had a history of an ischemic cardiomyopathy and a left bundle branch block. At electrophysiologic testing, he had inducible ventricular tachycardia as well as evidence for infra-Hisian block. An ICD was placed with back-up ventricular pacing. Driving was restricted for 6 months then, as he remained without symptoms, driving was allowed.

Only eight states have specific regulations regarding syncope resulting from ventricular arrhythmias.

Driving restrictions

Linzer *et al.* [150] showed that syncope leads to restriction in daily activities in up to 76% of individuals. Sixty-four percent will have some restriction on driving, in part because of physician recommendations and in part because of self-restriction. This is appropriate if syncopal episodes are frequent and likely to occur unexpectedly while driving.

Recommendations for driving depend on the suspected cause for syncope. It may not be appropriate to restrict driving activities for a patient with an arrhythmic cause for syncope if the problem is completely treated. For example, if a patient had lost consciousness because of asystole from complete heart block but this problem is treated effectively with a pacemaker, after proper recovery from the implant further restriction appears unwarranted.

Case 2

A 56-year-old man has recurrent syncope associated with marked bradycardia (> 5 s pauses) and hypotension 1–2 weeks after prostate surgery. He has never had syncope before.

Should he be permitted to go back to work to drive children in his school bus?

The answer is still not clear but, if he lived in Maine, the law states: "School Bus Endorsement is necessary for an individual to drive a school bus carrying 10 or more passengers. This requires a doctor's certification that the person presents no risk. However, should such an individual have a seizure-related accident, the doctor may be held liable for any result." It is crucial that the physician know the law.

On the other hand, most patients who pass out have, at best, a suspected cause for syncope or a cause that is multifactorial. In such a case, it is prudent to have the patient not drive for a period to assess the adequacy of treatment. Firm recommendations regarding this time limit are difficult to quantitate and must be considered on a case-by-case basis.

Considering the diverse causes for syncope, precedents for driving restriction focus on specific clinical situations. Often, data are lacking to substantiate even these recommendations. Some recommendations are based on guidelines for patients with seizure disorders; others are based on data for patients with malignant arrhythmias.

What are the medical data?

Lurie *et al.* [151] queried physicians who specialize arrhythmia management from nine countries regarding their approach to the evaluation and treatment of vasovagal syncope. Sixty-six physicians responding to the survey had treated > 11,500 patients with vasovagal syncope. Tilt table testing was used by 98% of physicians. The mean recommended without driving was 54 ± 10 days (range 0–365 days; median 7 days). Most physicians (82%) ultimately allowed driving, but driving privileges would need to be considered on a case-by-case basis. Approximately 20% indicated a 6–12-month event-free period before allowing driving. They were more cautious for commercial drivers. Nine respondents followed at least one patient who had at least one accident resulting from recurrent syncope after initial evaluation. In only 17 instances were accidents caused by syncope after starting therapy (prevalence among treated patients 0.1–0.2%).

Current AHA/NASPE recommendations for persons with vasovagal syncope range from grade "A" (no restriction) to "C" (driving prohibited) based on symptom severity and whether the patient operates a private or commercial vehicle [4].

Case 3

An 82-year-old man has episodes of profound fatigue and near-syncope. An electrocardiogram (ECG) shows complete heart block with a response rate of 35 b min^{-1}. A permanent pacemaker was placed. He quickly becomes pacemaker-dependent. Is it safe for him to drive?

It would be safe for this patient to drive after it is clear that the pacemaker lead is stable. It may be worth restricting this patient for a few weeks at most.

Case 4

A 17-year-old female athlete has just started college. She has recurrent syncope without an obvious prodrome. A tilt table test is positive at 10 min reproducing her symptoms. She wants to drive like all her friends. What do you recommend?

Consider a young patient with vasodepressor syncope. For one episode of loss of consciousness, driving restriction may be harsh and inappropriate, but there is a spectrum to consider in this regard. For a patient with "malignant" neurocardiogenic syncope in whom a tilt table test is positive, and the episodes occur without obvious cause, driving restriction, at least temporarily, may be appropriate.

Patients with a single unexplained episode of syncope, despite a complete and appropriate evaluation, have a low incidence of recurrence, perhaps < 20% in the next several years. Such a patient cannot be restricted from driving unless episodes recur and are relatively frequent.

Case 5

A 55-year-old truck driver, after a hard night of drinking, falls face first into his oatmeal. A tilt table test was markedly positive at 5 min. He undergoes therapy with a beta-blocker. He drives toxic waste around the city in a truck as part of his job. Do you let him drive . . . ever? He has been taking disopyramide and β-adrenergic blocker for 5 years, continues to drive as part of his job, and has never passed out again.

Perhaps a 3–6-month period of driving restriction would seem to be appropriate for patients with recurrent neurocardiogenic syncope, but this depends on the clinical situation. The risk of recurrence of syncope is rare considering the recurrence rate and the time behind the wheel. The patient was allowed to return to work after 6 months with no syncope. He has been driving in Chicago for the past 10 years without recurrence. The issue now is can the medications be stopped?

Case 6

A 78-year-old man has syncope, a dilated cardiomyopathy, and undergoes an electrophysiology test that shows inducible sustained ventricular tachycardia. An ICD is implanted but a recommendation is made that he wait 6 months to drive. He does not drive for 6 months but then starts driving. He receives an occasional ICD shock without loss of consciousness. Then, 6 years later, he loses consciousness while driving followed by an ICD shock. He drives into a tree, narrowly missing children sledding down a hill nearby.

This case highlights the fact that patients with ICDs are always at risk of passing out even after a 6-month window in which they appear stable. The medical conditions can change and by change alone an episode of ventricular tachycardia can occur while driving. In retrospect, the patient should have been allowed to drive but the issue of driving after

the episode must be considered very carefully. It is unlikely that this patient will be able to drive safely for quite some time. However, this depends on the evaluation. A complete evaluation showed that the patient had developed severe three-vessel coronary artery disease and worsening left ventricular function. Likely, this was the cause for the episode. Only if the problems can be resolved can the patient be allowed to drive.

The American Medical Association has adopted "H-140.925: Impaired Drivers and Their Physicians," which states that physicians have an ethical responsibility to assess physical or mental impairments that might affect driving. If necessary, physicians should use their best judgment when deciding when to report a patient to the Department of Motor Vehicles [152].

The European task force guidelines for driving and heart disease state that a person with recurrent syncope should be advised not to drive until a cause has been identified and symptoms are controlled. This poses a problem not only for the 13–41% of patients in whom the cause of syncope cannot be established, but also for most other patients because the accuracy of risk estimates and the treatment options are rather limited [149,153,154].

What are the legal data?

Driving restrictions vary from state to state. Rarely is the term "syncope" used to explicitly restrict driving. Most states use the terms, "seizure," "loss of consciousness or loss of voluntary control," "blackouts or loss of consciousness or body control," "lapses of consciousness," "episodes of marked confusion," or "loss of consciousness or any loss of ability to control a motor vehicle." These terms also vary by country (cerebral ischemia is used in the Canadian literature).

It is important for physicians caring for patients to know what the local laws are and what their responsibilities are concerning individual patients. These laws are continuously subject to change. Between 1988 and 2000, 28 states changed their restrictions on driving for patients with seizures. They generally liberalized their restrictions or adopted specific seizure-free intervals when none existed previously. Thirteen states reduced their seizure-free restrictions from 12 months to 3 months (four states) or 6 months (nine states) [6].

In some states, it is considered an imposition of the right to privacy for a physician to notify the Motor Vehicle Bureau about a patient who may pass out behind the wheel, or be likely to sustain a motor vehicle accident because of an underlying heart, or other, medical condition. In other states, however, it is mandatory that the physician report the patient to the Department of Motor Vehicles even without specific permission from a patient.

Alternatively, there have been no prosecutions of physicians for negligence in reporting an individual who may be at risk to drive a car. Further, no specific guidelines exist regarding syncope or transient loss of consciousness even though there are guidelines for patients who have seizure disorders and these guidelines are becoming less stringent.

Reporting disorders that could cause syncope vary from state to state. In most cases, a driver at risk needs to have a form completed by a physician if the driver is considered a risk for driving based on temporary lapses in consciousness. For most states, it is not the physician's responsibility to report a driver without the permission or knowledge of the driver, but the laws are not completely clear on this in all states.

In Illinois, the law (the Motor Vehicle Code) states that it is the duty of every driver who has a medical condition likely to cause loss of consciousness or has any loss of ability to safely operate a motor vehicle driver, within 10 days of becoming aware of such a condition, to report this to the Illinois Department of Motor Vehicles. Then a form is sent to the responsible physician who must fill it out. A review board assesses the ability of the driver to continue to drive. While under no obligation, and at no risk to him or herself, a physician may report an individual patient in Illinois who may be at risk of driving.

In California, the law is:

> "103900. Every physician and surgeon shall report immediately to the local health officer in writing, the name, date of birth, and address of every patient at least 14 years of age or older whom the physician and surgeon has diagnosed as having a case of a disorder characterized by lapses of consciousness. However, if a physician and surgeon reasonably and in good faith believes that the reporting of a

patient will serve the public interest, he or she may report a patient's condition even if it may not be required under the department's definition of disorders characterized by lapses of consciousness pursuant to subdivision."

In Ontario, an episode of syncope leads to a 1-month driving suspension, but if episodes recur in a year driving is suspended for 12 months [155]. A physician is obligated to provide a report on any patient who has a condition that could make it unsafe to drive. In Canada, legislation in seven of 10 provinces and all three territories requires that all physicians must report to the regulatory authorities all patients who may pose a risk on the road because of their medical condition (the remaining jurisdictions have discretionary reporting systems) [94].

There are several concerns with the present laws voiced regarding seizure but also applicable to patients with syncope [156]:

1 Seizure is often equated to syncope even though the conditions are not the same. Issues regarding epilepsy and driving are better addressed and more easily addressed than issues related to syncope [121].

2 Legalities regarding the role of the physician to allow or not allow a patient to drive with syncope are not completely clear in any venue. Licensing is not in the purview of the physician and yet the physician is often strapped with making legal decisions about patients.

3 It is not clear that physicians should step outside their roles to make binding legal decisions and take responsibility for what may happen if a patient drives.

4 Patients should be required to report syncope to the motor vehicle department; the physician should have the right to report, with immunity, a patient who has not reported him or herself and is putting the public at risk.

5 Physicians should have immunity for reporting or not reporting a patient. The right and need for a physician to report a patient against his or her will or without his or her knowledge may impair confidentiality and have an impact on the physician–patient relationship.

Restrictions vary substantially between Europe and the USA. Whether similar guidelines can be applied to other patients with syncope is uncertain but probably inappropriate.

Table 20.3 Driving recommendations for syncope patients. (Data from [131] and [132].)

Condition	Private driving	Commercial driving
Single episode of syncope	No restriction	No restriction
Diagnosed/treated cause, i.e., pacer for bradycardia	Waiting period 1 week	Waiting period 1 month
Situational syncope, avoidable trigger, e.g., micturition	Successful treatment of underlying condition	Successful treatment of underlying condition
Reversible cause, e.g., hemorrhage, dehydration	Waiting period 1 week	Waiting period 1 week
Single episode of unexplained syncope	Waiting period 1 month	Waiting period 12 months
Recurrent vasovagal syncope (within 12 months)		
Recurrent unexplained syncope (within 12 months)	Waiting period 12 months	Waiting period 12 months
Documented or inducible tachyarrhythmia	Depends on arrhythmia and treatment	Depends on arrhythmia and treatment

Table 20.4 Permanent pacemakers. (Data from [131] and [132].)

Private driving	Commercial driving
Waiting period 1 week	Waiting period 1 month
No cerebral ischemia after implant	No cerebral ischemia after implant
Normal sensing and capture on ECG	Normal sensing and capture on ECG
No evidence of pacemaker malfunction	No evidence of pacemaker malfunction

ECG, electrocardiogram.

Most physicians do not know their local state laws [127].

Recommendations

It is hard to find a well-constructed series of guidelines for patients who are at risk for having syncope while driving and what the proper restrictions should be. The Canadian authorities have devised an excellent (perhaps the best) series of guidelines that should be considered reasonable for any driver and any country, based on the most updated information. The Canadian Consensus is also updated regularly. It is useful to consult this information when considering restrictions for patients. The most recent information from the Canadian Consensus is included in Tables 20.3–20.9 [131,132].

Are restrictions followed by patients?

Maas *et al.* [157] brought to bear the reality that restriction guidelines will have no impact if they are not followed. Of 104 syncope patients, 95 were counseled not to drive (82 of 95 remembered this 6 months later) but continued to drive. Three of 104 had syncope while driving and one had a minor crash. After having syncope, only seven of 104 drivers stopped driving themselves and two stopped based on doctor recommendations. Within 1 year, syncope recurred in 19 after a median of 59 days. Syncope resulted in injury to one patient and another had syncope while driving but no crash. It appears that patients rarely follow driving recommendations and, even though they do not and continue to drive, risk remains low. Other studies confirm these data [158].

What are the specifics from the Department of Motor Vehicles?

When considering documentation sent to the Department of Motor Vehicles in the USA, several issues exist. In six states, physicians are required to report drivers to the licensing agency, and in three of these physicians who fail to report can be held

Table 20.5 Implantable cardioverter defibrillators (ICDs). (Data from [131] and [132].)

Condition	Private driving	Commercial driving
Primary prophylaxis. NYHA Functional Class I–III	Waiting period 4 weeks	Disqualified
Secondary prophylaxis for VT/VF with associated cerebral ischemia. NYHA Functional Class I–III	Waiting period 6 months	Disqualified
ATP therapy delivered by the ICD, not associated with cerebral ischemia if ATP does not speed VT and total VT duration < 30 s	No additional restriction	Disqualified
ATP therapy associated with cerebral ischemia or ATP speeding VT or ATP fails to stop VT in < 30 s or ICD shock delivery	Additional 6 month restriction	Disqualified

ATP, antitachycardia pacing; ICD, implantable cardioverter defibrillator; NYHA, New York Heart Association; VF, ventricular fibrillation; VT, ventricular tachycardia.

Table 20.6 Ventricular arrhythmia. (Data from [131] and [132].)

Condition	Private driving	Commercial driving
VF	Waiting period 6 months	Disqualified
VT with associated cerebral ischemia	Waiting period 6 months	Disqualified
VF resulting from a reversible cause	Successful treatment of underlying condition	Successful treatment of underlying condition
Sustained VT with no associated cerebral ischemia; LVEF < 0.40	Waiting period 3 months	Disqualified
Sustained VT with no associated cerebral ischemia; LVEF ≥ 0.40	Satisfactory control	Waiting period 3 months
Non-sustained VT with no associated cerebral ischemia; LVEF ≥ 0.40	No restriction	No restriction
Non-sustained VT with no associated cerebral ischemia; LVEF > 0.40	No restriction	Disqualified

LVEF, left ventricular ejection fraction; VF, ventricular fibrillation; VT, ventricular tachycardia.

Table 20.7 Other tachyarrhythmia conditions. (Data from [131] and [132].)

Condition	Private driving	Commercial driving
Brugada's syndrome, Long QT syndrome, Arrhythmogenic RV cardiomyopathy	Appropriate evaluation/treatment by a cardiologist. Waiting period 6 months after any event causing cerebral ischemia	Disqualified
S/p catheter ablation EPS with no inducible sustained ventricular tachyarrhythmias	Waiting period 48 h	Waiting period 1 week

EPS, electrophysiologic study; RV, right ventricle.

Table 20.8 Supraventricular arrhythmias (supraventricular tachycardia, atrial flutter, atrial fibrillation). (Data from [131] and [132].)

Condition	Private/commercial driving
With associated cerebral ischemia	Satisfactory control
Without associated cerebral ischemia	No restriction

Table 20.9 Canadian reporting regulations: unfit drivers and protection for physicians. (Data from [131] and [132].)

Jurisdiction	Reporting	MD Reporting
Alberta	Discretionary	Protected
British Columbia	Mandatory*	Not protected
Manitoba	Mandatory	Protected
New Brunswick	Mandatory	Protected
Newfoundland and Labrador	Mandatory	Protected
Northwest Territories	Mandatory	Protected[†]
Nunavut	Mandatory	Protected[†]
Nova Scotia	Discretionary	Protected
Ontario	Mandatory	Protected
Prince Edward Island	Mandatory	Protected
Quebec	Discretionary	Protected
Saskatchewan	Mandatory	Protected
Yukon	Mandatory	Protected

* Mandatory if unfit driver has been warned not to but continues to drive.
† Unless acting maliciously or without reasonable grounds.

liable. In one (Pennsylvania), failure to report can lead to conviction of a summary offense. In 30 states, physicians are immune from legal action from patients but in 20 (including Washington, DC), they are not. Most states do not accept anonymous letters. Reporting recommendations differ in other countries. Those from Canada are shown in Table 20.9. The 2003 Canadian Cardiovascular Society Consensus Conference: Assessment of the Cardiovascular Patient on the Fitness to Fly and Drive is excellent (see: www.ccs.ca/society/conferences/index.asp) [94]. Another website to view recent recommendations is: www.bcepilepsy.com/pdf/DriveFitness.pdf.

Thirty states provide training for their personnel on how to observe applicants for impairing conditions. Thirty-one (including Washington, DC) do not. Very few states provide specialized training for licensing personnel relating to older drivers.

The licensing agency does not provide counseling to drivers with functional impairments (41 versus 10). Every state (and Washington, DC) allows demented drivers to drive! Almost every state will accept an unfavorable physician report to terminate the driving privileges of a demented driver.

Board members of 35 states include physicians from several subspecialties. The most common subspecialties are ophthalmologists and neurologists. These board members are most commonly volunteer consultants who are in private practice.

The number of individuals referred annually to each state board varies widely from 13,000 in Maryland and 36,000 in North Carolina to < 5 in Arizona. The number of licenses denied annually varies from an unknown number in some states to 1271 in 2002 in Maryland, to one in Nebraska.

Further information can be obtained at: www.aamva.org/Documents/drvSummaryOfMedicalAdvisoryBoardPractices.pdf.

Conclusions

Drivers with recurrent syncope pose a challenge to the medical profession and to themselves. They are at risk to become injured, to injure others, and to die in a traffic accident if they have transient loss of consciousness behind the wheel. The risks for most syncope patients are small but risks vary by medical condition, cause for syncope, and chance of recurrence while driving. Recommendations are often ignored with few consequences. Guidelines regarding driving and its restriction remain vague, non-specific, and are often not followed and not applicable. In part, this is related to the multitude of causes for syncope and the wide variation in presentations.

Based on present data, physicians should be assured that the legal risks regarding driver recommendation for syncope are minimal, as long as the issues are discussed (and documented) with the patient and, if necessary, through proper legal channels. Physicians should become familiar with legal laws regarding driving.

For the patient, it is best to concentrate efforts on proper treatment of the cause for syncope, and while prudent guidelines for driving can be established based on common sense, recommendations must be individualized for each patient. It does not appear that this will change in the near future.

References

1 Petch MC. Driving and heart disease. *Eur Heart J* 1998;**19**:1165–77.

2 Linzer M, Pontinen M, Gold DT, Divine GW, Felder A, Brooks WB. Impairment of physical and psychosocial function in recurrent syncope. *J Clin Epidemiol* 1991; **44**:1037–43.

3 Akiyama T, Powell JL, Mitchell LB, Ehlert FA, Baessler C. Resumption of driving after life-threatening ventricular tachyarrhythmia. *N Engl J Med* 2001;**345**: 391–7.

4 Epstein AE, Miles WM, Benditt DG, *et al.* Personal and public safety issues related to arrhythmias that may affect consciousness: implications for regulation and physician recommendations. A medical/scientific statement from the American Heart Association and the North American Society of Pacing and Electrophysiology. *Circulation* 1996;**94**:1147–66.

5 Blumenthal RBJ, Connolly H, Epstein A, Gersh BJ, Wittels EH. *Cardiovascular Advisory Panel Guidelines for the Medical Examination of Commercial Motor Vehicle Drivers.* FMCSA-MCP-02-002, US Department of Transportation, October 2002.

6 Krauss GL, Ampaw L, Krumholz A. Individual state driving restrictions for people with epilepsy in the US. *Neurology* 2001;**57**:1780–5.

7 Littler WA, Honour AJ, Sleight P. Direct arterial pressure and electrocardiogram during motor car driving. *BMJ* 1973;**2**:273–7.

8 Taggart PI, Gibbons D, Somerville W. Some effects of motor car driving on the normal and abnormal heart. *Br Heart J* 1969;**31**:386–7.

9 Falkner F. The stress of racing driving. *Lancet* 1971;**1**:650.

10 Taggart P, Carruthers M. Hyperlipidaemia induced by the stress of racing driving. *Lancet* 1971;**1**:854.

11 Lauwers P, Aelvoet W, Sneppe R, Remion M. Effect of car driving on the electrocardiogram of patients with myocardial infarction and an ECG at rest devoid of dysrhythmia and repolarization abnormalities: comparison with the ECG changes obtained during exercise. *Acta Cardiol* 1973;**28**:27–43.

12 Kushnir B, Fox KM, Tomlinson IW, Portal RW, Aber CP. Primary ventricular fibrillation and resumption of work, sexual activity, and driving after first acute myocardial infarction. *BMJ* 1975;**4**:609–11.

13 Wielgosz AT, Azad N. Effects of cardiovascular disease on driving tasks. *Clin Geriatr Med* 1993;**9**:341–8.

14 Somerville W. Heart disease and fitness to drive motor vehicles. *Med Leg J* 1970;**38**:42–50.

15 McCue H. Cardiac arrhythmias in relation to automobile driving. Presented at the Scientific Conference on Personal and Public Safety Issues Related to Arrhythmias; January 12–13, 1995; Washington DC.

16 Somerville W. Emotions, catecholamines and coronary heart disease. *Adv Cardiol* 1973;**8**:162–73.

17 Bellet S, Roman L, Kostis J, Slater A. Continuous electrocardiographic monitoring during automobile driving: studies in normal subjects and patients with coronary disease. *Am J Cardiol* 1968;**22**:856–62.

18 Cocco G, Iselin HU. Cardiac risk of speed traps. *Clin Cardiol* 1992;**15**:441–4.

19 Sartory GRW, Kopell ML. Psychophysiological assessment of driving phobia. *J Psychophysiol* 1992;**6/4**:311–20.

20 Greco C. Riverdale man guilty of road-rage slaying. *Chicago Tribune*, January 28, 2004.

21 Hijar M, Carrillo C, Flores M, Anaya R, Lopez V. Risk factors in highway traffic accidents: a case control study. *Accid Anal Prev* 2000;**32**:703–9.

22 Cummings P, Koepsell TD, Moffat JM, Rivara FP. Drowsiness, counter-measures to drowsiness, and the risk of a motor vehicle crash. *Inj Prev* 2001;**7**:194–9.

23 Stutts J, Feaganes J, Rodgman E, *et al.* The causes and consequences of distraction in everyday driving. *Annu Proc Assoc Adv Automot Med* 2003;**47**:235–51.

24 Redelmeier DA, Tibshirani RJ. Association between cellular-telephone calls and motor vehicle collisions. *N Engl J Med* 1997;**336**:453–8.

25 Braver ER, Solomon MG, Preusser DF. Toll road crashes of commercial and passenger motor vehicles. *Accid Anal Prev* 2002;**34**:293–303.

26 Buttner A, Heimpel M, Eisenmenger W. Sudden natural death "at the wheel": a retrospective study over a 15-year time period (1982–96). *Forensic Sci Int* 1999;**103**:101–12.

27 Voigt J. Road traffic deaths from natural causes. International Association for Accident and Traffic Medicine. *Proceedings of the Third Triennial Congress on Medical and Related Aspects of Motor Vehicle Accidents.* 5/29–6/4, University of Michigan Highway Safety Research Institute, Ann Arbor, 1969: 71.

28 Peterson BJPC. Sudden natural death among automobile drivers. *J Forensic Sci* 1962;**7**:274–84.

29 Hossack DW. Death at the wheel: a consideration of cardiovascular disease as a contributory factor to road accidents. *Med J Aust* 1974;**1**:164–6.

30 Myerburg RJ, Davis JH. The medical ecology of public safety. I. Sudden death due to coronary heart disease. *Am Heart J* 1964;**68**:586–95.

31 Bowen DA. Deaths of drivers of automobiles due to trauma and ischaemic heart disease: a survey and assessment. *Forensic Sci* 1973;**2**:285–90.

32 Gillum RF. Sudden coronary death in the United States: 1980–85. *Circulation* 1989;**79**:756–65.

33 Baker SP. Natural disease as cause of fatal auto accident. *N Engl J Med* 1970;**283**:937.

34 Schmidt P, Haarhoff K, Bonte W. Sudden natural death at the wheel: a particular problem of the elderly? *Forensic Sci Int* 1990;**48**:155–62.

35 Parsons M. Fits and other causes of loss of consciousness while driving. *Q J Med* 1986;**58**:295–303.

36 Kerwin AJ. Sudden death while driving. *CMAJ* 1984; **131**:312–4.

37 Ostrom M, Eriksson A. Natural death while driving. *J Forensic Sci* 1987;**32**:988–98.

38 Christian MS. Incidence and implications of natural deaths of road users. *BMJ* 1988;**297**:1021–4.

39 Waller JA. Cardiovascular disease, aging, and traffic accidents. *J Chronic Dis* 1967;**20**:615–20.

40 Norman LG. Medical aspects of road safety. *Lancet* 1960;**1**:1039–45.

41 Herner B, Smedby B, Ysander L. Sudden illness as a cause of motor-vehicle accidents. *Br J Ind Med* 1966; **23**:37–41.

42 West I, Nielsen GL, Gilmore AE, Ryan JR. Natural death at the wheel. *JAMA* 1968;**205**:266–71.

43 Baker SP, Spitz WU. An evaluation of the hazard created by natural death at the wheel. *N Engl J Med* 1970; **283**:405–9.

44 Copeland AR. Sudden natural death "at the wheel": revisited. *Med Sci Law* 1987;**27**:106–13.

45 Natural death at the wheel. *BMJ* 1969;**1**:332.

46 Brouwer WH, Ponds RW. Driving competence in older persons. *Disabil Rehabil* 1994;**16**:149–61.

47 Brandaleone H, Katz R, Tebrock HE, Wheatley GM. Study of the relationship of health impairments and motor vehicle accidents. *J Occup Med* 1972;**14**:854–9.

48 Antecol DH, Roberts WC. Sudden death behind the wheel from natural disease in drivers of four-wheeled motorized vehicles. *Am J Cardiol* 1990;**66**:1329–35.

49 Hossack DW. Medical catastrophe at the wheel. *Med J Aust* 1980;**1**:327–8.

50 Williams AF, Preusser DF, Ulmer RG, Weinstein HB. Characteristics of fatal crashes of 16-year-old drivers: implications for licensure policies. *J Public Health Policy* 1995;**16**:347–60.

51 Preusser DF, Williams AF, Ferguson SA, Ulmer RG, Weinstein HB. Fatal crash risk for older drivers at intersections. *Accid Anal Prev* 1998;**30**:151–9.

52 McLean AJ. Death at the wheel. *N Engl J Med* 1970; **283**:1234.

53 Retchin SM, Anapolle J. An overview of the older driver. *Clin Geriatr Med* 1993;**9**:279–96.

54 Baldwin RW, Schoolman LR, Whittlesey P, *et al.* Medical conditions constituting a hazard in driving. *Md State Med J* 1966;**15**:55–8.

55 Waller JA. Medical conditions: what role in crashes? *N Engl J Med* 1970;**283**:429–30.

56 Waller PF. The older driver. *Hum Factors* 1991;**33**:499–505.

57 Levitt SD, Porter J. Sample selection in the estimation of air bag and seat belt effectiveness. NBER Working Paper No. w7210. National Bureau of Economic Research, issued July 1999.

58 http://216.239.57.104/search?q=cache:-OxZQUBKpBUJ: www.psych.upenn.edu/~baron/900/risk.htm+seat+belt+ life+year+saved+%2469&h.

59 Grimmond BB. Suicide at the wheel. *N Z Med J* 1974;**80**:90–4.

60 Simon F, Corbett C. Road traffic offending, stress, age, and accident history among male and female drivers. *Ergonomics* 1996;**39**:757–80.

61 Sorock GS, Ranney TA, Lehto MR. Motor vehicle crashes in roadway construction workzones: an analysis using narrative text from insurance claims. *Accid Anal Prev* 1996;**28**:131–8.

62 Mayou R, Simkin S, Threlfall J. The effects of road traffic accidents on driving behaviour. *Injury* 1991;**22**:365–8.

63 Pakola SJ, Dinges DF, Pack AI. Review of regulations and guidelines for commercial and non-commercial drivers with sleep apnea and narcolepsy. *Sleep* 1995; **18**:787–96.

64 Ray WA, Thapa PB, Shorr RI. Medications and the older driver. *Clin Geriatr Med* 1993;**9**:413–38.

65 Knight B. The drinking driver. *Practitioner* 1972; **209**:294–301.

66 Knight KK, Fielding JE, Goetzel RZ. Correlates of motor-vehicle safety behaviors in working populations. *J Occup Med* 1991;**33**:705–10.

67 Logan BK, Fligner CL, Haddix T. Cause and manner of death in fatalities involving methamphetamine. *J Forensic Sci* 1998;**43**:28–34.

68 Logan BK, Couper FJ. Zolpidem and driving impairment. *J Forensic Sci* 2001;**46**:105–10.

69 Logan BK, Couper FJ. 3,4-Methylenedioxymethamphetamine (MDMA, ecstasy) and driving impairment. *J Forensic Sci* 2001;**46**:1426–33.

70 Logan BK, Case GA, Gordon AM. Carisoprodol, meprobamate, and driving impairment. *J Forensic Sci* 2000;**45**:619–23.

71 Logan BK. Methamphetamine and driving impairment. *J Forensic Sci* 1996;**41**:457–64.

72 Drickamer MA, Marottoli RA. Physician responsibility in driver assessment. *Am J Med Sci* 1993;**306**:277–81.

73 Marottoli RA, Drickamer MA. Psychomotor mobility and the elderly driver. *Clin Geriatr Med* 1993;**9**:403–11.

74 Marshall C, Boyd KT, Moran CG. Injuries related to car crime: the joy-riding epidemic. *Injury* 1996;**27**:79–80.

75 Hanning CD, Welsh M. Sleepiness, snoring and driving habits. *J Sleep Res* 1996;**5**:51–4.

76 Hemenway D, Solnick SJ. Fuzzy dice, dream cars, and indecent gestures: correlates of driver behavior? *Accid Anal Prev* 1993;**25**:161–70.

77 Corfitsen MT. Enhanced tiredness among young impaired male nighttime drivers. *Accid Anal Prev* 1996;**28**:155–62.

78 Corfitsen MT. Fatigue in multiple-car fatal accidents. *Forensic Sci Int* 1989;**40**:161–9.

79 Deichmann WB. Backward driving. *JAMA* 1972;**221**:1517.

80 Gillberg M, Kecklund G, Akerstedt T. Sleepiness and performance of professional drivers in a truck simulator: comparisons between day and night driving. *J Sleep Res* 1996;**5**:12–5.

81 Gregersen NP, Brehmer B, Moren B. Road safety improvement in large companies: an experimental comparison of different measures. *Accid Anal Prev* 1996;**28**:297–306.

82 Gregersen NP, Bjurulf P. Young novice drivers: towards a model of their accident involvement. *Accid Anal Prev* 1996;**28**:229–41.

83 Gregersen NP, Berg HY, Engstrom I, Nolen S, Nyberg A, Rimmo PA. Sixteen years age limit for learner drivers in Sweden: an evaluation of safety effects. *Accid Anal Prev* 2000;**32**:25–35.

84 Gregersen NP, Berg HY. Lifestyle and accidents among young drivers. *Accid Anal Prev* 1994;**26**:297–303.

85 Gregersen NP. Young drivers' overestimation of their own skill: an experiment on the relation between training strategy and skill. *Accid Anal Prev* 1996;**28**:243–50.

86 Brown ID. Driver fatigue. *Hum Factors* 1994;**36**:298–314.

87 Brown ID, Tickner AH, Simmonds DC. Effects of prolonged driving upon driving skill and performance of a subsidiary task. *Ind Med Surg* 1966;**35**:760–5.

88 Schenck CH, Mahowald MW. A polysomnographically documented case of adult somnambulism with long-distance automobile driving and frequent nocturnal violence: parasomnia with continuing danger as a non-insane automatism? *Sleep* 1995;**18**:765–72.

89 Rutley KS, Mace DG. Heart rate as a measure in road layout design. *Ergonomics* 1972;**15**:165–73.

90 Rehm CG, Ross SE. Syncope as etiology of road crashes involving elderly drivers. *Am Surg* 1995;**61**:1006–8.

91 Rehm CG, Ross SE. Elderly drivers involved in road crashes: a profile. *Am Surg* 1995;**61**:435–7.

92 Norman LG. The health of bus drivers: a study in London transport. *Lancet* 1958;**2**:807–12.

93 Raffle PA. Fitness to drive. *Trans Med Soc Lond* 1974;**90**:197–205.

94 Simpson C, Ross D, Dorian P, *et al.* CCS Consensus Conference 2003: assessment of the cardiac patient for fitness to drive and fly – executive summary. *Can J Cardiol* 2004;**20**:1313.

95 Grattan E, Jeffcoate GO. Medical factors and road accidents. *BMJ* 1968;**1**:75–9.

96 Halinen MO, Jaussi A. Fatal road accidents caused by sudden death of the driver in Finland and Vaud, Switzerland. *Eur Heart J* 1994;**15**:888–94.

97 Weibel MA, Suter PM. Causes of death in road traffic injuries: a comparison between 1970 and 1976 (author's translation). *Rev Chir Orthop Reparatrice Appar Mot* 1978;**64**:205–11.

98 Hu P. *Crash Prediction Models for Older Adults: a Panel Data Analysis Approach.* Center for Transportation Analysis Oak Ridge National Laboratory Building 3156, MS-6073 P.O. Box 2008 Oak Ridge, Tennessee 37831-6073, USA. David A. Trumble Accustat, Inc. 2401 Caspian Drive Knoxville, Tennessee 37932, USA.

99 Hu PS, Gray C. *1990 National Personal Transportation Survey Data Book, FHWA-PL-94-010A.* Oak Ridge, TN: Oak Ridge National Laboratory for Federal Highway Administration, 1993.

100 Hu PS, Lu A, Trumble D. *Driving Decisions and Vehicle Crashes Among Older Drivers.* Oak Ridge, TN: Oak Ridge National Laboratory, 1995.

101 Miaou SPHP, Wright T, Davis SC, Rathi A. Development of relationship between truck accidents and geometric design: phase 1. *Federal Highway Administration Report, FHWA-RD-91-124.* Washington, DC: Oak Ridge National Laboratory for Federal Highway Administration, 1993.

102 Stewart RB, Marks MMT, May R, Hale G. *Driving Cessation and Accidents in the Elderly: An Analysis of Symptoms, Diseases, Cognitive Dysfunction and Medications.* Washington, DC: AAA Foundation for Traffic Safety, 1993.

103 Hale WE, Marks RG, Stewart RB. The Dunedin program, a Florida geriatric screening process: design and initial data. *J Am Geriatr Soc* 1980;**28**:377–80.

104 Marottoli RA, Cooney LM Jr, Wagner R, Doucette J, Tinetti ME. Predictors of automobile crashes and moving violations among elderly drivers. *Ann Intern Med* 1994;**121**:842–6.

105 Koepsell TD, Wolf ME, McCloskey L, *et al.* Medical conditions and motor vehicle collision injuries in older adults. *J Am Geriatr Soc* 1994;**42**:695–700.

106 Hansotia P, Broste SK. The effect of epilepsy or diabetes mellitus on the risk of automobile accidents. *N Engl J Med* 1991;**324**:22–6.

107 Foley DJ, Wallace RB, Eberhard J. Risk factors for motor vehicle crashes among older drivers in a rural community. *J Am Geriatr Soc* 1995;**43**:776–81.

108 Cornoni-Huntley JBD, Ostfeld AM, Taylor JO, Wallace RB. *Established Populations for Epidemiologic Studies of the Elderly*. NIH Publication No. 86-2443. Washington, DC: National Institute on Aging, US Department of Health and Human Services, 1980.

109 Leveille SG, Buchner DM, Koepsell TD, McCloskey LW, Wolf ME, Wagner EH. Psychoactive medications and injurious motor vehicle collisions involving older drivers. *Epidemiology* 1994;**5**:591–8.

110 Ray WA, Gurwitz J, Decker MD, Kennedy DL. Medications and the safety of the older driver: is there a basis for concern? *Hum Factors* 1992;**34**:33–47; discussion 49–51.

111 Ray WA, Fought RL, Decker MD. Psychoactive drugs and the risk of injurious motor vehicle crashes in elderly drivers. *Am J Epidemiol* 1992;**136**:873–83.

112 McCloskey LW, Koepsell TD, Wolf ME, Buchner DM. Motor vehicle collision injuries and sensory impairments of older drivers. *Age Ageing* 1994;**23**:267–73.

113 Waller JA. Research and other issues concerning effects of medical conditions on elderly drivers. *Hum Factors* 1992;**34**:3–15; discussion 17–24.

114 Reed D, Satariano WA, Gildengorin G, McMahon K, Fleshman R, Schneider E. Health and functioning among the elderly of Marin County, California: a glimpse of the future. *J Gerontol A Biol Sci Med Sci* 1995;**50**:M61–9.

115 Kenny RA. Syncope in the elderly: diagnosis, evaluation, and treatment. *J Cardiovasc Electrophysiol* 2003;**14**: S74–7.

116 Lundberg C, Johansson K, Ball K, et al. Dementia and driving: an attempt at consensus. *Alzheimer Dis Assoc Disord* 1997;**11**:28–37.

117 Trobe JD, Waller PF, Cook-Flannagan CA, Teshima SM, Bieliauskas LA. Crashes and violations among drivers with Alzheimer disease. *Arch Neurol* 1996;**53**:411–6.

118 Taylor J, Chadwick D, Johnson T. Risk of accidents in drivers with epilepsy. *J Neurol Neurosurg Psychiatry* 1996;**60**:621–7.

119 Gustavsson P, Alfredsson L, Brunnberg H, et al. Myocardial infarction among male bus, taxi, and lorry drivers in middle Sweden. *Occup Environ Med* 1996;**53**:235–40.

120 Spudis EV, Penry JK, Gibson P. Driving impairment caused by episodic brain dysfunction: restrictions for epilepsy and syncope. *Arch Neurol* 1986;**43**:558–64.

121 Consensus conference on driver licensing and epilepsy. Proceedings of American Academy of Neurology, American Epilepsy Society, and Epilepsy Foundation of America. Washington, DC: May 31–June 2, 1991. *Epilepsia* 1994;**35**:662–705.

122 Stock MS, Burg FD, Light WO, Douglass JM. Licensing the driver with alterations of consciousness. *Arch Neurol* 1970;**23**:210–1.

123 Krumholz A, Fisher RS, Lesser RP, Hauser WA. Driving and epilepsy: a review and reappraisal. *JAMA* 1991; **265**:622–6.

124 Cambre S, Silverman ME. Is it safe to drive with an automatic implantable cardioverter defibrillator or a history of recurrent symptomatic ventricular arrhythmias? *Heart Dis Stroke* 1993;**2**:179–81.

125 Beauregard LA, Barnard PW, Russo AM, Waxman HL. Perceived and actual risks of driving in patients with arrhythmia control devices. *Arch Intern Med* 1995; **155**:609–13.

126 Anderson MH, Camm AJ. Legal and ethical aspects of driving and working in patients with an implantable cardioverter defibrillator. *Am Heart J* 1994;**127**:1185–93.

127 Strickberger SA, Cantillon CO, Friedman PL. When should patients with lethal ventricular arrhythmia resume driving? An analysis of state regulations and physician practices. *Ann Intern Med* 1991;**115**:560–3.

128 Larsen GC, Stupey MR, Walance CG, et al. Recurrent cardiac events in survivors of ventricular fibrillation or tachycardia: implications for driving restrictions. *JAMA* 1994;**271**:1335–9.

129 Conti JB, Woodard DA, Tucker KJ, Bryant B, King LC, Curtis AB. Modification of patient driving behavior after implantation of a cardioverter defibrillator. *Pacing Clin Electrophysiol* 1997;**20**:2200–4.

130 Curtis AB, Conti JB, Tucker KJ, Kubilis PS, Reilly RE, Woodard DA. Motor vehicle accidents in patients with an implantable cardioverter-defibrillator. *J Am Coll Cardiol* 1995;**26**:180–4.

131 Assessment of the cardiac patient for fitness to drive: 1996 update. *Can J Cardiol* 1996;**12**:1164–70; 1175–82.

132 Assessment of the cardiac patient for fitness to drive. *Can J Cardiol* 1992;**8**:406–19.

133 Decter BM, Goldner B, Cohen TJ. Vasovagal syncope as a cause of motor vehicle accidents. *Am Heart J* 1994;**127**:1619–21.

134 Haffner HT, Graw M. Cough syncope as a cause of traffic accident. *Blutalkohol* 1990;**27**:110–5.

135 Dhala A, Bremner S, Blanck Z, et al. Impairment of driving abilities in patients with supraventricular tachycardias. *Am J Cardiol* 1995;**75**:516–8.

136 Blitzer ML, Saliba BC, Ghantous AE, Marieb MA, Schoenfeld MH. Causes of impaired consciousness while driving a motorized vehicle. *Am J Cardiol* 2003;**91**: 1373–4.

137 Li H, Weitzel M, Easley A, Barrington W, Windle J. Potential risk of vasovagal syncope for motor vehicle driving. *Am J Cardiol* 2000;**85**:184–6.

138 Sheldon R, Koshman ML. Can patients with neuromediated syncope safely drive motor vehicles? *Am J Cardiol* 1995;**75**:955–6.

139 Sowton E. Driving licences for patients with cardiac pacemakers. *Br Heart J* 1972;**34**:977–80.

140 Brandaleone H. Motor vehicle driving and cardiac pace-makers. *Ann Intern Med* 1974;**81**:548–50.

141 Kou WH, Calkins H, Lewis RR, *et al.* Incidence of loss of consciousness during automatic implantable cardioverter-defibrillator shocks. *Ann Intern Med* 1991; **115**:942–5.

142 DiCarlo LA Jr, Morady F, Schwartz AB, *et al.* Clinical significance of ventricular fibrillation-flutter induced by ventricular programmed stimulation. *Am Heart J* 1985;**109**:959–63.

143 Bansch D, Brunn J, Castrucci M, *et al.* Syncope in patients with an implantable cardioverter-defibrillator: incidence, prediction and implications for driving restrictions. *J Am Coll Cardiol* 1998;**31**:608–15.

144 Hickey K, Curtis AB, Lancaster S, *et al.* Baseline factors predicting early resumption of driving after life-threatening arrhythmias in the Antiarrhythmics Versus Implantable Defibrillators (AVID) Trial. *Am Heart J* 2001;**142**:99–104.

145 Brandaleone H. Driving and the coronary patient. *J Rehabil* 1966;**32**:97.

146 Highway travel and angina pectoris. *CMAJ* 1973; **108**:1095.

147 Douglass JM, Stock MS, Light WO, Burg FD. Licensing the driver with cardiovascular dysfunction. *Am Heart J* 1970;**80**:197–201.

148 Stock MS, Light WO, Douglass JM, Burg FD. Licensing the driver with musculoskeletal difficulty. *J Bone Joint Surg Am* 1970;**52**:343–6.

149 Jung W, Anderson M, Camm AJ, *et al.* Recommendations for driving of patients with implantable cardioverter defibrillators. Study Group on "ICD and Driving" of the Working Groups on Cardiac Pacing and Arrhythmias of the European Society of Cardiology. *Eur Heart J* 1997;**18**:1210–9.

150 Linzer M, Varia I, Pontinen M, Divine GW, Grubb BP, Estes NA III. Medically unexplained syncope: relationship to psychiatric illness. *Am J Med* 1992;**92**:18S–25S.

151 Lurie KG, Iskos D, Sakaguchi S, Fahy GJ, Benditt DG. Resumption of motor vehicle operation in vasovagal fainters. *Am J Cardiol* 1999;**83**:604–6; A8.

152 Council on Ethical and Judicial Affairs AMA. *American Medical Association CEJA Report 4-A-99*. Chicago, IL, 2000.

153 Brignole M, Alboni P, Benditt D, *et al.* Task force on syncope, European Society of Cardiology. Part 2. Diagnostic tests and treatment: summary of recommendations. *Europace* 2001;**3**:261–8.

154 Brignole M, Alboni P, Benditt D, *et al.* Task force on syncope, European Society of Cardiology. Part 1. The initial evaluation of patients with syncope. *Europace* 2001;**3**:253–60.

155 http://www.londoncardiac.ca/pages/bfs.html.

156 Ott BR, Mernoff ST. Driving policy issues and the physician. *Med Health R I* 1999;**82**:428–31.

157 Maas R, Ventura R, Kretzschmar C, Aydin A, Schuchert A. Syncope, driving recommendations, and clinical reality: survey of patients. *BMJ* 2003;**326**:21.

158 Akiyama T, Powell JL, Mitchell LB, Ehlert FA, Baessler C. Resumption of driving after life-threatening ventricular tachyarrhythmia. *N Engl J Med* 2001;**345**:391–7.

159 Medtronic. *When May Patients with Implanted Defibrillators Drive?* Follow-up Forum Winter 1995–96;**1**:8–10.

CHAPTER 21

Legal considerations in the management of patients with syncope

Mark J. Zucker, MD, JD, FACC, *& Gerald J. Bloch,* JD

Introduction

It is well recognized that syncope, regardless of etiology, may pose a risk not only to the patient but also to third parties. For this reason, physicians should naturally be concerned with the accuracy and implications of their diagnoses and treatment plans, including the consequences of either permitting or restricting the patient from participating in certain activities. Medical professionals can derive some comfort, however, from the knowledge that as long as a decision, made by the practitioner, is based upon solid medical reasoning and made in good faith, the medicolegal implications should be minimal.

The most significant medicolegal concern in the management of the patient presenting with syncope is the possibility that the failure to restrict a patient from performing certain activities may result in injury or death to the patient or to an innocent third party. Although this is of particular concern for physicians treating competitive athletes, drivers of motor vehicles, pilots of aircraft, operators of heavy equipment, handlers of hazardous materials, and the elderly, there are a myriad of circumstances in which the failure to prevent or warn about potential, recurring incapacity can prove disastrous.

While the medical evaluation and treatment of syncope can be tedious and frequently unrewarding, the medicolegal principles addressing the issues surrounding loss of consciousness are fairly straightforward. In the absence of specific statutes or regulations governing the reporting of these conditions, the liability of a physician is based solely upon the common law rules of negligence.

Negligence law addresses "conduct" and embraces both acts of commission as well as omission; i.e., what an individual did or failed to do. In general, the law imposes on an individual a duty to conduct oneself in a manner that does not expose others to an unreasonable risk of harm. If one breaches that duty, and that breach causes harm, liability may result. Basic to any consideration of negligence is the idea or concept that the harm was "foreseeable" [1]. However, foreseeability, although a key factor in determining whether a duty exists, is not the only factor. The question of duty in a negligence action should also take into account the likelihood of injury, the magnitude of the burden of guarding against it, and the consequences of placing that burden on the defendant [2–4].

A physician is thus charged with the duty of providing care and treatment in a manner that does not "unreasonably" threaten the safety of the patient or others. Unreasonably may be defined as conduct that falls below the standard established by law for the protection of others against unreasonable risk of harm [5]. What is reasonable depends upon the state of medical knowledge and the unique characteristics and factors associated with a particular patient.

Medical considerations – standard of care

The differential diagnosis of syncope includes both cardiovascular and non-cardiovascular etiologies. History and physical examination alone, however, can provide a diagnosis in only about half of cases [6]. Unfortunately, establishing a definitive diagnosis is critical to the prediction of recurrence. Liability exists only when the physician, presented with a patient who has had a loss of consciousness, fails to meet the reasonable standard of care, described in detail elsewhere in this treatise. However, a brief restatement of the work-up, focusing on documentation, is in order.

Particular attention should be paid to the patient's history, physical examination, and observations by individuals who may have witnessed the event. At a minimum, the history must include a chronologic record from the initial onset of symptoms until presentation for medical evaluation. Documentation of premonitory symptoms (such as palpitations, dizziness, and lightheadedness), association with activity or positional changes, existence of triggers, changes in dietary habits and/ or medications, and the presence or absence of emotional stress should be included. Further, a thorough inquiry into any prior medical illnesses that might be relevant to the present loss of consciousness (such as cardiac, neurologic, and/or vascular disorders) should be conducted. In many cases, obtaining an adequate history in a patient with syncope may require going beyond interviewing the patient; information available from family and friends is sometimes crucial [7–9].

Obtaining a detailed and accurate medical history can be a time-consuming and admittedly frustrating process. The use of a checklist or outline may facilitate the process. The history and physical examination are essential to ensuring that a proper diagnosis is made, appropriate laboratory evaluations are ordered, proper referrals are made, and correct therapy is instituted. The failure to order a test generally considered critical to the work-up may represent a breach of the standard of care and may constitute negligence, unless the physician has determined that the yield is unacceptably low, the test will not provide the needed information, or the test is not safe for the particular patient [10].

The importance of adequate documentation in the medical record cannot be overemphasized, as documentation represents the only credible evidence that logical and appropriate questions were asked in order to differentiate between those in need of an extensive work-up and those in whom the syncope was of a benign origin and highly unlikely to recur.

Statutory and administrative considerations

Typically, patients initially seek guidance from their physician with respect to activity restrictions. For this reason, a physician should be familiar with the applicable statutory or administrative requirements of his or her own jurisdiction that may apply to the operation of motor vehicles, aircraft, or any other activity that requires state licensing.

Familiarizing oneself with applicable state regulations generally requires either a telephone call to the appropriate licensing agency or a visit to the American Association of Motor Vehicle Agencies' website (www.aamva.org). Interestingly, a 1990s survey revealed that only 26% of randomly sampled cardiologists correctly understood their state's restrictions on driving. Moreover, although 44% of arrhythmia specialists were familiar with their state's regulations, the same could be said of only 8% of general cardiologists [11].

More recent data regarding physician familiarity with state regulations is not particularly encouraging. Two studies, both from the UK, again demonstrated that physicians' knowledge regarding regulatory or statutory driving restrictions was incomplete. Of 102 British emergency department physicians who responded to a 2003 survey, only 7.8% knew that the Driver and Vehicle Licensing Agency guidelines required either temporary or permanent driving restrictions after a syncopal episode [12]. Likewise, of 50 physicians questioned in Northern Ireland regarding their government's regulations with respect to driving with five specific medical conditions, only nine knew the correct driving restrictions for epilepsy, five for myocardial infarction, four for stroke, 22 for abdominal aortic aneurysm, and eight for diabetes [13]. In practice, most physicians probably rely upon their own observations and the prevailing standard of care in their community.

Although there are dozens of medical conditions that may interfere with the safe operation of a motor vehicle, the one condition that is specifically regulated by statute in all 50 states is epilepsy. However, the specific regulations setting forth the seizure-free interval required prior to securing or resecuring driving privileges vary greatly from state to state, ranging from less than 3 months to upwards of 12 months. Moreover, not only do the statutes vary from state to state, but even within a state the restrictions may change from year to year [14].

In some states, physicians are required to report, in good faith, patients who have a physical or mental condition that, in the physician's judgment, impairs the patient's ability to exercise reasonable and ordinary control over a motor vehicle. The report may be made without the patient's informed consent. By way of example, see Wisconsin Statute s. 146.82(3), which provides in pertinent part:

> Reports made without informed consent. (a) Notwithstanding sub. (1), a physician who treats a patient whose physical or mental condition in the physician's judgment affects the patient's ability to exercise reasonable and ordinary control over a motor vehicle may report the patient's name and other information relevant to the condition to the Department of Transportation without the informed consent of the patient.

A 1992 study by the Department of Transportation revealed that reports by physicians are considered confidential in 34 states. Twenty-seven states will grant a physician immunity from liability for either reporting or failing to report, in good faith, a physical and/or mental condition that did or did not, in the physician's judgment, impair the patient's ability to operate the motor vehicle [15]. For example, see Wisconsin Statute 448.03(5)(b), which states:

> (b) No physician shall be liable for any civil damages for either of the following:
> 1 Reporting in good faith to the Department of Transportation under s. 146.82(3)

a patient's name and other information relevant to a physical or mental condition of the patient which in the physician's judgment impairs the patient's ability to exercise reasonable and ordinary control over a motor vehicle.
> 2 In good faith, not reporting to the Department of Transportation under s. 146.82(3) a patient's name and other information relevant to a physical or mental condition of the patient which in the physician's judgment does not impair the patient's ability to exercise reasonable and ordinary control over a motor vehicle.

Note that the Wisconsin Statute would not provide immunity to a physician for failing to report an individual whose ability to exercise reasonable care and ordinary control is, in the physician's judgment, impaired. Liability under these circumstances would be subject to the defense of "good faith."

Notwithstanding the fact that most states provide immunity from criminal and/or civil liability to a healthcare provider who reports in good faith, most reports are actually made by law enforcement officials, with medical providers accounting for less than 10% of filed reports in Florida, 22% in Wisconsin, and 37% in Oregon [15].

In summary, maintaining familiarity with the inconsistent and ever-changing standards can be quite challenging for a busy practicing physician. Nevertheless, physicians must recognize that the physician–patient privilege is not absolute. Even after the adoption of the newly published Federal regulations, effective April 2004, exceptions to the privilege in the interest of "public health and welfare" or to comply with statutory or administrative regulations are permitted, if not occasionally required. Failure to comply with these mandatory reporting requirements can, in rare circumstances, subject the physician to fines or civil liability to the individual or even to injured third parties [16].

Syncope and the athlete

Syncope in the competitive athlete represents a unique and difficult problem [8,9,17]. The physician caring for such an athlete with a history of syncope or, for that matter, any significant cardiovascular disorder, may be subjected to enormous pressure from the individual, institution, family, and friends to provide a "clean" bill of health, thereby permitting a return to the prior activity. No cases highlight the problem better than those of basketball players Hank Gathers and Reggie Lewis. In each instance, the athlete obtained medical clearance (by one or more physicians) despite an initial diagnosis of a cardiac condition.

Gathers, playing for Loyola Marymount, first collapsed on December 9, 1989. Seventeen days later, physicians had him play one-on-one basketball with a Holter monitor attached to his heart. 188 episodes of ventricular tachycardia with rates of almost 200 b min^{-1} were recorded. Gathers was started on a beta-blocker (propranolol) and the Holter monitor repeated. The frequency and complexity of the ventricular ectopic activity was greatly reduced. Unfortunately, because of side-effects, and reportedly upon Gathers's request, the dosage of propranolol was decreased gradually from 240 to 40 mg day^{-1}. The last dosage change occurred 6 days before his death, and was made with the understanding that he would return 2 days later to see if the lower dosage was safe and effective prior to playing in an upcoming postseason game. Gathers did not appear for the appointment, dodged calls from the physician, and ultimately convinced the physician to delay the test until after the game. Gathers died during that postseason game.

An autopsy listed the cause of Gathers's death as cardiomyopathy of unknown etiology. His death, at age 23, reverberated among team physicians and athletic directors who imagined themselves on the damage end of a lawsuit where the claim involved the loss of earnings of someone who was likely to be a professional athlete capable of commanding an astronomically high salary.

Indeed, Gathers's mother, minor son, and other heirs subsequently filed a multimillion dollar suit against Loyola Marymount, the coach, the trainers, and seven physicians involved with the case [18]. Not only did the plaintiffs contend that the physicians' treatment was negligent, but claimed further that the defendants had conspired and fraudulently failed to inform Gathers of the seriousness of his heart condition and the dangers associated with continuing to play competitive basketball. Finally, the plaintiffs alleged that the dosage reduction was made to ensure that Gathers's playing ability and stamina were not compromised [19–21].

The Gathers suit was eventually settled out of court for $2.4 million. Other lawsuits along these lines, although infrequent, have occurred. In 1986, Anthony Penny, a Central Connecticut State University basketball player, was diagnosed with hypertrophic cardiomyopathy. His physician recommended that he discontinue playing competitive basketball and imposed a restriction of 2 years. Not satisfied with that recommendation, he sought additional opinions, and ultimately was permitted to remain on the university's team. After completing his college basketball career, he filed a malpractice suit questioning the competence of the cardiologist who first made the diagnosis [22]. Penny claimed damages of $1,000,000, based in part upon the lost future income from professional basketball and the lost enjoyment of life resulting from the 2-year restriction imposed upon him by the physician. Penny subsequently died during a competitive basketball game in England. The lawsuit was voluntarily dismissed.

Perhaps no lawsuit has created as much publicity in this area as that of Reggie Lewis, captain of the Boston Celtics, who died in May 1993 while shooting baskets at a gymnasium. Two months earlier, Lewis had fainted during a Celtics game. A "team" of 12 cardiologists assembled by the Celtics' physician diagnosed his condition as "cardiomyopathy" and recommended that he not play competitive basketball again. A second medical opinion, requested by Lewis, concluded that he had the heart of a normal athlete and that the syncopal episode was caused by a benign neurologic condition. A third consultant found evidence to support each of the former consultant's opinions. An autopsy confirmed the diagnosis of cardiomyopathy [23,24]. After the death of her husband, Donna M. Harris-Lewis filed a malpractice suit against four of the treating physicians. At trial, the jury rendered a verdict in favor of two of the defendant physicians, a third having previously settled the matter for $500,000. No decision could be reached with respect to the fourth physician. The case was retried against the remaining defendant physician and the jury entered a verdict for the defendant. Upon appeal, the trial court decision was eventually affirmed in February 2004 [25].

Physicians should recognize that there are also statutes intended to prevent discrimination against handicapped individuals which may also potentially provide legal redress for athletes precluded from participation in competitive sports. Section 504(a) of the Rehabilitation Act (29 USCA 794 [West Supp. 1992]) states in pertinent part that:

> No otherwise qualified individual with handicaps in the United States, as defined in 706(8) of this title, shall, solely by reason of her or his handicap, be excluded from the participation in, be denied the benefits of, or be subjected to discrimination under any program or activity receiving Federal financial assistance.

Most high schools and colleges receive some federal funding, making these institutions subject to the rules and regulations of the Act. Likewise, the Amateur Sports Act of 1978 (36 USC 371 et seq. [1988]) also ensures equal opportunities in athletics programs for handicapped individuals.

It is at least arguable that ventricular arrhythmias and/or syncope constitute a "handicap" that under specific circumstances may invoke the protection of these statutes. In such cases, the court will be charged with striking a balance between the statutory rights of the athlete and the desire of the school or team not to permit the "handicapped" athlete to play. How a court will rule is fact-sensitive and will depend upon whether the plaintiff can establish that his or her handicap constitutes the type of physical "impairment" contemplated by the Act. In *Larkin* v. *Archdiocese of Cincinnati*, for example, the federal district court upheld a private high school's refusal to permit an athlete with hypertrophic cardiomyopathy to play football [26,27].

The Gathers, Lewis, Penny, and Larkin cases demonstrate that providing medical clearance for sports participation and treating athletic injuries may involve not only complex medical issues, but complex legal issues as well. Not surprisingly, the number of reported judicial opinions involving litigation between team physicians, the specialists to whom the athletes are referred, and the competitive athlete is small [27–29].

Standards for athletic participation

Physicians involved in the treatment of athletes, whether primary care providers, team or sports medicine physicians, or specialists, often have the responsibility for medically clearing athletes prior to their returning to play. Coincident with the responsibility for the medical decision-making is the potential legal responsibility for injury that might occur to the athlete if proper medical practices are not followed.

In contrast to the "normal" patient, the competitive athlete is psychologically and economically intent upon returning to the game. The team's treating or consulting physician may find him or herself under extreme pressure from the coach, management, friends, or the athlete to "clear" the athlete [30]. Nowhere is the documentation of advice and the reasons behind the advice more important. If the athlete is properly advised such that he or she understands the risks and benefits, and chooses to disregard the physician's recommendation, legal liability will probably be avoided. At the least, the defenses of contributory negligence and assumption of risk can be raised.

It must be recognized that competitive athletes are often young and occasionally lacking in understanding. The conveyance of information must be made in a form capable of being understood and acknowledged. Options should be provided and opportunities to minimize risk discussed.

In 1985, the American College of Cardiology convened the 16th Bethesda Conference, which formulated recommendations for sports participation by athletes with cardiovascular abnormalities. The participants at that conference appreciated that "many decisions regarding disqualification from sports involve circumstances in which definitive scientific answers are conspicuously lacking." Nevertheless, the Bethesda Conference's nationally accepted recommendations provided, for the first time, guidance to physicians charged with the responsibility for making eligibility decisions [31].

Nine years later, at the 26th Bethesda Conference, the ethical, legal, and practical considerations affecting medical decision-making in competitive athletes were readdressed. Updated, objective, evidence-based, consensus recommendations were published in October 1994 and are now accepted as the medical standard of care [32]. It is likely that these recommendations would constitute substantial evidence to be used by a court in resolving malpractice claims or athletic participation disputes.

In the final analysis, the physician should provide a participation recommendation consistent with his or her best medical judgment. Nonmedical factors should not influence that decision. The physician must act reasonably, in good faith, and in such a manner as not to create an unreasonable risk of harm to the patient. If reasonable care dictates that an athlete with a potentially lethal condition not be allowed to play, then it is the physician's obligation to so inform the patient [33].

Whether the physician must inform others is situation-specific and probably depends upon whether the physician is the athlete's physician or the team physician. Certainly, in the former case, the law would be quite protective of the patient–physician relationship. Whether a team physician may assert the physician–patient privilege, however, is less clear-cut. Hence, a prudent team physician should disclose prior to starting an examination that he or she is also acting on behalf of the team and obtain permission to release pertinent medical information to team officials [33].

While it may be true that competitive athletes are motivated, stoic, and driven to succeed, most athletes will act reasonably in response to a trusted physician's recommendation regarding athletic participation. Winning that trust is as much a function of "bedside manner" as it is imparting the scientific and medical information.

Fortunately, there have been very few cases of cardiac death involving a high profile athlete that have ever created judicial precedent. The few cases that have been brought were either settled, dismissed, or ended in a verdict in favor of the defendant. Thus, in the absence of "on-point" appellate case law, physician liability remains based upon the traditional rules of law, that is, did the physician exercise reasonable care under the circumstances? Physicians are held to no greater standard than this.

Syncope and driving

Syncope, whether neurally mediated or cardiovascular, also compromises the safety of activities such as flying and driving. In recognition of this, the US Federal Aviation Administration (FAA) has promulgated guidelines that are used by the FAA Aeromedical Certification Division when evaluating an applicant with known supraventricular or ventricular arrhythmias [34]. Similar comprehensive medical standards addressing eligibility for flying were also adopted by the Joint Aviation Authorities in 1996, an international agency encompassing 26 European nations.

In contrast to flying, medical criteria for driving fitness are less formal, probably less strict, and generally determined by the individual states. The published guidelines that are available, such as those from the Canadian Cardiovascular Society, the joint statement from the American Heart Association (AHA) and the North American Society for Pacing and Electrophysiology (NASPE), and the European Society of Cardiology are generally based upon limited data [35–37]. Moreover, the guidelines tend to be fairly conservative and often recommend driving cessation for longer periods than may be medically indicated based upon current data [38]. For example, the AHA/NASPE scientific statement on safety issues related to arrhythmias recommended that non-commercial drivers with implantable cardioverter defibrillators (ICDs) refrain from driving for a minimum of 6 months after device implantation. Commercial driving should be prohibited permanently. Unfortunately, however inadequate the existing guidelines may be, practitioners who depart from these published guidelines may find themselves liable in the event of an injury to a third party.

For the most part, a distinction should be made between personal driving and commercial operators such as bus drivers and truckers. Whereas the former are licensed solely by the state, the latter are regulated, in part, by the US Department of Transportation through the Federal Motor Carrier Safety Regulation: "It is the intent of the Federal Motor Carrier Safety Regulation to disqualify a driver who has a current cardiovascular disease which is accompanied by and/or likely to cause symptoms of syncope, dyspnea, collapse, or congestive heart failure" [39]. Interestingly, current Federal regulations do not specifically require the driver or the examining physician to notify anyone if the applicant fails the fitness examination [40].

Although the actual incidence of medically

related automobile accidents is not known, at least two facts are well accepted. First, syncope, recurrent syncope, and/or sudden death while driving is rare [38,41–44]. Second, impairment of driving ability appears to increase with age and the concomitant increased prevalence of underlying medical disorders. By way of example, an analysis of 67 motor vehicle accidents in New Jersey occurring in patients aged 60 years and over revealed 12 instances attributable to syncope [45]. A follow-up study by the same investigators demonstrated a positive work-up for syncope in 25 of 33 elderly drivers where no external cause for the road crash could be found. Thirteen drivers had a prior history of syncope [46].

Loss of consciousness during driving has been reported in 19–36% of patients with supraventricular tachyarrhythmias [47]. Moreover, so-called "benign" events such as vasovagal syncope, bradyarrhythmias, and transient heart block have also resulted in motor vehicle accidents, prompting some physicians to advise their patients with these diagnoses not to drive because of the possibility of a recurrence despite treatment [48]. Not unexpectedly, compliance with physician recommendations is low, with only nine of 104 consecutively treated patients (during the period 1998–2000) admitting to following their physician's advice after experiencing a syncopal episode [49].

The rhythm disturbances of greatest concern are ventricular tachycardia and ventricular fibrillation. Treatment of these rhythm abnormalities increasingly includes implantation of a cardioverter defibrillator. The degree of risk posed by allowing individuals with ICDs to drive must be addressed. Certainly, across the board, driving restrictions, as prescribed by many electrophysiologists, may be inappropriate [41]. Instead, each patient should be evaluated individually with respect to risk of arrhythmia recurrence and risk of post-shock syncope. Fortunately, most patients do not experience syncope after implantation of an ICD; unfortunately, there are no historical or clinical variables that can be used to predict loss of consciousness. In fact, nearly two-thirds of those who lost consciousness during or after an ICD shock had never experienced a syncopal episode with previous shocks [50].

In general, most hemodynamically significant rhythm disturbances occur in the first month after ICD implantation [51]. The hazard rate then remains moderate until 7 months, after which it decreases substantially [52]. Even at that, spontaneous shocks have been reported to occur during driving in up to 18% of patients with ICDs [53].

Regardless of physician driving recommendations, the majority of patients receiving ICDs do not modify their driving habits [41,44,54,55]. Recent data from the Antiarrhythmics Versus Implantable Defibrillators Trial reconfirmed this observation [56]. Of 627 patients resuscitated from near-fatal ventricular arrhythmias, 78% had resumed driving by 6 months. Thankfully, the annualized rate of motor vehicle accidents in this patient population was only 3.4%, less than the national average of 7.1%. This finding was consistent with previously published data in which the injury and fatality rates in patients with ventricular arrhythmias, ICDs, and/or supraventricular arrhythmias were found to be at least comparable to that seen in the general US population [44,47,55,57].

The above observations notwithstanding, a review of the reported case law as of April 2004 revealed no published cases involving a physician's failure to impose driving restrictions on a patient with a pacemaker or defibrillator. That such cases will occur is perhaps inevitable.

Liability of a physician for injury or death of a third party – case law

Section 315 of the Restatement of Torts 2d provides that there is no duty to control the conduct of a third person so as to prevent him or her from causing physical harm to another unless either a special relationship exists between the actor and the third person that imposes a duty on the actor to control a third person's conduct, or a special relationship exists between the actor and the other which gives the other a right to protection [58].

As to a physician, it was historically held at common law that no duty existed that would extend liability beyond that of the patient. During the past 20 years, however, this traditional analysis has been revisited, most notably in *Tarasoff* v. *Regents of University of California* [59]. The court in *Tarasoff* imposed a duty on psychotherapists to protect third parties from harm. The court's holding was grounded on Section 319 of the Restatement of Torts, which provides that one who "takes charge" of a person whom he or she knows or should know to be likely to cause bodily harm to others if not controlled is under a duty to exercise reasonable care to control that person to prevent him or her from doing harm to others. The application of Section 319 to physicians is now generally accepted and several jurisdictions have since allowed a cause of action by a third party against a physician for negligence in the treatment of a patient [60].

The possibility of physician liability for injury to a third party can be inferred from existing case law. In *Freese* v. *Lemon* [61], the Iowa Supreme Court, in a 5–4 decision, addressed the responsibility of a physician treating a patient with a seizure disorder. In that case, the court held that if a pedestrian could prove that the physician had negligently failed to advise his patient not to drive an automobile, the physician could be held liable for injuries sustained by the pedestrian and that allegations to this effect sustained a cause of action against the physician. The case was subsequently tried and resulted in a verdict for the physician. It must be noted, however, that the trial court verdict, ultimately sustained by the Iowa Supreme Court, was based primarily on the grounds that the injured party failed to prove the applicable standard of care. In theory, at least under the *Freese* analysis, had the plaintiff met the burden of proof, physician liability could have been found.

The holding in *Freese* was revisited by the Iowa Supreme Court in 2003 in the case of *Schmidt* v. *Mahoney* [62]. In *Schmidt*, the plaintiff was injured when the driver of an approaching vehicle lost control of her vehicle secondary to a seizure. The defendant, the driver's treating physician, was sued not only for medical malpractice, but also for the negligent failure to control the conduct of a third person based upon the Restatement (Second) of Torts Section 315 alleging that the defendant physician should have warned the driver of the dangers associated with driving a vehicle with a known seizure disorder. The district court ruled that "there is no duty running from a doctor to a member of the general public to control the conduct of a patient as to prevent her from causing a motor vehicle accident." Upon appeal to the Iowa Supreme Court, the justices reversed their holding in *Freese*,

observing that "it is an unwarranted intrusion on the relationship between healthcare providers and their patients to recognize a right of action in favor of the general public based on actions of a healthcare provider in directing the activities of a patient." Clearly, the court recognized that permitting liability to members of the general public would prompt physicians to make overly restrictive recommendations to minimize liability and "would not be in their patients' best interests."

Using a somewhat different analysis, the Missouri Court of Appeals in *Young* v. *Wadsworth* [63] reached a conclusion similar to that of the Iowa Supreme Court with respect to the liability of a physician to non-patient third parties. In *Young*, the defendant physician had seen and evaluated an individual for syncope. The patient was scheduled for ambulatory electrocardiographic monitoring and given a prescription for alprazolam. On the way home from the clinic visit, reportedly prior to ingesting any medication, the patient lost consciousness and was involved in a motor vehicle accident in which the driver of the other vehicle was killed and the passengers injured. The estate of the driver and the surviving passengers sued the treating physician, alleging that the failure to warn the patient regarding the risks of driving constituted negligence. The court held that it was not necessary to address the issue of physician responsibility to members of the general public. Rather, the case could be decided simply based upon the common law rules of negligence. First, there was no allegation that the patient/driver was of other than normal intelligence. Second, the patient/driver knew he was having blackout spells. Third, common sense would suggest that someone who is prone to loss of consciousness should not be operating a motor vehicle. Fourth, "there is no duty to warn of danger that is open and obvious." Ultimately, the proximate cause of the accident was that the patient/driver elected to operate a motor vehicle, not the failure of the physician to warn of the dangers.

Clearly, as suggested in *Young*, a history of recurrent syncope can (and probably will) impact on the final analysis. In *Simmons* v. *Aldi-Brenner Company* [64], an Illinois court addressed the admissibility of "prior occurrences" to establish notice of a dangerous condition. Store customers and relatives of a deceased victim brought a negligence action against a motorist who lost consciousness and drove her car through a storefront. The etiology of the defendant's syncopal episode was AV block. Plaintiffs argued that the existence of vertigo in the past should have placed the defendant on notice that it was negligent for her to drive. The court, relying upon *Grant* v. *Joseph J. Duffy Co.* [65], observed that the crucial factor to determine admissibility of prior episodes is whether those episodes are "reasonably" similar. In *Simmons*, the court noted that there was no suggestion from plaintiff's counsel of a clear connection between an episode of syncope related to AV block and the previous episodes of vertigo.

By way of contrast, in a State of Washington case, *Kaiser* v. *Suburban Transportation Systems* [66], the plaintiff was successful. Mrs. Kaiser, a passenger on a Suburban Transportation System bus, was injured when the driver lost consciousness and the bus struck a telephone pole. The lapse of consciousness was attributed to the side-effects of a drug (pyribenzamine), which had been prescribed by the driver's physician for treatment of a nasal condition. The driver testified that the doctor gave him no warning of the possible side-effects of the drug and that he had taken the first pill on the morning of the accident. Four doctors, including the defendant, testified that, in view of the known side-effect, a warning should be given when the drug is prescribed.

A similar fact pattern was presented to the Texas courts in *Gooden* v. *Tips* [67], a claim by a third party vehicular accident victim against a physician for failure to warn a patient about the risks of driving under the influence of a drug prescribed by the physician. Relying upon decisions from other jurisdictions, the Texas court upheld the victim's right to sue the physician stating, in pertinent part, that the duty being imposed was not a duty to control the patient's actions, but rather a duty to warn the patient that his or her driving ability might be impaired and in what manner. The court in *Gooden* went on to note that while the third party's suit could not be maintained as a malpractice action because of the absence of a patient–physician relationship, the suit could be maintained as an ordinary negligence action.

The *Gooden* holding was later reconsidered by the Texas Supreme Court in *Praesel* v. *Johnson* [68],

a wrongful death and survival action against the physicians and clinic responsible for the treatment of a patient who, as a result of a seizure, caused an automobile accident in which Terri-Lynn Praesel was fatally injured. This time, however, the court ruled that while there may be circumstances where a physician has a duty to warn an "identifiable" third party, the consequences of expanding that duty to include the entire general public were significant and would impose substantial liability on physicians whose warnings may be ineffective anyway. As the court aptly observed, ultimately, the responsibility for the safe operation of an automobile remains with the driver.

Recent court rulings tend towards limiting physician liability to third parties. In *Weigold* v. *Patel* [69], the plaintiff, as husband and administrator of his wife's estate, first brought a wrongful death action against the driver of the motor vehicle that struck and killed his wife. After the defendant testified that she had been prescribed medication that made her prone to daytime somnolence, the plaintiff expanded the lawsuit to include the treating psychiatrist and psychologist. Upon motion for summary judgment, both healthcare practitioners were dismissed from the case and the plaintiff appealed to the Connecticut Supreme Court. In affirming the trials court's decision to grant the motions for summary judgment, the Supreme Court pondered the issue of causation, ultimately concluding (as did the court in *Praesel*) that neither the defendant psychiatrist nor psychologist was in a position to control the behavior of their mutual patient. Rather, the proximate cause of the decedent's injuries was the driver's decision to operate her motor vehicle despite her knowledge that the medications resulted in daytime somnolence.

Not infrequently, physicians are called upon to conduct physical examinations of airline pilots, truck drivers, fire-fighters, police officers, etc. and to certify these individuals as being physically fit to perform the duties of their employment. In that regard, the Tennessee Supreme Court, in *Wharton Transport Corp.* v. *Bridges* [70], was asked to determine whether a third party could assert a claim against a physician for the failure to identify bilateral chorioretinitis, which severely impaired a commercial trucker's depth perception and resulted in injury to the plaintiffs. The court held that the injuries suffered, in the manner in which they occurred, were reasonably foreseeable to the physician who negligently performed the pre-employment examination and the Court reversed a directed verdict for the defense.

To summarize, although the facts in each of the above cases are similar, subtle differences existed which were sufficient to justify different conclusions, often by the same court. Seemingly, the courts have been reluctant to expand the "duty to warn" to unidentifiable third parties in cases in which the driver suddenly lost consciousness because of a naturally occurring medical condition in which the risks associated with operating a motor vehicle were obvious (e.g., seizure disorders, recurrent syncope). On the other hand, the courts have occasionally allowed third party actions to proceed against physicians in cases in which the physician's actions, such as the prescription of sedating medications, were, at least in part, associated with the subsequent automobile accident. How a court will rule on the issue of physician liability to a third party in the event that an individual with an ICD becomes involved in a fatal automobile accident remains to be seen.

Arguably, the body of law creating a basis for imposing liability on a physician for foreseeable injuries to third parties remains unsettled [71]. Nevertheless, it would be prudent for the physician to assume that if there is negligence in the failure to properly diagnose, treat or restrict the activities of patients with syncope, the potential liability may well extend to injuries or death caused by the patient. While such exposure properly should be of concern to a physician treating patients with syncope, the fact remains that historically such cases appear to be few and far between.

Conclusions

Physicians involved in the treatment of patients with syncope or other similar disorders should always be cognizant of the activities in which the patient engages and must carefully assess whether continuation of those activities will place the patient or others at an unreasonable risk of harm. Such assessment requires knowledge of applicable rules, regulations, and statutes as well as maintaining familiarity with current practice modalities and

guidelines. Reasoned and appropriate care will greatly minimize, and perhaps most likely eliminate, physician liability in these cases.

References

1 Prosser and Keeton; *Law of Torts*, 5th edn. 1984.

2 *Lance v. Senior* (1967) 36 Ill 2d 516, 224 NE 2d 231.

3 *Kirk v. Michael Reese Hospital and Medical Center* (1987) 117 Ill 2d 507, 111 Ill Dec. 944, 513 NE 2d 387, cert. den. (US) 99 L Ed 2d 236.

4 Margolis MR. Do physicians of potentially dangerous patients owe a duty to third parties? http://www.law.uh.edu/healthlawperspectives/Tort/980615DoPhysicians.html.

5 Speiser, Krause and Gans; *American Law of Torts*, 1985.

6 Manolis AS, Linzer M, Salem D, Estes III M. Syncope: current diagnostic evaluation and management. *Ann Intern Med* 1990;**112**:850–63.

7 Benditt DG, Remole S, Milstein S, Bailin S. Syncope: causes, clinical evaluation, and current therapy. *Ann Rev Med* 1992;**43**:283–300.

8 Link MS, Homoud MK, Wang PJ, Estes M. Syncope in athletes. *Cardiovasc Rev Rep* 2002;**23**:625–32.

9 Zipes DP, Garson A Jr. 26th Bethesda conference: recommendations for determining eligibility for competition in athletes with cardiovascular abnormalities. Task Force 6: arrhythmias. *Med Sci Sports Exerc* 1994;**26**:S276–83.

10 Pegalis SE, Wachsman HF, Kellet E. *American Law of Medical Malpractice*, 2nd edn. 1993.

11 Strickberger SA, Cantillon CO, Friedman PL. When should patients with lethal ventricular arrhythmias resume driving? *Ann Intern Med* 1991;**115**:560–3.

12 Frampton A. Who can drive home from the emergency department? A questionnaire based study of emergency physicians' knowledge of DVLA guidelines. *Emerg Med J* 2003;**20**:526–30.

13 Kelly R, Warke T, Steele I. Medical restrictions to driving: the awareness of patients and doctors. *Postgrad Med J* 1999;**75**(887):537–9.

14 Krauss GL, Ampaw L, Krumholz A. Individual state driving restrictions for people with epilepsy in the US. *Neurology* 2001;**57**:1780–5.

15 Sterns HL, Sterns R, Aizenberg R, Anapole J. Family and friends concerned about an older driver: final report. National Highway Traffic Safety Administration, US Department of Transportation 2001; DOT HS 809 307.

16 *Health Insurance Portability and Accountability Act of 1996* (45 CFR Parts 160, 162 and 164).

17 Williams CC, Bernhardt DT. Syncope in athletes. *Sports Med* 1995;**19**:223–34.

18 *Gathers v. Loyola Marymount University*. No. C 759027 (Los Angeles, CA, Super. Ct., filed Apr. 20, 1990).

19 Hudson MA. Gathers collapse is issue. *Los Angeles Times* August 16, 1992.

20 Hudson MA. A legacy on court, in court. *Los Angeles Times* October 6, 1992.

21 Maron BJ. Sounding board: sudden death in young athletes – lessons from the Hank Gathers affair. *N Engl J Med* 1993;**329**:55–7.

22 *Penny* v. *Sands*. No. H89-280 (D. Conn, filed May 3, 1989).

23 Fainaru S. Legal advice given: Lewis side told suit not worth it. *Boston Globe* August 10, 1993.

24 Johnson WO. Heart of the matter. *Sports Illustrated* May 24, 1993.

25 *Harris-Lewis* v. *Mudge*. Nos. 00-P-1759 and 01-P-1649 (Suffolk, Mass, Sept 11, 2003–Feb 20, 2004).

26 Partial Transcript of Proceedings at 25–26, *Larkin* v. *Archdiocese of Cincinnati*, No. C-1-90-619 (SD Ohio, filed Aug 31, 1990).

27 Mitten MJ. Team physicians and competitive athletes: allocating legal responsibility for athletic injury. *Univ Pitt L Rev* 1993;**55**:129–60.

28 Mitten MJ. Amateur athletes with handicaps or physical abnormalities: who makes the participation decision? *Neb L Rev* 1992;**71**:987–1032.

29 Altman LK. The doctor's world: an athlete's health and a doctor's warning. *The New York Times* March 13, 1990.

30 Manno A. A high price to compete: the feasibility and effect of waivers used to protect schools from liability for injuries to athletes with high medical risks. *Ky L J* 1991;**79**:867.

31 Mitchell JH, Maron BJ, Epstein SE. 16th Bethesda Conference: cardiovascular abnormalities in the athlete: recommendations regarding eligibility for competition. *J Am Coll Cardiol* 1985;**6**:1186–232.

32 Maron BJ, Mitchell JH. 26th Bethesda Conference: recommendations for determining eligibility for competition in athletes with cardiovascular abnormalities. *J Am Coll Cardiol* 1994;**24**:846–99.

33 Maron BJ, Brown RW, McGrew CA. Ethical, legal, and practical considerations affecting decision making in competitive athletes. *J Am Coll Cardiol* 1994;**24**:854–60.

34 *Federal Aviation Regulations* 14 CFR 67.

35 Epstein AE, Miles WM, Benditt DG, *et al*. Personal and public safety issues related to arrhythmias that may affect consciousness: implications for regulation and physician recommendations. *Circulation* 1996;**94**:1147–66.

36 Assessment of the cardiac patient for fitness to drive: 1996 update. *Can J Cardiol* 1996;**12**:1164–70; 1175–82.

37 Jung W, Anderson M, Camm AJ, *et al*. Recommendations for driving of patients with implantable cardioverter-defibrillators. *Eur Heart J* 1997;**18**:1210–9.

38 Bleakley JF, Akiyama T. Driving and arrhythmias: implications of new data. *Card Electrophysiol Rev* 2003;**7**:77–9.

39 Medical regulatory criteria for evaluation. Section 391.41(b)(4). *Federal Register*. November 23, 1977; amended October 1983.

40 Carmody CJ. *Remarks for the public meeting on motorcoach safety*, April 30, 2002. National Highway Traffic Safety Administration, US Dept of Transportation; remarks available at http://www.ntsb.gov/speeches/carmody/cc020430.htm

41 Curtis AB, Conti JB, Reilly RE, Tucker KJ. Implantable cardioverter defibrillators: should patients be allowed to drive? *J Am Coll Cardiol* 1994;**23**:206A.

42 Epstein, AE, Miles WM. Personal and public safety issues related to arrhythmias that may affect consciousness: implications for regulation and physician recommendations. *Circulation* 1996;**94**:1147–66.

43 Bhatia A, Dhala A, Blanck Z, Deshpande S, Akhtar M, Sra AJ. Driving safety among patients with neurocardiogenic (vasovagal) syncope. *Pacing Clin Electrophysiol* 1999;**22**: 1576–80.

44 Curtis AB, Conti JB, Tucker KJ, Kubulis PS, Reilly RE, Woodward DA. Motor vehicle accidents in patients with an implantable cardioverter-defibrillator. *J Am Coll Cardiol* 1995;**26**:180–4.

45 Rehm CG, Ross SE. Elderly drivers involved in road crashes: a profile. *Am Surg* 1995;**61**:435–7.

46 Rehm CG, Ross SE. Syncope as etiology of road crashes involving elderly drivers. *Am Surg* 1995;**61**:1006–8.

47 Dhala A, Bremner S, Blanck Z, *et al*. Impairment of driving abilities in patients with supraventricular tachycardias. *Am J Cardiol* 1995;**75**:516–8.

48 Decter BM, Goldner B, Cohen TJ. Vasovagal syncope as a cause of motor vehicle accidents. *Am Heart J* 1994; **127**:1619–21.

49 Maas R, Ventura R, Kretzschmar C, Aydin A, Schuchert A. Syncope, driving recommendations, and clinical reality: survey of patients. *BMJ* 2003;**326**:21.

50 Kou WH, Calkins H, Lewis RR, *et al*. Incidence of loss of consciousness during automatic implantable cardioverter defibrillator shocks. *Ann Intern Med* 1991;**115**:942–5.

51 Larsen GC, Stupey MR, Walance CG, *et al*. When should survivors of ventricular tachycardia/fibrillation resume driving? *Circulation* 1990;**82**(Suppl. 3):83.

52 Larsen GC, Stupey MR, Walance CG, *et al*. Recurrent cardiac events in survivors of ventricular fibrillation or tachycardia: implications for driving restrictions. *JAMA* 1994;**271**:1335–9.

53 Zilo P, Luceri RM, Vardeman LL. Driving after implantation of a cardioverter defibrillator. *PACE* 1994;**17**(II):781.

54 Tucker KJ, Conti JB, King LC, Reilly RE, Curtis AB. Driving behavior after implantation of cardioverter defibrillators. *PACE* 1994;**17**(II):781.

55 Akiyama T, Powell JL, Mitchell LB, Ehlert FA, Baessler C. Resumption of driving after life-threatening ventricular tachyarrhythmi. *N Engl J Med* 2001;**345**:391–7.

56 The Antiarrhythmics Versus Implantable Defibrillators (AVID) Investigators. A comparison of anti-arrhythmic drug therapy with implantable defibrillators in patients resuscitated from near-fatal ventricular arrhythmias. *N Engl J Med* 1997;**337**:1576–83.

57 Trappe HJ, Wenzlaff P, Grellman G. Should patients with implantable defibrillators be allowed to drive? Observations in 291 patients from a single center over an 11-year period. *J Interv Card Electrophysiol* 1998;**2**:193–201.

58 *Restatement of Torts 2d*, 1964.

59 *Tarasoff* v. *Regents of University of California* (1976) 17 Cal 3d 425, 131 Cal Rptr 14, 551 P 2d 334.

60 Sarno GG. Liability of physician, for injury to or death of third party, due to failure to disclose driving related impairment. 43 ALR 4th 153.

61 *Freese* v. *Lemon* (1973) 210 NW 2d 576.

62 *Schmidt* v. *Mahoney* (2003) 659 NW 2d 552.

63 *Young* v. *Wadsworth* (1996) 916 SW 2d 877.

64 *Simmons* v. *Aldi-Brenner Co.* (1987) 162 Ill App 3d 238, 515 NE 2d 403.

65 *Grant* v. *Joseph J. Duffy Co.* (1974) 20 Ill App 3d 669, 314 NE 2d 478.

66 *Kaiser* v. *Suburban Transportation Systems* (1965) 65 Wash 2d 461, 398 P 2d 14.

67 *Gooden* v. *Tips* (1983) 651 SW 2d 364.

68 *Praesel* v. *Johnson* (1998) 41 Tex Sup Ct J 630, 967 SW 2d 391.

69 *Weigold* v. *Jayantkumar* (2004) AC23289. *Connecticut Law Journal*, February 3, 2004.

70 *Wharton Transport Corp.* v. *Bridges* (1980) 606 SW 2d 521.

71 Dickens BM. Malpractice liability implications of pacemaker and defibrillator guidelines in Canada. *Card Electrophysiol Rev* 2003;**7**:36–9.

Inspire me with love for my art (medicine)
And for thy creatures. In the sufferer
Let me see only the human being . . .

Maimonides
Oath for the Physician
1200 CE

The good physician knows his patients through and through,
And his knowledge is bought dearly. Time, sympathy,
And understanding must be lavishly dispensed, but the reward
Is to be found in that personal bond which forms the greatest
Satisfaction of the practice of medicine. One of the essential
Qualities of the clinician is interest in humanity, for the secret
Of the care of the patient is in caring for the patient.

Dr. Francis Weld Peabody
Lecture to the Harvard Medical Students
1927 CE

Index

Printed and bound by CPI Group (UK) Ltd, Croydon, CR0 4YY

16/04/2025

14658828-0005